Emmanuel Apergis

Fracture-Dislocations of the Wrist

Foreword by Hisao Moritomo

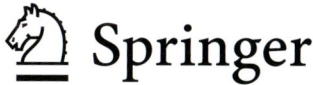 Springer

Emmanuel Apergis
Red Cross Hospital
Athens
Greece

ISBN 978-88-470-5327-4   ISBN 978-88-470-5328-1   (eBook)
DOI 10.1007/978-88-470-5328-1
Springer Milan Heidelberg New York Dordrecht London

Library of Congress Control Number: 2013932455

This volume is partially based on Καταγματα–εξαρθρηματα του καρπου, First edition, by Emmanuel Apergis, 360 pages, Copyright 2004, with permission from Konstantaras Medical Books.

Printed on acid-free paper

Springer is part of Springer Science+Business Media (www.springer.com)

Dedicated to Alexandra, Marianna and Dafni

Foreword

I met Dr. Emmanuel 'Manos' Apergis for the first time at a lunch reception of the International Federation of Societies for Surgery of the Hand (IFSSH) meeting in Australia in 2007. We had been exchanging emails regarding common work in IFSSH Committee but had never met each other; hence, he placed a white flower on the lapel of his jacket so that I would recognize him. In spite of this being the first time we met, he was frank and we get along well immediately. We enjoyed a "manic" discussion about the wrist.

I, who was at that time the chairman of the wrist biomechanics committee of IFSSH, had asked him to write about the wrist dart-throwing motion for the IFSSH Committee Report. He was enthusiastic and prepared a wonderful contribution. Dr. Marc Garcia-Elias had recommended nominating him as a member of the wrist biomechanics committee of IFSSH. Dr. Garcia-Elias informed me that Manos had written a wonderful book about wrist fracture-dislocation (Dr. Garcia-Elias wrote a chapter on wrist biomechanics in that book). Manos kindly sent the first edition of this book to me in 2007. Because it was written in Greek, his native language, I could not read the text; however, I enjoyed browsing through the many beautiful photographs and figures included in the book.

To enlarge its readership, Dr. Garcia-Elias and I persuaded him to translate this book into English. Finally, the English version of this book, with additional photographs and figures, was completed. In this book, Manos explains the fracture dislocation of a wrist joint as well as normal anatomy and biomechanics of wrist joint using a considerable number of photographs and figures. The difficulty in completing such a great work almost single handedly exceeds my imagination (particularly for those whose native language is not English). He must surely have been encouraged by his wise wife, Alex.

Manos has very deep discernment, abundant knowledge, and great clinical experience on the wrist joint. In the 2007 IFSSH Committee Report, he wrote his manuscript not only from a clinical point of view but also from anthropological and physical points of view, which added depth to the report. On the occasion of the 2013 committee report update, I readily asked him to write a sentence again. He accepted willingly and provided a great contribution that once more met my expectations.This book is a monograph that specifically focused on wrist fracture-dislocation and was written almost entirely by one experienced wrist surgeon, who is well aware of anatomy and biomechanics of wrist joint. There is probably no other book similar to this one nor there will be one in the future. This book can undoubtedly teach many people about the complicated wrist disorders. The medical contribution of this book is vast. I sincerely appreciate the input of Manos and Alex.

Hisao Moritomo, MD, PhD

Professor, Department of Physical Therapy
Osaka Yukioka college of Health Science
Yukioka Hospital Hand Center, Japan
Professor, The center for Advanced Medical
Engineering and Informatics
Osaka University, Japan

Preface

The wrist surgeon is expected to know the current treatment options to address a specific wrist problem for a particular patient and often has the ability to apply the most suitable treatment or refer the patient to someone with more expertise. However, knowledge of and ability to apply treatment options are not enough; we must also be able to achieve for each patient the *maximum benefit with the minimum intervention*. If no intervention is best for the patient, then let it be so. If only a K-wire or a complex combination of materials or approaches can restore the wrist to almost its original state, then that should be our course of action. Achieving this goal is still a work in progress.

We may disagree on the optimal treatment, but we should all agree that before anything else, we must identify the problem. There is an unacceptably high percentage of cases in which fracture-dislocations of the wrist are missed on clinical and radiographic examination. Therefore the main purpose of this book is to facilitate recognition of the problem and the patterns with which it emerges.

Dislocations and fracture–dislocations of the wrist are mainly high-energy injuries; therefore the completion of this book was facilitated by the following main factors: (a) *the hospital*, which for the last 20 years has constituted mainly a trauma center in Athens, (b) *the considerable case material*, due to the high rate of road accidents in Greece and the significant number of patients with intricate wrist complications referred to me by colleagues. Two more factors also contributed in writing this book: (a) *the extensive documentation* of the material comprising operative photographs, x-rays, and sufficient follow-up and (b) the author's "*addiction" to wrist injuries*, which commenced as early as his residency era.

I am greatly indebted to all my patients for their trust. I wish to thank all those distinguished wrist surgeons worldwide who, with their writings, publications, and lectures, inspired me to focus on and care for the enigmatic and puzzling wrist joint. I would also like to thank Dr. Marc Garcia-Elias, whose chapter on the Biomechanics of the Wrist contributed to the completion of this book and who has offered valuable support throughout this project.

I would like to express my gratitude to John Konstantaras, the publisher of the previous book of mine, which was released in the Greek language and which laid the foundation for this volume. I am much obliged to the Springer staff, Antonella Cerri, Juliette Ruth Kleemann, Roberto Garbero, and Sundari for their cooperation, useful advice, and assistance in the completion of this edition. Finally, the contribution of my daughter Marianna in bringing this project to fruition has been extraordinary.

Emmanuel Apergis

Contents

Part IV   Other Carpal Dislocations

10   Axial Dislocations or Fracture-Dislocations   275

11   Isolated Dislocations of the Carpal Bones   289

Introduction

Carpal dislocations can be divided into five separate groups: perilunate, radiocarpal, axial, carpometacarpal, and isolated carpal bone dislocations. The most frequent traumatic carpal dislocations are perilunate dislocations or fracture-dislocations. Less common are the radiocarpal, axial, and carpometacarpal dislocations, while isolated pure carpal bone dislocations are the most unusual of wrist injuries. They share many common features: all are rare injuries, most often occurring from high-energy trauma, they are usually seen in young males between their second and fourth decades of life, and they could all be initially missed or underestimated.

Rarely is a wrist surgeon fortunate or unfortunate enough (depends on the perspective), to come across an injured patient who suffers from almost all of the above dislocations or fracture-dislocations simultaneously (Fig. 1.1a–k).

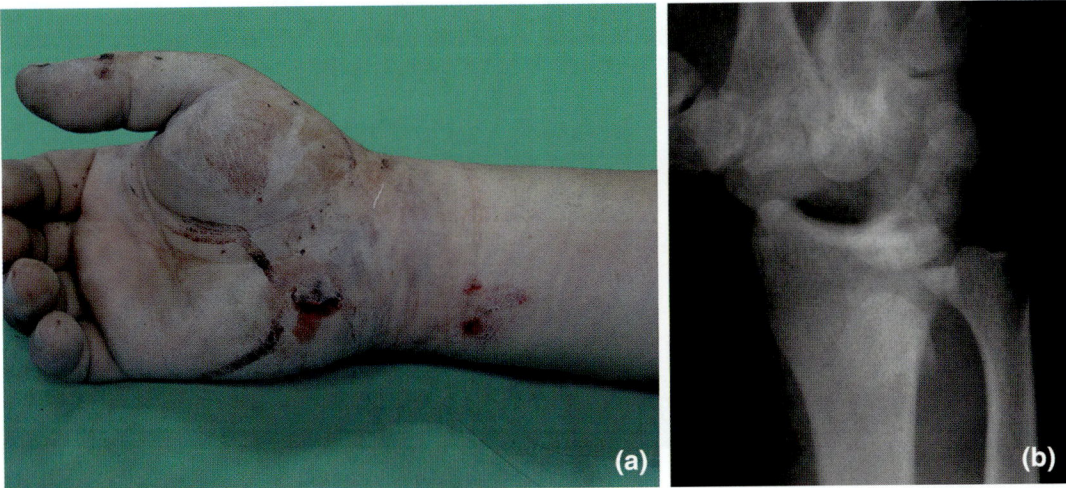

Fig. 1.1 The admitted hand (**a**); the initial X-rays (**b**, **c**); the distraction view (**d**); volar approach, the volarly dislocated capitate and lunate (**e**); the proximal scaphoid remained volarly dislocated after the reduction of lunocapitate complex (*PS* Proximal scaphoid) (**f**); dorsal approach, absence of bones (*H* Hamate, *DS* Distal scaphoid, *R* Radius) (**g**); dorsal approach, comminution of the volar radial rim (**h**); dorsal approach, fracture of the dorsal part of the lunate (*asterisk*) (**i**); postoperative X-rays (**j**, **k**)

E. Apergis, *Fracture-Dislocations of the Wrist*,
DOI: 10.1007/978-88-470-5328-1_1, © Springer-Verlag Italia 2013

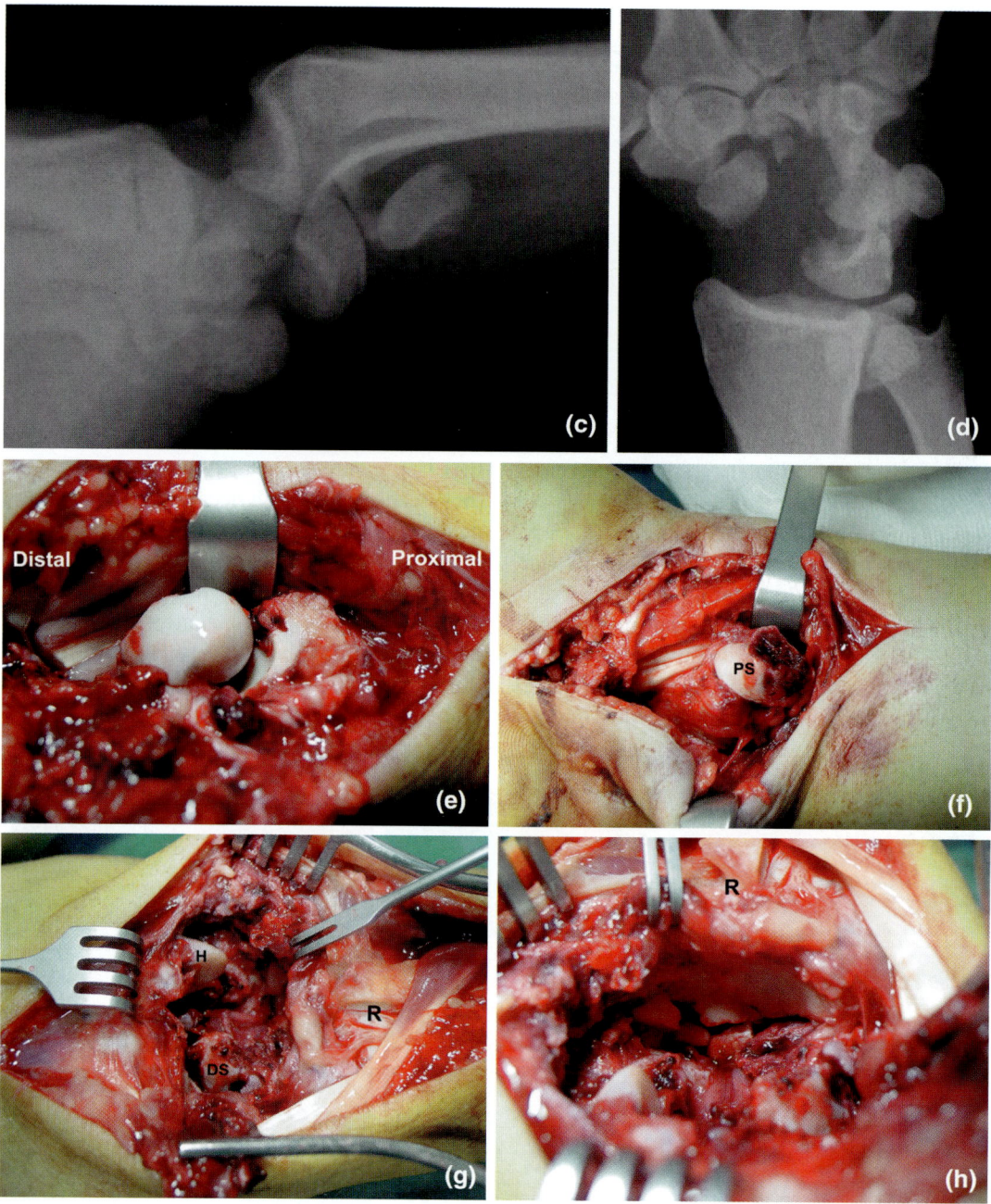

Fig. 1.1 (continued)

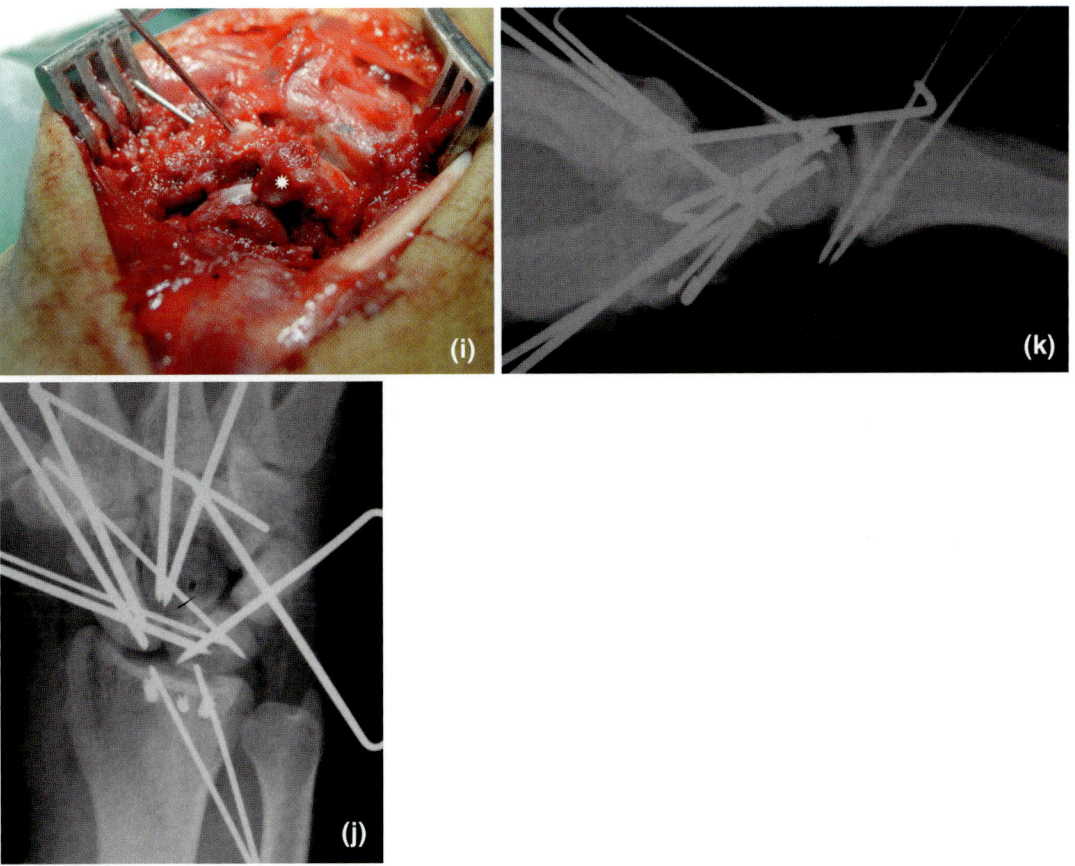

Fig. 1.1 (continued)

Part I
General Aspects

Wrist Anatomy

2.1 Ligaments of the Wrist and their Functional Significance

2.1.1 Overview of Carpal Ligament Organization

The ligaments of the wrist can be categorized by generic divisions (intrinsic vs. extrinsic), by location (palmar versus dorsal, radiocarpal versus midcarpal), or by function (guiding, constraining) [1]. The differentiation of the wrist ligaments into intrinsic (intra-articular or interosseous) and extrinsic (capsular) is based on histological criteria. Moreover, the intrinsic ligaments originate and insert on the carpal bones, while extrinsic ligaments course between the carpal bones and the radius or the metacarpals [2]. Both intrinsic and extrinsic ligaments consist of relatively parallel groups of densely packed, highly organized collagen fibers called *fascicles*. The fascicles are surrounded by regions of poorly organized connective tissue, called *perifascicular* spaces. Near the periphery of the ligament, the perifascicular spaces coalesce to form the *epiligamentous sheath*. The superficial surface of a capsular ligament forms the *fibrous stratum* of the epiligamentous sheath, while on the deep, or joint surface of the ligament, the epiligamentous sheath forms a continuous layer called the *synovial stratum* of the epiligamentous sheath. Intrinsic (intra-articular) ligaments are covered entirely by a synovial stratum, whereas extrinsic (capsular) ligaments have the synovial stratum only on their deep or joint surface [1].

A third category of ligaments has been described [1, 3] by the term *meniscocapsular* ligaments referring to a synovial capsular structure containing massive concentrations of blood vessels and nerves. A typical example of such a structure is the radioscapholunate ligament (RSL).

There is some degree of function overlap between the intrinsic and extrinsic ligaments leading to a temporary counterbalance after an individual ligament injury. That equilibrium may be exceeded with cyclic loading following an injury and this progressively leads to insufficiency of the secondary ligamentous constraints and an initially normal radiographic image becomes over time diagnostic of the instability. A typical example of this progressively evolving instability is the scapholunate and lunotriquetral dissociation. Berger in 1997 [4] prophetically argued what was in recent years confirmed: "We tend to look upon the carpal ligaments as passive bands of collagen constraining the action of the bones that they connect. The rich innervation of the ligaments, however, may introduce an entirely new consideration of function for the ligaments as end organs of mechanoreception. It is possible that the wrist is stabilized by a mixture of static structures such as ligaments and dynamic structures such as muscles. As such, the ligaments may play roles as both static support and sensory organs".

E. Apergis, *Fracture-Dislocations of the Wrist*,
DOI: 10.1007/978-88-470-5328-1_2, © Springer-Verlag Italia 2013

Table 2.1 The ligaments of the wrist and their acronyms used in the book

Extrinsic or capsular ligaments		
Radiocarpal (RC) joint	Palmar	Radioscaphocapitate (RSC)
		Long radiolunate (LRL)
		Short radiolunate (SRL)
		Radioscapholunate (RSL)
	Dorsal	Dorsal radiocarpal (Dorsal RC)
Midcarpal (MC) Joint	Palmar	Scapho-trapezium-trapezoid (STT)
		Scaphocapitate (SC)
		Capitate trapezium (CTm)
		Triquetrocapitate (TC)
		Triquetrohamate (TH)
		Palmar scaphotriquetral (Palmar ST)
	Dorsal	Dorsal intercarpal (DIC)
		Dorsal scaphotriquetral (Dorsal ST)
Ulnocarpal (UC) joint		Ulnolunate (UL)
		Ulnotriquetral (UT)
		Ulnocapitate (UC)
Distal radioulnar joint (DRUJ)		Triangular fibrocartilage complex (TFCC)
		Dorsal radioulnar (DRU)
		Palmar radioulnar (PRU)
		Meniscus homologue (MH)
Intrinsic or intra-articular or interosseous ligaments		
Proximal carpal row		Scapholunate interosseous (SLI)
		Lunotriquetral interosseous (LTI)
Distal carpal row		Trapeziotrapezoid (TT)
		Trapeziocapitate (TC)
		Capitohamate (CH)

To date, the detailed carpal ligament nomenclature and classification by Berger is the most commonly cited and most detailed of all [5], therefore this is mainly used in this book.

Table 2.1 shows aggregately all the wrist ligaments and the acronyms described in this book.

2.1.2　Extrinsic or Capsular Ligaments: Volar Surface

2.1.2.1　Radiocarpal Joint

The palmar radiocarpal ligaments originate from the palmar rim of the distal radius, attaching approximately 1–2 mm proximal to the articular surface and coursing distally, attach to one or more carpal bones (Figs. 2.1 and 2.2). These ligaments constitute the main stabilizing structures of the radiocarpal joint and are best viewed from an intra-articular perspective.

Radioscaphocapitate ligament (RSC ligament)

The RSC ligament is the most radial of the palmar radiocarpal ligaments that originates proximally from a roughened area on the palmar and radial aspects of the radial styloid process [4]. It courses distally and ulnarly and attaches partially to the radial surface of the waist of the scaphoid and to the proximal cortex of the distal scaphoid pole

Fig. 2.1 Schematic (**a**) and cadaveric (**b**) depiction of palmar radiocarpal ligaments: radioscaphocapitate (*1*), long radiolunate (*2*), radioscapholunate (Testut) (*3*), short radiolunate (*4*)

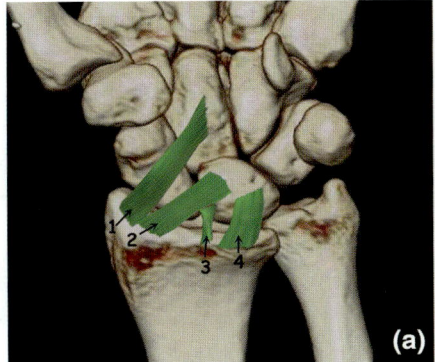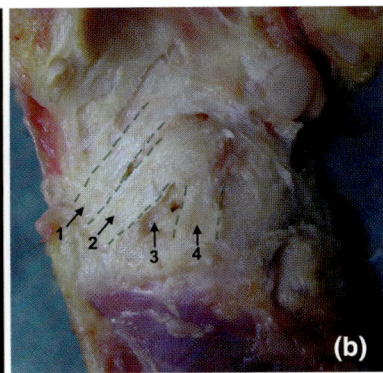

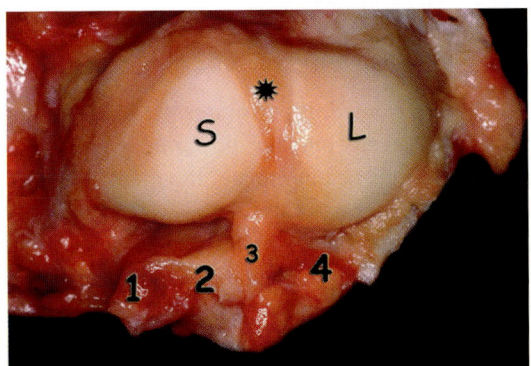

Fig. 2.2 Palmar radiocarpal ligaments: Radioscaphocapitate (*1*), Long radiolunate (*2*), Radioscapholunate (Testut) (*3*), short radiolunate (*4*). The *asterisk* indicates scapholunate ligaments. Scaphoid (*S*), lunate (*L*). With permission from [157]

together with the palmar scaphotriquetral ligament (Palmar ST ligament) [6, 7]. The majority of its fibers pass anterior to the waist of the scaphoid to form the palmar capsule of the midcarpal joint. The percentage of fibers that attach to the capitate neck varies. Berger [1, 4] estimated that only 10 % of its fibers actually insert into the palmar cortex of the capitate. The remaining fibers course ulnarly interdigitating with fibers from the ulnocapitate and triquetrocapitate ligaments to form the *arcuate (deltoid or V) ligament* [4, 8]. In contrast to these findings, Buijze et al. [5, 6] found that the bulk of fibers seem to insert mostly on the capitate and do not seem to interdigitate predominantly with fibers arching toward the ulna and triquetrum.

The RSC is separated from the LRL ligament by a deep division called the interligamentous sulcus, which is more obvious intraarticularly. This sulcus, between lunate and capitate, constitutes a weak area of the joint capsule known as *space of Poirier*. The RSC ligament is approximately 1.4 mm thick, 29.8 mm long, and 5.1 mm wide [6].

A number of functions have been attributed to this ligament: (a) Some of its fibers form a radial collateral ligament [9], which is a controversial ligament as its existence is disputed. The greatest controversy is whether it is a separate ligament or the most radial bundle of the RSC ligament, (b) provides resistance to passive pronation of the radiocarpal joint [10], (c) along with the other palmar radiocarpal ligaments provides restraint to dorsal translation of the carpus [11], (d) constrains ulnar translation of the carpus [4, 12, 13], (e) stabilizes the distal pole of the scaphoid [4, 10], and (f) acts as a fulcrum around which the scaphoid rotates [14].

The force required for rupture of the radial collateral region is approximately 100 N, compared with approximately 150 N for rupture of the radiocapitate region. Strain rates at rupture average approximately 125 % and 75 %, respectively [4, 15].

Styloidectomy, depending on the size and morphology, affects in different degrees the origin of the palmar radiocarpal ligaments [16]. Great care must be taken to avoid damage to this ligament in cases of scaphoid excision (proximal row carpectomies, SLAC wrists) [17, 18].

Long Radiolunate Ligament (LRL ligament) (Palmar Radiolunotriquetral Lig., Palmar Radiotriquetral Lig.)

The LRL is a large capsular ligament that originates proximally from the palmar rim of the scaphoid fossa of the distal radius, just ulnar to the RSC ligament. The length, width, and thickness of the LRL are approximately 16, 5.8, and 1.2 mm, respectively [19]. The proximal attachment of the LRL is partially overlapped by the radioscaphocapitate ligament [20, 21] (Fig. 2.3). It courses obliquely distally and ulnarly anterior to the proximal pole of the scaphoid and anterior to the SL joint, overlapping completely the volar scapholunate interosseous ligament (SLI Ligament), to insert widely on the palmar horn of the lunate [3]. The degree of attachment to the lunate may vary between individuals. Some authors [7, 22] have suggested that this ligament continues ulnarly inserting to the palmar surface of the triquetrum, between the insertion of the palmar ulnotriquetral ligament (UT ligament) proximally and the insertion of the Palmar ST ligament distally, forming the radiolunotriquetral ligament. It has been supported that only the fibrous stratum of the joint capsule continues toward the triquetrum and not the fibers of the ligament, thus the designations of the radiolunotriquetral and radiotriquetral ligaments are misleading [3, 4].

Functions attributed to this ligament are: (a) along with the short radiolunate, it functions as a primary restraint to ulnar translocation of the lunate [4, 23], (b) participates in the formation of the antipronation sling, which is responsible for the control of intracarpal pronation [10, 24].

Material property testing of the LRL ligament shows that it ruptures at approximately 110 N of applied force, with approximately 125 % strain at rupture [15].

Radioscapholunate ligament (RSL ligament) (Testut or Testut and Kuenz Ligament)

It is located between the LRL and short radiolunate ligament (SRL) ligaments, originating from the prominence between the scaphoid and lunate articular facets on the distal articular surface of the radius (Figs. 2.1, 2.2, and 2.3).

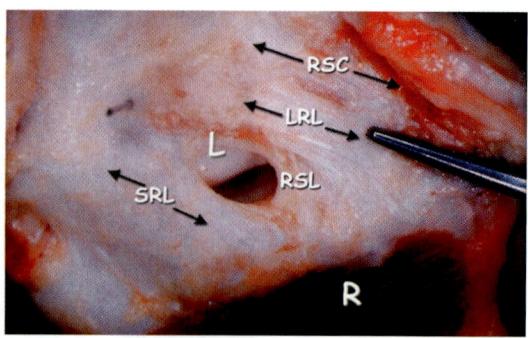

Fig. 2.3 Palmar radiocarpal ligaments: radioscaphocapitate (*RSC*), long radiolunate (*LRL*), radioscapholunate (*RSL*), short radiolunate (*SRL*). *R* radius. With permission from [157]

Vertically oriented, it perforates the palmar joint capsule inserting into the proximal and palmar aspects of the scapholunate ligament [20, 25, 26]. It is approximately 0.7–1.2 mm thick, 8.3–9 mm long, and 2.5–4.8 mm wide [6, 20]. Its arthroscopic appearance is characterized as intra-articular fat pad [27, 28].

Various studies showed that this ligament presents a number of particularities:

(a) The RSL is morphologically distinguished from the other palmar radiocarpal ligaments by its loosely organized collagen fibers and relatively high degree of vascularity [25]. The vessels originate from the radial carpal arch, which is an anastomotic vessel between the anterior interosseous and radial arteries while the nerve fibers are terminal branches of the anterior interosseous nerve [4]. It is probably not a true ligament but a neurovascular conduit to the SLI Ligament with little mechanical integrity [29].

(b) The ligament possibly constitutes a fetal remnant of a septum that temporarily divides the radiocarpal joint into radioscaphoid and radiolunate clefts [4].

(c) Biomechanical studies showed that it is a rather weak ligament failing at approximately 40 N of applied load, but with substantial elastic behavior and higher strain at failure—approximately 175 % [15].

(d) Although its mechanical contribution is disputed, it may be important to the functional integrity of the wrist [26]. There is increasing evidence that it plays a role as a mechano-receptor monitoring the SL relationship, with afferents through the anterior interosseous nerve [4]. It is also a likely source for synovial filtration, producing synovial fluid and possibly resorbing metabolic waste.

Short Radiolunate Ligament (SRL ligament)

This ligament originates from the ulnopalmar edge of the distal radius and inserts at the junction of the proximal articular surface and the nonarticular palmar horn of the lunate, proximal to the insertion of the ulnolunate ligament (UL ligament) [3] (Fig. 2.4). The length, width, and thickness of the SRL are approximately 7.5, 10.6, and 1.2 mm, respectively [20]. The orientation of its fibers is changed from fan shaped in palmar flexion to longitudinal in dorsiflexion of the lunate [3, 4]. Although its functional role has not been fully clarified, it seems that it stabilizes the lunate (and hence the proximal carpal row) and prevents its volar, dorsal, and ulnar translation. The deficiency of the SRL is mainly responsible for the dorsal subluxation of the radiocarpal joint during the dorsal stress test of the wrist, (Fig. 2.5a, b) while the SRL has been considered the primary soft tissue restraint against volar translation of the carpus [9]. Consequently, fracture of the volar radial rim where the SRL ligament is attached, could destabilize the carpus leading to volar subluxation of the wrist (Fig. 2.6).

The SRL and LRL ligaments remain intact during a perilunate or lunate dislocation of the wrist, except in cases where the lunate is extirpated to the volar surface of the radius.

2.1.2.2 Ulnocarpal Joint

The ulnocarpal ligaments form the anterior and ulnar aspects of the ulnocarpal joint capsule [4]. These ligaments are responsible for maintaining the stability of the ulnocarpal joint, ensuring a correct axial alignment between the ulna and the ulnar side of the wrist [30] and also play an important role in the antero–posterior stability of the ulnar carpus [31, 32] or a significant restraint

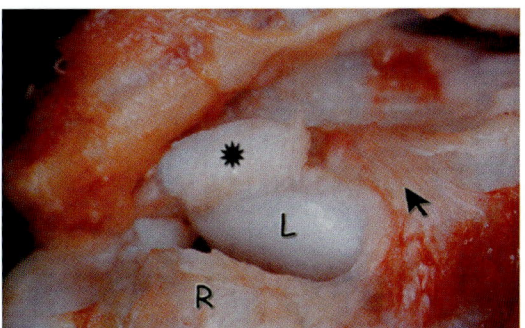

Fig. 2.4 The SRL ligament has been inverted from the volar radial rim (*asterisk*). *Arrow* indicates the LRL ligament (*R* radius, *L* lunate). With permission from [157]

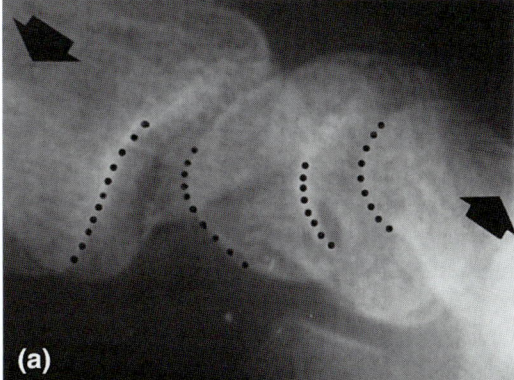

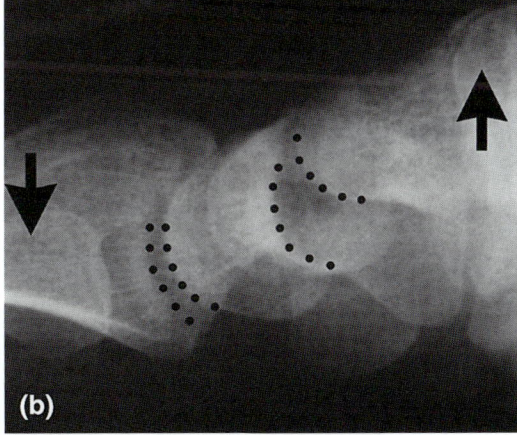

Fig. 2.5 A lax or insufficient SRL ligament could be responsible for dorsal subluxation of the radiolunate joint (**a**), while slacking of the arcuate ligament leads to subluxation of the lunocapitate joint during dorsal stress test (**b**). With permission from [157]

to dorso–palmar translation of the radiocarpal joint [11]. In addition, being part of the

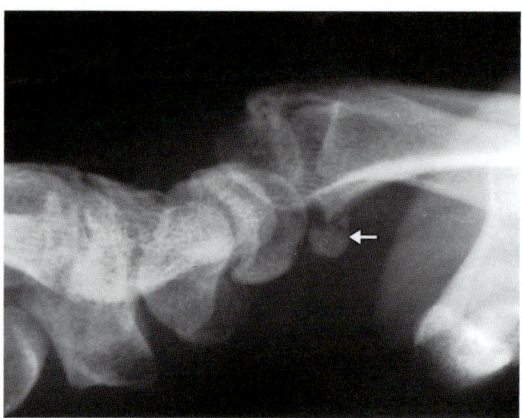

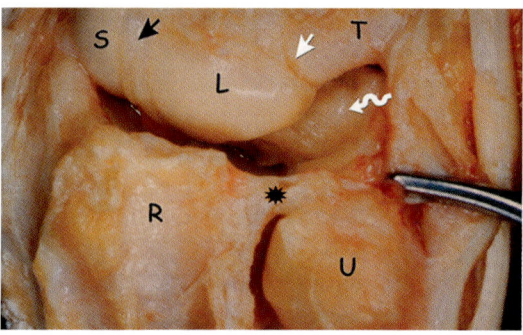

Fig. 2.8 The ulnocarpal ligaments from the dorsal side (*wavy arrow*), scapholunate ligament (*black arrow*), lunotriquetral ligament (*white arrow*), dorsal radioulnar ligament (*asterisk*) (*S* scaphoid, *L* lunate, *T* triquetrum, *R* radius, *U* ulna). With permission from [157]

Fig. 2.6 Fracture of the ulnovolar radial rim, where the SRL ligament attaches, could destabilize the wrist

ligamentous components of the TFCC, they contribute to the stability of the distal radioulnar joint (DRUJ) [23, 33] (Figs. 2.7 and 2.8).

Rupture or elongation of the ulnocarpal ligaments may lead to supination deformity of the ulnar carpus [34]. In perilunate dislocations, the infrequent finding of ruptured ulnocarpal ligaments probably indicates a reverse path of injury namely from ulnar to radial, while in cases of radiocarpal dislocations the rupture of ulnocarpal ligaments leeds to progression of the injury from ulnar translocation to multidirectional instability [35].

Ulnolunate Ligament (UL ligament)

It is located in continuity with the SRL ligament joining the formation of the volar capsule,

ulnarly of the lunate fossa. It originates from the radial-most region of the volar radioulnar ligament and coursing directly distally, attaches on the volar edge of the lunate. This ligament shows similar changes in shape as the SRL ligament during dorsiflexion and palmarflexion of the wrist. The precise function of the UL ligament is not known, but it is reasonable to assume that it mirrors the function of the SRL ligament, proximally stabilizing the lunate during all phases of wrist motion [4].

Material property studies reveal that the UL ligament fails at approximately 175 N of applied load at approximately 125 % strain [15]. The length, width, and thickness of the UL ligament are approximately 18, 2.3, and 0.7 mm, respectively [20].

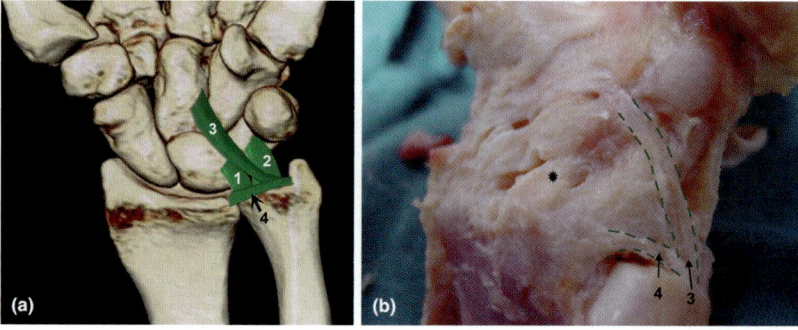

Fig. 2.7 Schematic (**a**) and cadaveric (**b**) depiction of ulnocarpal ligaments: Ulnolunate (*1*), Ulnotriquetral (*2*), Ulnocapitate (*3*), Volar radioulnar ligament (*4*) (*asterisk* short RL ligament)

Ulnotriquetral Ligament (UT ligament)

It is located ulnar to UL ligament and takes origin from the volar radioulnar ligament. It courses directly distally to insert into the proximal and palmar surface of the triquetrum. Two perforations have been found to its substance: one distally, found in more than 70 % of normal adults, leading to the pisotriquetral joint (pisotriquetral orifice) and one proximally, called the prestyloid recess that communicates with the ulnar styloid process [1] (Fig. 2.9). These two perforations constitute areas of ligamentous weakness, which can lead to longitudinal split tears of the UT ligament [36]. The medial border of the UT ligament forms the ulnar and dorsal wall of the ulnocarpal joint and the deep surface of the ECU tendon sheath as it traverses the ulnocarpal joint.

There is no clear delineation between the ulnolunate and ulnotriquetral ligaments, the division between the two being made only by their distal attachments [1].

Ulnocapitate Ligament (UC ligament)

The UC ligament is the only ulnocarpal ligament that attaches directly to the fovea region of the ulnar head. It passes distally across the ulnocarpal joint, superficial to the UT and UL ligaments. It is therefore not visible from an intraarticular perspective. Passing distally and anterior to the junction between the other ulnocarpal ligaments, at the level of lunotriquetral joint it interdigitates with fibers from the palmar region of the LT interosseous ligament. It courses around the distal margin of the palmar horn of the lunate, interdigitating with fibers from the RSC ligament, forming an "arcuate" (deltoid) ligament [4, 36]. As with the RSC ligament, only approximately 10 % of the fibers of the UC ligament actually attach to the body of the capitate [1]. Proximal to the apex of the arcuate ligament an area of weakness is located (space of Poirier), through which the midcarpal joint dislocates in perilunate injuries. The UC ligament may serve to reinforce the ulnocarpal joint capsule and the LT joint, while disruption of the UC ligament may have implications in the stability of the DRU joint [4].

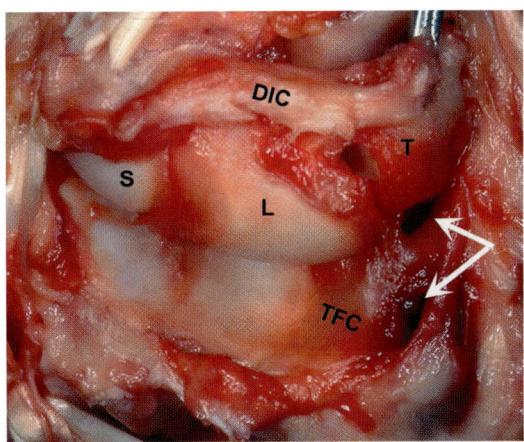

Fig. 2.9 The radiocarpal and ulnocarpal joints from the dorsal side. *White arrows* indicate the prestyloid recess (proximally) and the pisotriquetral orifice (distally). (*DIC* Dorsal intercarpal ligament, *S* scaphoid, *L* lunate, *T* triquetrum, *TFC* triangular fibrocartilage disk). In this specimen, rupture of the proximal LT ligament is evident. With permission from [157]

There has been some confusion regarding the origin of the ulnocarpal ligaments. Berger [1, 3] argued that UL and UT ligaments take origin from the volar radioulnar ligament, while the UC ligament originates directly from the fovea of the ulnar head. On the contrary, Moritomo et al. [33] stated that all ulnocarpal ligaments originate together at the fovea of the ulnar head and at the base of the ulnar styloid process. He supports that the discrepancy is due to the perspective view of the ligaments. Inspecting the ligaments arthroscopically, their origin appears to be along the volar radioulnar ligament. When inspected from the palmar side on cadavers, the ulnocarpal ligaments appear to converge into the fovea. Probably arthroscopically seeing, only part of the ligaments is visible and in fact the fibers of these ligaments extend proximally toward the fovea, although some fibers of the ligaments blend with the volar radioulnar ligament. However, it has been argued that the attachment of the ulnocarpal ligaments to the periphery of the TFC constitutes a phylogenic modification, which is necessary in order to increase the range of pronosupination without impairing the ulnocarpal joint stability [1, 30].

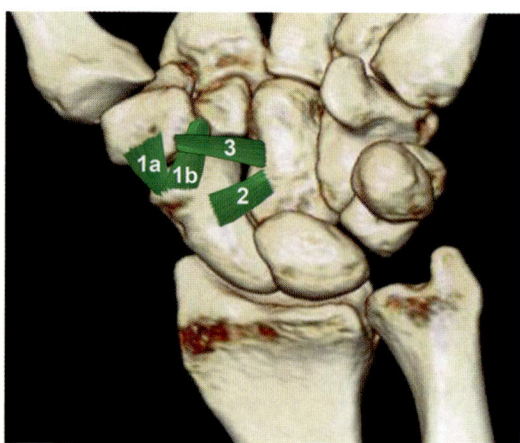

Fig. 2.10 Volar ligaments on the radial side of the midcarpal joint. Scapho-trapezium-trapezoid ligament (STT ligament) with its radial (*1a*) and ulnar band (*1b*); scaphocapitate ligament (*2*) and capitate–trapezium ligament (*3*)

2.1.2.3 Midcarpal Joint

Scapho-Trapezium-Trapezoid Ligament (STT ligament)

The STT ligament originates proximally from the radiovolar aspect of the scaphoid tuberosity, distal to the attachment of the RSC ligament. Coursing distally, it fans out to form two variably evident bands: the radial (scaphotrapezium) band forms a V-shaped structure, which attaches to the palmar and radial aspects of the trapezium. The ulnar (scaphotrapezoid) band attaches to the palmar surface of the trapezoid [1, 21, 37] (Fig. 2.10). It is the main stabilizing structure of the STT joint and is closely related to the sheath of the flexor carpi radialis tendon. Many authors [4, 38–40] studied clinically, experimentally and, biomechanically the STT ligamentous complex and made the following observations: (a) The predominant role of the distal ligamentous complex of the scaphoid over the SL ligament, which is thought to be half as strong as the distal ligamentous complex of the scaphoid, has been experimentally shown [38]. The existence of an intact STT ligament explains the absence of rotatory subluxation of the scaphoid in cases of scapholunate dissociation. (b) Scaphoid tuberosity fractures are equivalent to avulsion of the scaphotrapezial ligament [39]. (c) The axis of motion of the distal pole of the scaphoid passes through the origin of the scaphotrapezial ligament [39, 40]. (d) Although the exact function of the STT ligament remains unclear, it is believed that its principal function is to assist in maintaining the scaphoid in a palmar-flexed attitude preventing it from lying horizontally (with SL complex intact) [38], while it simultaneously minimizes excessive scaphoid flexion [39]. (e) It has been identified as an important secondary stabilizer of the scaphoid [41, 42].

Material property studies demonstrate yield strength of the STT ligament of approximately 150 N and a strain of failure at approximately 275 % [15].

Scaphocapitate Ligament (SC ligament)

The SC ligament is a strong band that obliquely crosses the palmar midcarpal joint, coursing immediately distal to the RSC ligament. It originates from the ulnar and volar side of the distal pole of the scaphoid and inserts to the radial and volar side of the capitate [4, 21] (Fig. 2.10). The SC ligament functions as a stabilizer of the distal pole of the scaphoid [4] and it may also contribute as a constraint of midcarpal pronation participating to the formation of the antipronation sling [24, 43]. A line connecting the origin of the scaphotrapezium ligament and the SC ligament is perpendicular to the interfacet ridge of the distal scaphoid, indicating that they function as collateral ligaments of a monoaxial articulation [44], and consequently, are the only ligaments guiding dart-throwing motion [45, 46]. The SC ligament is approximately 2.2 mm thick, 14 mm long, and 6.7 mm wide. It is the thickest ligament attached to the scaphoid and has the largest attachment surface area of all scaphoid ligaments [6]. Material property studies have shown average yield strength of the SC ligament of approximately 100 N and a strain of failure at approximately 200 %.

Capitate–Trapezium Ligament (CTm ligament)

The C–Tm ligament was found to originate from the radiovolar aspect of the trapezium, just under the flexor carpi radialis sheath and inserts directly

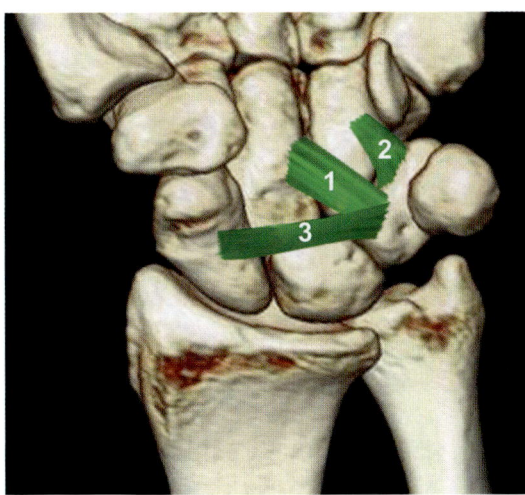

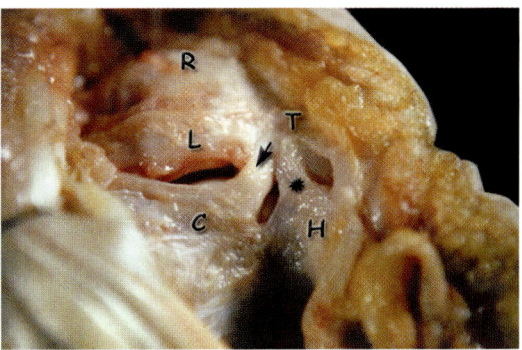

Fig. 2.12 Anatomical specimen indicating: triquetro-capitate ligament (*arrow*); triquetrohamate ligament (*asterisk*); (*C* capitate, *L* lunate, *T* triquetrum, *H* hamate, and *R* radius). With permission from [157]

Fig. 2.11 Volar ligaments on the ulnar side of the midcarpal joint: triquetrocapitate (*1*), triquetrohamate (*2*), palmar scaphotriquetral (*3*)

onto the volar waist of the capitate without any attachment to the trapezoid (Fig. 2.10). The anatomical description and its functional significance were made by Moritomo et al. [37]. This ligament appears to deepen the socket of the STT joint and serves as a labrum for the distal pole of the scaphoid, reinforcing the palmar aspect of the STT joint capsule. It was found to be highly variable in its development. The width of the C–Tm ligament ranges from 0 to 7.7 mm (average length, 3.3 mm). The development of C–Tm ligament was directly correlated to the range of scapholunate angle and the prevalence of degenerative changes in the STT joint [37].

Triquetrocapitate Ligament (TC ligament)

The TC ligament attaches proximally to the volar and radial edges of the triquetrum. It passes obliquely distally and radially to contribute to the ulnar half of the midcarpal joint capsule before attaching to the proximal and ulnar half of the capitate body (Figs. 2.11 and 2.12). Insufficiency of the TC ligament contributes to the development of ulnar or anteromedial midcarpal instability (CIND type) [47]. It may also contribute to the constraint of midcarpal supination [4], while

it is involved in the formation of the antisupination sling [43]. The yield strength has been estimated at approximately 110 N, with a yield strain at approximately 60 %.

Triquetrohamate Ligament (TH ligament)

The TH ligament is the ulnar-most ligament of the palmar midcarpal joint, originating proximally from the distal margin of the palmar cortex of the triquetrum, just ulnar to the TC ligament. It courses distally to attach to the palmar cortex of the body of the hamate, just radial to the base of the hamulus [48], with no substantial insertion onto the proximal pole of the hamate [3] (Figs. 2.11 and 2.12). The fibers of the TC and TH ligaments are interdigitated with the fibers of the UC ligament and together form the ulnar limb of the arcuate ligament. Nakamura et al. [49] described the anatomic relation of the TC and the TH ligaments as dependent on the type of lunate, whereby in type I there is no medial hamate facet and in type II there is a medial hamate facet. The relation between the TC and the TH ligaments was classified into three types. In type A, the TC ligament is completely separate from the TH ligament; in type B, the TC ligament overlaps the TH ligament; and in type C, the TC ligament has an additional ligament from the triquetrum to the proximal pole of the hamate. Eighty-two

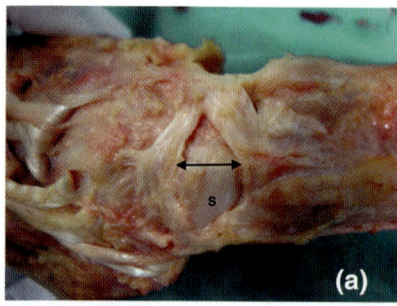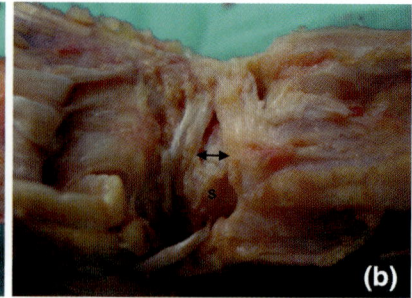

Fig. 2.13 Change in the configuration of the dorsal V ligament (dorsal radiocarpal and midcarpal ligaments) during wrist palmarflexion (**a**) and dorsiflexion (**b**), provides indirect stability to the scaphoid [52] (*S* scaphoid)

percent of type I lunates are associated with a type A relation between the TC and the TH ligaments, and 96 % of type II lunates are associated with a type C relation between the TC and the TH ligaments.

Palmar scaphotriquetral ligament (Palmar ST ligament)

There were reports of the existence of this ligamentous structure by Gunther in 1841 and Poirier et.al in 1908, (quoted by Sennwald [8]), while a more accurate description was made by Sennwald et al. [50].

Its attachment to the triquetrum is substantial and more distinct and lies between the attachments of the TC and LT interosseous ligaments. It courses horizontally spanning the midcarpal joint and inserts to the scaphoid with a thin and fan-shaped attachment, with its fibers interdigitating with those of the RSC ligament (Fig. 2.11). The palmar ST ligament may be considered an integral part of the midcarpal arcuate ligament formed by the RSC and UC ligaments [4]. With the wrist in dorsiflexion the palmar ST ligament tightens, while in palmarflexion it slackens. Radioulnar deviation does not alter the tension of the ligament. Although its function needs further investigation, it is postulated that it supports the head of the capitate during dorsiflexion of the wrist, acting as volar labrum for the lunocapitate joint [51]. It is also speculated that widening of the SL joint during dorsiflexion of the wrist, may only be possible when the palmar ST ligament is torn [50].

2.1.3 Extrinsic or Capsular Ligaments: Dorsal Surface

Until recently, emphasis was given to the description and functional significance of the palmar ligaments of the wrist. In addition, the dorsal ligaments of the wrist were generally neither preserved nor repaired during or after a dorsal approach to the wrist joint [21]. In recent years, much interest has been focused on anatomic varieties and functional significance of dorsal carpal ligaments. The dorsal radiocarpal joint is reinforced by a single ligament which bridges the ulnar half of the dorsal capsule, while the radial half of the radiocarpal joint capsule lacks any ligament reinforcement, thus leaving the proximal pole of the scaphoid and scapholunate joint uncovered. Viegas et al. [52, 53] described the "lateral V configuration" of the dorsal intercarpal and dorsal radiocarpal (DRC) ligaments. They stated that these two ligaments together act effectively as a dorsal radioscaphoid ligament that has the ability to vary its effective length threefold by changing the angle between the two arms of the V, such that the intersection angle between them at the triquetrum is acute in extension and becomes almost orthogonal in wrist palmarflexion. This ligamentous arrangement allows normal carpal kinematics while maintaining its indirect dorsal stabilizing effect on the scaphoid throughout the range of motion of the wrist. (Fig. 2.13a, b). Both dorsal ligaments, (DRC and DIC), have also been described as the dorsal V ligament [8].

2.1.3.1 Radiocarpal Joint

Dorsal Radiocarpal Ligament (DRC ligament) (Dorsal Radiotriquetral Lig., Dorsal Radiolunotriquetral Lig.)

The DRC ligament originates from the ulnar and dorsal portions of the distal end of the radius just distal and ulnar to the Lister's tubercle. It courses obliquely distally and ulnarly and inserts on the dorsal tubercle of the triquetrum. During its course it was found to have an osseous attachment onto the distal ulnar aspect of the dorsal lunate and dorsal portion of the lunotriquetral interosseous ligament (LTI ligament) [4, 20, 21]. The DRC ligament forms the floor of the fourth, fifth, and sixth extensor tendon compartments [3].

The DRC ligament morphology presents itself with many anatomical varieties [5]. It has been described as being formed by two components: a superficial radiotriquetral band and a deep radiolunotriquetral ligament, which intermingles with fibers of the lunotriquetral ligament [54]. Shaaban and Lees [55] showed that the DRC ligament consisted of two distinct parts. The ulnar part is more superficial and arises from the distal part of the interosseous border of the radius. It runs obliquely distally and ulnarward, over the distal ulna to attach to the lunate and triquetrum. On its course, the DRC ligament blends with the underlying dorsal radioulnar ligament. The radial part of the DRC ligament is deeper and arises from the posterior edge of the distal border of the radius and runs nearly horizontally and ulnarwards to attach to the lunate and triquetrum.

Mizuseki and Ikuta [56] and subsequently Viegas et al. [52, 53] classified the DRC ligament into four subtypes according to its morphology, while Smith [57] using three-dimensional Fourier transform MR imaging techniques, differentiated the DRC ligament into two subtypes. A common feature of all these subtypes is that there are forms of DRC ligament with deltoid fibers covering the dorsal aspect of the proximal scaphoid, which may offer some dorsal support to the scaphoid (Fig. 2.14).

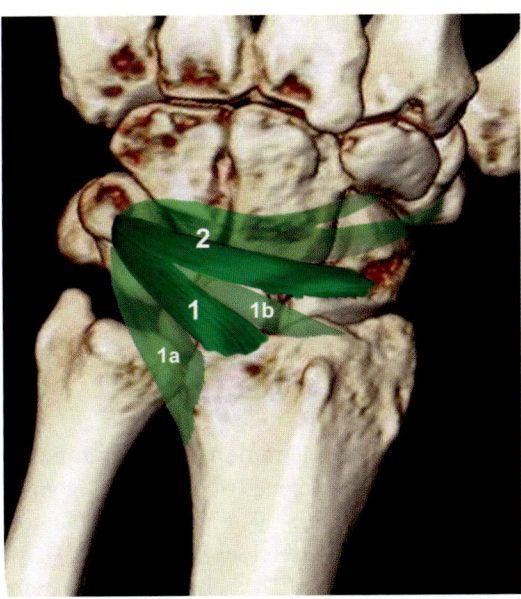

Fig. 2.14 The dorsal carpal ligaments: Dorsal radiocarpal ligament (*1*). The faint ligamentous drawings on either side of the main ligament have been described as variations: (*1a*) [55] and (*1b*) [53, 56]. Dorsal intercarpal ligament (*2*): It is consisted of a proximal thicker part (dorsal scaphotriquetral ligament) which is attached consistently to the dorsal lunate and scaphoid and a thinner distal part with inconsistent osseous attachments to the capitate, trapezoid, and trapezium [52, 57]

The reported functions of the DRC are:

(a) The DRC ligament having an oblique direction (like the palmar RC ligaments) serves to constrain ulnar translocation of the carpus [4, 13].

(b) It functions as a stabilizer and pronator of the wrist. When the forearm pronates, the DRC ligament draws the attached carpus and hand passively into pronation [22].

(c) It has been stated that the DRC ligament provides resistance to passive supination of the radiocarpal joint [10], thus participating in the formation of the antisupination sling.

(d) Sectioning the DRC ligament alters scaphoid and lunate kinematics during dynamic wrist motion and this angular change in carpal kinematics can vary up to 8° [58].

(e) The attenuation or disruption of the DRC ligament have been implicated in the development of a static VISI deformity, either as a CIND instability [59] or as a complex instability (combination of CID and CIND instabilities), when associated with rupture of the LTI ligament [59, 60].

(f) The superficial ulnar part of the dorsal radiocarpal ligament may play a role in the stabilization of DRUJ and supporting its capsule, especially in extreme pronation [55].

2.1.3.2 Midcarpal Joint

Dorsal Intercarpal Ligament (DIC ligament)
The osseous attachments of the DIC ligament have been described by a number of authors using anatomical dissections [3, 4, 52, 54], 3-D Fourier transform MRI techniques [57] or a combination of dissection, CT imaging, and a 3-D digitization technique [20, 61]. Depending on the size of development, osseous attachments, and morphology, Viegas et al. [52] identified three types of DIC, while Smith [57] recognized four types which are comparable. The fact is that the DIC ligament originates from the dorsal surface of the triquetrum interdigitating with the fibers of DRC ligament. Coursing radially, it is constituted of a thicker portion, which inserts on the dorsal groove of the scaphoid and a thinner arm, which inserts onto the dorsal trapezium and trapezoid. The proximal thicker branch augments the dorsal regions of the LT and SL interosseous ligaments, also having osseous attachments to the dorsal lunate and scaphoid. This proximal thicker band is called *dorsal scaphotriquetral ligament* [4] and probably has an important role in the transverse stabilization of the proximal carpal row [3, 54]. It may also function as a labrum for the head of the capitate and the proximal pole of the hamate dorsally, deepening the midcarpal joint, just as the Palmar ST ligament does volarly [3, 4] (Fig. 2.14). The width of this ligament is inconstant, causing it to be frequently confused with the DIC ligament [62]. Recently, the osseous attachment of the DIC ligament on the scaphoid gained particular functional significance [63]. The most dorsal and ulnar nonarticulating part of

the scaphoid, where the dorsal SL interosseous ligament and the proximal fibers of the DIC ligament attach, is called *scaphoid apex*. It is argued that carpal instability following scaphoid nonunion is closely related to whether the fracture line passes distal or proximal to the scaphoid apex [64]. Moritomo et al. [19] stated that there are two clear patterns of the interfragmentary motions of the scaphoid, based on the fracture location: the unstable (mobile) type scaphoid nonunion, where the fracture is located distal to the scaphoid apex and the stable type, where the fracture is located proximal to the scaphoid apex [19].

Its dimensions were calculated, using CT and an imaging cryomicrotome, and it was found to be approximately 1.2 mm thick, 32.6 mm long, and 6.3 mm wide [6].

Viegas et al. [52] suggested that the mechanical strength of the DIC ligament is 115.0 ± 57.2 N and that the combined mechanical properties of the DIC and the dorsal SLI Ligament have mechanical strength (162.4 ± 64.7 N) comparable with the DRC (143.3 ± 41.5 N).

Significant observations related to the DIC ligament are the following:

(a) The utilization of the DIC ligament for dorsal capsulodesis of the scaphoid in cases of scapholunate dissociation, as opposed to the traditional Blatt's capsulodesis which tethers the scaphoid to the distal radius and predictably leads to limitations in wrist flexion. The DIC ligament capsulodesis has been used by detaching the ligament off its insertion on the trapezoid and trapezium and tied to a bony trough on the dorsal surface of the distal pole of the scaphoid [65, 66]. The technique assumes that a substantial part of the DIC ligament is attached to the trapezio-trapezoid bones. Alternatively, the proximal part of the DIC ligament could be detached from the triquetrum and transferred to the distal radius after the reduction of the scaphoid malalignment [67]; (b) the need to reattach the DIC ligament to the dorsal pole of the scaphoid and lunate as well as the dorsal portion of the SL ligament in cases of static DISI [52, 68, 69]; (c) the surgical approach to the dorsum of the wrist that spares both the dorsal radiocarpal and intercarpal ligaments [4, 70] or the concomitant ligament and nerve sparing approach [71]; and (d) having an important role in the transverse stabilization of the proximal carpal row and being part of the ligamentous arrangement which constitutes the antipronation sling, there is often a need for substitution of the DIC ligament, using tendon grafts [24].

2.1.4 Intrinsic Ligaments

2.1.4.1 Interosseous Ligaments of the Proximal Carpal Row

The scapholunate and lunotriquetral interosseous ligaments of the proximal carpal row are both C-shaped spanning the dorsal, proximal, and palmar margins of their respective joint spaces [48]. Their integrity is essential for maintenance of normal carpal kinematics. The thickest and strongest region of the scapholunate ligament is located dorsally, while that of the lunotriquetral ligament is located palmarly [72, 73]. This construction seems to support the "balanced lunate" concept [73], meaning that the lunate is under the influence of two opposite moments (scaphoid flexion and triquetral extension) which counteract each other (Fig. 2.15).

Scapholunate interosseous ligament (SLI ligament)

The SLIL has been described as consisting of three regions on the basis of macroscopic and histological criteria: dorsal, proximal, and palmar regions (Fig. 2.16). Bone insertions on both the scaphoid and the lunate are limited to the most proximal and superior parts of the articular surface between the two bones [62]. The dorsal and palmar regions have histologic organizations consistent with true capsular ligaments, while the proximal region is composed of fibrocartilage, with few collagen fascicles [4]. The dorsal region is the thickest of the three regions, it has a trapezoidal shape and is composed of transversely oriented collagen fascicles surrounded by connective tissue, through which course vascular and nervous bundles. It measures approximately

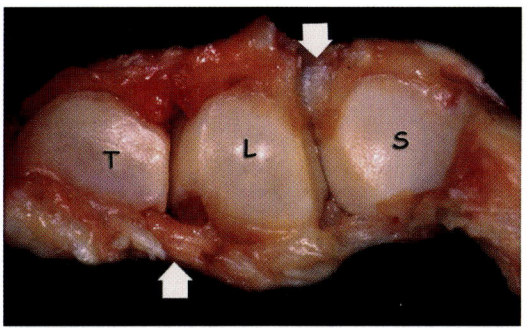

Fig. 2.15 The distal articular surfaces of the proximal carpal row bones as seen from the midcarpal joint. The distal parts of the scapholunate and lunotriquetral joint spaces remain free from ligamentous attachments. *White arrows* indicate the strongest regions of the scapholunate (dorsal) and the lunotriquetral (volar) ligaments. (*S* scaphoid, *L* lunate, *T* triquetrum). With permission from [157]

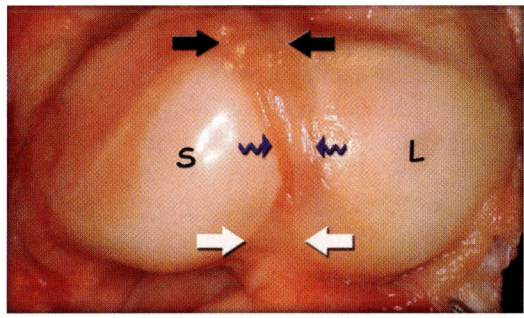

Fig. 2.16 The scapholunate interosseous ligament as seen from the radiocarpal joint. Dorsal region (*black arrows*); Volar region (*white arrows*); proximal fibrocartilaginous region (*wavy blue arrows*) (*S* scaphoid, *L* lunate). With permission from [157]

5–6 mm in proximal—distal length, 3–5 mm long, and 2–4 mm thick. It is contiguous distally to the dorsal scaphotriquetral ligament and merges proximally and indiscernibly with the proximal region of the SL ligament. The proximal region of the SL ligament can extend into the scapholunate joint space with a triangular cross-section, much like a knee meniscus. The proximal region is composed almost entirely of fibrocartilage. It is approximately 1 mm thick, 4 mm long, and 11 mm wide [20]. The continuity of the proximal and palmar regions of the SL ligament is interrupted by the RSL ligament [3]. The dimensions of the palmar region vary

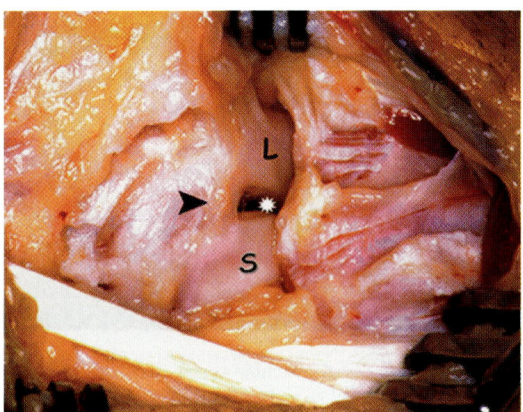

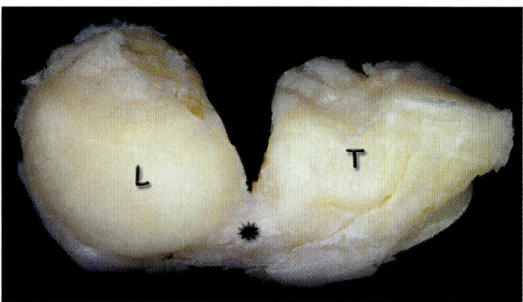

Fig. 2.18 The lunate and triquetral bones from the dorsal side. Lunotriquetral ligament (*asterisk*). With permission from [157]

Fig. 2.17 Surgical finding of a patient, who reported pain during loading of the wrist in dorsiflexion. Watson test was negative. The dorsal SL ligament was intact (*arrow*), while the proximal region was absent due to chronic rupture (*asterisk*). (*S* scaphoid, *L* lunate). With permission from [157]

between 1 and 2 mm in thickness, 3–5 mm in length, and 4–7 mm in width [20, 25, 62]. Its fibers are obliquely oriented from the palmar rim of the proximal scaphoid to the palmar rim of the palmar horn of the lunate. This region of the ligament is not visible because the LRL ligament covers its palmar surface, while proximally and dorsally it is covered by the RSL ligament.

The SLIL is a strong ligament often requiring up to 300 N of distraction force to rupture. The majority of distraction strength is found in the dorsal region, the palmar region fails with 150 N stress, and the proximal region can withstand only a 25–50 N stress [4, 74]. Biomechanical studies showed that the dorsal region is the most critical for resistance to palmar–dorsal translation and distraction, but the palmar region is the most important rotational constraint [62, 74]. The proximal fibrocartilage region appears appropriate to accept compression and shear loads (Fig. 2.17). Less than 20° of motion is possible at the SL joint [29]. A number of biomechanical studies have emphasized the importance of the SLIL as the primary stabilizer of the SL articulation and that its disruption alters scaphoid and lunate kinematics, i.e., scaphoid flexion, scaphoid pronation, and lunate extension [75, 76].

It is known that the dorsal and proximal regions of the SLI ligament are the most accessible regions through a dorsal wrist arthrotomy, while it is impossible to approach the palmar region of the scapholunate ligament without compromising the palmar radiocarpal ligaments through a palmar wrist arthrotomy [74]. Regardless of the above, some authors, believing that the palmar region of the SLI ligament plays an important role in the stability of the SL complex, suggested the reconstruction of the palmar part of the ligament alone [77] or in combination with the dorsal part of the SLI ligament [78] or substituted the palmar part with tendon graft in cadavers [79]. Berger [74, 80] suggested that for scapholunate dissociation, the operation is unlikely to be successful with reconstruction of the dorsal SLIL alone. In addition, there are reports upgrading the mechanical [81] and sensory [82] importance of the palmar SLI ligament.

Lunotriquetral interosseous ligament (LTI ligament)

The LT ligament is divided histologically into three regions, in a manner similar to the SL ligament (Figs. 2.15 and 2.18). The dorsal and palmar regions are composed of true ligaments, with collagen fascicles, perifascicular spaces, small blood vessels, and nerves. The proximal region is composed of avascular fibrocartilage [4]. The palmar subregion of the LT ligament is the thickest subregion (2.3 ± 0.3 mm) and the proximal region is the thinnest (1.0 ± 0.2 mm); the

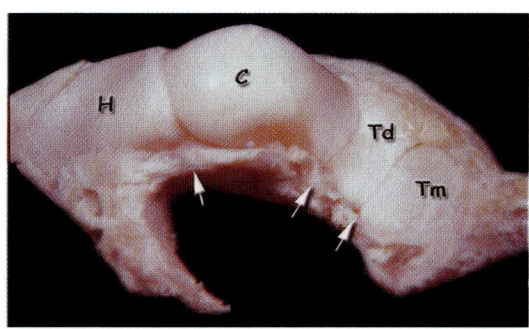

Fig. 2.19 The proximal articular surfaces of the distal carpal row. *Arrows* indicates the volar interosseous ligaments of the distal carpal row. (*H* hamate, *C* capitate, *Td* trapezoid, *Tm* trapezium). With permission from [157]

dorsal subregion is intermediate (1.4 ± 0.2 mm) [73]. The dorsal region is often reinforced with fibers of the DRC and dorsal scaphotriquetral ligaments.

The palmar region is strongly reinforced and interdigitating with fibers from the UC ligament. The proximal region, like the SLIL, resembles a knee meniscus, often with a distally directed apex extending into the LT joint space.

The material and constraint properties have shown that the palmar component failure force was 301 ± 36 N; the dorsal, 121 ± 4 2 N; and the proximal, 64 ± 14 N [73].

Contrary to the SLIL, the palmar region of the LTI is the most critical in constraining mutual translation of the lunate and triquetrum, whereas the dorsal region is the most important rotational constraint.

Published reports have shown that isolated complete sectioning of the LT ligament alters the kinematics of the LT complex, but the classic VISI deformity does not occur until both the dorsal radiotriquetral (RT) and scaphotriquetral (ST) ligaments are compromised [4, 83].

2.1.4.2 Interosseous Ligaments of the Distal Carpal Row

The four bones of the distal carpal row form three interposed joints: trapezium-trapezoid, trapezo-capitate, and capito-hamate joints. These joints are principally constrained by ligaments that simply span the joint space of two adjacent

bones. These joints are bridged by interosseous ligaments and adjoin each other especially on the palmar side (Fig. 2.19). These ligaments do not span the entire proximal–distal dimension of the joint, having only dorsal and palmar portions, which tend to interdigitate with fibers from the adjacent carpometacarpal joints [4].

It has been stated that the interosseous ligaments (especially their palmar regions) connecting the bones of the distal carpal row, are crucial in providing transverse carpal stability and that the flexor retinaculum has small contribution to the transverse carpal stability [84].

Trapeziotrapezoid ligament (TT ligament)

The TT ligament is composed of dorsal and palmar regions transversely spanning the dorsal and palmar edges of the trapezium-trapezoid joint space. Both regions are 1–2 mm thick and up to 5 mm wide in the proximal–distal direction. The dorsal region forms the floor for the ECRL tendon. The material properties of the dorsal and palmar regions have been studied, revealing yield strengths of 150 and 125 N, respectively [15].

Trapeziocapitate Ligament (TC ligament)

The TC ligament is composed of dorsal, palmar, and deep regions. The dorsal and palmar regions are composed of flat sheets of true capsular ligament (1–2 mm thick, 3–5 mm wide), spanning the space between the two bones.

The deep region is situated entirely within the joint space; it is cylindrical in shape and covers the "notch" created in the articular surface of the trapezoid and capitate. The deep component substantially enhances the structural integrity of the joint. Material property testing of the dorsal and palmar regions of the TC ligament reveal failure occurring at approximately 125 N individually [15, 84].

Capitohamate Ligament (CH ligament)

The CH ligament, like the TC ligament, can be divided into three regions—dorsal, palmar, and deep. The dorsal region is thick (1–2 mm) and broad and is transversely oriented, spanning the distal part of the capitohamate joint. The proximal part of the joint is devoid of ligamentous connections. The dorsal region was found to be the principal stabilizing structure for palmar rotation and palmar translation, as well as for proximal and distal translation of the capitate relative to the hamate. The palmar region is similar to the dorsal, but is more continuous with the other palmar interosseous ligaments. The deep region was found to be short and very strong while, because of its central location to the joint, it acts as a pivot point for rotation at the CH joint. It is most important in constraining dorsal rotation and dorsal translation of the capitate relative to the hamate. The coherence between capitate and hamate was investigated by Ritt [83], who found that the dorso–palmar translational displacement averaged 0.9 and 0.5 mm, respectively, proximal–distal translational displacement averaged 0.8 and 0.4 mm, respectively, and distractional displacement averaged 0.3 mm. Material property studies reveal that the deep ligament was strongest at 289 N, followed by the palmar at 171 N and the dorsal at 133 N [83].

Therefore, the CH ligament and especially the combined palmar and deep regions exhibit the greatest strength contributing substantially to the transverse stability of the distal row.

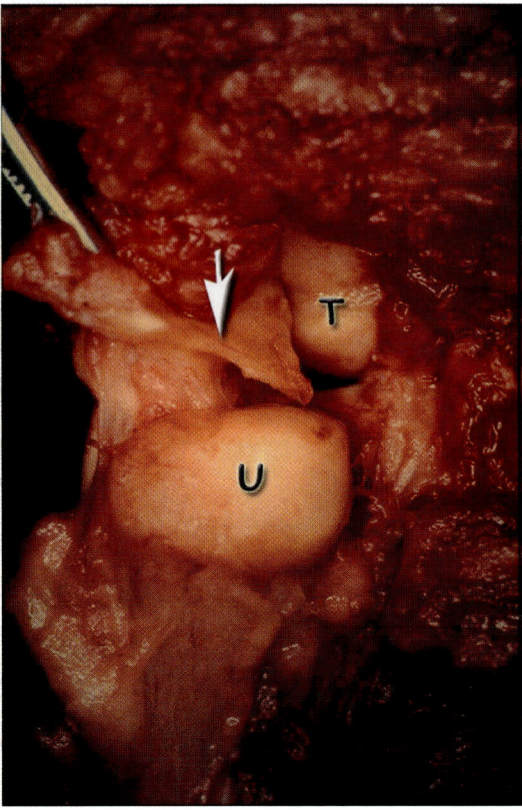

Fig. 2.20 The distal radioulnar joint. The *arrow* indicates the articular disk, which has been cut from the sigmoid notch and lifted up. *U* ulnar head, *T* triquetrum. With permission from [157]

2.1.5 Ligaments of the Distal Radioulnar Joint

2.1.5.1 Triangular Fibrocartilage Complex

The triangular fibrocartilage complex (TFCC) separates DRUJ from the radiocarpal joint. The term "TFCC" was invented by Palmer and Werner [85]. The complex includes: the articular disk (discus articularis) (Fig. 2.20), the dorsal and palmar radioulnar ligaments, the meniscus homologue (MH), and the extensor carpi ulnaris sheath (the floor of which is often called the ulnar collateral ligament) (Fig. 2.21). The TFCC originates from the distal rim of the radial sigmoid notch and inserts on the fovea of the ulnar head and the base of the ulnar styloid. The articular

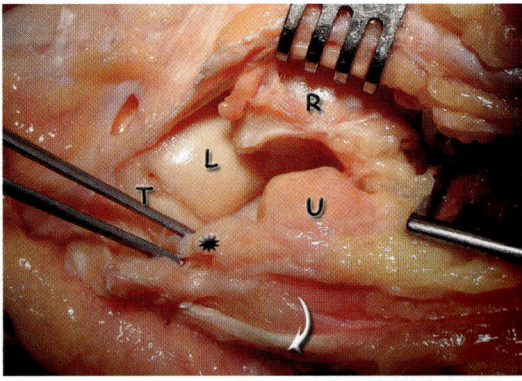

Fig. 2.21 DRUJ from the dorsal side. The picture indicates the close relationship of the ECU sheath with the TFCC. The ECU tendon has been dislocated from its sheath (*curved arrow*). The *asterisk* indicates the TFC that has been lifted off its radius attachment. *T* triquetrum, *L* lunate, *U* ulnar head, *R* radius. With permission from [157]

disk is a fibrocartilaginous biconcave structure, interposed between the ulnar dome and the ulnar aspect of the carpus. Although it has been determined that the thickness of the articular disk proper is generally 1–2 mm, the thickness varies inversely with positive ulnar variance [86].

The dorsal (DRU) and palmar (PRU) radioulnar ligaments are composed of longitudinally oriented bundles of collagen fibers that originate and insert directly into the bone, while the central articular disk is composed of fibrocartilage that originates from the hyaline cartilage of the distal radiolunate fossa [87, 88].

The DRU and PRU ligaments, contribute to the formation of the extensor carpi ulnaris subsheath and the ulnocarpal ligament complex, respectively [3]. The DRU ligament is also reinforced with ligamentous fibers originating from the ulnar aspect of the distal radius. These ligamentous fibers have been described as a separate ligament (dorsal radial metaphyseal arcuate ligament [48]), a component of the dorsal radiocarpal ligament [55], or part of the interosseous ligament of the forearm [89].

The DRU and PRU ligaments consist of *superficial* components inserting directly onto the ulna styloid and *deep* components inserting more lateral, into the fovea adjacent to the articular surface of the pole of the distal ulna [90] (Fig. 2.22). The fibers of the superficial component form an acute angle as they converge on the ulna styloid from the medial radius. This acute angle of attachment gives the superficial TFC a poor mechanical advantage for guiding the radio-carpal unit through an arc of pronosupination. The deep components of the TFC form an obtuse angle of attachment, much more mechanically advantageous in stabilizing rotation of the radius around the fixed ulna. The deep components of the TFC have been referred to by wrist investigators as the *Ligamentum subcruentum* [30, 90, 91].

Two independent studies, that of Af Ekenstam and Hagert [92], Schuind et al. [93], have created confusion in the scientific community as to which fibers (those of DRU or PRU ligament) tighten in pronation and which tighten in supination, because the results of their study were exactly the

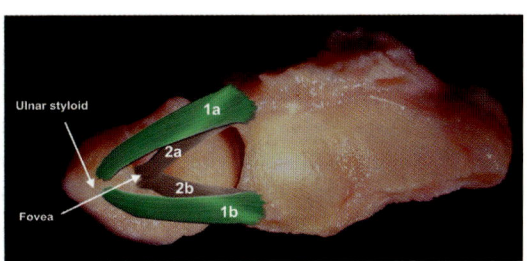

Fig. 2.22 The superficial components of the dorsal (*1a*) and volar (*1b*) radioulnar ligaments that are inserted to the ulnar styloid; the deep components of the dorsal (*2a*) and volar (*2b*) radioulnar ligaments, which are inserted to the fovea of the ulnar head. Both components (*1a* and *2a*) constitute the dorsal radioulnar ligament, while both (*2a* and *2b*) components constitute the volar radioulnar ligament

opposite. The conflict ended in 1994 when Hagert [94] recognized that both research groups were correct but that each was examining a different piece of the puzzle. Af Ekenstam and Hagert [92] examined the deep fibers, while Schuind [93] examined the superficial fibers of the ligaments. Hagert [94] clearly stated that in forearm pronation, the dorsal superficial fibers of the TFC must tighten for stability, as do the deep palmar fibers of the Ligamentum subcruentum. Conversely, in supination, the palmar superficial TFC radioulnar fibers (to the ulna styloid) tighten, as do the deep dorsal fibers of the Ligamentum subcruentum, making both theories correct.

The radius of curvature of the sigmoid notch is 15 mm and its center correlates to the ulnar styloid, while the radius of curvature of the ulnar head is 10 mm and its center correlates to the region of the fovea. This difference in the radius of curvatures leads to both rotational and sliding motions in the normal joint.

Hagert and Hagert [95] recently presented a new perspective on the stability of the joint which is correlated to the structural principle named *Tensegrity (A term derived from combining the words tension and integrity; means that the integrity of a structure depends on the balance of tension and compression within it).* The analogue of this principle to the stability of DRUJ is that "the radioulnar ligaments have a spiral configuration as they insert into a surface area, not one single point, on the ulnar head. The helicoidal bundles, in conjunction with the combined centric and epicentric insertions of the deep and superficial radioulnar portions respectively, lead to a continuous shift in the tension of various portions of the ligaments. This continuous shift in tension and compression constitutes the core of DRUJ stability and is the essence of tensegrity".

The Meniscus Homologue (MH) is the soft-tissue structure that emerged after the recession of the ulnar styloid in hominoids [30]. The MH has been described as a triangular soft tissue structure located in the space between the medioproximal aspect of the triquetrum and the ulnar styloid process and the articular disk. It is formed by well vascularized, loose connective tissue, the inner surface of which is lined by synovial cells. Although it has been considered as an extension of the TFC [96] or as a true collateral ligament [97], Berger [3] stated that the impression of a "meniscus" is derived from paracoronal sections of cadaver wrists, where the section cuts were through the prestyloid recess, where the UT ligament appears to form a distal "lip" covering the recess and that in any case it does not denote any functional significance or anatomic difference from surrounding tissue.

According to Ishii et al. [91]. the MH and the prestyloid recess (the cavity adjacent to the ulnar styloid) can be seen in three anatomic variations: the narrow opening type in 74 % of specimens, the wide opening type in 11 %, and the no opening type in 15 %.

The TFC receives its blood supply from: (1) the ulnar artery through its palmar and dorsal radiocarpal branches and (2) the dorsal and palmar branch of the anterior interosseous artery [87, 98]. Interosseous vessels from the ulnar head also enter the TFCC through the foveal area. Small vessels penetrate the TFCC in a radial fashion from the palmar, ulnar, and dorsal attachments of the joint capsule and supply the peripheral 10–20 % of the TFC. The central 80–85 % is avascular, with no vessels entering the articular disk from the radius [87, 99]. Therefore, tears that occur in the center and along the radial attachment of the disk, are not likely to heal [98, 99].

The TFCC has been shown to have three major functions:

1. The central part (articular disk) functions as a cushion for the ulnar carpus carrying approximately 20 % of the axial load of the forearm.
2. The peripheral part (ligamentous) is the major stabilizer of the DRUJ.
3. The ulnocarpal ligaments and the sheath of the ECU contribute to the stability between the ulnar head and the ulnar carpus.

2.1.6 Morphology and Ligamentous Restraints of the Scaphoid

Many authors clearly demonstrated the variations in morphology of the carpal bones and their articulations [100–102]. Normal carpal kinematics relies on the complex interplay between the arrangement of carpal ligaments and carpal bone morphology [103], while the ligamentous attachments of the scaphoid and the shape of the bones with which it articulates, play an important role [104, 105].

The morphological and morphometric features of the scaphoid have been described in radiographs [106], and in cadavers [107, 108]. Although the ligament attachments cover 9 ± 0.9 % of the total scaphoid surface area, there is a lack of consensus on the anatomy of the ligaments attaching to the scaphoid, while interindividual variability of ligament insertions and morphology, exists [5].

In vivo kinematic studies had previously identified two distinct types of scaphoid motion [109–111], which constitute two major theories of carpal mechanics (row and column). In both theories, the scaphoid is considered an essential structure [104, 112], but the patterns observed have not been related to anatomical variations in the reviewed literature [113]. Fogg [113] in his thesis correlated the anatomic variation in morphology of the scaphoid and of the ligaments attached to it, with the kinematic behavior of the scaphoid. The two types of scaphoid are summarized in Table 2.2.

Table 2.2 Osseous and ligamentous characteristics of the two types of scaphoid

	Type 1 scaphoid rotating/translating. Row theory	Type 2 scaphoid flexing/extending. Column theory
Osseous morphology		
Dorsal crest	Single dorsal high crest	Three dorsal low crests
Distal articular surface	Large and elongated	Small
Ulnar surface to capitate	Large, elongated, and shallow	Short and deep; Acts as fulcrum about which the scaphoid is moved
Ulnar surface to lunate	Smaller	Larger
Length of scaphoid	Longer	Shorter
Tuberosity	Prominent tuberosity	Less distinct tuberosity
Ligamentous patterns		
STT ligament	V-shape with proximal apex	V-shape with distal apex
Scaphocapitate lig	Long and thin; radial scaphoid attachment	Short and wide; ulnar scaphoid attachment
Dorsal intercarpal lig	Trapeziotrapezoid radial attachment	Scaphoid radial attachment
Radiocapitate lig.	No scaphoid attachment (Radiocapitate lig.)	Scaphoid attachment (Radioscaphocapitate lig.)

It is widely accepted that the ligamentous restraints stabilizing the scaphoid are classified into primary and secondary [41, 42, 58, 114–116]. There is no consensus as to which ligaments are the primary and which are the secondary stabilizers. SLIL is considered as *the primary stabilizer* of the SL joint and is surrounded by several secondary stabilizers, each insufficient to cause instability after isolated disruption, but each is important in the maintenance of normal SL kinematics and vulnerable to attritional wear after complete disruption of the SLIL [116]; this is thought to be the etiology for delayed development of dorsal intercalated segment instability (DISI) after isolated disruption of the SLIL. The relative importance of each of these ligaments to SL stability has not conclusively been established; however, the status of the secondary stabilizers is particularly important in choosing the method to treat the SL instability.

As *Scaphoid secondary stabilizers* or the second line of defense, the following have been reported: the STT, RSC, SC, and the unique V-arrangement of the DIC and DRC ligaments. Probably the insertions of the DIC (dorsal scaphotriquetral ligament) to the dorsal SLIL and its osseous attachments to the dorsal lunate and scaphoid should also be considered as primary stabilizers of the scaphoid.

In clinical settings, there are cases of rupture or insufficiency of the primary ligamentous restraints, while the secondary restraints are intact. Such cases manifest with *SL dissociation without rotary subluxation of the scaphoid (RSS)* (widening of the SL space, rupture of the dorsal SL ligament, and normal SL angle) (Fig. 2.23a, b, c). At the other end of the spectrum, there are cases with insufficiency mainly of the secondary stabilizers, while the primary stabilizers remain relatively intact. Such cases manifest with *RSS without SL dissociation* (foreshortened scaphoid on posteroanterior radiographs with a positive ring sign, increased SL angle, and the dorsal SL ligament macroscopically intact) (Fig. 2.24a, b, c). Finally, there are cases of concurrent injury of the primary and secondary stabilizers which is manifested *with SL dissociation and RSS* resulting

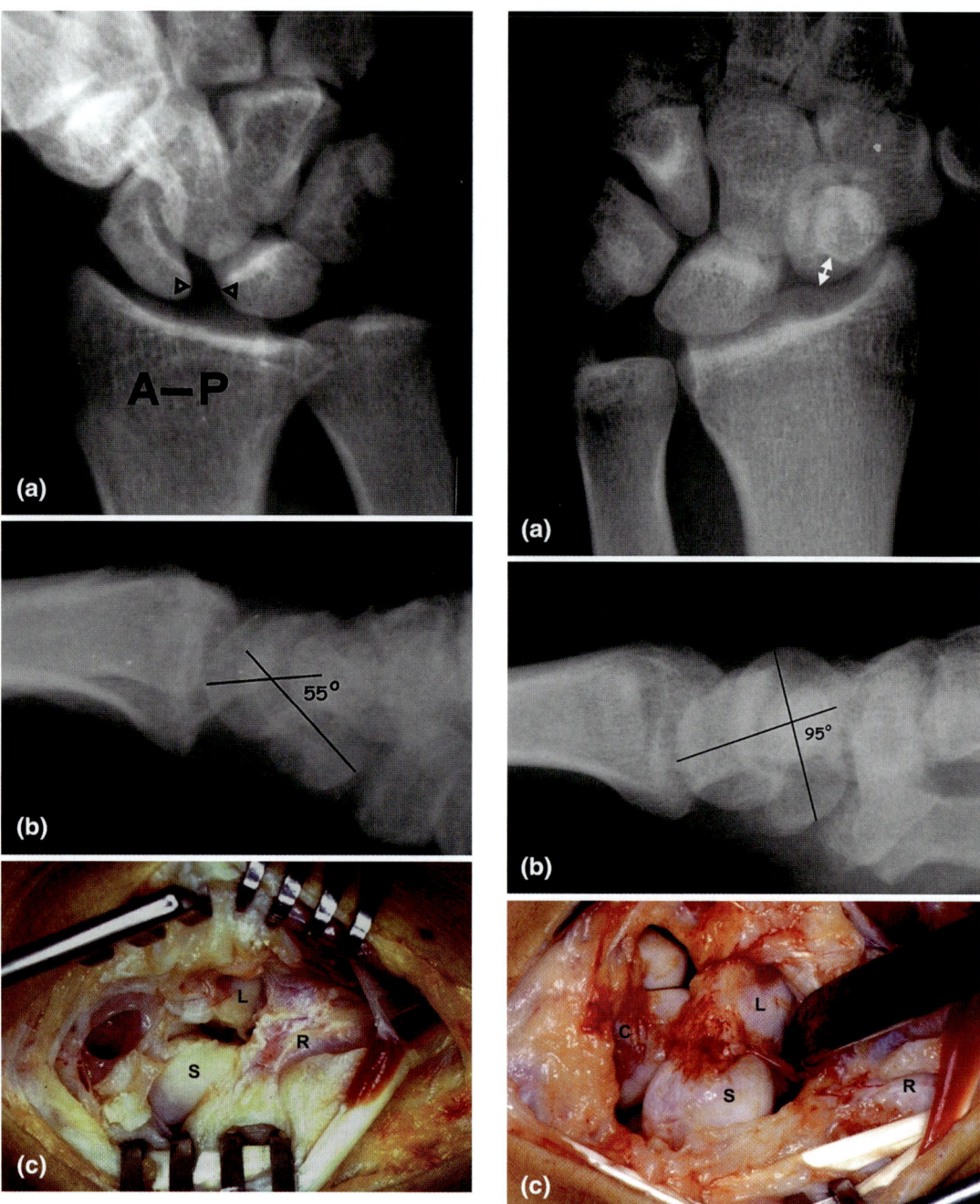

Fig. 2.23 An example of injury of the primary ligamentous restraints of the scaphoid, while secondary restraints are intact. Widening of the SL space (**a**), normal SL angle (**b**), complete rupture of the dorsal SL ligament (**c**)

Fig. 2.24 A case with insufficiency of the secondary stabilizers while the primary stabilizers remain relatively intact. Foreshortened scaphoid on P-A radiographs with a positive ring sign (**a**), increased SL angle (**b**) and a macroscopically intact dorsal SL ligament (**c**)

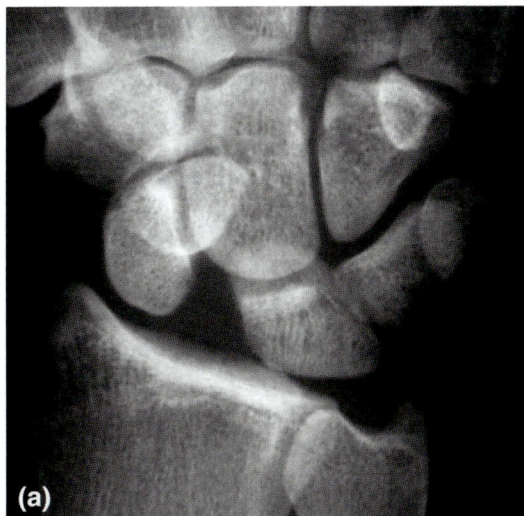

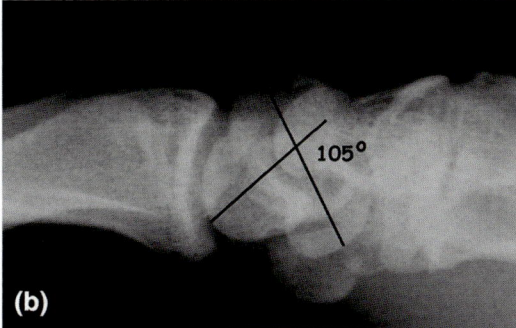

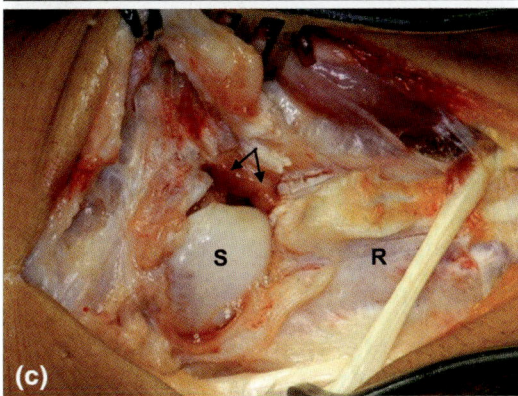

Fig. 2.25 A case of concurrent injury of the primary and secondary stabilizers of the scaphoid. SL dissociation (**a**), rotatory subluxation of the scaphoid (**b**) and complete rupture of the SL ligament (**c**)

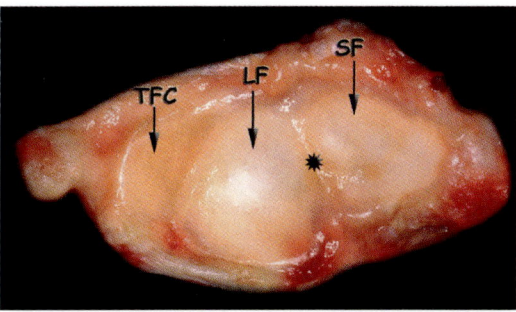

Fig. 2.26 The proximal part of the radiocarpal joint. Scaphoid fossa (*SF*), lunate fossa (*LF*), triangular fibrocartilage disk (*TFC*), interfacet prominence (*asterisk*). With permission from [157]

2.2 Anatomy of the Joints

2.2.1 Radiocarpal Joint

The radiocarpal joint is a glenoid type of articulation consisting of two elements: (a) the antebrachial glenoid, formed by the distal articular surface of the radius in conjunction with the TFC (Fig. 2.26) and (b) the carpal condyle, formed by the convex proximal articular surfaces of the proximal carpal row bones.

The articular surface of the distal radius is grossly triangular in shape with its apex toward the radial styloid and its base next to the articular cavity for the head of the ulna (sigmoid notch). The radius has two articular facets (the scaphoid and lunate fossae), separated by a cartilaginous saggital ridge (the interfacet prominence). The biconcave scaphoid fossa is triangular or oval shaped and has a smaller radius of curvature than that of the lunate fossa. The orientation of the scaphoid fossa is 11° volar and 21° ulnar relative to the long axis of the radius [14]. The lunate fossa is quadrangular in shape, biconcave although shallower, and less inclined toward the ulnar side (15° average) than the scaphoid fossa (30°). The volar lunate facet projects approximately 3 mm anterior to the flat volar surface of the distal radius with narrow width (on average <5 mm) [48]. The fracture of this bone protrusion (to which the SRL ligament attaches)

either because the initial injury is extensive or because to the initial limited ligamentous injury, attritional wear or slackening of the remaining ligaments is added (Fig. 2.25a, b, c).

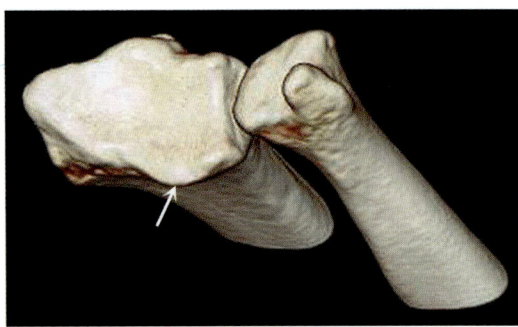

Fig. 2.27 The projection of the volar lunate facet

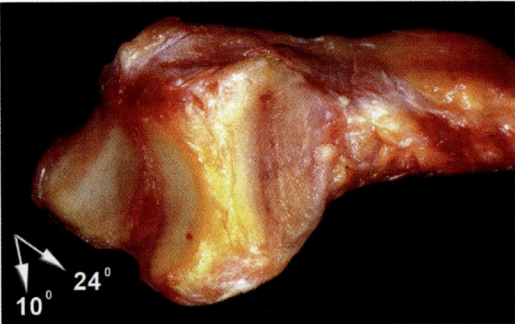

Fig. 2.28 The ulnovolar inclination of the distal radius. With permission from [157]

destabilizes the wrist, while its fixation is difficult with the usual volar plates (Fig. 2.27). The radioulnar and the dorso–palmar diameters of the two articular surfaces are 4–5 and 1.5–2 cm, respectively. The distal articular surface of the distal radius is tilted in two planes. In the saggital plane, there is an average 10° of tilt and in the frontal plane there is an ulnar inclination averaging 24° (19°–29°) [117] (Fig. 2.28).

The bones of the proximal row are joined at their proximal edges by the interosseous ligaments forming a smooth biconvex surface. Communication through these ligaments becomes a normal feature at advanced ages [96].

The thickness of the articular cartilage of the distal articular surface of the radius ranges between 0.7 and 1.2 mm. There is a significant difference in the size of the articular surfaces and the degree of curvature between the opposing articular surfaces of the radiocarpal joint. The proximal articular surfaces of the scaphoid and

lunate are 60 % larger than the distal articular surface of the radius. The curvature of the proximal carpal row is 1.5 times greater than that of the distal articular surface of the radius.

It has been postulated that differences in bony anatomy of the radioscaphoid articulation may affect the scaphoid stability after soft-tissue injury. Larger curvatures of the scaphoid fossa and proximal scaphoid as well as a deeper scaphoid fossa and a greater volar tilt of the radius, are factors preventing instability despite any ligamentous tears [118].

The joint capsule is reinforced by palmar and dorsal capsular ligaments the inner side of which appears resurfaced by synovial tissue. A number of recesses, varying in size and shape, have been described: (a) recessus prestyloideus, located just palmar to the ulnar styloid process, (b) recessus prescaphoideus, located proximal and palmar to the scaphoid, (c) recessus preradialis, located in front of the RSL ligament, and (d) recessus pretriquetralis which acts as communication with the pisotriquetral joint.

2.2.2 Midcarpal Joint

From an anatomic point of view the midcarpal joint may have the most complicated joint shape in the human body. In a broad sense there are three articulations: (a) the STT joint, (b) the scapholuno-capitate joint, and (c) the triquetro-hamate joint. The former is convex proximally whereas the latter two are concave.

2.2.2.1 Scapho-Trapezium-Trapezoid Joint

It is a glenoid type of joint that is formed from the convex articular surface of the scaphoid and the concave joints of trapezium-trapezoid. Moritomo et.al [37] depending on the shape, recognized three types of joint surfaces of the distal scaphoid and in most cases (81 %) they found an interfacet ridge on the joint surface of the distal scaphoid, which is oriented in line with the trapezio-trapezoid articulation (Fig. 2.29). This ridge was classified into three categories according to its

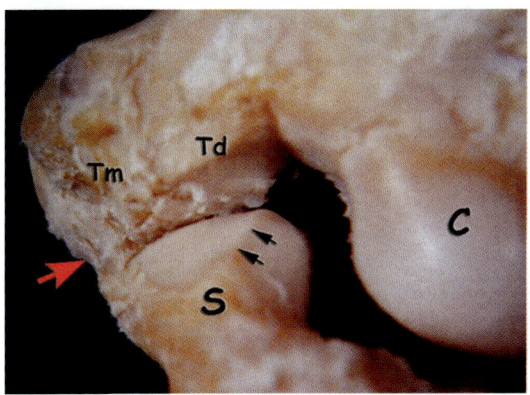

Fig. 2.29 The radial side of the midcarpal joint. The STT ligament (*red arrow*); The interfacet ridge of the distal scaphoid (*double black arrows*); (*C* capitate, *S* scaphoid, *Tm* trapezium, *Td* trapezoid). With permission from [157]

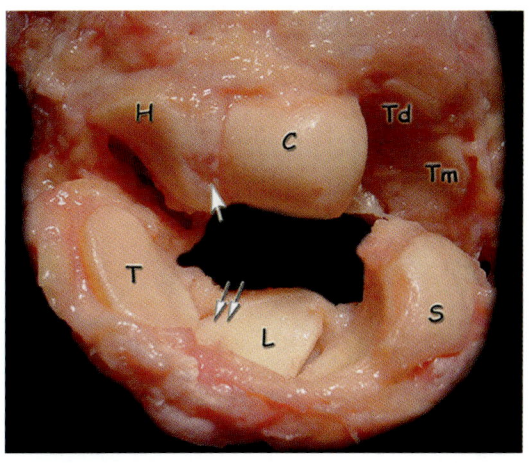

Fig. 2.30 The midcarpal joint. A lunate type II is apparent (*double arrows*) with arthritic changes of the proximal hamate (*white arrow*) (*T* triquetrum, *L* lunate, *S* scaphoid, *H* hamate, *C* capitate, *Tm* trapezium, *Td* trapezoid). With permission from [157]

development or lack of development and runs obliquely from radiodorsal to ulnopalmar dividing the distal surface of the scaphoid into two facets [37]. They suggested that the orientation of this obliquely oriented ridge guides STT joint motion and coincides with the plane of dart-throwing motion. On the contrary, it has been suggested that the ridge is merely cartilaginous, and therefore cannot resist such forces and they considered the ridge as a result of wrist motion, not a factor influencing motion [113].

2.2.2.2 Scapholunocapitate Joint

It is a ball and socket joint, formed by the concave articular surfaces of the lunate and scaphoid proximally and the convex articular surface of the capitate and sometimes the proximal pole of the hamate, distally. Two types of articular surfaces of the scaphoid that articulate with the lunate and capitate have been identified. A large lunate facet is coupled with a small, distal capitate facet, while a small lunate facet is coupled with a large, proximal capitate facet [106, 113].

In the MC joint, two types of lunates have been identified based on their distal articular surface: In type I lunates there is no medial facet, while type II lunates have a medial facet that articulates with the hamate. This is a distinctive facet with a ridge on the hamate

separating it from the triquetrohamate joint and a ridge on the lunate separating it from the capitolunate joint [100]. The lunate type was determined using capitate–triquetrum (C-T) distance. A type I lunate was defined as a C-T distance ≤2 mm. A type II lunate was defined as a C-T distance ≥4 mm [119].The size of the medial facets in type II lunates ranges from 1 to 6 mm [120] and its incidence has been reported to range from 46 to 73 % [100, 102, 120].

The clinical significance of the wrists with type II lunates has been described by many authors: (a) the kinematics of a type II lunate are different from those of a type I lunate during radial-ulnar deviation of the wrist [110, 121] and the condylar double-facet midcarpal articulation permits only flexion and extension of the proximal carpal row, restricting radial translation [151]; (b) arthritic changes at the proximal pole of the hamate were more commonly associated with the type II lunates (49 %) [49], while these arthritic changes were also associated with LTI ligament tears [100] (Fig. 2.30); (c) variations in scaphoid motion of the wrists with lunate type II may contribute to the development of STT arthritis [119]; (d) type II lunates constitute an anatomical factor predisposing to Kienbock's disease, because the loads applied to the

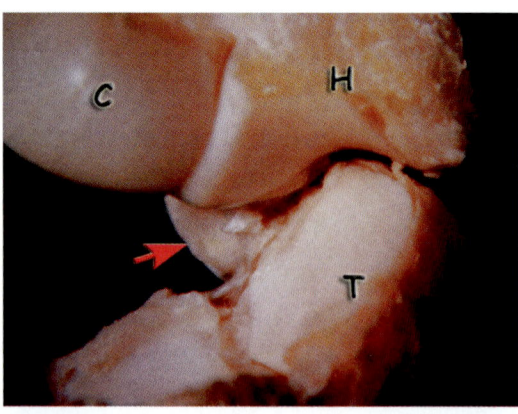

Fig. 2.31 The ulnar side of the midcarpal joint. The helicoidal shape of the articular surface of the hamate is apparent. The volar triquetrocapitate ligament (*red arrow*) (*C* capitate, *H* hamate, *T* triquetrum). With permission from [157]

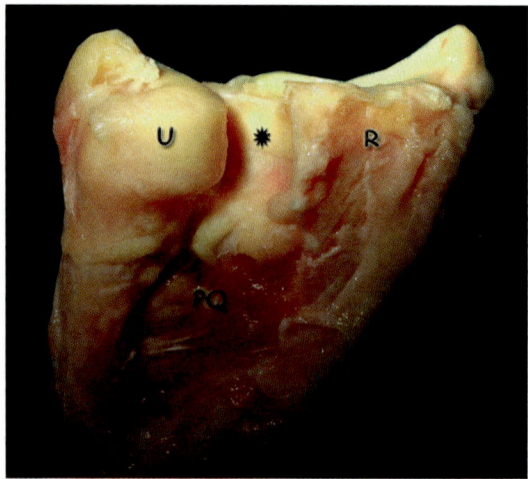

Fig. 2.32 The DRUJ from the dorsal side. (*U* ulnar head, *R* radius). Sigmoid notch (*asterisk*). With permission from [157]

radiolunate joint are supposed to be greater in type II lunates than in type I [123], and (e) type II lunate morphology is associated with significantly decreased incidence of DISI deformity in cases of established scaphoid nonunion [122].

2.2.2.3 Triquetrohamate Joint

It is a helicoid or screw shape joint, formed by the distal surface of the triquetrum and the proximal surface of the hamate (Fig. 2.31). McLean et.al [124] suggested the existence of two distinct TqH joint patterns, which have been termed TqH-1 and TqH-2. A TqH-1 joint is a helicoidal configuration. It is double faceted, with the hamate and the triquetrum articular surfaces possessing complementary concave and convex parts. A TqH-2 joint has a predominantly oval convex shape, whereas the primarily concave triquetrum is better described as a dish for the flatter hamate. It has no hamate groove or distal ridge. There appears to be a spectrum of variation between these two identifiable types.

2.2.3 Distal radioulnar joint (DRUJ)

DRUJ is a trochoid articulation, formed by the ulnar head and the sigmoid notch of the distal radius. The articular surface of the radius that

articulates with the ulna is called the sigmoid notch. The sigmoid notch has a triangular shape with a distal, a dorsal, and a palmar rim. The distal rim separates the lunate fossa from the sigmoid notch and is the site of insertion of the triangular fibrocartilage disk. The portion of the ulnar head that articulates with the sigmoid notch is referred to as the "seat" and the articular surface in juxtaposition to the proximal (undersurface) of the TFCC is the "pole" (Fig. 2.32).

The arc of curvature of the sigmoid notch ranges from 47° to 80°. Articular cartilage covers a much greater arc of the ulnar head, ranging from 90° to 135°. The radius of curvature of the sigmoid notch is 15 mm, compared to 10 mm for the seat of the ulna. Thus, the ulnar head and the sigmoid notch are obviously not congruent. This incongruity between the radius of curvature of the sigmoid notch and the ulnar head results in: (a) *Reduced articular contact between the articular surfaces*. At the neutral position, approximately 60 % of the cartilage surfaces are in contact, whereas at the extremes of prono-supination only about 10 %, corresponding to an area of 1–2 mm, are in contact [95]; (b) *The inherent instability of the joint* necessitating the existence of different stabilizing mechanisms through intrinsic (intracapsular) as well as extrinsic (extracapsular) structures. The intrinsic stability is provided by the dorsal and palmar radioulnar ligaments. Extrinsic stability is provided principally by the ECU tendon and sheath, the superficial and deep heads of the pronator quadratus and the interosseous ligament of the mid-forearm [90]. The distal interosseous ligament has variable thickness, ranging from 0.4 to 1.2 mm and when fully developed, constitutes the distal oblique band (DOB), which has a significant impact on DRUJ stability. Moritomo [125] in a recent anatomical study found that the DOB existed in 40 % of specimens and when present, it originates from the distal one-sixth of the ulnar shaft and runs distally to insert on the inferior rim of the sigmoid notch of the radius; (c) *The combined motion of rotation and translation* at the DRUJ, the articulating surfaces of which allow 150° of motion in pronation and supination of the forearm [87, 126, 127]. Bowers [128] and Pirela-Cruz [129] documented a mean palmar and dorsal translational motion of 2.2 mm, while the passive motion of the joint in a dorso–palmar direction causes a translational motion of 5.4 mm for palmar direction and 2.8 mm for dorsal direction. The translational motion is dorsal in pronation and palmar in supination [127], while according to Adams and Holley [130], the translation occurs mostly at the extremes of pronosupination.

In addition to the motions described, there also exists an abduction–adduction movement referred to, by Pirela-Cruz et al. [129], as diastatic motion. This motion occurs because of the cam-effect of the elliptical nature of the ulnar head as rotation takes place. Finally, one other motion of the DRUJ is the pistoning-type effect that is observed during rotation of the forearm and loading of the joint. Relative to the radius, the ulna moves distally with pronation and proximally with supination. With stress loading of the wrist the ulna moves distally relative to the radius [127].

The orientation of the articular surfaces of the ulnar head and the sigmoid notch is also of major clinical importance. Sagerman et al. [131] have radiographically shown that the inclination of these opposing articular surfaces is almost never parallel, and is usually much different. Relative to the long axis to the ulna, the ulnar seat inclination averages 21° (range, −13.8° to 40.5°), while the sigmoid notch inclination averages 7.7° (range, −24.3° to 26.8°). Consequences of this observation are: (a) The component of translation movement that accompanies the rotation of the forearm can be attributed, to some degree, to a difference in the degree of inclination, apart from the difference in the radii of curvature of the opposing articular surfaces; (b) Because of the wide variation between the inclination of the sigmoid notch and ulnar seat, symptomatic articular incongruity can occur following joint leveling procedures. Tolat [132] reports three basic configurations of the DRUJ, depending on the orientation of the articular surfaces: The vertical type (I) (38 %), the oblique type (II) (50 %), and the reverse type (III) (12 %) (Fig. 2.33a, b, c).

The role of the DRUJ capsule has been clarified by Kleinman and Graham [133]. They observed that the inferior capsule is strong and durable and may be involved in the stability of the joint. The volar and dorsal aspects of the capsule are compliant and accept the ulna head as the radiocarpal unit rotates and translates through the pronosupination arc. The contraction of this part of the capsule plays an important role in limiting the rotation of the forearm.

Ishii et al. [134] measured the pressure distribution within the DRUJ with axial loads applied to the wrist in varying degrees of forearm rotation. They found that: (a) by increasing application of an axial load across the wrist, the average area of the sigmoid notch in contact with the ulnar head also increased, and (b) In pronation, there is compressive loading between the dorsal sigmoid notch and the ulnar head; in supination there is compressive loading between the palmar sigmoid notch and the ulnar head. This was confirmed by Bowers [135] who claimed that on the extreme positions of pronation-supination, part of the stability of the joint can be attributed to the compression of the dorsal or volar rim of the sigmoid notch and the ulnar head.

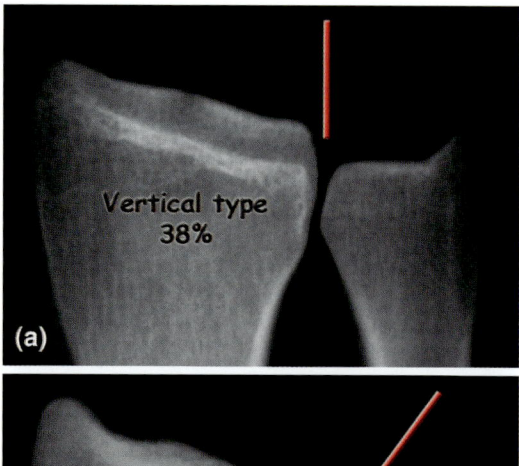

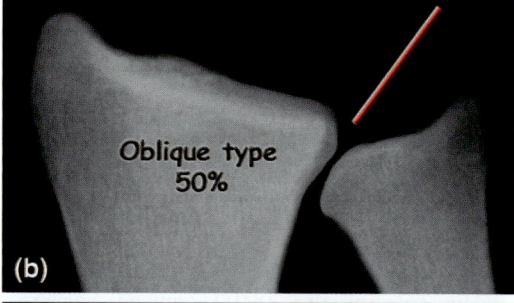

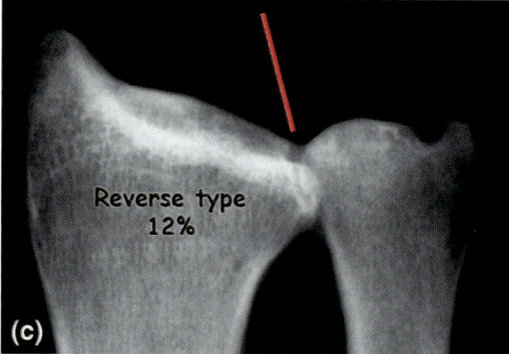

Fig. 2.33 The three basic configurations of the DRUJ depending on the orientation of the articular surfaces, according to Tolat [132] (**a, b, c**). With permission from [157]

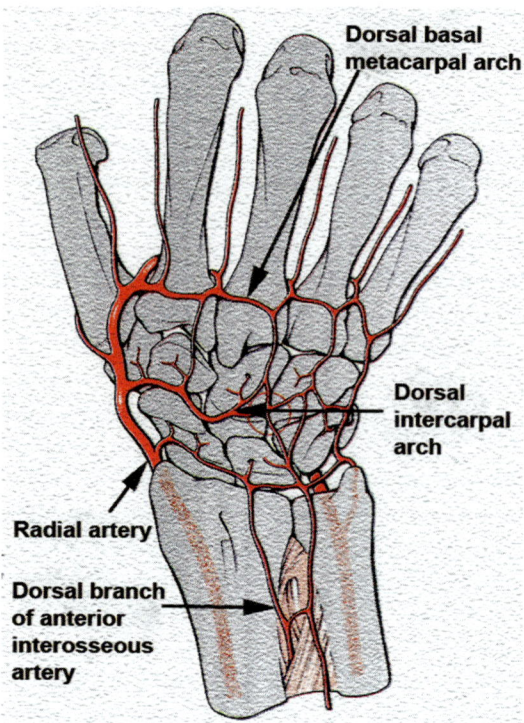

Fig. 2.34 Schematic drawing of the dorsal arterial network. With permission from [157]

(a) The dorsal and palmar radiocarpal arches;
(b) The dorsal and palmar intercarpal arches; and
(c) The dorsal basal metacarpal and the deep palmar arches (Figs. 2.34 and 2.35).

Gelberman et al. [136–138] found that on the dorsal surface, the largest and most consistent arch is the intercarpal arch, which provides the major blood supply to the distal carpal row and contributes to the vascularity of the lunate and the triquetrum. The next largest arch, the radiocarpal arch, was present in 75–80 % of the specimens. It supplies the distal radial metaphysic, as well as the lunate and the triquetrum from the dorsum. The basal metacarpal arch was often tenuous and was present in only 27 % of the specimens.

On the palmar surface, both the palmar radiocarpal arch and the deep palmar arch were present in 100 % of all specimens while the intercarpal arch was present in only 53 %. The

2.3 Vascularity of the Wrist

The blood supply to the wrist is provided by an extrinsic and an intrinsic vascular system. The extrinsic blood supply is developed through branches of the radial, ulnar, and anterior interosseous arteries, which form an arcade of anastomosing branches that produce three dorsal and three palmar arches:

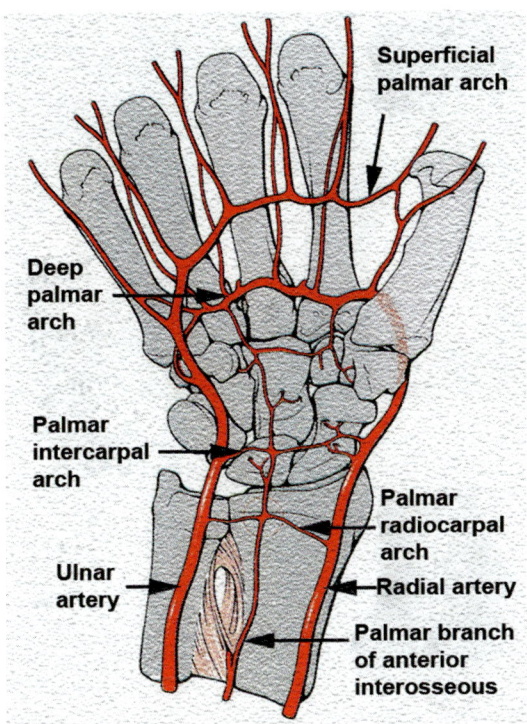

Superficial palmar arch

Deep palmar arch

Palmar intercarpal arch

Palmar radiocarpal arch

Ulnar artery

Radial artery

Palmar branch of anterior interosseous

Fig. 2.35 Schematic drawing of the volar arterial network. With permission from [157]

palmar radiocarpal arch provides the major blood supply both to the lunate and to the triquetrum from the palmar surface. The deep palmar arch supplies the distal carpal row by way of radial and ulnar recurrent arteries (present in 100 %) and via the accessory ulnar recurrent artery (in 27 %). The intercarpal arch is small and inconsistent, and in no case does it make a significant contribution to the carpal bones.

The superficial palmar arch and the posterior interosseous artery do not appear to provide any substantial contribution to the vascular supply of the wrist. However, with their multiple vascular anastomoses, they provide significant collateral circulation to the wrist [136, 137].

The radial artery forms the lateral border and the ulnar artery forms the medial border of this system. The anterior interosseous artery has a palmar and dorsal division that form at the proximal border of the pronator quadrates. The dorsal division extends distally on the interosseous membrane to the carpus, where it joins the

dorsal carpal arch that provides vascular supply to the proximal carpal row. The palmar division continues deep into the pronator quadrates and bifurcates into branches that communicate with the palmar radiocarpal arch supplying the lunate and the triquetrum, and finally enters the RSL ligament [139].

All but three carpal bones receive blood vessels directly from the dorsal and palmar arches: the scaphoid, pisiform, and trapezium have direct blood supply from the radial and ulnar arteries.

Panagis et al. [140] and Gelberman and Gross [137] classified the carpal bones into three groups on the basis of the number and location of nutrient vessels, the presence or absence of intraosseous anastomoses, and the dependence of large areas of bone on a single vessel. The clinical significance of the various groups is based on the risk of posttraumatic avascular necrosis for the bones in each group:

Group I (Scaphoid, Capitate, and 8 % [137] or 20 % [139] of the lunates). Includes carpal bones which either have vessels entering from only one surface, or large areas of bone that are dependent on a single vessel. This group is the most vulnerable to posttraumatic avascular necrosis.

Group II (Hamate, Trapezoid). Includes carpal bones, which have two or more areas of vessel entry but lack significant anastomoses within the entire or a major part of the bones. Specific injuries can compromise their blood supply.

Group III (Trapezium, triquetrum, pisiform, and 80 % [139] or 92 % [137] of the lunates). Includes carpal bones, which have two or more areas of vessel entry and consistent intraosseous anastomoses.

Vascularity of the scaphoid [136, 141]: The scaphoid receives its vascular supply mainly from the radial artery. Vessels enter dorsally and palmarly in the limited areas that are nonarticular of ligamentous attachment.

The *palmar vascular supply* is responsible for 20–30 % of the internal vascularity, all in the region of the distal pole. The palmar vascular supply is provided by: (a) the superficial palmar branch, which at the level of the radioscaphoid joint is giving off the radial artery and (b) several smaller branches that are coursing distal to the origin of the superficial palmar branch to enter through the region of the tubercle. In 75 % of specimens, these arteries arise directly from the radial artery and in the remainder, they arise from the superficial palmar branch of the radial artery.

The *dorsal vascular supply* to the scaphoid accounts for 70–80 % of the internal vascularity of the bone, and supplies the waist and the proximal pole of the bone. The major dorsal vessels to the scaphoid enter the bone through small foramina located on the dorsal ridge. At the level of the intercarpal joint, the radial artery gives off the intercarpal artery, which participates in the formation of the dorsal intercarpal arch. Just proximal to the origin of the intercarpal artery, at the level of the styloid process of the radius, a vessel is given off to enter the scaphoid through its waist along the dorsal ridge. In 70 % of specimens, the dorsal vessel arises directly from the radial artery. In 23 %, the dorsal branch has its origin from the common stem of the intercarpal artery. In 7 %, the scaphoid receives its dorsal blood supply directly from the branches of the intercarpal artery and the radial artery. In all specimens, there are consistent major communications between the dorsal scaphoid branch of the radial artery and the dorsal branch of the anterior interosseous artery. It has been stated [38] that the vessels enter through the dorsal ridge in 79 %, distal to the waist in 14 %, and proximal to the waist in 7 % of specimens. The fact that in 14 % of specimens the blood supply enters distal to the waist means that approximately one out of seven specimens would have shown a significant loss of blood supply to the proximal pole following a fracture through the waist [2, 142].

Vascularity of capitate [139, 141]: The capitate receives its vascularity from dorsal and palmar sources. Most arteries enter the capitate distally and follow a retrograde proximal course to supply the rest of the bone. The main (dorsal) vascularity originates from vessels of the dorsal

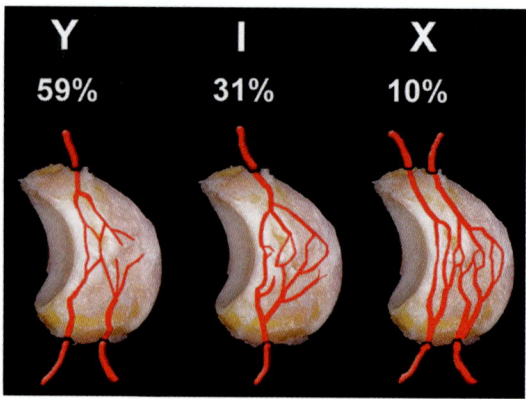

Fig. 2.36 Patterns of intraosseous vascularity of the lunate and the frequency of their appearance according to Gelberman et al. [143]. With permission from [157]

intercarpal and dorsal basal metacarpal arches. The palmar vascular supply arises from anastomosing branches of the recurrent ulnar artery, palmar radiocarpal arch, and deep palmar arch. In the majority of specimens (67 %) the dorsal vessels supply the major part of the capitate. In 33 % of specimens, the vascularity to the capitate head originates entirely from the palmar surface. There are notable anastomoses between the dorsal and the palmar blood supplies in 30 % of specimens. In the remainder there are no anastomoses seen.

Vascularity of the lunate [141, 143]: The lunate receives its blood supply from both palmar and dorsal sources or from the palmar aspect alone. The vessels entering the dorsal surface are from branches of the dorsal radiocarpal arch, the dorsal intercarpal arch, and occasionally from smaller branches of the dorsal branch of the anterior interosseous artery. In 80 % of specimens, the lunate receives nutrient vessels from the palmar and dorsal surfaces. In 20 % of specimens, it receives nutrient vessels from the palmar surface alone. There are three major intraosseous patterns, which are formed in the shape of the letters Y, I, or X. (Fig. 2.36).

The Y pattern is the most common, occuring in 59 % of specimens studied. The stem of the Y occurs dorsally or palmarly, with equal frequency.

The I pattern occurs in 31 % of specimens, and consists of one dorsal and one palmar vessel that anastomose in a straight line.

The X pattern occurs in 10 % of specimens, consisting of two dorsal and two palmar vessels that anastomose in the center of the lunate.

Vascularity of the trapezoid [140]: The trapezoid is supplied by branches of the dorsal intercarpal, the basal metacarpal, and the radial recurrent artery. The nutrient vessels enter the trapezoid through its two nonarticular surfaces on the dorsal and palmar surfaces. Three or four small vessels enter the dorsal surface to supply the dorsal 70 % of the bone. These dorsal vessels provide the primary vascularity of the trapezoid. From the palmar surface one or two small vessels supply the palmar 30 % of the bone. The palmar vessels do not anastomose with the dorsal vessels.

Vascularity of the hamate [2, 141]: The vascularity of the hamate is supplied by the dorsal intercarpal arch, the ulnar recurrent artery of the deep palmar arch, and the ulnar artery. The vessels enter through the three nonarticular surfaces of the hamate, which include the dorsal, the palmar, and the medial surface through the hook of the hamate. The dorsal surface receives three to five vessels from the dorsal intercarpal arch which supply the dorsal 30–40 % of the bone. The palmar surface usually receives one large vessel that enters through the radial base of the hook. It then branches and anastomoses with the dorsal vessels in 50 % of the specimens studied. The hook of the hamate receives one or two small vessels that enter through the medial base and tip of the hook. These vessels anastomose with each other but usually not with the vessels to the body of the hamate.

Vascularity of the trapezium: The vascularity of the trapezium is by vessels from the distal branches of the radial artery. Nutrient vessels enter the trapezium through its three nonarticular surfaces: dorsal, radial, and palmar. Dorsally, the vascular supply predominates and one to three vessels enter and supply the entire dorsal aspect of the bone. Palmarly, one to three vessels enter and anastomose with the vessels entering through the dorsal surface. Radially, three to six small vessels penetrate the lateral

surface and anastomose with the dorsal and palmar vessels.

Vascularity of the triquetrum: The triquetrum receives its blood supply from branches from the ulnar artery, the dorsal intercarpal arch, and the palmar intercarpal arch. Nutrient vessels enter through its two nonarticular surfaces on the dorsal and palmar aspects. Two to four vessels enter the dorsal ridge of the bone and supply the dorsal 60 % of the triquetrum. From the volar surface, one or two vessels enter proximal and distal to the facet that articulates with the pisiform and supply the palmar 40 % of the bone. The dorsal vessels provide the primary vascularity for the triquetrum in 60 % of the specimens while the palmar vessels constitute the main vascularity in 20 % of specimens. Significant anastomoses between the dorsal and palmar vascular networks have been found to be present in 86 % of specimens studied.

Vascularity of the pisiform: The pisiform receives one to three small vessels directly from the ulnar artery entering the bone at the proximal and distal poles. Vessels anastomose with each other just beneath the articular surface of the pisiform, assuming a vascular ring pattern that is consistently seen in all specimens.

2.4 Innervation of Wrist Ligaments

The innervation of the wrist joint capsule has been identified largely by reports associated with surgical denervation of the wrist for chronic pain [144–147].

The main innervation to the wrist capsule derives from the anterior interosseous nerve, lateral antebrachial cutaneous nerve, and posterior interosseous nerve. Other minor sources of capsular innervation include: The palmar cutaneous branch of the median nerve, the deep branch of the ulnar nerve, the superficial branch of the radial nerve, and the dorsal branch of the ulnar nerve [148].

The terminal branch of the *posterior interosseous nerve* innervates the dorsal capsules of the radiocarpal and midcarpal joints as well as the dorsal wrist ligaments. It also innervates the dorsal capsules of the second, third, and fourth CMC joints [149]. It is considered to be the major dorsal source of innervation of the wrist. Minor contributions are also provided by the terminal branches of the dorsal sensory radial and ulnar nerves [71].

The terminal branch of the *anterior interosseous nerve* innervates the central two-thirds of the volar wrist capsule. Buck-Gramcko [149], however, defined this zone of innervation extending distally to include the palmar midcarpal joint and the central CMC joints.

The *lateral antebrachial cutaneous nerve* innervates the radial aspects of the radiocarpal and midcarpal joints and the first CMC joint [148, 150]. Other branches contributing less to the volar capsular innervation include the volar cutaneous branch of the median nerve and the deep branches from the ulnar nerve [71, 148].

The innervation to DRUJ and TFCC appears to be threefold, with the dorsal region (dorsal DRUJ capsule, DRU ligament, and dorsal ulnocarpal capsule) primarily innervated by branches of the posterior interosseous nerve, the ulnar region (MH, foveal attachment of the TFC, prestyloid recess, and UT ligament) primarily by articular extensions of the dorsal sensory branches of the ulnar nerve, and the volar region (volar DRUJ capsule, PRU ligament, and UL ligaments) by branches from the ulnar nerve [151, 152].

Recent investigations disputed the role of carpal ligaments as simple passive restraints. The microscopic innervation of the extrinsic and intrinsic wrist ligaments has been studied, to reveal a variable degree of sensory innervation by highly specialized nerve endings, called mechanoreceptors. The mechanoreceptors embedded into the ligaments, receive the mechanical signals and transform them into afferent nerve stimuli to influence periarticular muscles. In a recent study, Hagert et al. [153] made clear for the first time the existence of ligamento–muscular reflexes initiating in the carpal ligaments.

The innervation pattern of the wrist ligaments reflects in structural differences between the ligaments. Ligaments with limited innervation consisted mostly of densely packed collagen fibers. In the ligaments with abundant innervation, mechanoreceptors and nerve fascicles were consistently found in the loose connective tissue of the superficial region of the ligaments (epifascicular region), while the density of innervation was greatest close to the ligament insertions into bone [71]. Hagert et al. [154] found a pronounced innervation in the dorsal wrist ligaments (dorsal radiocarpal, dorsal intercarpal, scaphotriquetral, dorsal scapholunate interosseous), an intermediate innervation in the volar triquetral ligaments (palmar lunotriquetral interosseous, triquetrocapitate, triquetrohamate), and only limited/occasional innervation in the remaining volar wrist ligaments. They state that wrist ligaments are regarded as either mechanically or sensory important ligaments. The mechanically important ligaments are ligaments with densely packed collagen bundles, limited innervation, and are located primarily in the radial, force-bearing column of the wrist. The sensory important ligaments, by contrast, are richly innervated although less dense in connective tissue composition and are related to the triquetrum, which is the key element in the generation of the proprioceptive information.

Mataliotakis et al. [82] in a cadaver study investigated the sensory innervation of the subregions of the SLI ligament and found that the palmar subregion, apart from its major mechanical role, contains the greatest amount of neural structures and mechanoreceptors. The dorsal subregion, with densely packed collagen fibers and limited innervation, functions mainly to constrain the scaphoid-lunate relative motion.

Other studies evaluated the distribution of mechanoreceptors on the dorsal radiocarpal ligament [155], where the nerve endings predominate the superficial layer and the ligament insertions to the bone, or on the TFCC [156], where the nerve endings were distributed at the periphery of TFC and showed different concentrations of each type of mechanoreceptors per topographic area.

References

1. Berger RA (2001) The anatomy of the ligaments of the wrist and distal radioulnar joints. Clin Orthop 383:32–40

2. Taleisnik J (1985) The wrist. Churchill Livingstone, New York

3. Berger RA (2010) Wrist anatomy. In: Cooney W (ed) The wrist. Diagnosis and operative treatment, 2nd edn. Lippincott Williams & Wilkins, Philadelphia, pp 25–76

4. Berger RA (1997) The ligaments of the wrist: a current overview of anatomy with considerations of their potential functions. Hand Clin 13:63–82

5. Buijze GA, Lozano-Calderon SA, Strackee SD et al (2011) Osseous and ligamentous scaphoid anatomy: part I. A systematic literature review highlighting controversies. J Hand Surg [Am] 36:1926–1935

6. Buijze GA, Dvinskikh NA, Strackee SD et al (2011) Osseous and ligamentous scaphoid anatomy: part II. Evaluation of ligament morphology using three-dimensional anatomical imaging. J Hand Surg [Am] 36:1936–1943

7. Theumann NH, Pfirrmann CWA, Gregory AE et al (2003) Extrinsic carpal ligaments: normal MR arthrographic appearance in cadavers. Radiology 226:171–179

8. Sennwald S (1987) Anatomical approach: The wrist. Springer, Berlin, pp 13–46

9. Berger RA, Landsmeer JM (1990) The palmar radiocarpal ligaments: a study of adult and fetal human wrist joints. J Hand Surg [Am] 15:847–854

10. Ritt MJPF, Stuart PR, Berglund LJ et al (1995) Rotational stability of the carpus relative to the forearm. J Hand Surg [Am] 20:305–311

11. Katz DA, Green JK, Werner FW et al (2003) Capsuloligamentous restraints to dorsal and palmar carpal translation. J Hand Surg [Am] 28:610–613

12. Rayhack JM, Linscheid RL, Dobyns JH et al (1987) Posttraumatic ulnar translation of the carpus. J Hand Surg [Am] 12:180–189

13. Viegas SF, Patterson RM, Ward K (1995) Extrinsic wrist ligaments in the pathomechanics of ulnar translation instability. J Hand Surg [Am] 20:312–318

14. Watts AC, Mclean JM, Fogg Q et al (2011) Scaphoid anatomy. In: Slutsky DJ, Slade JF III (eds) The scaphoid. Thieme, New York, pp 3–10

15. Nowak MD (1991) Material properties of ligaments. In: An KN, Berger RA, Cooney WP (eds) Biomechanics of the wrist Joint. Springer, New York, pp 139–156

16. Siegel DB, Gelberman RH (1991) Radial styloidectomy: an anatomical study with special reference to radiocarpal intracapsular ligamentous morphology. J Hand Surg [Am] 16:40–44

17. Kwon BC, Choi SJ, Shin J et al (2009) Proximal row carpectomy with capsular interposition arthroplasty for advanced arthritis of the wrist. J Bone Joint Surg Br 91:1601–1606

18. Scobercea RG, Budoff JE, Hipp JA (2009) Biomechanical effect of triquetral and scaphoid excision on simulated midcarpal arthrodesis in cadavers. J Hand Surg [Am] 34:381–386

19. Moritomo H, Apergis E, Herzberg G et al (2011) Committee report on wrist biomechanics and instability: Carpal instability following scaphoid fracture. IFSSH Ezine 4: 14–17 Nov

20. Nagao S, Patterson RM, Buford WL et al (2005) Three-dimensional description of ligamentous attachments around the lunate. J Hand Surg [Am] 30:685–692

21. Kijima Y, Viegas S (2009) Wrist anatomy and biomechanics. J Hand Surg [Am] 34:1555–1563

22. Bogumill G (1988) Anatomy of the wrist. In: Lichtman D (ed) The wrist and its disorders. WB Saunders, Philadelphia, pp 14–26

23. Cardoso R, Szabo RM (2010) Wrist anatomy and surgical approaches. Hand Clin 26:1–19

24. Chee KG, Chin AYH, Chew EM, Garcia-Elias M (2012) Antipronation spiral tenodesis—a surgical technique for the treatment of perilunate instability. J Hand Surg [Am] 37:2611–2618

25. Berger RA, Blair WF (1984) The radioscapholunate ligament: a gross and histologic description. Anat Rec 210(2):393–405

26. Hixson ML (1990) Microvascular anatomy of the radioscapholunate ligament of the wrist. J Hand Surg [Am] 15:279–282

27. Cooney WP (1998) Arthroscopic anatomy of the wrist. In: Linscheid RL, Dobyns JH (eds) Cooney WP. The wrist. diagnosis and operative treatment. Mosby, Missouri, pp 169–187

28. Whipple TL (1995) The role of arthroscopy in the treatment of scapholunate instability. Hand Clin 11:37–40

29. Berger RA, Kauer JMG, Landsmeer JMF (1991) Radioscapholunate ligament: a gross anatomic and histologic study of fetal and adult wrists. J Hand Surg [Am] 16:350–355

30. Garcia-Elias M (1998) Soft-tissue anatomy and relationships about the distal ulna. Hand Clin 14(2):165–176

31. Wiesner L, Rumelhart C, Pham E et al (1996) Experimentally induced ulno-carpal instability. a study on 13 cadaver wrists. J Hand Surg [Br] 21(1): 24–29

32. Munk B, Jensen SL, Olsen BS et al (2005) Wrist stability after experimental traumatic triangular fibrocartilage complex lesions. J Hand Surg [Am] 30:43–49

33. Moritomo H, Murase T, Arimitsu S et al (2008) Change in the length of the ulnocarpal ligaments during radiocarpal motion: possible impact on triangular fibrocartilage complex foveal tears. J Hand Surg [Am] 33:1278–1286

34. Bos K (1996) Instability of the distal radioulnar joint. In: Büchler U (ed) Wrist instability. Martin Dunitz, London, pp 45–54

35. Ilyas AM, Mudgal CS (2008) Radiocarpal fracture-dislocations. J Am Acad Orthop Surg 16:647–655

36. Tay S-C, Berger RA, Parker WL (2010) Longitudinal split tears of the lunotriquetral ligament. Hand Clin 26:495–501

37. Moritomo H, Viegas SF, Nakamura K et al (2000) The scaphotrapezio-trapezoidal joint. Part 1: an anatomic and radiographic study. J Hand Surg [Am] 25:899–910

38. Boabighi A, Kuhlmann JN, Kenesi C (1993) The distal ligamentous complex of the scaphoid and the scapho-lunate ligament. An anatomic, histological and biomechanical study. J Hand Surg [Br] 18:65–69

39. Drewniany JJ, Palmer AK, Flatt AE (1985) The scaphotrapezial ligament complex: an anatomic and biomechanical study. J Hand Surg [Am] 10:492–498

40. Masquelet AC, Strube F, Nordin JY (1993) The isolated scapho-trapezio-trapezoid ligament injury. Diagnosis and surgical treatment in four cases. J Hand Surg [Br] 18:730–735

41. Kuo CE, Wolfe SW (2008) Scapholunate instability: current concepts in diagnosis and management. J Hand Surg [Am] 33:998–1013

42. Short WH, Werner FW, Green JK et al (2007) Biomechanical evaluation of the ligamentous stabilizers of the scaphoid and lunate: part III. J Hand Surg [Am] 32(3):297–309

43. Heras-Palou C (2009) Midcarpal instability. In: Slutsky DJ, Osterman AL (eds) Fractures and injuries of the distal radius and carpus. The cutting edge. Saunders, Philadelphia, pp 417–423

44. Moritomo H, Goto A, Sato Y et al (2003) The triquetrum-hamate joint: an anatomic and in vivo three-dimensional kinematic study. J Hand Surg [Am] 28:797–805

45. Moritomo H, Murase T, Goto A et al (2004) Capitate-based kinematics of the midcarpal joint during wrist radioulnar deviation: an in vivo three-dimensional motion analysis. J Hand Surg [Am] 29(4):668–675

46. Moritomo H, Apergis E, Herzberg G et al (2007) 2007 IFSSH Committee report of wrist biomechanics committee: Biomechanics of the so-called dart-throwing motion of the wrist. J Hand Surg [Am] 32:1447–1453

47. Garcia-Elias M (2008) The non-dissociative clunking wrist: a personal view. J Hand Surg [Eur] 33(6):698–711

48. Andermahr J, Lozano-Calderon S, Trafton T et al (2006) The volar extension of the lunate facet of the distal radius: a quantitative anatomic study. J Hand Surg [Am] 31:892–895

49. Nakamura K, Patterson RM, Moritomo H et al (2001) Type I versus type II lunates: ligament anatomy and presence of arthrosis. J Hand Surg [Am] 26:428–436

50. Sennwald GR, Zdravkovic V, Oberlin C (1994) The anatomy of the palmar scaphotriquetral ligament. J Bone Joint Surg Br 76:147–149

51. Sennwald G, Zdravkovic V, Fischer M (1996) Wrist arthroscopy: can you see instability? In: Büchler U (ed) Wrist instability. Martin Dunitz, London, pp 56–60

52. Viegas SF, Yamaguchi S, Boyd NL et al (1999) The dorsal ligaments of the wrist: anatomy, mechanical properties, and function. J Hand Surg [Am] 24:456–468

53. Viegas SF (2001) The dorsal ligaments of the wrist. Hand Clin 17(1):65–75

54. Berger RA, Garcia-Elias M (1991) General anatomy of the wrist. In: Kai-Nan A, Berger RA, Cooney WP III (eds) Biomechanics of the wrist joint. Springer, Berlin, pp 1–22

55. Shaaban H, Lees VC (2006) The two parts of the dorsal radiocarpal (radiolunotriquetral) ligament. J Hand Surg [Br] 31(2):13–215

56. Mizuseki T, Ikuta Y (1989) The dorsal carpal ligaments: their anatomy and function. J Hand Surg [Br] 14:91–98

57. Smith DK (1993) Dorsal carpal ligaments of the wrist: normal appearance on multiplanar reconstructions of three-dimensional fourier transform MR imaging. Am J Roentgen 161:119–125

58. Short WH, Werner FW, Green JK et al (2002) The effect of sectioning the dorsal radiocarpal ligament and insertion of a pressure sensor into the radiocarpal joint on scaphoid and lunate kinematics. J Hand Surg [Am] 27:68–76

59. Viegas SF, Patterson RM, Peterson PD et al (1990) Ulnar-sided perilunate instability: an anatomic and biomechanic study. J Hand Surg [Am] 15:268–278

60. Horii E, Garcia-Elias M, An KN et al (1991) A kinematic study of luno-triquetral dissociations. J Hand Surg [Am] 16:355–362

61. Nanno M, Patterson RM, Viegas SF (2006) Three-dimensional imaging of the carpal ligaments. Hand Clin 22:399–412

62. Sokolow C, Saffar P (2001) Anatomy and histology of the scapholunate ligament. Hand Clin 17:77–81

63. Moritomo H, Murase T, Oka K et al (2008) Relationship between the fracture location and the kinematic pattern in scaphoid nonunion. J Hand Surg [Am] 33:1459–1468

64. Moritomo H, Viegas SF, Elder KW et al (2000) Scaphoid nonunions: a 3-dimensional analysis of patterns of deformity. J Hand Surg [Am] 25:520–528

65. Slater RR, Szabo RM (1999) Scapholunate dissociation: treatment with the dorsal intercarpal ligament capsulodesis. Techn Hand Upper Extrem Surg 3:222–228

66. Slater RR, Szabo RM, Bay BK et al (1999) Dorsal intercarpal ligament capsulodesis for scapholunate dissociation: biomechanical analysis in a cadaver model. J Hand Surg [Am] 24:232–239

67. Walsh JJ, Berger RA, Cooney WP (2002) Current status of scapholunate interosseous ligament injuries. J Am Acad Orthop Surg 10:32–42

68. Mitsuyasu H, Patterson RM, Shah MA et al (2004) The role of the dorsal intercarpal ligament in dynamic and static scapholunate instability. J Hand Surg [Am] 29:279–288

69. Viegas SF, Dasilva MF (2000) Surgical repair for scapholunate dissociation. Techn Hand Upper Extrem Surg 4:148–153

70. Berger RA, Bishop AT, Bettinger PC (1995) New dorsal capsulotomy for the surgical exposure of the wrist. Ann Plast Surg 35:54–59

71. Hagert E, Ferreres A, Garcia-Elias M (2010) Nerve-sparing dorsal and volar approaches to the radiocarpal joint. J Hand Surg [Am] 35:1070–1074

72. Gelberman RH, Cooney WP, Szabo RM (2000) Carpal instability. J Bone Joint Surg Am 82:578–594

73. Ritt MJPF, Bishop AT, Berger RA et al (1998) Lunotriquetral ligament properties: a comparison of three anatomic subregions. J Hand Surg [Am] 23:425–431

74. Berger RA, Imeada T, Berglund L et al (1999) Constraint and material properties of the subregions of the scapholunate interosseous ligament. J Hand Surg [Am] 24:953–962

75. Ruby LK, An K-N, Linscheid RL et al (1987) The effect of scapholunate ligament section on scapholunate motion. J Hand Surg [Am] 12:767–771

76. Short WH, Werner FW, Fortino MD et al (1995) A dynamic biomechanical study of scapholunate ligament sectioning. J Hand Surg [Am] 20:986–999

77. Conyers DJ (1990) Scapholunate interosseous reconstruction and imbrication of palmar ligaments. J Hand Surg [Am] 15:690–700

78. Marcuzzi A, Acciaro AL, Caserta G et al (2006) Ligamentous reconstruction of scapholunate dislocation through a double dorsal and palmar approach. J Hand Surg [Br] 31(4):445–449

79. Dunn MJ, Johnson C (2001) Static scapholunate dissociation: a new reconstruction technique using a volar and dorsal approach in a cadaver model. J Hand Surg [Am] 26:749–754

80. Berger RA, Blair WF, Crowninshield RD et al (1982) The scapholunate ligament. J Hand Surg [Am] 7(1):87–91

81. Nikolopoulos F, Apergis E, Poulilios A et al (2011) Biomechanical properties of the scapholunate ligament and the importance of its portions in the capitate intrusion injury. Clin Biomech 26:819–823

82. Mataliotakis G, Doukas M, Kostas I et al (2009) Sensory innervation of the subregions of the scapholunate interosseous ligament in relation to their structural composition. J Hand Surg [Am] 34:1413–1421

83. Ritt MJPF, Berger RA, Bishop AT et al (1996) The capitohamate ligaments. J Hand Surg [Br] 21(4):451–454

84. Garcia-Elias M, An KN, Cooney WP III et al (1989) Stability of the transverse carpal arch: an experimental study. J Hand Surg [Am] 14:277–282

85. Palmer AK, Werner FW (1981) The triangular fibrocartilage complex of the wrist-anatomy and function. J Hand Surg [Am] 6:153–162

86. Palmer AK, Glisson RR, Werner FW (1984) Relationship between ulnar variance and triangular fibrocartilage complex thickness. J Hand Surg [Am] 9:681–682

87. Chidgey LK (1995) The distal radioulnar joint: problems and solutions. J Am Acad Orthop Surg 3:95–109

88. Nakamura T, Takayama S, Horiuchi Y et al (2001) Origins and insertions of the triangular fibrocartilage complex: a histological study. J Hand Surg [Br] 26(5):446–454

89. Gabl M, Zimmermann R, Angermann P et al (1998) The interosseous membrane and its influence on the distal radioulnar joint. An anatomical investigation of the distal tract. J Hand Surg [Br] 23:179–182

90. Kleinmann W (2007) Stability of the distal radioulnar joint: biomechanics, pathophysiology, physical diagnosis, and restoration of function. What we have learned in 25 Years. J Hand Surg [Am] 32(7):1086–1106

91. Ishii S, Palmer AK, Werner FW et al (1998) An anatomic study of the ligamentous structure of the triangular fibrocartilage complex. J Hand Surg [Am] 23:977–985

92. Af Ekenstam F, Hagert CG (1985) Anatomical studies on the geometry and stability of the distal radio ulnar joint. Scand J Plast Reconstr Surg 19:17–25

93. Schuind F, An KN, Berglund L et al (1991) The distal radioulnar ligaments: a biomechanical study. J Hand Surg [Am] 16:1106–1114

94. Hagert CG (1994) Distal radius fracture and the distal radioulnar joint—anatomical considerations. Handchir Mikrochir Plast Chir 26:22–26

95. Hagert E, Hagert CG (2010) Understanding stability of the distal radioulnar joint through an understanding of its anatomy. Hand Clin 26:459–466

96. Mikic ZD (1978) Age changes in the triangular fibrocartilage of the wrist joint. J Anat 126:367–384

97. Nakamura T, Yabe Y, Horiuch IY (1996) Functional anatomy of the triangular fibrocartilage complex. J Hand Surg [Br] 21(5):581–586

98. Thiru-Pathi RG, Ferlic DC, Clayton ML et al (1986) Arterial anatomy of the triangular fibrocartilage of the wrist and its surgical significance. J Hand Surg [Am] 11:258–263

99. Bednar MS, Arnoczky SP, Weiland AJ (1991) The microvasculature of the triangular fibrocartilage complex: Its clinical significance. J Hand Surg [Am] 16:1101–1105

100. Burgess RC (1990) Anatomic variations of the midcarpal joint. J Hand Surg [Am] 15:129–131

101. Canovas F, Roussanne Y, Captier G et al (2004) Study of carpal bone morphology and position in three dimensions by image analysis from computed tomography scans of the wrist. Surg Radiol Anat 26(3):186–190

102. Viegas SF (2001) Advances in the skeletal anatomy of the wrist. Hand Clin 17(1):1–11

103. Moojen TM, Snel JG, Venema HW et al (2003) In Vivo analysis of carpal kinematics and comparative review of the literature. J Hand Surg [Am] 28:81–87

104. Craigen MAC, Stanley JK (1995) Wrist kinematics. Row, column or both? J Hand Surg [Br] 20(2):165–170

105. Garcia-Elias M, Ribe M, Rodriguez J et al (1995) Influence of joint laxity on scaphoid kinematics. J Hand Surg [Br] 20(3):379–382

106. Compson JP, Waterman JK, Heatley FW (1994) The radiological anatomy of the scaphoid. Part 1: osteology. J Hand Surg [Br] 19:183–187

107. Ceri N, Korman E, Gunal I et al (2004) The morphological and morphometric features of the scaphoid. J Hand Surg [Br] 29(4):393–398

108. Heinzelmann AD, Archer G, Bindra RR (2007) Anthropometry of the human scaphoid. J Hand Surg [Am] 32:1005–1008

109. Moojen TM, Snel JG, Ritt MJPF et al (2002) Scaphoid kinematics in vivo. J Hand Surg [Am] 27:1003–1010

110. Moritomo H, Viegas S, Elder K et al (2000) The scaphotrapezio-trapezoidal joint. Part 2: a kinematic study. J Hand Surg [Am] 25:911–920

111. Wolfe SW, Neu C, Crisco J (2000) In vivo scaphoid, lunate, and capitate kinematics in flexion and in extension. J Hand Surg [Am] 25:860–869

112. Berger RA (2001) The anatomy of the scaphoid. Hand Clin 17:525–532

113. Fogg Q (2004) Scaphoid variation and an anatomical basis for variable carpal mechanics. Department of Anatomical Sciences, University of Adelaide. Thesis

114. Garcia-Elias M, Lluch AL, Stanley JK (2006) Three-ligament tenodesis for the treatment of scapholunate dissociation: Indications and surgical technique. J Hand Surg [Am] 31:125–134

115. Short WH, Werner FW, Green JK et al (2005) Biomechanical evaluation of the ligamentous stabilizers of the scaphoid and lunate: Part II. J Hand Surg [Am] 30:24–34

116. Wolfe SW (2001) Scapholunate instability. J Am Soc Surg Hand 1(1):45–60

117. Schuind FA, Linscheid RL, An K-N et al (1992) A normal data base of posteroanterior roentgenographic measurements of the wrist. J Bone Joint Surg Am 74(9):1418–1429

118. Werner FW, Short WH, Green JK et al (2007) Severity of scapholunate instability is related to joint anatomy and congruency. J Hand Surg [Am] 32:55–60

119. Mclean JM, Turner PC, Bain GI et al (2009) An association between lunate morphology and scaphoid–trapezium–trapezoid arthritis. J Hand Surg [Eur] 34(6):778–782

120. Viegas SF, Wagner K, Patterson R et al (1990) Medial (hamate) facet of the lunate. J Hand Surg [Am] 15:564–571

121. Nakamura K, Beppu M, Patterson RM et al (2000) Motion analysis in two dimensions of radial–ulnar deviation of type I versus type II lunates. J Hand Surg [Am] 25:877–888

122. Haase SC, Berger RA, Shin AY (2007) Association between lunate morphology and carpal collapse patterns in scaphoid nonunions. J Hand Surg [Am] 32:1009–1012

123. Nakamura K, Beppu M, Matsushita K et al (1997) Biomechanical analysis of the stress force on midcarpal joint in Kienbock's disease. Hand Surg 2:101–115

124. Mclean J, Bain G, Eames M et al (2006) An anatomic study of the triquetrum– hamate joint. J Hand Surg [Am] 31:601–607

125. Moritomo H (2012) The distal interosseous membrane: current concepts in wrist anatomy and biomechanics. J Hand Surg [Am] 33(7):1501–1507

126. Imbriglia JE, Clifford JW (2001) Management of the painful distal radioulnar joint. Lippincott Williams & Wilkins, Philadelphia

127. Loftus JB, Palmer AK (1997) Disorders of the distal radioulnar joint and triangular fibrocartilage complex: an overview. In: Lichtman DM, Alexander AH (eds) The wrist and its disorders, 2nd edn. WB Saunders Co, Philadelphia, pp 385–414

128. Bowers WH (1993) The distal radial ulnar joint. In: Green DP (ed) Operative hand surgery, 3rd edn. Churchill Livingstone, Philadelphia, pp 973–1019

129. Pirela-Cruz MA (1991) Stress computed tomography analysis of the distal radioulnar joint: a diagnostic tool for determining translational motion. J Hand Surg [Am] 16:75–81

130. Adams BD, Holley KA (1993) Strains in the articular disk of the triangular fibrocartilage complex: a biomechanical study. J Hand Surg [Am] 18:919–925

131. Sagerman SD, Zogby RG, Palmer AK et al (1995) Relative articular inclination of the distal radioulnar joint: a radiographic study. J Hand Surg [Am] 20:597–601

132. Tolat AR (1992) The gymnast's wrist: acquired positive ulnar variance following chronic epiphyseal injury. J Hand Surg [Br] 17:678–681

133. Kleinman WB, Graham TJ (1998) The distal radioulnar joint capsule: clinical anatomy and role in posttraumatic limitation of forearm rotation. J Hand Surg [Am] 23:588–599

134. Ishii S, Palmer AK, Werner FW et al (1996) Pressure distribution in the distal radioulnar joint. In: Presented at the 51st annual meeting of the American society for surgery of the hand nashville, TN

135. Bowers WH (1991) Instability of the distal radioulnar articulation. Hand Clin 7:311–328

136. Gelberman RH, Menon J (1980) The vascularity of the scaphoid bone. J Hand Surg [Am] 5(5):508–513

137. Gelberman RH, Gross MS (1986) The vascularity of the wrist. Identification of arterial patterns at risk. Clin Orthop 202:40–49

138. Gelberman RH, Botte MJ (1997) Vascularity of the carpus. In: Lichtman DM, Alexander AH (eds) The wrist and its disorders. WB Saunders Co, Philadelphia, pp 34–47

139. Cooney WP (1998) Vascular and neurologic anatomy of the wrist. In: Cooney WP, Linscheid RL, Dobyns JH (eds) The wrist. Diagnosis and operative treatment. Mosby, Missouri, pp 106–123

140. Panagis JS, Gelberman RH, Taleisnik J (1983) The arterial anatomy of the human carpus. Part II: the intraosseous vascularity. J Hand Surg [Am] 8:375–382

141. Freedman DM, Botte MJ, Gelberman RH (2001) Vascularity of the carpus. Clin Orthop 383:47–59

142. Schmidt H-M, Lanz U (2004) Surgical anatomy of the Hand. Georg Thieme Verlag, New York

143. Gelberman RH, Bauman TD, Menon J et al (1980) The vascularity of the lunate bone and Kienbock's disease. J Hand Surg [Am] 5(3):272–278

144. Braga-Silva J, Román JA, Padoin AV (2011) Wrist denervation for painful conditions of the wrist. J Hand Surg [Am] 36:961–966

145. Ferreres A, Foucher G, Suso S (2002) Extensive denervation of the wrist. Techn Hand Upper Extrem Surg 6(1):36–41

146. Grechenig W, Mahring M, Clement HG (1998) Denervation of the radiocarpal joint. J Bone Joint Surg Br 80:504–507

147. Wilhelm A (1965) Denervation of the wrist [in German]. Hefte Unfallheilkd 81:109–114

148. Van de Pol GJ, Koudstaal MJ, Schuurman AH et al (2006) Innervation of the wrist joint and surgical perspectives of denervation. J Hand Surg [Am] 31:28–34

149. Buck-Gramcko D (1977) Denervation of the wrist joint. J Hand Surg [Am] 2:54–61

150. Fukumoto K, Kojima T, Kinoshita Y et al (1993) An anatomic study of the innervation of the wrist joint and Wilhelm's technique for denervation. J Hand Surg [Am] 18(3):484–489

151. Gupta R, Nelson SD, Baker J et al (2001) The innervation of the triangular fibrocartilage complex: nitric acid maceration rediscovered. Plast Reconstr Surg 107(1):135–139

152. Shigemitsu T, Tobe M, Mizutani K et al (2007) Innervation of the triangular fibrocartilage complex of the human wrist: quantitative immunohistochemical study. Anat Sci Int 82(3): 127–132

153. Hagert E, Persson JKE, Werner M et al (2009) Evidence of wrist proprioceptive reflexes elicited after stimulation of the scapholunate interosseous ligament. J Hand Surg [Am] 34:642–651

154. Hagert E, Garcia-Elias M, Forsgren S et al (2007) Immunohistochemical analysis of wrist ligament innervation in relation to their structural composition. J Hand Surg [Am] 32:30–36

155. Tomita K, Berger EJ, Berger RA et al (2007) Distribution of nerve endings in the human dorsal radiocarpal ligament. J Hand Surg [Am] 32:466–473

156. Cavalcante MLC, Rodrigues CJ, Rames M (2004) Mechanoreceptors and nerve endings of the triangular fibrocartilage in the human wrist. J Hand Surg [Am] 29:432–435

157. Apergis E (2004) καταγματα-εξαρθρήματα του καρπου. Konstantaras Medical Books, Athens

Wrist Biomechanics

3

Marc Garcia-Elias

3.1 Introduction

In order to facilitate hand function, the upper limb must be mobile, but also stable. If the proximal articulations of the upper extremity lack mobility, the hand will not be properly positioned where it is needed. If those joints are unstable, the hand will not be able to carry heavy objects. To understand wrist biomechanics, therefore, one needs to learn kinematics (how joints move) and kinetics (how do they resist loads without yielding or suffering injury) [1, 2].

The wrist is often described as the least important articulation of the upper limb; a joint that can be fused without generating great distress to the patient. This is only partly true. Unquestionably, patients with a fused wrist may cope effectively with stressful activities, but they have substantial limitations in daily activities such as washing one's back, turning a door knob, or rotating the steering wheel [3, 4]. Without a mobile wrist, there is no precision in placing the hand where is required to manipulate an object. Without the wrist, the hand is less effective [5]. The wrist, indeed, is an important articulation.

Several mechanical models have been hypothesized to explain wrist function: the wrist as two interconnected rows (proximal and distal),

as three interdependent columns (lateral, central, and medial), or as a ring of four linked units (distal row, scaphoid, lunate and triquetrum) [6, 7]. Although certainly useful for teaching purposes, none of these models can fully explain how the wrist is allowed to move and yet be able to transfer substantial amount of loads. Wrist function is not only the result of a perfect mechanical interaction between moving bones and soft tissue constraints (Fig. 3.1), but also the consequence of a complex system of ligament-muscle reflexes mediating its dynamic muscle stabilization [8, 9]. Most of these factors have been largely ignored or underestimated in the past. Furthermore, most descriptions of carpal bone kinematics have been based on observations made on a limited number of specimens or in vivo determinations using 3-D reconstructions of CT scans [10–14]. Being the number of observations small, some perspective may have been lost in terms of individual variations of normality, both in terms of anatomy as in mechanics [15–17]. In short, carpal kinematics is not yet a fully understood issue, and needs more thorough investigations for us to be efficient in coping with its dysfunctions.

The wrist is not only a complicated composite joint allowing large range of motion; the wrist is also a load bearing articulation [18]. The carpus has a self-locking mechanism allowing transmission of large amount of forces [18–20]. Albeit certain wrist positions are better prepared than others to bear loads [21, 22], the normal wrist does not need to be placed in one particular position to grasp, push, or pull an object.

M. Garcia-Elias (✉)
Institute Kaplan, Passeig de la Bonanova,
9, 2 on 2a, 08022 Barcelona, Spain
e-mail: garciaelias@institut-kaplan.com
www.institut-kaplan.com

E. Apergis, *Fracture-Dislocations of the Wrist*,
DOI: 10.1007/978-88-470-5328-1_3, © Springer-Verlag Italia 2013

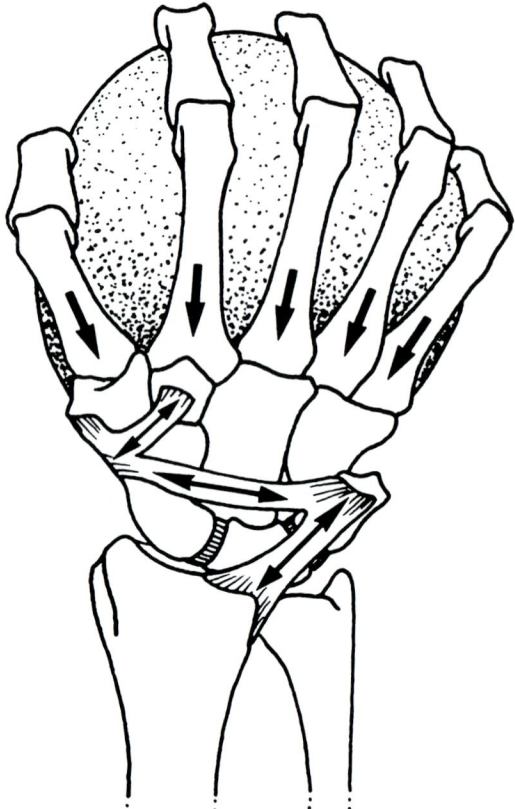

Fig. 3.1 The wrist is a very mobile, load bearing articulation, which stability is based upon an adequate interaction between the different articular surfaces and soft tissue constraints. With permission from [64]

Aside from its role as a mobile self-stabilizing load bearing articulation, the wrist is also an important pulley to enhance finger function [5, 23, 24]. The so called "carpal pulley", which is basically composed of the distal carpal row and their transverse ligament interconnections, can be oriented at will for an optimal finger function. This chapter will analyze the wrist joint and the carpal pulley from a kinematic and a kinetic perspective.

3.2 Carpal Kinematics

Carpal bone motion has been traditionally described as a combination of three rotations (Eulerian angles) and three translations (antero-posterior, mediolateral and proximodistal)

around and along three orthogonal axes, taking the distal radius as a reference (Table 3.1). Wrist rotation along the sagittal plane (Y axis) corresponds to flexion–extension, rotation along the coronal plane (X axis) determines abduction (radial deviation) or adduction (ulnar deviation), and rotation along the axial or transverse plane (Z axis) corresponds to pronation-supination. The first and second types of rotation (flexion–extension and radial-ulnar deviation) may be either the result of a passive external force, or be actively contracting the muscles which tendons cross the wrist. Active rotation along the axial plane of pronosupination only happens if the two other rotations (flexion–extension and radio-ulnar deviation) are constrained in neutral position (isometric type of loading); a typical example of this type of rotation is when the hand makes a closed fist: it does not move from a slightly extended position, but it rotates an average 1.9° supination [25].

The unconstrained wrist seldom rotates in a pure flexion–extension or radial-ulnar deviation mode. Most activities of daily living require the wrist to move along an oblique plane, from extension-radial deviation to flexion-ulnar deviation. It is one of the most utilized planes of wrist motion (using a hammer, fly fishing, throwing, pushing or holding a heavy object). Although known by Corson [26] in 1897, the so-called "physiologic flexion–extension" motion was not properly addressed until recently. Fisk [27], in 1980, was the first to use the term "dart throwing " to refer to this type of rotation, and Saffar and Seumaan [28], in 1994, were the first to investigate it from a biomechanical perspective. Since then, multiple studies have emphasized its peculiar kinematics [12, 14, 29].

3.2.1 Flexion–Extension

Wrist flexion is a rotation around the Y axis, located proximal to the head of the capitate, near the lunate, and parallel to the palmar surface of the distal radial metaphysis. Flexion brings the palm towards the volar aspect of the forearm. Extension of the wrist is also a rotation about

Table 3.1 Individual carpal bone rotation (average Eulerian angles) relative to the radius during wrist movements, according to the kinematic study by Kobayashi et al. [10]

	Wrist flexion 60°	Wrist extension 60°	Wrist radial deviation 15°	Wrist ulnar deviation 30°
Scaphoid (n: 22)	Flx 40°, UD 8°	Ext 52°, UD 4°	RD 4°, Flex 8°	Ext 17°, UD 14°, Pron 7°
Lunate (n: 22)	Flx 23°, UD 11°	Ext 30°, UD 4°	RD 2°, Flex 7°	Ext 22°, UD 15°, Pron 4°
Triquetrum (n: 22)	Flx 30°, UD 10°	Ext 39°	RD 5°, Flex 4°	Ext 17°, UD 18°
Trapezium (n: 13)	Flx 54°, UD 3°	Ext 59°	RD 14°, Sup 5°	UD 32°, Flx 10°, Pron 16°
Capitate (n: 22)	Flx 63°, UD 3°	Ext 60°	RD 15°, Sup 4°	UD 31°, Flx 6°, Pron 12°

Flx Flexion, *Ext* Extension, *RD* Radial deviation, *UD* Ulnar deviation, *Pron* Pronation, *Sup* Supination

this axis, but in the reverse direction: the back of the hand approximates the dorsal aspect of the forearm. All tendons located palmar to the Y-axis contribute to wrist flexion, while extension results from contraction of muscles located dorsal to this axis [30]. The most active wrist flexors are the flexor carpi radialis (FCR), the flexor carpi ulnaris (FCU) and palmaris longus, while the extensor carpi radialis brevis and longus (ECRB-L), and extensor carpi ulnaris (ECU) are active extensors. Aside from those, any tendon crossing the wrist to mobilize the fingers also has an influence on the wrist. The mean range of active flexion–extension of normal wrists is 59° and 79° respectively [31].

Regardless the direction of wrist motion, the trapezoid, capitate and hamate bones move synchronously (in about the same direction) as if they were connected by synostoses. In fact, only the trapezium-trapezoid joint exhibits some minor, but detectable mobility [10]. Consequently, the internal dimensions of the carpal tunnel change little during wrist motion [32]. The bones of the proximal carpal row, by contrast, appear less strongly connected to each other. Substantial differences in sagittal rotation exist between the three row bones. For a total 120° of wrist flexion–extension, the average rotation of the scaphoid, lunate and triquetrum are 92°, 53°, and 69° respectively (Table 3.1) [10]. The different radii of curvatures of their proximal convexities explains why the three bones move differently. To coordinate such complex mobility, a complex arrangement of

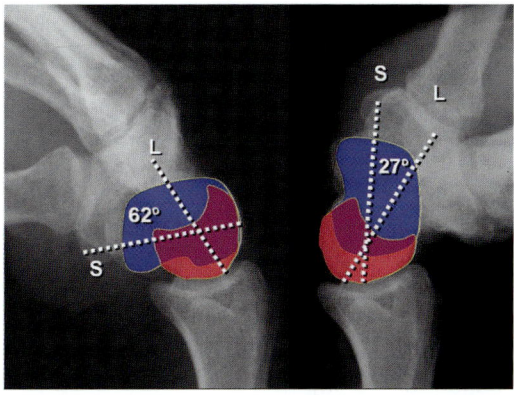

Fig. 3.2 Outlines of the scaphoid and lunate bones obtained from radiographs of a wrist in flexion (*left*) and extension (*right*). The scapholunate angle shows substantial variation from one position to another. This demonstrates that, unlike the distal row bones, there is substantial rotational motion between the bones of the proximal row. In particular, at the scapholunate joint, this rotation occurs around a dorsally located axis represented by the dorsal scapholunate ligament. With permission from [64]

scapholunate (SL) and lunotriquetral (LTq) ligaments is necessary. In the SL joint, there is a "scissor-like" type of rotation around a transverse axis which coincides quite well with the dorsal SL ligament. (Fig. 3.2) [33]. By contrast, the LTq joint axis of flexion–extension coincides with the palmar LTq interosseous ligament [34].

The relative contribution of the radiocarpal and midcarpal joints to the total wrist flexion–extension is controversial. It varies substantially from one column to another. In the central column (radius-lunate-capitate) about a 50 % of the overall flexion–extension occurs at the

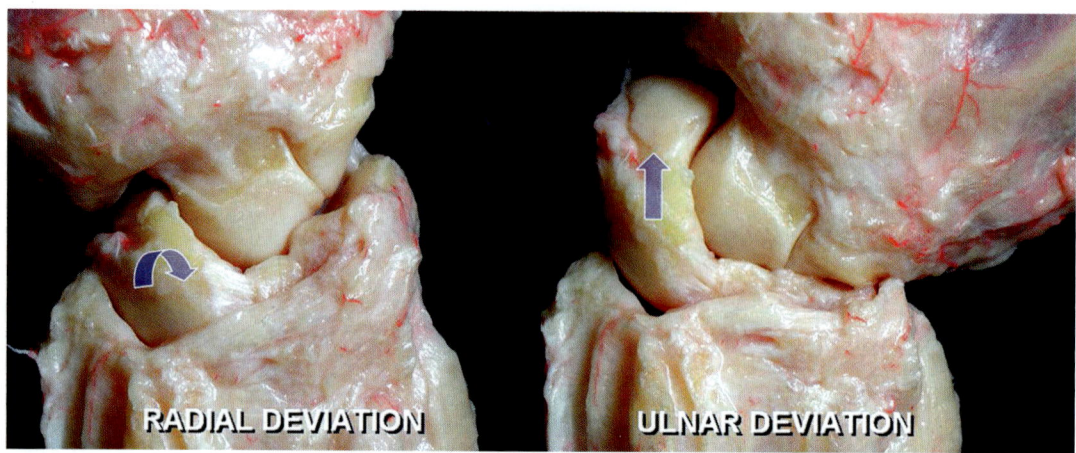

Fig. 3.3 Dorsal view of a dissected specimen demonstrating the two major components of motion exhibited by the proximal carpal bones during radio-ulnar deviation. *Radial deviation* involves flexion and medial translation of the three bones of the proximal row. Contrarily, during wrist *ulnar deviation* the bones of the proximal row rotate into extension while displacing towards the radius. With permission from [64]

proximal radiolunate joint, while the other half occurs at the lunocapitate interval. In the scaphoid column (radius-scaphoid-trapezoid), by contrast, 75 % of flexion and 92 % of extension occurs at the radioscaphoid joint, the scaphoid-trapezium-trapezoid (STT) joint being much less mobile [10, 35, 36].

3.2.2 Radial-Ulnar Deviation

Ulnar deviation (adduction) of the wrist may be described as a rotation that approximates the ulnar aspect of the hand to the medial border of the forearm. The X axis around which this occurs is located at the centre of the head of the capitate, and it is perpendicular to the Y axis of flexion–extension. Radial deviation (abduction) is also a rotation about this axis, but in the reverse direction: the thumb gets closer to the radial aspect of the forearm. All tendons crossing the wrist radial to the X axis bring about a radial deviation, while the tendons located ulnarly are ulnar deviators [30]. The average range of active abduction–adduction is 21° and 38° respectively [31].

As stated for flexion–extension, during wrist radial-ulnar deviation there is almost no rotation between trapezoid, capitate and hamate. The trapezium-trapezoid joint is slightly more mobile, but only in a proximodistal direction: the trapezium tilts proximally when axially loaded by the first metacarpal [37]. This, however does not preclude the distal row to maintain its internal dimensions during motion.

At the level of the proximal row, there is substantial rotation between the three proximal carpal bones during abduction–adduction. From radial deviation to ulnar deviation there is a mean of 10° of SL rotation and 14° of LTq rotation [10] (Table 3.1). Despite differences in rotation, the direction of motion is similar for the three bones: they move synergistically from a flexed position in radial deviation to an extended position in ulnar deviation (Fig. 3.3).

The magnitudes of flexion–extension of the proximal row bones during radioulnar deviation vary between individuals: there is a spectrum of behaviours, all being normal. From wrists with a scaphoid exhibiting almost exclusively flexion–extension, to wrists in which the scaphoid only translates lateromedially, all combinations are possible (Fig. 3.4) [11]. The wrists with a predominant scaphoid flexion–extension component are called "column-type" while the ones with predominant mediolateral translation are "row-type" wrists [16]. The "column-type" wrist appears to be more lax, with a more prominent interfacet ridge than the "row-type"

Fig. 3.4 There are different patterns of wrist kinematics. The so-called "row wrists" exhibit little flexion–extension of the scaphoid during radioulnar deviation, while the "column wrists" have substantial out-of-plane motion. With permission from [64]

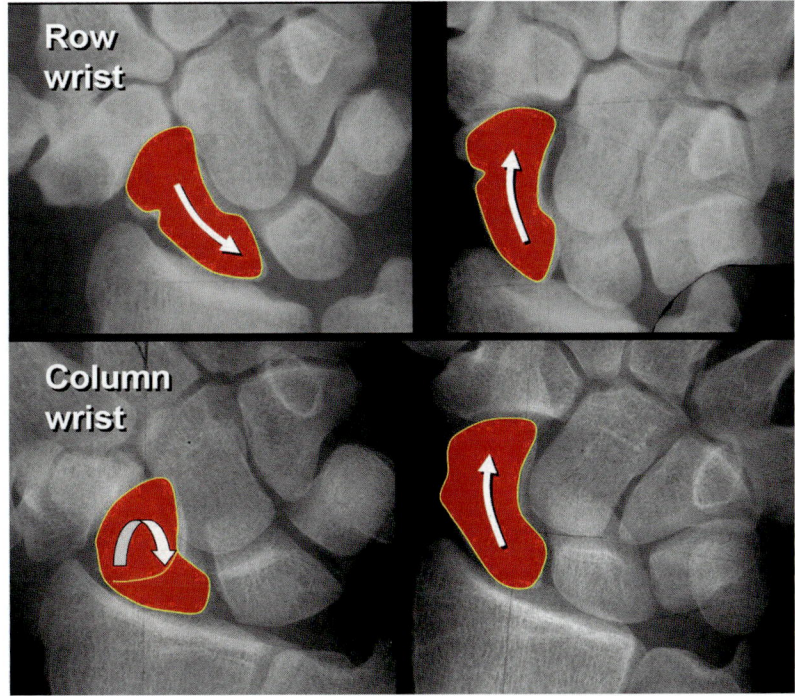

[38]. Such a complex kinematics is necessary to ensure joint congruency throughout the entire range of wrist motion.

3.2.3 "Dart-Throwing" Motion

It has long been known that the unconstrained wrist seldom rotates along the sagittal or coronal planes [26]. Most actions require a rotation from an extended-radial deviated position to a flexed-ulnar deviated position (Fig. 3.5) [27–29]. It is an oblique plane of motion commonly referred to as the "physiologic" plane of flexion–extension or "dart throwing" plane of rotation [27]. There are several reasons to explain why this oblique plane is so commonly utilized. First, because this rotation is produced by the most

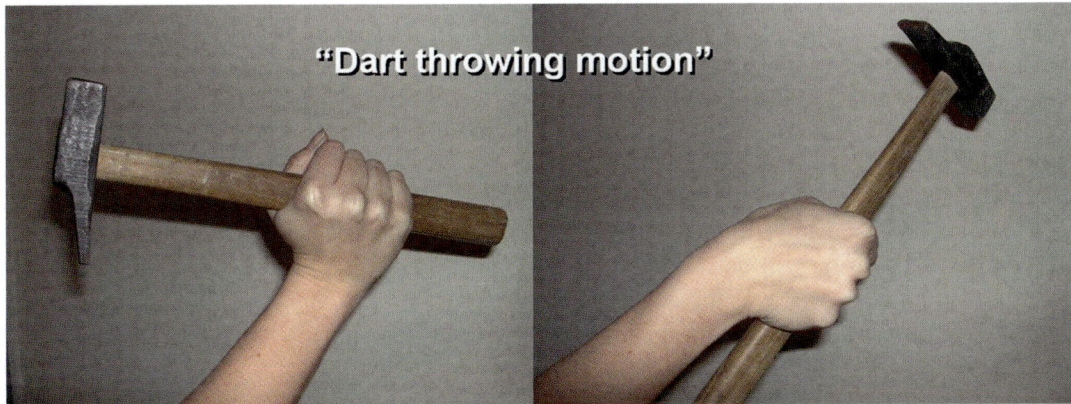

Fig. 3.5 The so-called "physiologic flexion–extension", also known as "dart-throwing" motion, is one of the most usual planes of rotation of the wrist: from extension-radial deviation to flexion-ulnar deviation. This motion mostly involves a rotation of the midcarpal joint. With permission from [64]

powerful muscles of the forearm, the ones with the highest tension fraction: the extensor carpi radialis (longus and brevis) and the FCU [28]. Second, because the midcarpal ball-and-socket articulation is not spherical but ovoid, with an oblique axis oriented towards the anteromedial corner of the wrist. And third, because the distal articular surface of the scaphoid has a ridge which is parallel to the plane of "dart throwing" [33], and guides the distal row towards the anteromedial corner of the wrist.

When the wrist rotates along the "dart throwing" plane, the radiocarpal joint does not move much [12, 14, 29]. When the wrist rotates from radial-extension to ulnar-flexion, the proximal row does not extend, but only translates laterally. The scaphoid does not flex in radial deviation because the concomitant wrist extension prevents that. During ulnar deviation, the proximal row does not extend because is constrained by the flexing distal row. In short: when the wrist rotates along the "dart throwing" plane [39], most motion occurs at the midcarpal level. One of the keys to understand why the proximal row does not move much during this type of motion is the STT ligamentous complex. During radial deviation, the scaphoid tends to rotate into flexion in order to allow the trapezium to approximate to the radial styloid. The STT ligament allows that because is not taut. However, in radial-extension, the trapezium slides down the dorsal slope of the scaphoid, thus pulling the scaphoid into extension by means of the STT ligaments. The equilibrium between the scaphoid flexion tendency and the tensile forces exerted by the STT ligaments explains why the scaphoid remains still during dart-throwing rotations. Likewise, when the wrist ulnarly deviates, the STT ligament becomes taut, thus inducing scaphoid extension. Such scaphoid extension will not happen if the wrist rotates into flexion, in which case the STT ligaments become loose. This may explain why radio-scaphoid-lunate stiffness is so well tolerated. Truly, radiocarpal arthrodeses tend to do better than midcarpal fusions.

3.2.4 Intracarpal Pronosupination Motion

When subjected to a torque along the axial plane, the wrist may be passively displaced in both directions of pronosupination [40]. When unloaded, the mean total rotational laxity of the wrist is 42° [41]. Under load, such displaceability is reduced proportionally to the amount of load being exerted across the wrist. Until recently, it was believed that the wrist could not be actively pronated or supinated, that the muscles with tendons across the wrist could only generate axial compressive forces to the distal row, which eccentricity explained wrist deviations along the coronal or sagittal plane. Recent investigations, however, have demonstrated in the cadaver that the wrist may be actively pronated or supinated depending upon the obliquity of the tendon at the level of the carpus [25]. Certainly, at the level of the carpus, some tendons have an oblique course towards their distal insertion. The abductor pollicis longus (APL), for instance, is located dorsally in the first extensor compartment, but inserts anterolaterally at the base of the first metacarpal. The ECU, by contrast, has an opposite obliqueness from the dorsum of the ulna to the anteromedial corner of the fifth metacarpal. They both are dorsal at the level of the radiocarpal joint, to diverge distally towards either the medial or lateral aspects of the wrist. When these muscles contract, its tendon obliquity is likely to generate pronation or supination moments to the distal row: the medially inserted tendons will induce pronation, while the laterally inserted tendons will induce supination to the distal row. The APL, the extensor carpi radialis longus (ECRL) and the FCU are intracarpal supinators, while the FCR and the ECU are distal row pronators. As it will be stated below, this active pronosupination capability may partly explain how the wrist achieves stability under load.

3.3 Carpal Kinetics

Kinetics is the branch of mechanics that deals with the effects of forces in producing or constraining motion of a mass. Carpal kinetics describes the mechanisms by which the wrist may sustain load without yielding; that is, the mechanisms of carpal stabilization. Unquestionably, most hand activities generate forces and torques that will be transferred proximally across the carpus. Stability is defined as the ability of carry on with such centripetal forces without suffering injury. Although some wrist positions are better prepared to bear loads than others (extension better than flexion) [20], the stable wrist is able to bear load in any given position. A stable wrist is prepared to develop self-locking strategies to facilitate proper transfer of loads. To better understand those strategies, it is important to discuss: (1) what is the magnitude of forces crossing the wrist, (2) how are they distributed among the different carpal articulations, (3) what is the role of ligaments as primary stabilizers, (4) what is the role of mechanoreceptors in the detection of ligaments at risk of being injured, and (5) what is the role of muscles as the ultimate wrist stabilizers.

3.3.1 Magnitude of Forces Transmitted Across the Wrist

The wrist is a load bearing articulation that sustains considerable compressive and shear forces [18]. Wrist loading not only derives from external forces being applied to the hand and transmitted across the wrist onto the forearm, but also from contraction of the muscles that control finger and carpal function. Reaction forces generated in the different stabilizing ligaments also contribute to this (Fig. 3.1). According to a series of mathematical and experimental laboratory studies, the amount of compressive forces that cross each carpometacarpal joint may be as high as 1.5–4.2 times the applied force at the tip of the corresponding fingers. These calculations have been recently validated by Rikli et al. [20] who inserted a pressure-sensor device in the radiocarpal joint space of volunteers. According to these experiments, during motion the pressure sustained by the distal articular surface of the radius varies from 54 N/cm^2 (Newtons per centimetre square) in maximal active extension to 26 N/cm^2 in maximum flexion.

3.3.2 Force Distribution Across the Wrist

Once in the distal row, the axial forces distribute among the different joints following specific patterns. These depend upon direction and point of application of the external loads, position of the wrist, and orientation and shape of the articular surfaces [6]. Most forces concentrate on the SL interval and from there into the radius. Viegas and Patterson [42] found that about 50 % of the load is transferred from the capitate into the scaphoid and lunate, while a 35 % goes across the STT joint. At the radiocarpal level, forces distribute as follows: radio-scaphoid joint, 50–56 %; radio-lunate joint, 29–35 %; and ulno-lunate joint 10–21 % [22, 42–44]. These percentages vary with wrist position, the radiolunate fossa being more loaded with ulnar deviation, while the scaphoid resisting more load with radial deviation [20].

3.3.3 Role of Ligaments in the Stabilization of the Carpus

For the wrist to be stable there is a need for a perfect interaction between articular surface geometries and soft-tissue constraints. Not only the ligaments are of importance for a stable function, but also tendons, muscles, capsule, and tendons sheaths contribute to stability. Indeed, carpal stability is a multifactor phenomenon. Of all structures involved, however, the ligaments are the first to react when a load is about to displace bones beyond normal limits. Undeniably, ligaments are the primary stabilizers, the first line of defence against any disturbing force. For the neutrally positioned wrist there are four groups of ligaments that are especially important in stabilizing the different levels of the joint [19]. What follows is a short description of the mechanisms by which these ligaments achieve primary stability:

3.3.3.1 Stabilizing Mechanism of the Distal Row

Once distally emerged from the carpal tunnel, the flexor digitorum tendons have divergent directions. When their corresponding muscles contract, the flexors of the little finger generate a tangential compressive force in an ulnar direction to the hook of the hamate. This force is opposite in direction to the force that generates the FCR to the inner surface of the trapezium. Such opposite forces would tend to open the palmar carpal concavity (the trapezium towards the radial side, the hamate towards the ulnar side) was if not for both the flexor retinaculum and the strong and taut transverse intercarpal ligaments [45]. Their annular disposition appears essential to maintain adequate transverse stability to the carpal pulley. Failure of any one of these structures is likely to create a particular type of instability, called "axial" or "longitudinal", with the tunnel splitting into two or more unstable columns, displacing in divergent directions [46].

3.3.3.2 Midcarpal Stabilizing Mechanism

Under axial load, the distal carpal row exerts an axial compressive force onto the proximal row bones. Because of its oblique orientation relative to the long axis of the forearm, the axially loaded scaphoid tends to rotate into flexion and pronation [10, 19]. If the ligaments connecting the scaphoid to the distal row, namely the anterolateral STT and the volar scaphocapitate (SC) ligaments [47], are intact, the flexion and

pronation moment by the scaphoid will be transmitted to the distal row. The more the trapezium is pulled forward by the STT-SC ligaments, the more the distal row pronates. Excessive distal row pronation, however, could be dangerous for the triquetrum-hamate (TqH) joint. Indeed, being the distal row a rigid structure, the more the capitate pronates, the more the hamate is displaced dorsally. Fortunately, the palmar TqH fascicle of the medial arcuate ligament is strong enough as to prevent such medial midcarpal subluxation. Indeed, the midcarpal crossing ligaments have opposite functions in this regard: the STT-SC ligaments induce pronation to the distal row; the TqH ligament counteracts such pronation vector. Should the latter be insufficient or torn, the distal row would be dragged by the scaphoid into an abnormal flexion-pronation pattern of carpal malalignment, known as "volar intercalated segment instability" (VISI) [7, 48].

3.3.3.3 Stabilizing Mechanism of the Proximal Row

If both the medial and lateral midcarpal crossing ligaments are intact, the proximal carpal row would be subjected to two opposite moments: the scaphoid flexion and pronation moment, and the extension-supination moment induced by the TqH ligament. On theory, if the two moments had equal magnitudes, and if the SL and LTq interosseous ligaments were intact, the scaphoid would rotate into flexion and the triquetrum into extension until a neutral equilibrium would be achieved. In reality, the scaphoid moment predominates over the extension moment of the triquetrum, for not only the scaphoid rotates into flexion and pronation, but also the lunate and triquetrum rotate into flexion and pronation [25, 49]. The scaphoid and triquetrum, however, are not equally constrained by the palmar crossing midcarpal ligaments: the scaphoid is allowed substantial rotation into flexion and pronation, while the triquetrum is tightly controlled by the TqH ligament. Consequently, there are decreasing magnitudes of rotation from lateral to medial. According to Kobayashi et al. [49],

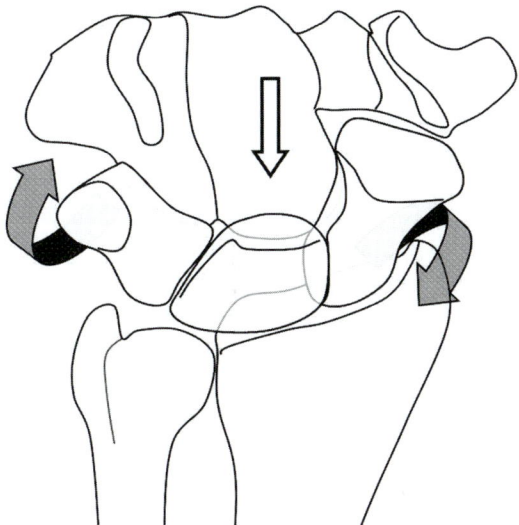

Fig. 3.6 Under axial load (*white arrow*) the proximal row has to cope with two opposite forces (*grey arrows*): one is caused by the scaphoid which tends to draw the entire proximal row into flexion; another is produced by the distal row which extension is transmitted to the triquetrum via the TqH portion of the arcuate ligament. The two opposite moments reach equilibrium provided the transverse inter-carpal scapholunate and lunotriquetral interosseous liga-ments are intact. With permission from [64]

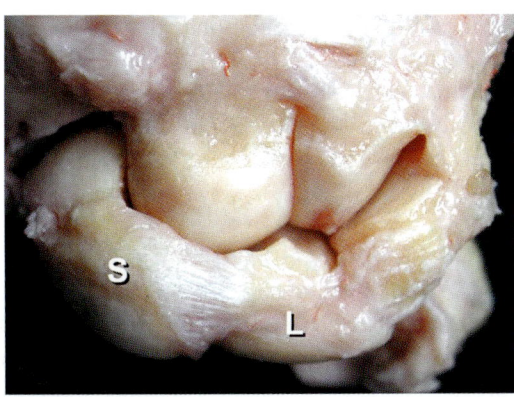

Fig. 3.7 Dorsal view of a dissected wrist demonstrating the obliquely oriented fibres of the dorsal scapholunate interosseous ligament, one important stabilizer of the scaphoid. Its oblique orientation is particularly well adapted to constrain the scaphoid tendency towards collapsing into flexion under load. *S* Scaphoid; *L* Lunate. With permission from [64]

when the carpus is isometrically loaded, the scaphoid rotates into flexion an average 5.1° relative to the radius, while the lunate rotates 4.2° and the triquetrum 3.8° [25, 49].

In short, the proximal row is subjected to two opposite moments: a flexion moment generated by the scaphoid and an extension moment transmitted to the triquetrum by the TqH fascicle of the ulnar arcuate ligament (Fig. 3.6). If both the palmar and dorsal SL and LTq ligaments are intact (Fig. 3.7), such opposite moments gener-ate increasing torques at both intercarpal levels resulting in a stable cooptation of the two SL and LTq joints. Such an increased cooptation further contributes to the proximal carpal row stability. Based on this, if the SL ligaments are completely torn, the scaphoid no longer is constrained by the rest of the proximal row, and tends to collapse into an abnormally flexed and pronated posture (the so called "rotatory subluxation of the scaphoid") [6] (Fig. 3.8), while the lunate and triquetrum, under the

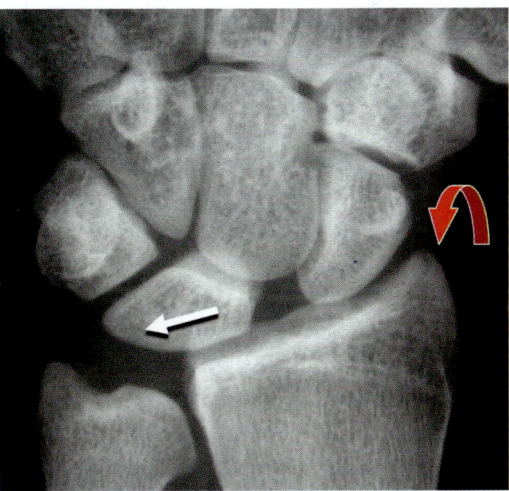

Fig. 3.8 Scapholunate instability resulting from com-plete rupture of the scapholunate interosseous ligaments. The scaphoid shows the typical rotary subluxation (*curved red arrow*) with increased scapholunate gap formation and slight ulnar translocation of the lunate (*white arrow*). With permission from [64]

influence of the ulnar part of the arcuate liga-ment, are pulled into an abnormal extension, known as a "dorsal intercalated segment insta-bility" (DISI) [47]. The consequence of all these changes is an alteration of the moment arms of all wrist motor tendons, and muscle imbalance [50]. By contrast, if it is not the SL ligaments, but the LTq ligaments the ones that have completely failed, the scaphoid and lunate tend to adopt an abnormal flexed posture VISI, while the triquetrum remains solidly linked to the distal row [34, 51].

3.3.3.4 Radiocarpal Stabilizing Mechanism

The proximal convexities of the scaphoid, lunate and triquetrum are proximally interconnected by fibrocartilaginous membranes, forming what has been called the carpal condyle. Such a biconvex structure does not articulate to a horizontal flat surface but to an ulnarly and palmarly inclined antebrachial glenoid, formed by the distal articular surface of the radius and the distal surface of the triangular fibrocartilage. In such circumstances, the loaded carpal condyle has an inherent tendency to slide down ulnarly and palmarly. This tendency is effectively constrained by both palmar and dorsal radiocarpal ligaments which oblique orientation appears ideal to resist such an ulnar and palmar translation tendency. Failure of these obliquely oriented ligaments is likely to result in a very dysfunctional ulnar and palmar translocation of the carpus relative to the radius [52].

3.3.4 Role of Mechanoreceptors in Carpal Stability

Until recently, all the above mechanisms of ligament stabilization were thought to be the essence of wrist stabilization [6]. Ligaments are the first to detect and react against excessive bone displacement; however, they cannot be the only stabilizers. If they were, they would disrupt easily. Indeed, ligaments are not strong enough to resist the magnitude of strains involved in carpal stabilization. The dorsal SL ligament, for instance, considered by many as one of the most resistant components of the SL ligamentous complex, yields at about 260 N of distraction. The palmar SL ligament fails at 118 N, and the proximal membrane at 63 N [53]. The palmar LTq ligament

is thicker and stronger than the dorsal ligament, but still it fails at a mean 301 N while the dorsal LTq ligament disrupts at 121 N [34].

If ligaments were the only means of keeping bones reduced, we would see ligament ruptures very frequently, particularly in certain sports, like gymnastics, where gymnasts land on their wrists after pirouetting in the air. In reality, ligament ruptures are nor that frequent because gymnast's wrists have adequate proprioception, and their sensorimotor system is warned well ahead of time when unusual ligament strains develop. When there is a risk for a ligament to disrupt, the system activates specific muscles that shelter the ligaments against rupture (Fig. 3.9). Indeed, ligaments are protected by muscles, but only if wrist proprioception is fully functional.

Wrist proprioception is more than just conscious perception of joint position. Wrist proprioception is both conscious and unconscious awareness of what occurs within the wrist capsule [8, 9]. Most carpal ligament contain mechanoreceptors able to detect unusually growing strains in the ligaments, and react by sending afferent stimuli to the spinal cord. One of the most active mechanoreceptors in the SL interosseous ligament is the Ruffini corpuscle, a slowly-adapting, low-threshold receptor, constantly active during joint motion, and particularly reactive to axial loading and tensile strain in the ligament, but not to perpendicular compressive load. The afferent stimuli sent by the Ruffini receptor is analyzed at different levels (local, spinal and supraspinal), this triggering the release of efferent (motor) stimuli to specific muscles which contraction will prevent ligament damage. There are different categories of response: from fast joint protective reflexes through monosynaptic spinal control, to more complex plurisynaptic supraspinal responses. In all cases, the faster the muscle response, the better. If the latency time, between ligament aggression and muscle response, is abnormally long, the ligament will suffer more extensive damage than if it is short. Thus, it is important to plan an adequate proprioception training of sportsmen and musicians: by reducing their latency time, injuries are prevented.

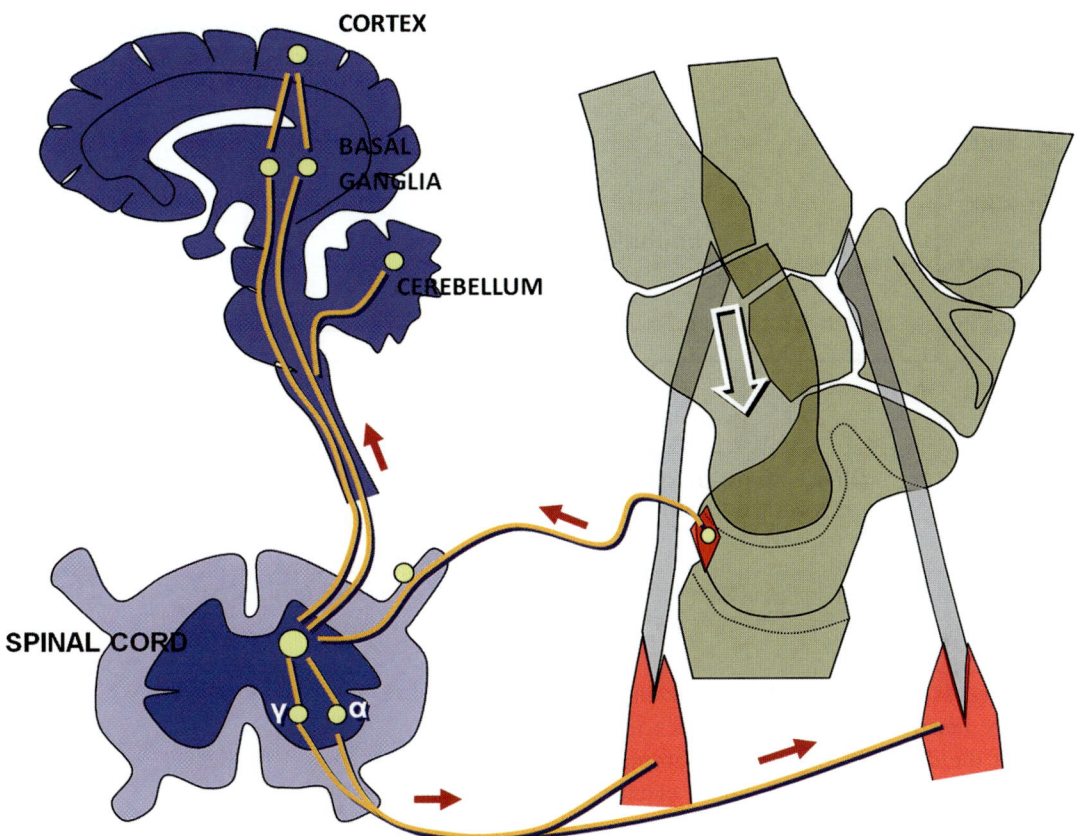

Fig. 3.9 Schematic representation of a ligament-muscle reflex. Under axial load (*white arrow*) the receptors within the dorsal SL ligament send an afferent stimulus (*red arrows*) to the *spinal cord*. The information is forwarded to the supraspinal levels; once analyzed, an efferent (motor) stimuli is sent to specific muscles which contraction will prevent ligament damage. With permission from [64]

Until 1997, it was thought that there were no mechanoreceptors within the carpal capsule. Petrie and associates were the first to demonstrate Golgi organs, Pacinian and Ruffini corpuscles within three palmar wrist ligaments [54]. Since then, several immuno-histo-chemical investigations have been published identifying, qualifying and quantifying sensory receptors in the carpal ligaments [55–57]. The distribution of receptor in the ligaments was not homogeneous: some ligaments are densely innervated while others have almost no innervation [55]. Interestingly enough, with the exception of the dorsal SL ligament, the most poorly innervated ligaments were the ones with the highest yield strength, while the richly innervated ligaments had poorly arranged collagen fibers [55]. In a way, it is reasonable to say that there are mechanically important ligaments, like cables holding bones reduced, and sensorially important ligaments with a predominant proprioceptive role. In general, most ligaments inserted into the triquetrum are richly innervated, while the ones about the scaphoid are mechanically important ligaments. Based on this, it has hypothesized that the triquetrum plays a special role in the detection of abnormal carpal bone displacements, that the triquetrum is the key element in wrist proprioception [55].

In order to prove the existence of ligament-muscle reflexes emanating from inside of the carpal joint, Hagert et al. [58] performed an

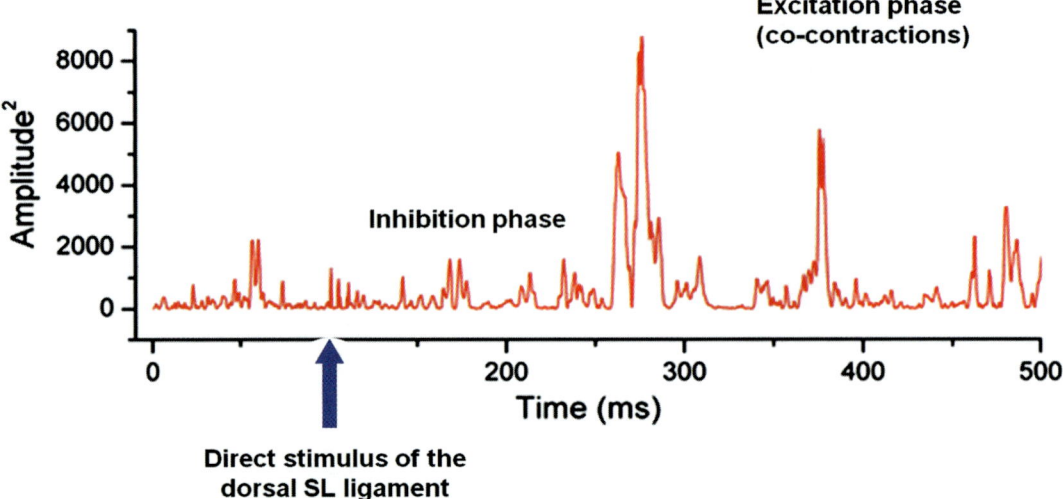

Fig. 3.10 Typical graph demonstrating the changes in muscle activity that occurs in the FCR muscle, 150 ms after the SL ligament was stimulated. Courtesy of Elisabet Hagert, Karolinska Institutet, Stockholm, Sweden. With permission from [64]

interesting experiment. Under ultrasound control, they inserted fine wire electrodes into the depth of the dorsal SL ligament of normal volunteers. The ligament was then electrically stimulated, while surface electromyography sensors documented activity changes in some forearm muscles. The results of that study were conclusive: ligament stimulation was always followed by a muscle response (Fig. 3.10) [58]. In the normal situation, the response was almost immediate (in less than 50 ms after the stimulus) and lasted for 500 ms or sometimes more. The early muscle reaction was interpreted as an attempt to protect the ligaments from suffering injury; while late muscle activity was thought to represent a more elaborated supraspinal response to carpal instability. In all circumstances, the muscle response was not restricted to one muscle, but to several: usually more than three muscles reacted positively for each wrist position. Most often, the response was in the form contraction, except when the muscle could have a destabilizing effect to the joint. In other words, the sensorimotor system is able to discriminate between potential muscle stabilizers and destabilizers; to the first, the system sends an order to contract; to the second, an inhibition

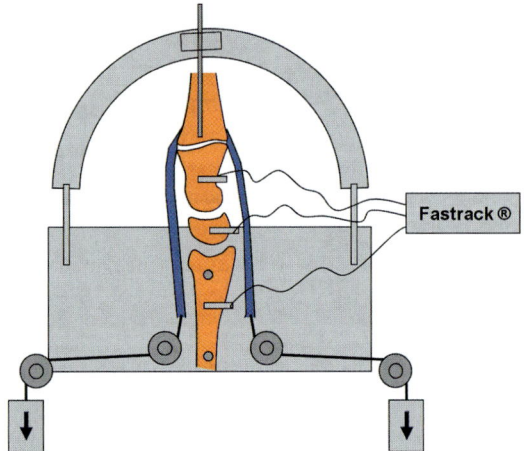

Fig. 3.11 Schematic representation of the experimental setup used by Salvà-Coll to investigate the effects of isometric contraction of muscles on carpal alignment [25, 62, 63]. With permission from [64]

order. When a disturbing load risks rupture of the SL ligament, only the muscles able to prevent that injury are asked to contract, while the potential destabilizers are inhibited.

Needless to say, for this to be possible, the nerves carrying afferent stimuli need to be intact. As demonstrated in vivo by Hagert et al. [58, 59] when the posterior interosseous nerve was

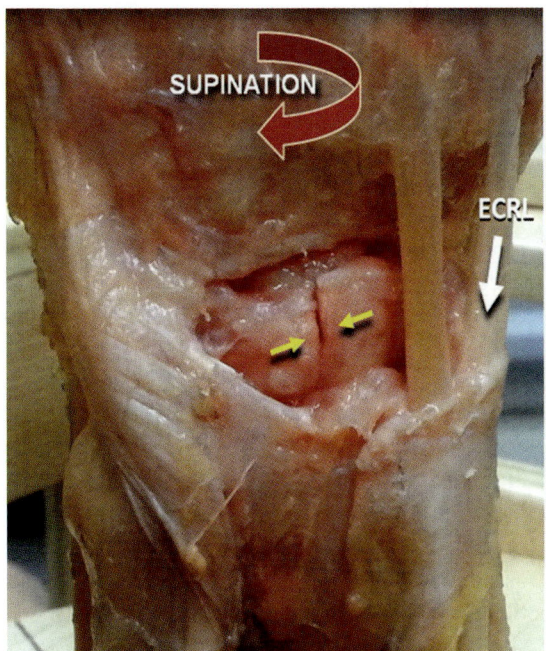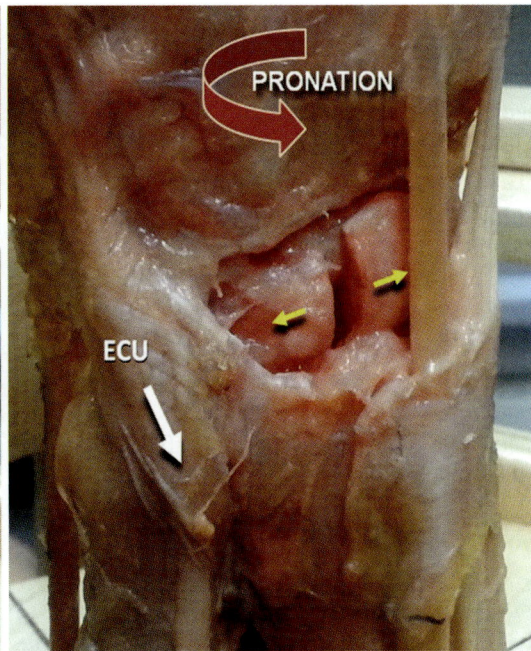

Fig. 3.12 Typical behaviour of the carpus when the SL ligament has been cut and the wrist is subjected to *supination* (*left*) or *pronation* (*right*) torques (*purple curved arrows*). The rotation is produced by pulling tendons with an oblique direction (*white arrows*). When the distal row is torque in supination (*left*), the SL joint becomes reduced (*yellow arrows*). By contrast, when the wrist is pronated, the SL gap increases. From the Department of Anatomy. University of Barcelona. With permission from [64]

anesthetized, stimulation of the SL ligament did not triggered any muscle response. Wrist denervation, therefore, may not influence conscious proprioception (joint position sense) [60, 61], but it may seriously impair unconscious neuromuscle control of carpal stability.

3.3.5 Role of Muscles in Carpal Stability

Until recently, muscles were assumed to have a negative effect on carpal stability [6]. The axial compressive forces generated by their contraction was said to contribute to carpal collapse. Now we know that, in the presence of adequate ligament-muscle reflexes, patients with substantial ligament disruptions may learn to activate unconsciously the beneficial muscles while inhibiting the ones that could destabilize the joint. Indeed, it is not rare to find asymptomatic ligament disruptions.

In order to clarify what muscles are potential stabilizers, in what circumstances and through what mechanism, a number of experiments were conducted by Salvá-Coll et al. [25, 62, 63]. Using a 3D motion tracking device in a cadaver model, the effects of isometric loading of specific wrist motor tendons on carpal bone alignment were analyzed (Fig. 3.11). Despite radius and ulna had been blocked in neutral forearm rotation, some muscles induced pronation to the distal row, while others induced supination. The mechanism by which some muscles are able to supinate or pronate the distal row has been explained above (see Sect. 3.2.4). Interestingly enough, when all forearm muscles contract at once, the distal row always supinates, a displacement that counteracts the natural tendency of the distal carpal row towards pronation (see Sect. 3.3.3.2) [25]. Certainly, if muscles are able to stabilize the carpus is because they are capable of resisting the pronation torque sustained by the carpus under axial load.

According to Salvá-Coll et al. [25] supinator muscles are particularly effective in controlling the symptoms in cases of a dynamic SL dissociation. Indeed, supination constrains the pronation tendency of the scaphoid, and closes the SL gap (Fig. 3.12). Pronator muscles, by contrast, are deleterious in those cases, because they pull the scaphoid away from the lunate, thus widening the SL gap. Certainly, after a dorsal SL ligament repair, contraction of the ECU, a strong pronator, may affect negatively the results by pulling the sutures apart. It is not surprising, therefore, that after stimulation of the SL ligament, the ECU muscle gets an efferent order to relax, to do not contract. Indeed, the ECU is a SL destabilizing muscle, a muscle that can make worse the symptoms of a SL deficient wrist.

As said above (Sect. 3.2.4), there are three muscles that consistently induce supination to the distal row: the ECRL, the APL, and the FCU, and two muscles that generate pronation: the ECU and the FCR. Interestingly enough, the supinator muscles are the ones that generate the "dart-throwing" type of rotation. This explains why patients with dynamic SL dissociation benefit from dart throwing exercises.

The FCR has long been assumed to be a dynamic scaphoid stabilizer [6]. Because the tendon angles around the scaphoid tuberosity, its contraction has been long believed to generate a dorsally directed force that would extend the scaphoid. Recent studies, however, have demonstrated that the FCR muscle does not induce extension to the scaphoid, but flexion and supination, the latter being what makes this muscle beneficial in SL deficient wrists [62]. Indeed, as said above, by supinating the scaphoid, the SL gap is closed.

structural stiffness of the carpal arch. As demonstrated by Garcia-Elias et al. [45], when the transverse carpal ligament (the deepest layer of the flexor retinaculum) is experimentally sectioned, the transverse diameter of the carpal arch increases an average 6 mm, whereas the resultant structural stiffness appears to decrease to no more than a 10 %. The role of the flexor retinaculum as a carpal arch stabilizer is minimal as compared to its function as a pulley, and particularly during wrist flexion.

As demonstrated by Kang et al. [23], and later confirmed by Netscher et al. [24], 30° extension of the wrist improves an average 16 % the work efficiency of the flexor tendons, whereas flexing the wrist produces the opposite effect. This is in accordance with the work by O'Driscoll and associates [21] and Li [5], who demonstrated that the most effective wrist position as far as grip strength is concerned involves about 20°–30° of extension and 5°–10° of ulnar deviation.

Section of the transverse carpal ligament tends not to modify the effectiveness of the finger flexor tendons if the wrist is in extension. By contrast, if the wrist is flexed, and the transverse carpal ligament has been removed, greater tendon excursion is required for the same amount of finger flexion to be obtained, mostly due to the bowstringing effect. Since the flexor digitorum muscles have scarce possibilities to increase their tendon excursion, their work efficiency is likely to decrease, as it has been both clinically and experimentally demonstrated. Indeed, section of the transverse carpal ligament results in an average 16 % weakening effect on finger flexion when the wrist is in flexion. The biomechanical importance of the transverse carpal ligament as a true pulley, therefore, cannot be neglected.

3.4   The Carpal Pulley

Stiffness of the distal carpal row against dorsopalmar compression is quite high provided that the short and stout transverse intercarpal ligaments are intact. In normal conditions, the flexor retinaculum contributes little to the overall

References

1. Garcia-Elias M (1999) Anatomy and biomechanics committee of the international federation of societies for surgery of the hand. Definition of carpal instability. J Hand Surg Am 24(4):866–867
2. Kijima Y, Viegas SF (2009) Wrist anatomy and biomechanics. J Hand Surg Am 34(8):1555–1563

3. Adey L, Ring D, Jupiter JB (2005) Health status after total wrist arthrodesis for posttraumatic arthritis. J Hand Surg Am 30(5):932–936
4. Nelson DL (1997) Functional wrist motion. Hand Clin 13(1):83–92
5. Li ZM (2002) The influence of wrist position on individual finger forces during forceful grip. J Hand Surg Am 27(5):886–896
6. Garcia-Elias M (2011) Carpal instability. In: Wolfe S, Hotchkiss R, Pederson W, Kozin S (eds) Green's operative hand surgery, 6th edn. Churchill, Livingstone, Elsevier, Philadelphia, pp 465–521
7. Lichtman DM, Schneider JR, Swafford AR, Mack GR (1981) Ulnar midcarpal instability—clinical and laboratory analysis. J Hand Surg 6(5):515–523
8. Riemann BL, Lephart SM (2002) The sensorimotor system, part I: the physiologic basis of functional joint stability. J Athl Train 37(1):71–79
9. Hagert E (2010) Proprioception of the wrist joint: a review of current concepts and possible implications on the rehabilitation of the wrist. J Hand Ther 23(1):2–16
10. Kobayashi M, Berger RA, Nagy L et al (1997) Normal kinematics of carpal bones: a three-dimensional analysis of carpal bone motion relative to the radius. J Biomech 30(8):787–793
11. Moojen TM, Snel JG, Ritt MJ, Venema HW, Kauer JM, Bos KE (2003) In vivo analysis of carpal kinematics and comparative review of the literature. J Hand Surg Am 28(1):81–87
12. Werner FW, Green JK, Short WH, Masaoka S (2004) Scaphoid and lunate motion during a wrist dart throw motion. J Hand Surg Am 29(3):418–422
13. Kaufmann R, Pfaeffle J, Blankenhorn B, Stabile K, Robertson D, Goitz R (2005) Kinematics of the midcarpal and radiocarpal joints in radioulnar deviation: an in vitro study. J Hand Surg Am 30(5):937–942
14. Crisco JJ, Coburn JC, Moore DC, Akelman E, Weiss AP, Wolfe SW (2005) In vivo radiocarpal kinematics and the dart thrower's motion. J Bone Joint Surg Am 87(12):2729–2740
15. Feipel V, Rooze M (1999) Three-dimensional motion patterns of the carpal bones: an in vivo study using three-dimensional computed tomography and clinical applications. Surg Radiol Anat 21(2):125–131
16. Craigen MAC, Stanley JK (1995) Wrist kinematics. Row, column or both? J Hand Surg Br 20(2):165–170
17. Galley I, Bain GI, McLean JM (2007) Influence of lunate type on scaphoid kinematics. J Hand Surg Am 32(6):842–847
18. An KN, Chao EY, Cooney WP, Linscheid RL (1985) Forces in the normal and abnormal hand. J Orthop Res 3(2):202–211
19. Garcia-Elias M (1997) Kinetic analysis of carpal stability during grip. Hand Clin 13(1):151–158
20. Rikli DA, Honigmann P, Babst R, Cristalli A, Morlock MM, Mittlmeier T (2007) Intra-articular pressure measurement in the radioulnocarpal joint using a novel sensor: in vitro and in vivo results. J Hand Surg Am 32(1):67–75
21. O'Driscoll SW, Horii E, Ness R et al (1992) The relationship between wrist position, grasp size, and grip strength. J Hand Surg Am 17(1):169–177
22. Majima M, Horii E, Matsuki H, Hirata H, Genda E (2008) Load transmission through the wrist in the extended position. J Hand Surg Am 33(2):182–188
23. Kang HJ, Lee SG, Phillips CS, Mass DP (1996) Biomechanical changes of cadaveric finger flexion: the effect of wrist position and of the transverse carpal ligament and palmar and forearm fasciae. J Hand Surg Am 21(6):963–968
24. Netscher D, Lee M, Thronby J, Polsen C (1997) The effect of division of the transverse carpal ligament on flexor tendon excursion. J Hand Surg Am 22(6):1016–1024
25. Salvà-Coll G, Garcia-Elias M, Leon-Lopez MT, Llusa-Perez M, Rodríguez-Baeza A (2011) Effects of forearm muscles on carpal stability. J Hand Surg Eur 36:553–559
26. Corson ER (1897) X-ray study of normal movements of the carpal bones and wrist. Proc Assoc Am Anat, Session 11th pp 67–92
27. Fisk GR (1980) La biomécanique de l'articulation du poignet. In: Tubiana R (ed) Traité de Chirurgie de la Main, Masson, Paris, pp 171–176
28. Saffar Ph, Seumaan I (1994) The study of the biomechanics of wrist movements in an oblique plain. In: Schuind F, An KN, Cooney WP, Garcia-Elias M (eds) Advances in the biomechanics of the hand and wrist. Plenum press, New York, pp 305–311
29. Moritomo H, Apergis EP, Herzberg G, Werner FW, Wolfe SW, Garcia-Elias M (2007) 2007 IFSSH committee report of wrist biomechanics committee: biomechanics of the so-called dart-throwing motion of the wrist. J Hand Surg Am 32(9):1447–1453
30. Brand PW, Hollister A (1993) Mechanics of individual muscles at individual joints. In: Brand PW, Hollister A (eds) Clinical mechanics of the hand, 2nd edn. St. Louis Mosby Year Book, pp 254–352
31. Ryu J, Cooney WP, Askew LJ, An KN, Chao EYS (1991) Functional ranges of motion of the wrist joint. J Hand Surg Am 16(3):409–419
32. Garcia-Elias M, Sanchez-Freijo JM, Salo JM, Lluch AL (1992) Dynamic changes of the transverse carpal arch during flexion-extension of the wrist: effects of sectioning the transverse carpal ligament. J Hand Surg Am 17(6):1017–1019
33. Kauer JMG (1986) The mechanism of the carpal joint. Clin Orthop Rel Res 202:16–26
34. Ritt MJPF, Linscheid RL, Cooney WP, Berger RA, An KN (1998) The lunotriquetral joint: kinematic effects of sequential ligament sectioning, ligament repair, and arthrodesis. J Hand Surg Am 23(3):432–445
35. Neu CP, Crisco JJ, Wolfe SW (2001) In vivo kinematic behaviour of the radio-capitate joint during wrist flexion-extension and radio-ulnar deviation. J Biomech 34(11):1429–1438

36. Kaufmann RA, Pfaeffle HJ, Blankenhorn BD, Stabile K, Robertson D, Goitz R (2006) Kinematics of the midcarpal and radiocarpal joint in flexion and extension: an in vitro study. J Hand Surg Am 31(7):1142–1148

37. Garcia-Elias M, Orsolini C (2011) Relationship between thumb laxity and trapezium kinematics. Chir Main 30(3):224–227

38. Garcia-Elias M, Ribe M, Rodriguez J, Cots M, Casas J (1995) Influence of joint laxity on scaphoid kinematics. J Hand Surg Br 20(3):379–382

39. Ishikawa JI, Cooney WP, Niebur G et al (1999) The effects of wrist distraction on carpal kinematics. J Hand Surg Am 24(1):113–120

40. Ritt MJPF, Stuart PR, Berglund LJ et al (1995) Rotational stability of the carpus relative to the forearm. J Hand Surg Am 20(2):305–311

41. Ritt MJPF, Stuart PR, Berglund LJ et al. (1996) Rotational laxity and stiffness of the radiocarpal joint. Clin Biomech (Bristol, Avon) 11(4):227–232

42. Viegas SF, Patterson RM (1997) Load mechanics of the wrist. Hand Clin 13(1):109–128

43. Hara T, Horii E, An KN et al (1992) Force distribution across wrist joint: application of pressure-sensitive conductive rubber. J Hand Surg Am 17(2):339–347

44. Werner FW, An KN, Palmer AK, Chao EYS (1991) Force analysis. In: An KN, Berger RA, Cooney WP (eds) Biomechanics of the wrist joint. Springer, New York, pp 77–97

45. Garcia-Elias M, An KN, Cooney WP et al (1989) Stability of the transverse carpal arch: an experimental study. J Hand Surg Am 14(2):277–281

46. Garcia-Elias M, Dobyns JH, Cooney WP et al (1989) Traumatic axial dislocations of the carpus. J Hand Surg Am 14(3):446–457

47. Short WH, Werner FW, Green JK, Masaoka S (2005) Biomechanical evaluation of the ligamentous stabilizers of the scaphoid and lunate. Part II. J Hand Surg Am 30(1):24–34

48. Linscheid RL, Dobyns JH, Beabout JM, Brian RS (1972) Traumatic instability of the wrist: diagnosis, classification and pathomechanics. J Bone Joint Surg Am 54(8):1612–1632

49. Kobayashi M, Garcia-Elias M, Nagy L et al (1999) Axial loading induces rotation of the proximal carpal row bones around unique screw-displacement axes. J Biomech 30(11–12):1165–1167

50. Tang JB, Ryu J, Omokawa S, Wearden S (2002) Wrist kinetics after scapholunate dissociation: the effect of scapholunate interosseous ligament injury and persistent scapholunate gaps. J Orthop Res 20(2):215–221

51. Shin AY, Battaglia MJ, Bishop AT (2000) Lunotriquetral instability: diagnosis and treatment. J Am Acad Orthop Surg 8(3):170–179

52. Rayhack JM, Linscheid RL, Dobyns JH, Smith JH (1987) Post-traumatic ulnar translation of the carpus. J Hand Surg Am 12(2):180–189

53. Berger RA, Imaeda T, Berglund L, An KN (1999) Constraint and material properties of the subregions of the scapholunate interosseous ligament. J Hand Surg Am 24(5):953–962

54. Petrie S, Collins J, Solomonow M, Wink C, Chuinard R (1997) Mechanoreceptors in the palmar wrist ligaments. J Bone Joint Surg Br 79(3):494–496

55. Hagert E, Garcia-Elias M, Forsgren S, Ljung BO (2007) Immunohistochemical analysis of wrist ligament innervation in relation to their structural composition. J Hand Surg Am 32(1):30–36

56. Lin YT, Berger RA, Berger EJ, Tomita K, Jew JY, Yang C, An KN (2006) Nerve endings of the wrist joint: a preliminary report of the dorsal radiocarpal ligament. J Orthop Res 24(6):1225–1230

57. Mataliotakis G, Doukas M, Kostas I, Lykissas M, Batistatou A, Beris A (2009) Sensory innervation of the subregions of the scapholunate interosseous ligament in relation to their structural composition. J Hand Surg Am 34(8):1413–1421

58. Hagert E, Persson JK, Werner M, Ljung BO (2009) Evidence of wrist proprioceptive reflexes elicited after stimulation of the scapholunate interosseous ligament. J Hand Surg Am 34(4):642–651

59. Hagert E, Persson JK (2010) Desensitizing the posterior interosseous nerve alters wrist proprioceptive reflexes. J Hand Surg Am 35(7):1059–1066

60. Patterson RW, Van Niel M, Shimko P, Pace C, Seitz WH Jr (2010) Proprioception of the wrist following posterior interosseous sensory neurectomy. J Hand Surg Am 35(1):52–56

61. Gay A, Harbst K, Hansen DK, Laskowski ER, Berger RA, Kaufman KR (2011) Effect of partial wrist denervation on wrist kinesthesia: wrist denervation does not impair proprioception. J Hand Surg Am 36(11):1774–1779

62. Salva Coll G, Garcia-Elias M, Llusá Pérez M, Rodriguez Baeza A (2011) The role of the flexor carpi radialis muscle in scapholunate instability. J Hand Surg Am 36(1):31–36

63. Salva Coll G, Garcia-Elias M, Leon Lopez M, lusá Pérez M, Rodriguez Baeza A (2012) Role of the extensor carpi ulnaris and its sheath on dynamic carpal stability. J Hand Surg Eur 37(6):544–548

64. Apergis E (2004) καταγματα-εξαρθρήματα του καρπου. Konstantaras Medical Books, Athens

Part II
Perilunate Fracture-Dislocations

Acute Perilunate Dislocations and Fracture-Dislocations

4

The first case of perilunate fracture-dislocation that appeared in the literature was from Malgaigne in 1855 and later from DeQuervain before the introduction of radiography. The first detailed description of these injuries was published 10 years after the discovery of X-rays, by Etienne Destot in 1905. The first series reporting perilunate fracture-dislocations was from Tavernier in 1906, who described in detail 22 cases [1]. The majority of these patients were victims of high-energy injuries of that era, caused by falls from horses.

Perilunate injuries affect both soft tissues and bony elements around the lunate and rarely the lunate itself. There is an almost endless array of injury patterns, which mainly concerns the fracture-dislocation group. The vast majority involves specific types of injuries, but in the literature isolated cases have been described in the most unlikely combination of fracture-dislocations.

Although perilunate injuries could be manifested in a multitude of radiographic images, the constant and defining feature of the perilunate dislocations is the dislocation of the capitate head from the concavity of the distal lunate (Fig. 4.1), while fracture-dislocations have additionally in common the fracture of one or more bones surrounding the lunate [2–4].

4.1 Incidence

Carpal dislocations and fracture-dislocations are uncommon injuries and represent approximately 5–7 % of all wrist injuries [5–8], or about 10 % of all carpal injuries according to others [1, 9]. The true incidence and prevalence of these injuries are difficult to define precisely because there is a belief that perilunate injuries in general are under-diagnosed or because high-energy injuries are increasing the last decades.

The population that is most frequently involved is young male individuals, in the second or third decade of life, who have sustained a sport, traffic, or work accident [5, 10]. However, the injury has also been described in children [11, 12].

Perilunate fracture-dislocations are twice as frequent as the pure ligamentous perilunate dislocations [2, 3]. Herzberg et al. [13] in a multicenter study of 166 perilunate injuries found that four types covered 94 % of cases: (a) the dorsal trans-scaphoid perilunate fracture-dislocations (Stage I) (49 %), (b) the dorsal trans-scaphoid perilunate fracture-dislocations (Stage II) (12 %), (c) the dorsal perilunate dislocations (Stage I) (17 %), and (d) the dorsal perilunate dislocations (Stage II) (palmar lunate dislocations) (16 %).

The increased incidence of trans-scaphoid perilunate fracture-dislocations (50–96 %) compared to all other perilunate fracture-dislocations, has been confirmed by several authors [3, 14, 15].

Dorsal displacement of the distal carpal row occurs in 97 % of cases, while palmar dislocations or fracture-dislocations are the less frequent types of perilunate injuries (2–3 %) with the greater arc variety being the most common [3, 5, 13].

E. Apergis, *Fracture-Dislocations of the Wrist*,
DOI: 10.1007/978-88-470-5328-1_4, © Springer-Verlag Italia 2013

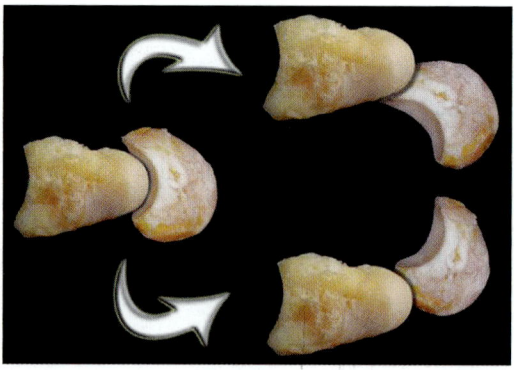

Fig. 4.1 Common characteristic of all perilunate injuries is the loss of articular contact between the lunate and capitate. With permission from [231]

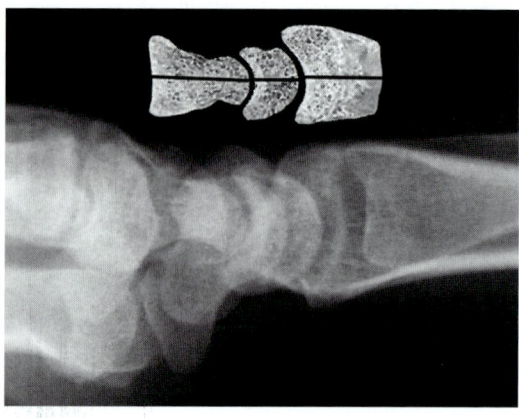

Fig. 4.2 In the L view, the longitudinal axis of the radius, lunate, and capitate should be in almost coaxial alignment. With permission from [231]

The vast majority are closed injuries while open cases represent less than 10 % [3]. Because they most frequently occur from high-energy trauma, the percentage of associated injuries reaches 61 % [16]. One out of four patients were polytraumas [13], while visceral or other extremity injuries were present in 65 % of patients [17]. In 11 % of the patients, an associated injury of the ipsilateral upper limb occurred [18–20].

These injuries are rarely seen in the older population, since without good bone quality the distal radius is most likely to fail before the carpal bones or ligaments. In the pediatric population, the hyperextension forces required to cause these injuries usually injure the weaker radial physis rather than the carpal ligaments [21].

4.2 Nomenclature

In order to name these complex injuries and to communicate with each other, it is usually sufficient to study the two classical X-ray projections, i.e., posteroanterior (PA) and lateral (L) view. In the L view, it is necessary to be acquainted with the radiological outline of the radius, lunate, and the head of the capitate, which should be in almost coaxial alignment (Fig. 4.2). Since a constant and defining feature of all perilunate dislocations and fracture-dislocations is the

dislocation of the capitate head from the concavity of the distal lunate, we are interested in clarifying: (a) Which of these two bones has lost its coaxial alignment and (b) In which direction it is displaced. If the capitate, which is an indicator of the distal carpal row, loses its alignment and is displaced, while the lunate remains in alignment with the radius, then this injury is called "perilunate dislocation". Depending on the direction of the displacement, the perilunate dislocation could be "dorsal" or "volar". Conversely, if the head of the capitate remains in alignment with the radius and the lunate is the displaced bone, then this injury is called "dislocation of lunate, dorsal or volar", depending on the direction of the displacement. In every case, the prefix "*trans-*" is applied to describe a fracture while the prefix "*peri-*" is applied to describe dislocations.

For the nomenclature of these injuries, three essential components are utilized.

The *first component* stems from the PA X-ray view and is used if the presence of a fracture is determined. The first component is formed by the prefix trans- followed by the name of the fractured bone(s). If no fracture is observed, the first component is omitted.

The lateral X-ray provides us with the other two components after, however, we have determined which bone has lost its axial alignment and toward which direction. Thus, *the second component* indicates the direction of the dislocated bones

Fig. 4.3 For the nomenclature, the first component is derived from the PA view and at the presence of a fracture, by applying the prefix "trans". With permission from [231]

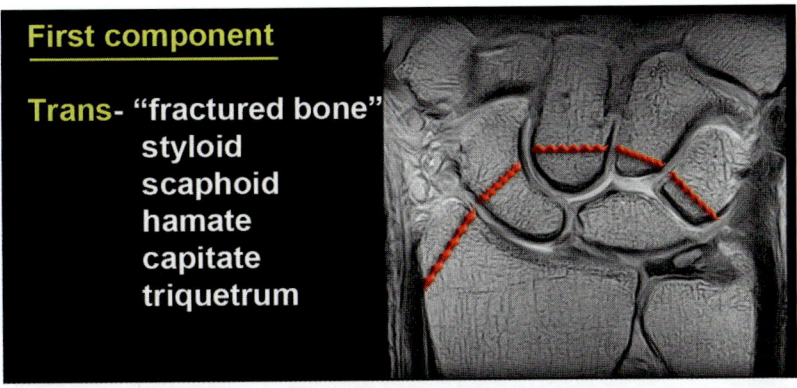

Fig. 4.4 The second component is derived from the L view and describes the direction of the dislocated bones (*dorsal* or *volar*). With permission from [231]

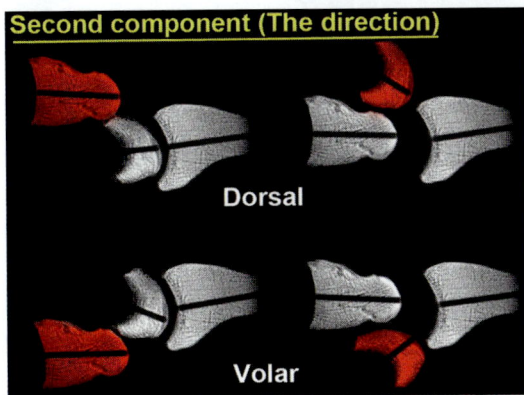

Fig. 4.5 The third component is also based on the L view and depends on the type of the dislocation (*perilunate* or *lunate*). With permission from [231]

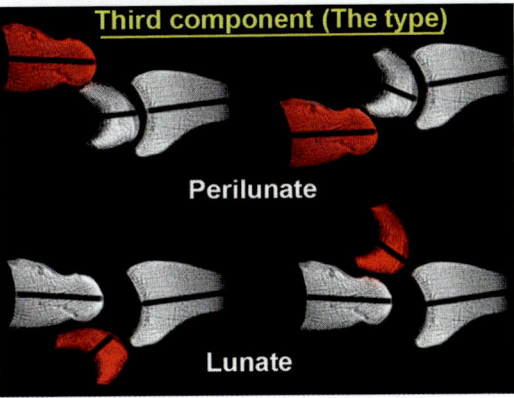

(dorsal or volar) and the *third component* describes the type of dislocation, i.e., if the dislocation is perilunate or lunate depending on the bone that has been misaligned (Figs. 4.3, 4.4, 4.5).

4.3 Classification

The classification of lunate and perilunate injuries is a difficult task. A classification no matter how comprehensive and detailed it is, there will always be unclassified cases since the spectrum of these injuries is unlimited. The good news is that unclassified cases are the vast minority, so even dedicated wrist surgeons may encounter few such cases in their careers. Moreover, despite their rarity, their treatment follows the general principles of the perilunate injuries treatment.

The close relationship between carpal instabilities and perilunate injuries is well known. Existing ligamentous instabilities could be considered as incomplete dislocations or as residual of a closed reduced dislocation [22]. This close relationship is shown in a number of classifications [23–25].

In terms of instability, since the derangement, in perilunate injuries, is both within and between carpal rows, these injuries are considered as carpal instabilities complex (CIC), which is a combination of dissociative (CID) and non-dissociative (CIND) instabilities.

Using the terminology that was popularized by Johnson [26], perilunate injuries could be classified as lesser and greater arc injuries depending on the path of injury around the lunate. Equally important is the separation of these injuries into

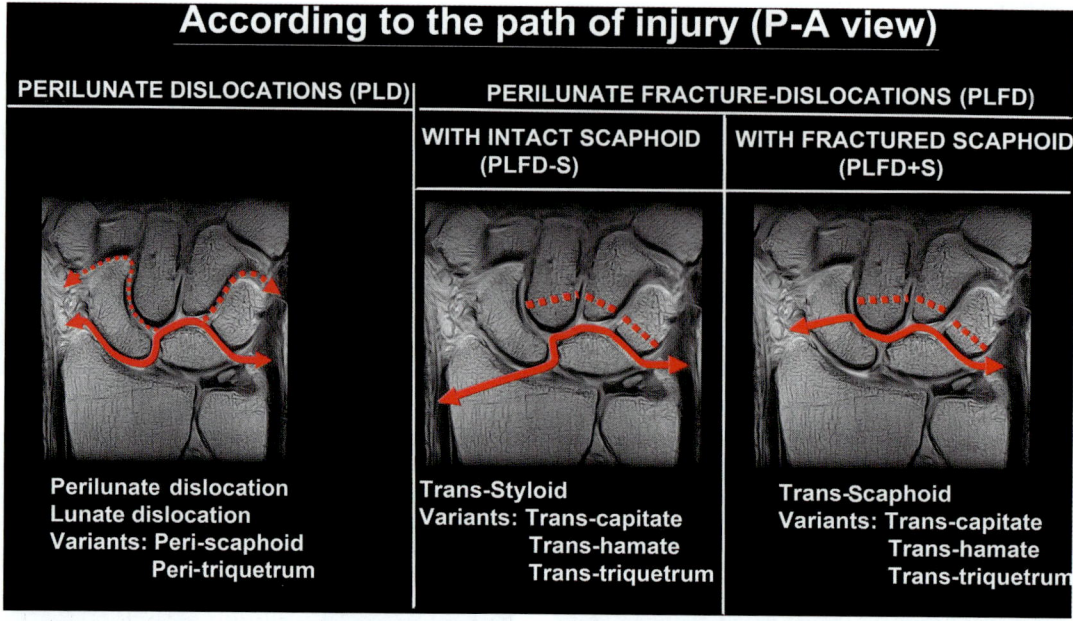

Fig. 4.6 The modified radiologic classification by Herzberg [2] and Herzberg and Forissier [27] based on the PA (according to the path of injury) view (see text for details). With permission from [231]

those with dorsal (most frequent) or volar displacement of the head of the capitate from the distal articular surface of the lunate.

Herzberg [2] and Herzberg and Forissier [27] proposed a radiologic classification of these injuries, which was obtained from the two standard PA and L views taken at the time of diagnosis (Figs. 4.6, 4.7).

The *PA view* demonstrates the path of trauma and defines two categories: *the perilunate dislocations (PLD)*, where the injury is primarily ligamentous and *perilunate fracture-dislocations (PLFD)*, where there is a combination of ligamentous and osseous injuries. The latter group includes fracture-dislocations with an intact *(PLFD−S)* or fractured scaphoid *(PLFD+S)*.

Fig. 4.7 The modified radiologic classification by Herzberg [2] and Herzberg and Forissier [27] based on the L view (according to the displacement of capitate) (see text for details). With permission from [231]

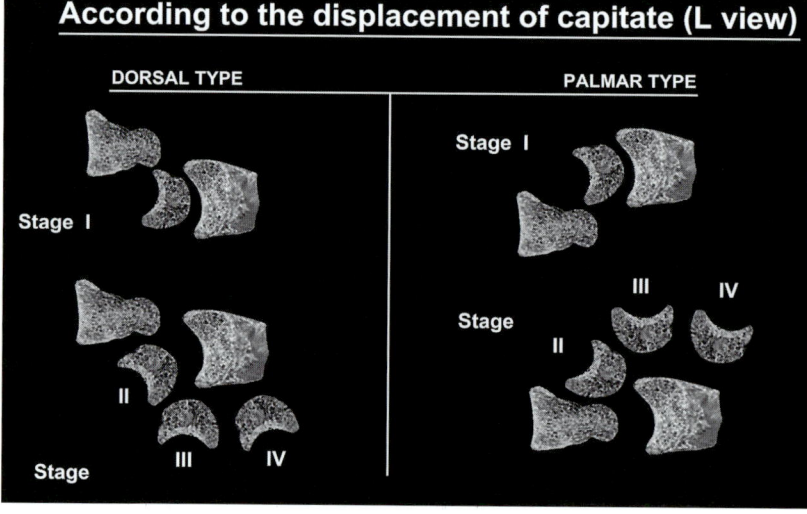

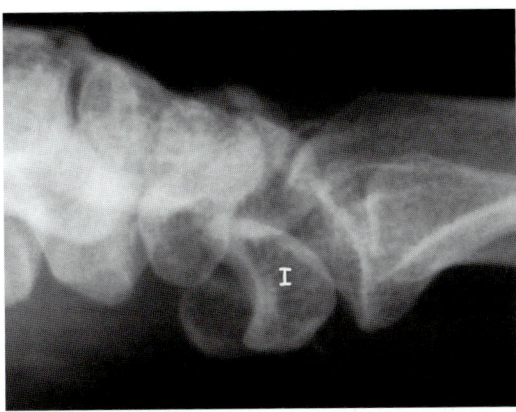

Fig. 4.8 A *type I* dorsal perilunate dislocation. With permission from [231]

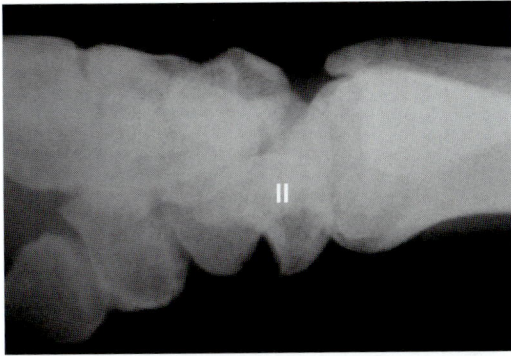

Fig. 4.9 A *type II* dorsal perilunate dislocation. With permission from [231]

In the PLD group, Herzberg et al. [13] recognized that instead of the classical path of trauma around the lunate, there could be variants: scaphotrapeziotrapezoid dislocation instead of scapholunate dislocation (periscaphoid perilunate dislocation) and/or a triquetrohamate instead of a triquetrolunate dislocation (peritriquetral perilunate dislocation).

In the PLFD group, the typical PLFD−S type involves the radial styloid or variants (transcapitate, trans-triquetrum, or combinations), while the PLFD+S type involves the scaphoid or variants (trans-styloid, trans-capitate, trans-triquetral, or combinations).

The **L view** demonstrates the alignment of the radius, lunate, and capitate and clarifies the displacement of the capitate with respect to the lunate. Based on this projection, two types of injuries are distinguished: In the *Dorsal type*, there is dorsal displacement and in the *Palmar type* there is palmar displacement of the capitate with respect to the lunate. In both types, the lunate may remain normally aligned relative to the radius (*Stage I*) or may appear partially (rotated palmarly less than 90°-*Stage II*) or totally displaced (rotated palmarly 90°-*Stage III*), invading the carpal canal. In stage III, the lunate is still attached by the palmar ligaments to the radius (mainly with the short radiolunate ligament), a fact which is certainly related to its viability. Witvoet and Allieu [28] described a stage IV of

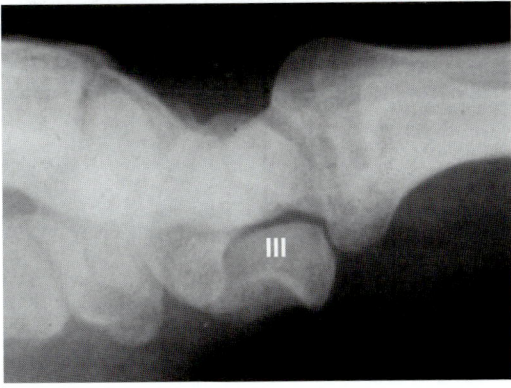

Fig. 4.10 A *type III* dorsal perilunate dislocation. With permission from [231]

lunate displacement, which is totally enucleated without any soft tissue connections, lying at the level of the distal forearm (Figs. 4.8, 4.9, 4.10, 4.11). (From Herzberg's original description [2, 27], we have modified the stages IIA and IIB as stages II and III, for educational purposes).

The presence of associated chip fractures is not sufficient to place the injury in the fracture-dislocation group [13]. Such fractures are the tip of the radial styloid, the osteochondral fragment from the head of the capitate, or an avulsion fragment from the proximal volar surface of the triquetrum [13, 25].

Avulsion fractures of carpal bones may be a subtle sign of carpal ligament injury that is manifested belatedly with carpal derangement or malalignment. Examples are the volar aspect of

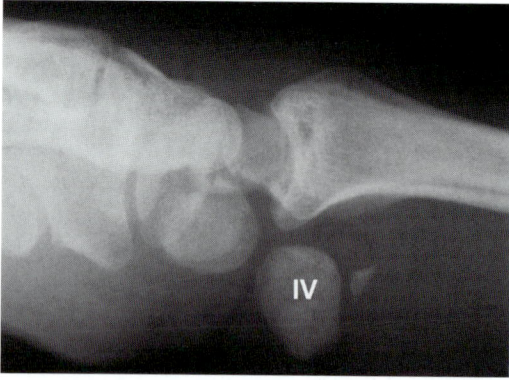

Fig. 4.11 A *type IV* dorsal perilunate dislocation. With permission from [231]

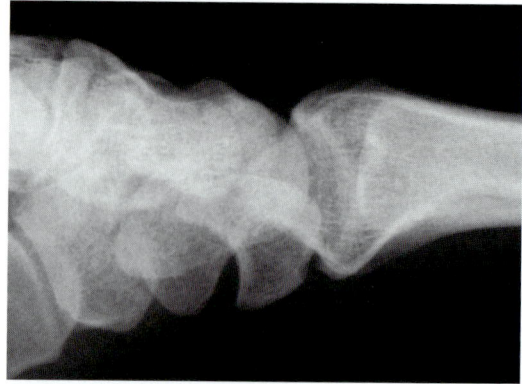

Fig. 4.13 A seemingly stage II dorsal perilunate dislocation. (continued)

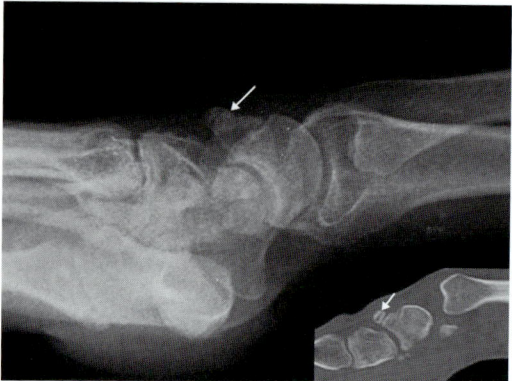

Fig. 4.12 *The arrows* indicate an avulsion fracture from the dorsal triquetrum, which could be responsible for VISI malalignment of the wrist

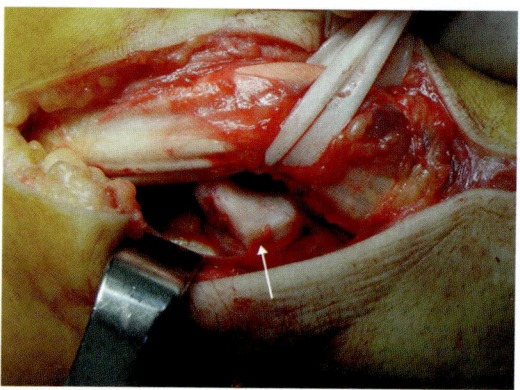

Fig. 4.14 After anesthesia, what seemed to be a stage II, becomes a stage III injury, with the lunate (*arrow*) compressing the median nerve

triquetrum [29], volar horn of the lunate [30], and dorsal triquetrum (Fig. 4.12).

Assuming that the rotation of the lunate is an indicator of the severity of the injury, two observations are important: (a) The distinction between stages II and III is often a matter of radiological interpretation and of the muscle spasm that is eliminated during anesthesia. In several cases in which the lunate was radiologically considered to be rotated less than 90° (Stage II), during the operation it was found to be palmarly dislocated and in direct contact with the median nerve (Stage III) (Figs. 4.13, 4.14), (b) Same type of injuries, based on the stage of the lunate rotation, may have totally different severity, if instead of the lunate, the displacement of the capitate (and therefore the distal carpal row) is taken into account (Figs. 4.15, 4.16).

Consequently, with the PA and L views, lunate and perilunate injuries could be classified into three stages of severity (concerning soft tissue injuries), according to the displacement of the capitate: In *stage I*, the capitate remains in approximately normal position; in *stage II,* it is displaced but still remains within the limits of the distal radius; and in *stage III*, it is displaced outside the limits of the distal radius (Figs. 4.17a, b, 4.18a, b).

Excessive displacements of perilunate injuries persuaded some authors to describe such injuries using informal nomenclature as for example "radial perilunar dislocation" [31].

A retrospective review of the medical records and roentgenograms of all patients treated for radiographically proven lunate and perilunate injuries was carried out during the period from

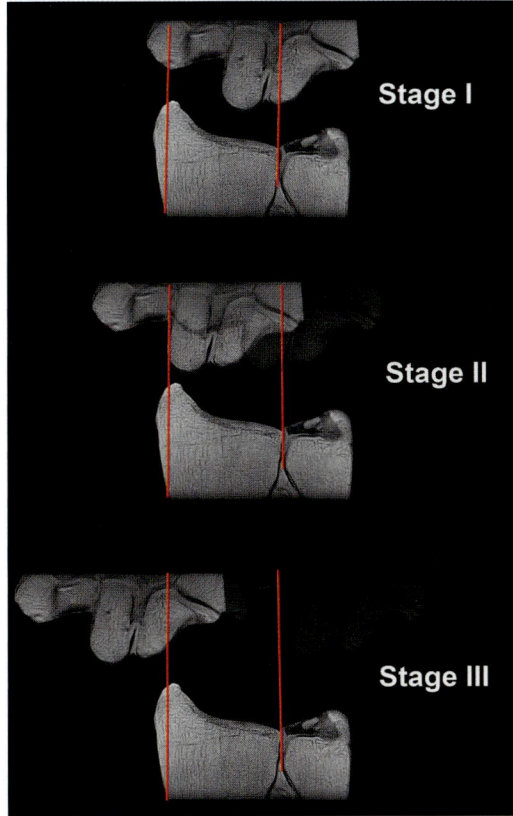

Fig. 4.15 Classification of wrist displacement into three stages (PA view), with the capitale as index, instead of the lunate

1985 to 2010 at the Red Cross Hospital of Athens. A total of 128 injuries in 126 patients were reviewed. There were 36 patients (38 cases) with PLD and 90 patients with PLFD, while 71 patients of the latter group had fractured scaphoids. Thirty patients (31 cases) were excluded, either because they were treated operatively at other institutions or because they

were treated conservatively after closed reduction. Thus, 97 patients (98 cases) with lunate and perilunate injuries were operatively treated. The distribution by type of perilunate dislocations or fracture-dislocations is shown in Table 4.1.

4.4   Disruption Mechanisms of the Wrist

It is clear that the understanding of wrist injuries based on different classifications which are often complex and difficult to remember, is not feasible. If the (seemingly) individual lesions are not a problem, it is not the same for complex injuries with limitless spectrum. The effort to integrate every wrist injury in a classification scheme and to deal accordingly depends essentially on our ability to correctly interpret the radiographic images. Thus, injury patterns have largely been characterized by the osseous injury profile and the consequential injuries of the soft tissues. There is a tendency to try to "fit" the apparent findings into the established category with which they best agree. This approach can underestimate the injury and potentially lead to under-treatment [32].

A different approach that will help us understand and deal more effectively with these complex injuries has to do with the knowledge of the path of injury and of the extent of tissue derangement, until the applied force is exhausted. Graham [32] supported that carpal instability is best considered either as compressive or transverse.

Thus, the wrist could be disrupted after: (a) Compressive or axial force transmission, which is responsible for axial dislocations or fracture-

Fig. 4.16 Classification of wrist displacement into three stages (L view), with the capitale as index, instead of the lunate

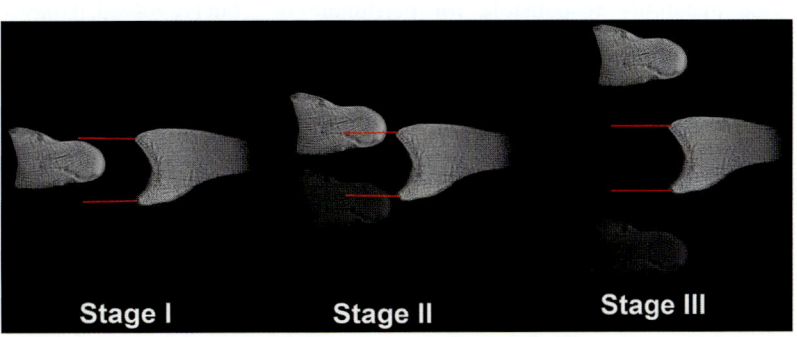

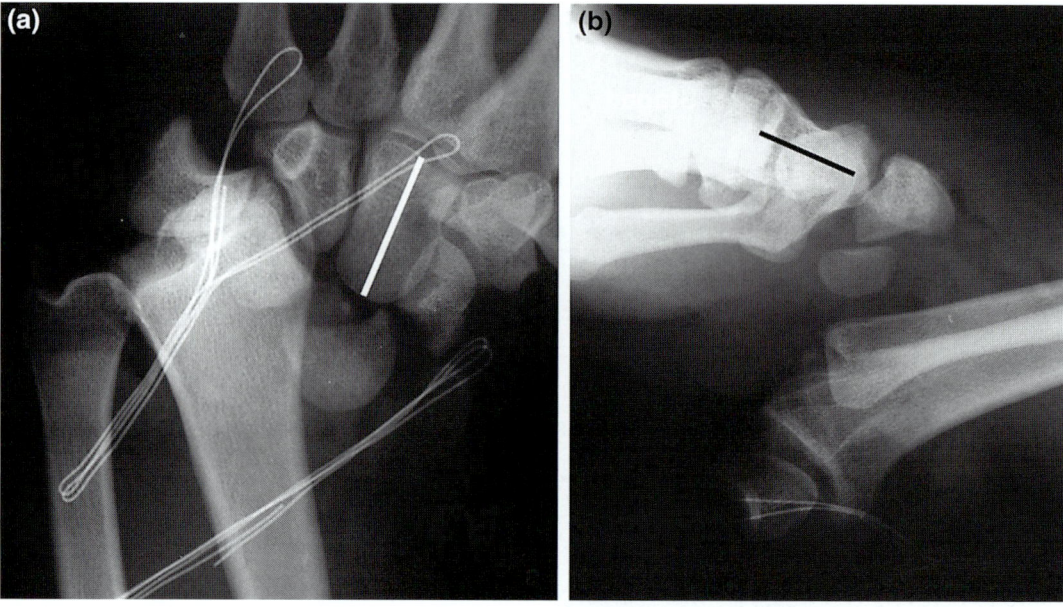

Fig. 4.17 **a, b** Based on the lunate displacement, this excessive wrist dislocation is deceptively characterized as stage I injury. When considering the displacement of capitate, it is characterized as stage III injury, where the capitate is displaced outside the limits of the distal radius

Fig. 4.18 **a, b** A stage I PLFD+S injury (based on lunate displacement), becoming a more serious stage II injury when considering the displacement of capitate

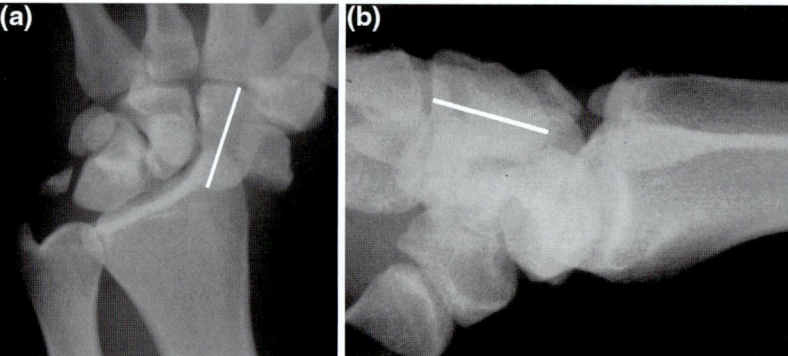

dislocations, but more commonly, after (b) Transverse force transmission that causes transverse instability responsible for perilunate or radiocarpal injuries.

4.4.1 Disruption Started from the Radial Side of the Wrist

The fractured scaphoid and the scapholunate dissociation are certainly injuries located in the radial side of the wrist. If the force that caused these injuries is not exhausted in these anatomical areas but is evolved, it may lead to more complex injuries such as perilunate or lunate injuries. The above injuries are the result of transverse force transmission and it is assumed that the disruptive force started from the radial side and propagated to the ulnar side of the wrist. It is known that the scaphoid acts as a stabilizing link between the proximal and distal carpal rows. In case of scaphoid nonunion, the wrist is particularly susceptible to injury [33, 34] (Fig. 4.19).

Table 4.1 Distribution by the type of injuries treated at the Red Cross Hospital in Athens

PLD		PLFD			
		PLFD+S		PLFD–S	
Type	N° of cases	Type	N° of cases	Type	N° of cases
Dorsal perilunate	15	Trans-S dorsal perilunate	34	Trans-Sty dorsal perilunate	12
Stage I (7)		Incomplete (1)		Stage I (3)	
Stage II (8)		Stage I (18)		Stage II (5)	
Palmar Lunate dislocation	16	Stage II (11)		Stage III (4)	
Stage III (16)		Stage III (3)		Trans-Sty-lunate dorsal perilunate	1
		Stage IV (1)		Stage III (1)	
		Trans-S-Triq., dorsal perilunate	4	Trans-Sty-Triq dorsal perilunate	1
		Stage I (1)		Stage II (1)	
		Stage II (1)		Peri-S, trans-C (reduced)	1
		Reduced (2)			
		Trans-Sty-S.. dorsal perilunate	4		
		Stage I (1)			
		Stage II (3)			
		Trans-Sty-S-Triq., dorsal perilunate	1		
		Stage I (1)			
		Scaphocapitate syndrome	8		
		Dorsal perilunate (7)			
		Palmar perilunate (1)			
		Unclassified	1		

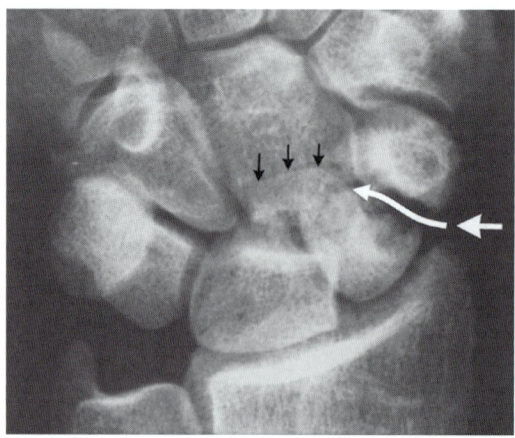

Fig. 4.19 Fracture of the head of the capitate with 180° rotation (*arrows*), following a preexisting scaphoid nonunion. With permission from [231]

The concept of a sequential pattern of intercarpal wrist instability was supported by the work of Mayfield [35] and Mayfield et al. [36] and resulted in the understanding of perilunate instability as a spectrum of injury termed "progressive perilunar instability", propagating from the radial to the ulnar side of the wrist, with the lunate dislocation representing the final stage of the injury.

Based on this fundamental work, four stages of perilunate instability have been described (Fig. 4. 20a–d) [5, 7, 10, 21, 35, 37, 38]:

Stage I. The failure is transmitted either through the body of the scaphoid or through the scapholunate ligament which ruptured volarly to dorsally, eventually resulting in a complete scapholunate dissociation. At this stage, rupture of the radioscaphocapitate ligament has been reported [8, 39], although others dispute it [40].

Stage II. The force continues on to the space of Poirier which is lying between the RSC and LRL ligaments and disrupts the lunocapitate joint. The dislocation of the capitate is followed by the rest of the distal carpal row and the entire (or the distal part in cases of fracture) scaphoid. If the violence is exhausted at

Fig. 4.20 a, b, c, and **d** The four stages of progressive perilunate instability (see text for description). With permission from [231]

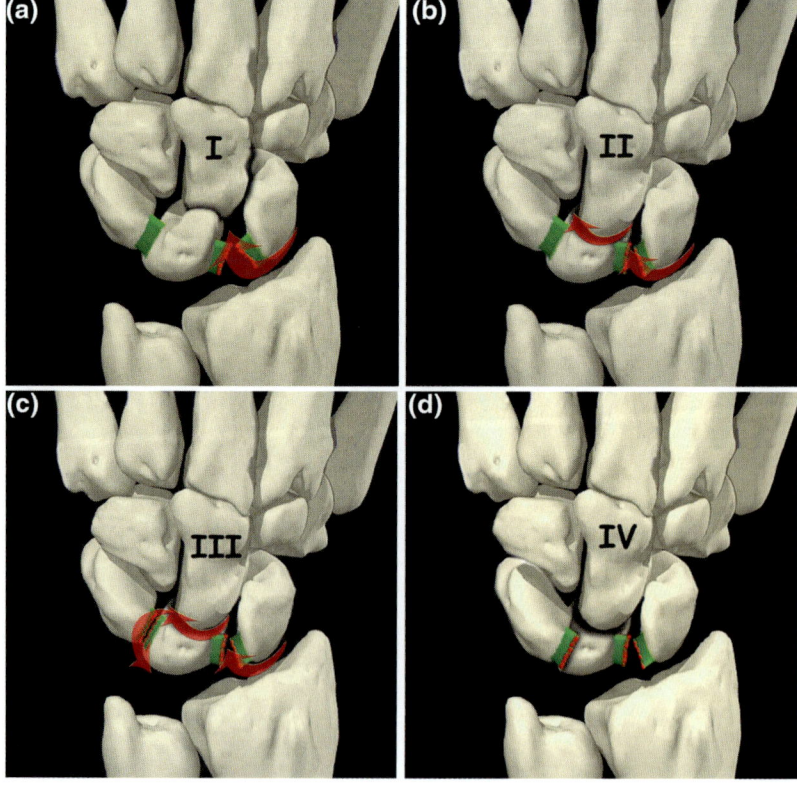

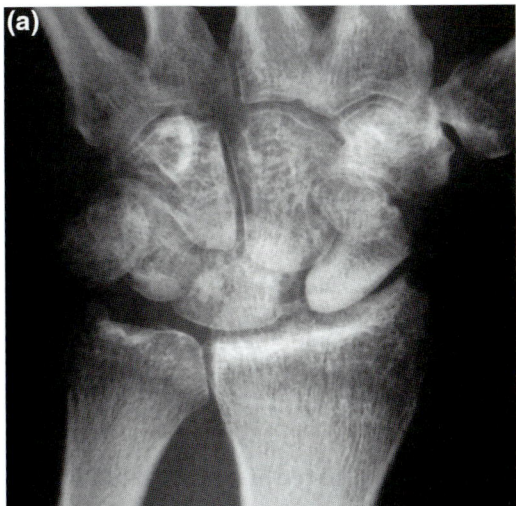

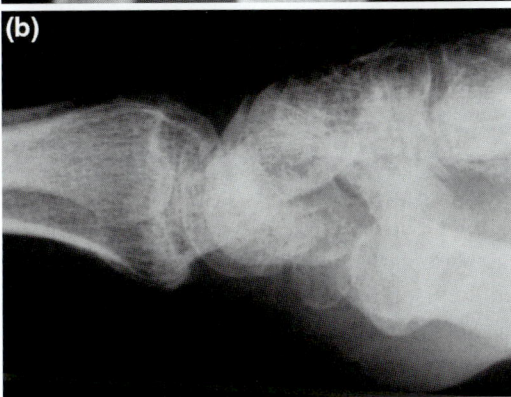

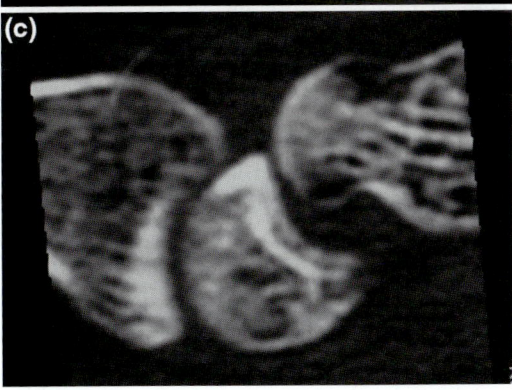

Fig. 4.21 **a**, **b**, and **c** A patient with incomplete perilunar instability with fractured scaphoid (stage I), dislocation of the capitate (stage II) and normal LT joint, who was undiagnosed and had been treated conservatively for 4 months

this stage, only the lunate and the triquetrum maintain their relations (Fig. 4.21a–c).

Stage III. The continuation of the force ulnarly usually disrupts the lunotriquetral ligament from palmar to dorsal (lunotriquetral dissociation) including the medial expansion of the long RL ligament, or rarely the TH and TC ligaments (triquetrohamate dislocation) [41] or both (Fig. 4.22a, b). At that stage, rupture of the ulnotriquetral ligament has been mentioned [39]. Alternatively, a triquetral avulsion fracture may result. The depletion of the force at this stage results in dorsal perilunate dislocation.

Stage IV. The dorsally displaced capitate is pulled proximally and volarly by muscle contraction, by an external force or by the intact RSC ligament and exerting pressure on the dorsum of the lunate forcing it to dislocate. At that stage, it is argued that the DRC ligament is torn [21, 37–39, 42, 43] allowing the lunate to dislocate into the carpal tunnel, using the intact palmar ligaments (SRL, UL) as a hinge. Lunate dislocation, therefore, is the end stage of a dorsal perilunate dislocation representing the most severe form and highest degree of instability.

According to Mayfield et al. [36], the trans-scaphoid fracture-dislocation constitutes Stage I injury, the trans-scaphoid, trans-capitate Stage II, and the trans-scaphoid, trans-capitate, and trans-triquetral Stage III injury, while the trans-styloid fracture-dislocation is considered as variant of the trans-scaphoid as both these fractures only rarely coexist.

It is generally accepted, that dorsal perilunate dislocations precede palmar lunate dislocations, and both are manifestations of the same injury and are produced by the same mechanism of injury.

Johnson [26] supported that most of the carpal fractures and dislocations, are confined to a "*vulnerable zone*", which is largely contained within a more proximal lesser arc and a more distal greater arc. A path of injury progressing around the lunate is purely ligamentous, leading to a perilunate or lunate dislocation and is called "*lesser arc injury*", while a path across the osseous structures around the lunate constitutes a "*Greater arc injury*" (Fig. 4.23). This separation

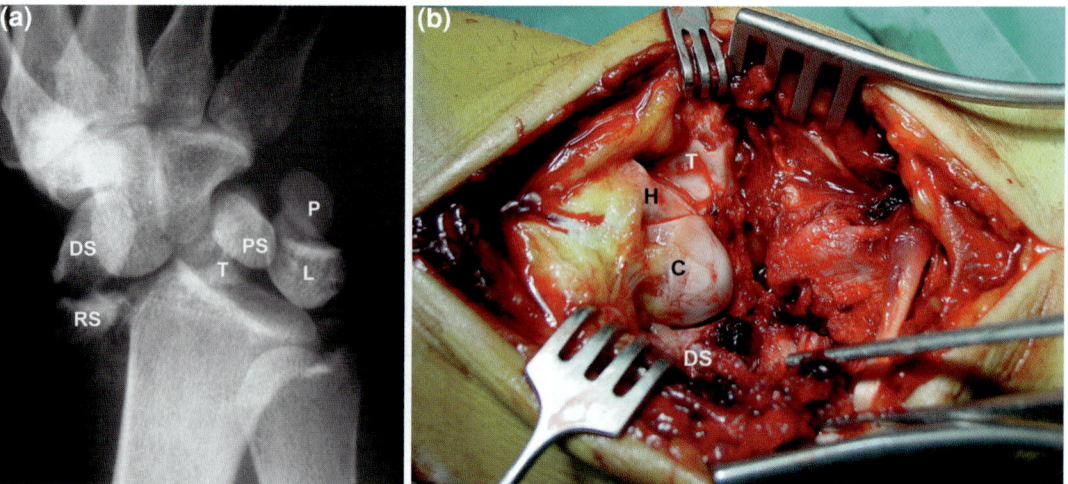

Fig. 4.22 A case of trans-styloid, trans-scaphoid, dorsal perilunate dislocation with disruption of both the LT and TH joints. Oblique view (**a**) and operative picture (**b**).

(*RS* Radial styloid, *DS* Distal scaphoid, *T* Triquetrum, *PS* Proximal scaphoid, *L* Lunate, *P* Pisiform, *C* Capitate, and *H* Hamate)

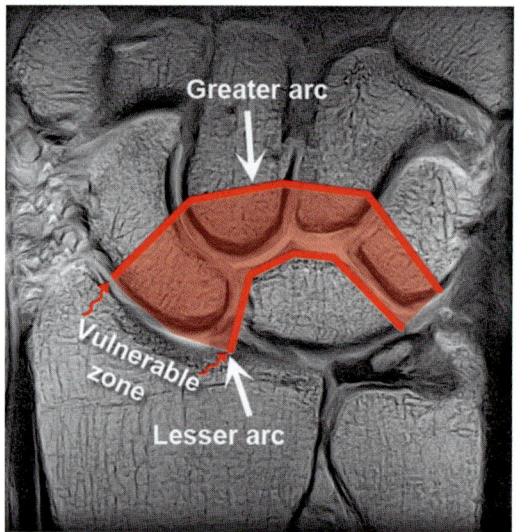

Fig. 4.23 The "vulnerable zone" [26], confined between the *greater* and *lesser arc*

into lesser and greater arc injuries, could be a rough classification of these injuries [44].

Usually, clinically seen lesser arc injuries are indeed purely ligamentous injuries and only in rare cases can be associated with fracture of the triquetrum [45] (Fig. 4.24). On the contrary, there is no consensus on the definition of greater arc injuries, because it is extremely rare to find a

case with all the bones fractured around the lunate. Some authors [46] consider a greater arc injury to be any fracture-dislocation involving the perilunar carpal bones; others [47] would require the presence of at least both the scaphoid and the capitate as the discerning feature of a greater arc lesion. Most common are osseoligamentous injuries, with one or two bones fractured around the lunate [48, 49], which only constitutes a partial greater arc injury (Fig. 4.25). Rarely, three bones around the lunate are involved [50–52]. The simplest and perhaps most common form of perilunate fracture-dislocation is the trans-scaphoid dorsal perilunate dislocation, which could be an "*intermediate arc injury*" (Fig. 4.26).

A pattern of injury in which the intercarpal region is spared and the lesion extends from radial to ulnar and through the radiocarpal joint, has been recently designated as an "*inferior arc injury*" [32, 53]. This path of injury is responsible for radiocarpal dislocations or fracture-dislocations (Fig. 4.27).

Graham [32] rationalized the reason why a transverse force propagating from the radial to the ulnar side of the wrist follows a prescribed path. He speculated that the force entering the

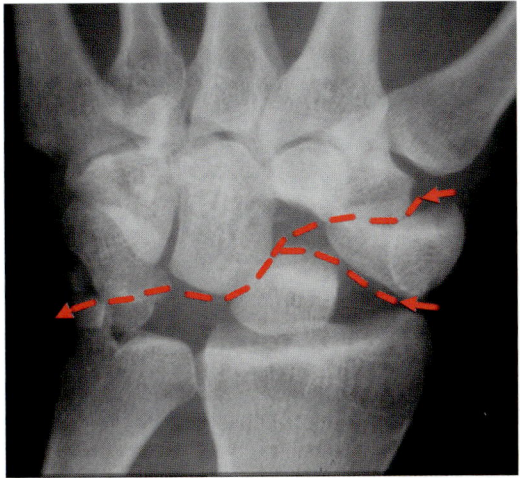

Fig. 4.24 A lesser arc injury, associated with scaphoid dislocation and fracture of the triquetrum. With permission from [231]

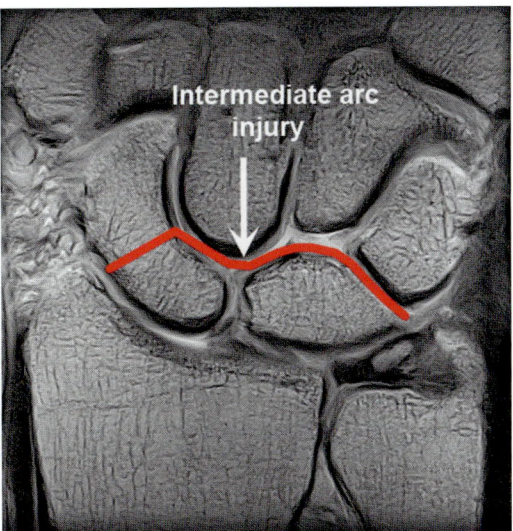

Fig. 4.26 The most common form of a perilunate fracture-dislocation is the trans-scaphoid perilunate fracture-dislocation. Although it is classified as greater arc injury, it represents *an intermediate arc injury*. With permission from [231]

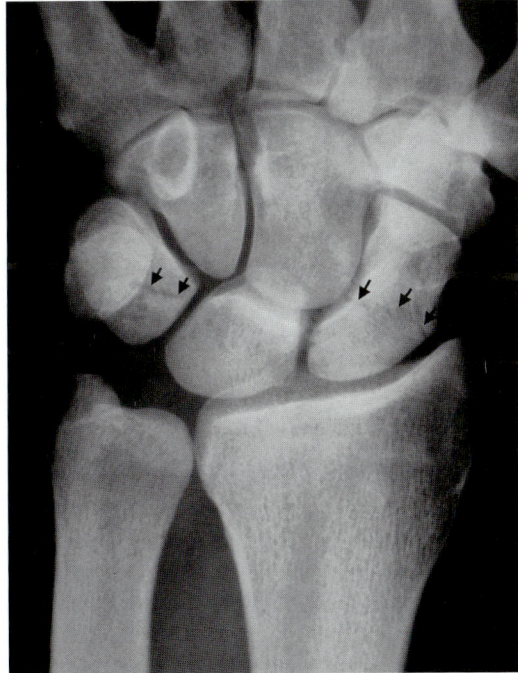

Fig. 4.25 Concomitant incomplete fractures of the scaphoid and triquetrum (*arrows*) probably constitute an incomplete greater arc injury. With permission from [231]

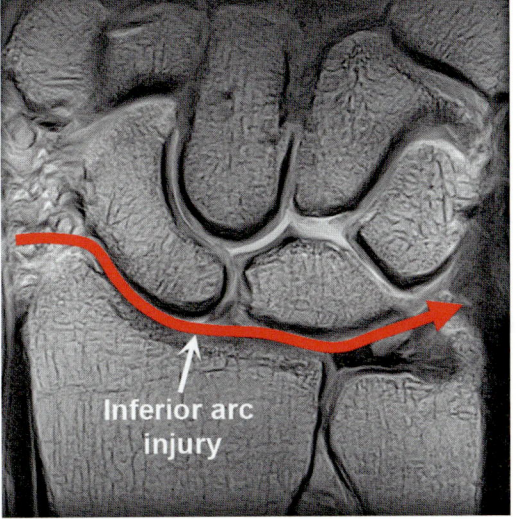

Fig. 4.27 The *inferior arc injury* according to Graham [32] and Graham et al. [53]

radial aspect of the carpus encounters a "stout deflector of forces", which is the LRL and is directed through the SL ligament.

The term *"translunate"* had been used early enough [54–57], to describe the rare, usually high-energy injury in which a lunate fracture was found in association with fractures of the

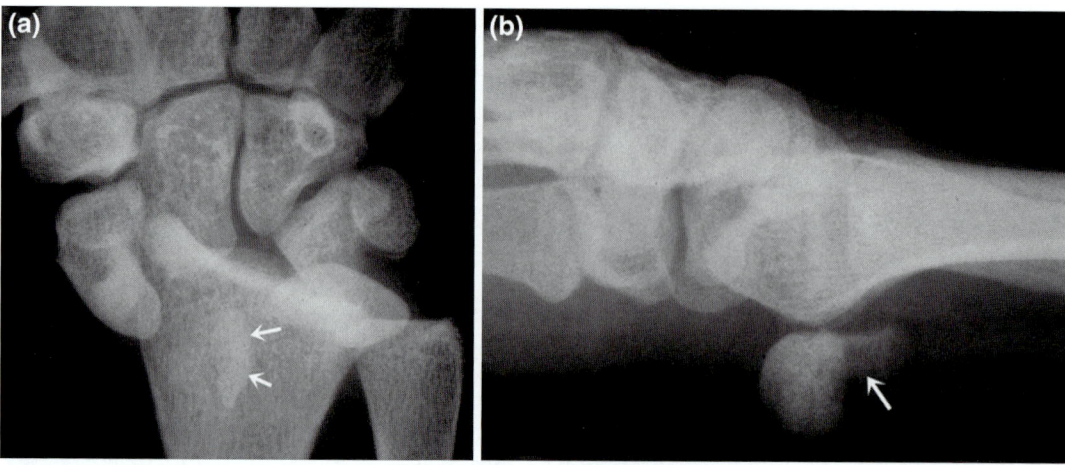

Fig. 4.28   A trans-lunate volar lunate dislocation. *Arrows* indicate the fractured lunate fragment in both PA (**a**) and L view (**b**)

surrounding bones. Recently, Bain et al. [42] proposed the term "*translunate arc injuries*" to include all trans-lunate fractures with perilunate injuries (Fig. 4.28a, b). He supported that the mechanism of injury in these cases did not fit Mayfield's classification system, and emphasized the destabilizing effect of all the ligaments attached to the fractured lunate (Fig. 4.29a–c). It has been reported, that a trans-lunate arc injury, could be dispersed from the radial to the ulnar side of the wrist [58, 59] or reverse from ulnar to radial side of the wrist [60]. It could also be complete but reduced [61], complete and dislocated [42, 56], or incomplete [62, 63].

To confirm the magnitude of these complex injuries, case reports have described uniquely followed paths, that show the unpredictable way that a high-energy trauma can break the wrist [64–74] (Fig. 4.30a–h).

4.4.2   Disruption Started from the Ulnar Side of the Wrist

One of the components of the three-dimensional mechanism of injury, proposed by Mayfield [35], is the intercarpal supination which implies loading on the thenar eminence. It is reasonable to assume that if the load is applied to the hypothenar area, an intercarpal pronation component is produced, which in combination with extension and radial deviation, can cause a gradually progressive instability; the first stage of which is located to the ulnar side of the wrist (probably the LT joint). One such possible mechanism is when falling backward on the outstretched internally rotated hand [5].

Different authors [44, 75, 76] have speculated that a progressive sequence of ligament disruption can occur on the ulnar side of the carpus, similar to what Mayfield [35] and Mayfield et al. [36] had described on the radial side. This would be the beginning of "*reverse perilunate instability*", which was first hypothesized by Reagan et al. [75] and was later confirmed in the laboratory by Viegas et al. [77]. However, instabilities starting from the ulnar side are less known, less understood, and probably less common. In such cases, the LT dissociation would be the first stage, the lunocapitate dislocation would be the second, and the SL dissociation would be the third stage of the reverse perilunar instability.

Viegas et al. [77] and Viegas [78], developed a staging system for ulnar-sided perilunate instability based on a series of cadaver dissections and load studies. The stages are as follows:

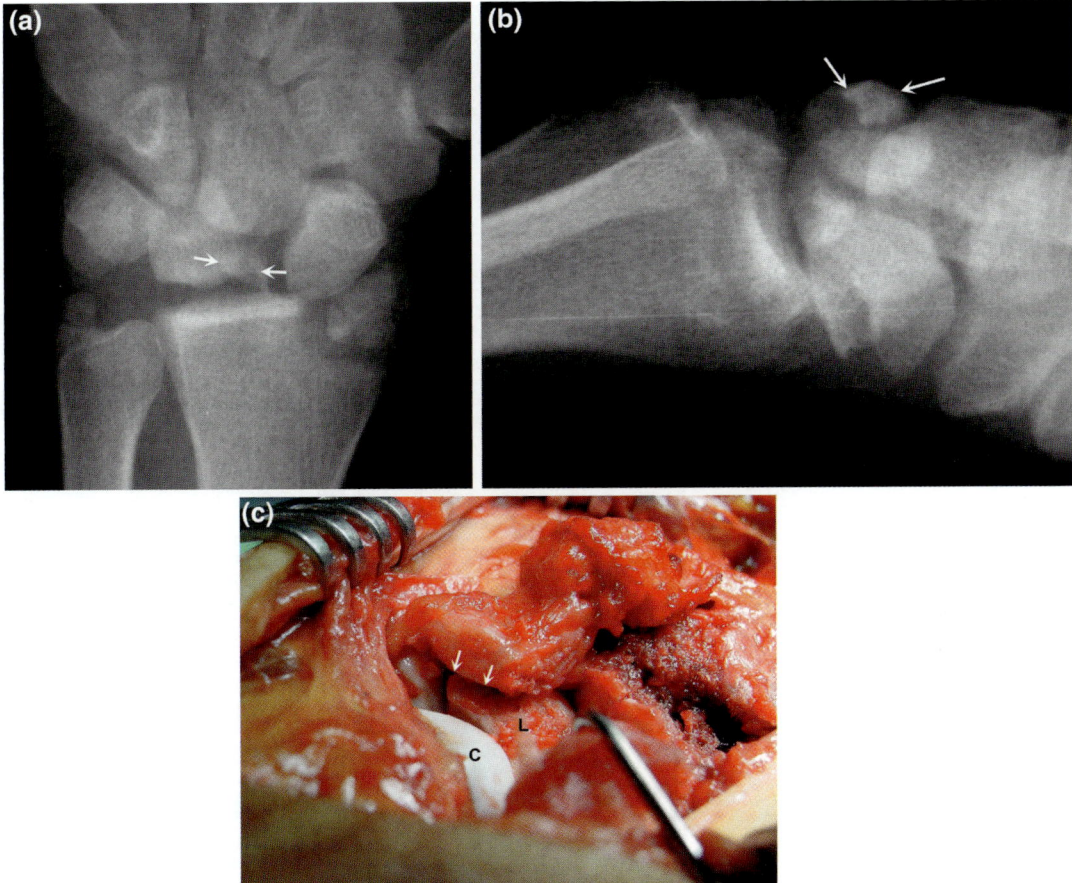

Fig. 4.29   A trans-styloid dorsal perilunate dislocation with an osseous fragment appearing in the PA (**a**) and L view (**b**) (*arrows*). Operatively, it is shown to derive from the dorsal pole of the lunate (*arrows*) (**c**) (*C* Capitate, *L* Lunate)

Stage I. Partial or complete disruption of the dorsal and central portion of the LT interosseous ligament (No clinical and/or radiological evidence of dynamic or static VISI deformity).

Stage II. Complete tear of the LT interosseous ligament including its palmar region (and the extension of LRL ligament to the triquetrum) (Clinical and/or radiographic evidence of dynamic VISI deformity).

Stage III. The above ligamentous disruption plus the attenuation or disruption of the DRC ligament (Clinical and/or radiographic evidence of static VISI deformity) (Fig. 4.31).

Melone and Nathan [79] described the surgical pathology in 42 cases with traumatic TFCC disruption as the initial injury and comprised a spectrum of injury resulting in five basic stages of increasingly severe ulnar wrist instability (Fig. 4.32).

Stage 1. Detachment of the articular disk from its insertion at the base of the ulnar styloid with associated partial peripheral detachment of the dorsal or volar radioulnar ligaments.

Stage 2. Disruption of the adjacent infraretinacular ECU sheath, resulting in subluxation of the unrestrained tendon.

Stage 3. Disruption of the UC ligaments.

Fig. 4.30 Examples of unique path of injuries: Capo et al. [65] (**a**); Mullan and Lloyd [230] (**b**); Healey et al. [69], Sarrafian and Breihan [73], Chalidis and Dimitriou [66] (**c**); Brown and Muddu [64], Komura et al. [70], Lee et al. [71], Yamabe et al. [74] (**d**); Fowler [68], Lundkvist et al. [72] (**e**); Christodoulou et al. [61] (**f**); Sabat et al. [50] (**g**); Amaravati et al. [58] (1 h), Noble and Lamb [54] (2 h)

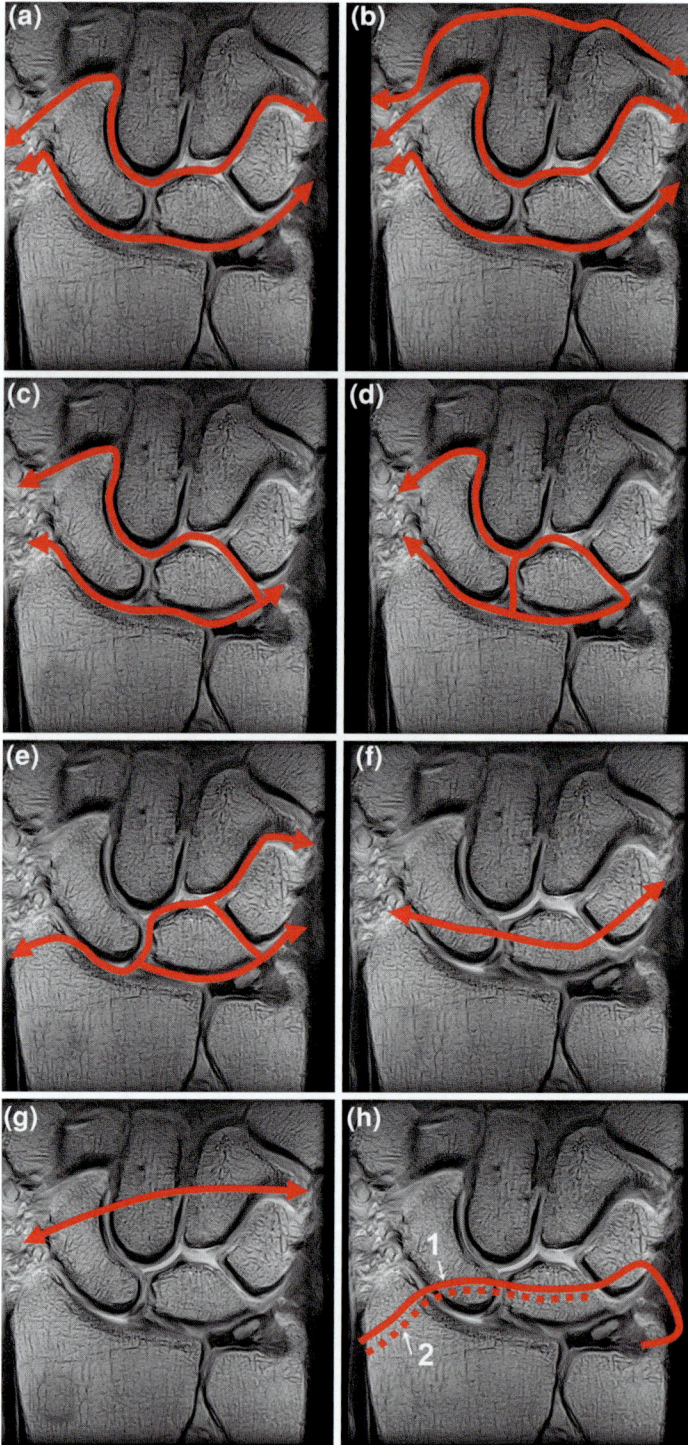

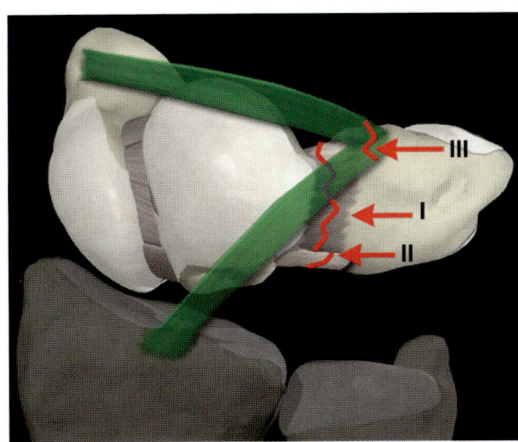

Fig. 4.31 A three-stage perilunar instability according to Viegas et al. [77] and, Viegas [78] (see text for details). With permission from [231]

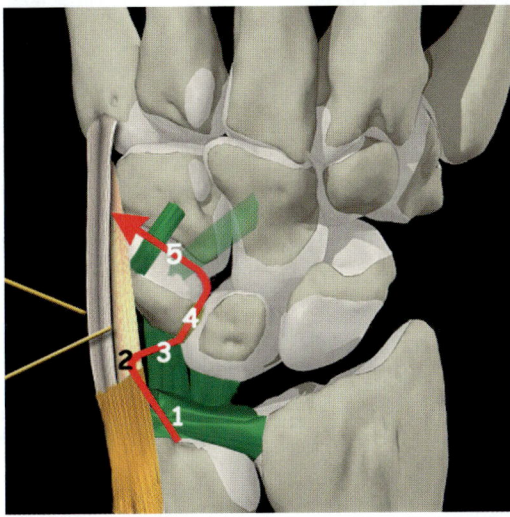

Fig. 4.32 The five stages of progressive ulnar wrist instability according to Melone and Nathan [79] (see text for details). With permission from [231]

Stage 4. Partial or complete rupture of the LT interosseous ligament.

Stage 5. Disruption of the triquetral-capitate and triquetral-hamate ligaments, which compromise the ulnar midcarpal joint.

Recently, Murray et al. [80] based on a cadaver loading model and six clinical cases, proposed a three-stage mechanism for ulnar-sided perilunate instability of the wrist: *Stage 1:* Disruption of the LTIL; *Stage 2:* Stage 1 plus disruption of the ulnolunate, ulnotriquetral, and ulnocapitate ligaments as well as disruption of the dorsal scaphotriquetral and radiotriquetral ligaments; and *Stage 3:* Stage 2 with progression of the injury through the midcarpal joint plus disruption of the scapholunate and radioscapholunate ligaments potentially resulting in a dorsal perilunate dislocation.

It has been reported [29, 80] that the volar triquetral avulsion fracture represents a subtle radiographic sign for ulnar-sided ligamentous injury, while rupture of the dorsal ligaments attached to the triquetrum [81, 82] and of the ulnocarpal ligaments which are in tension during extension and radial deviation of the wrist [83] are essential components of the reverse perilunar instability.

Cases of presumed ulnar-sided perilunate injury have been previously reported [41, 45, 60, 84] while the case reported by Nunn [85], where a fracture of the triquetrum was associated with dorsal perilunate dislocation without radial side injury, could represent an incomplete (Stage II) reverse perilunar instability.

It is known that in both PLD and PLFD a volarly constant finding is a transverse capsular derangement at the space of Poirier, in different degrees. This capsular rent typically curves proximally across the palmar LT ligament, where it is usually completed. From 96 patients (97 cases) with lunate and perilunate injuries that were operatively treated by the author, with combined (72 cases) or volar (4 cases) approach, we found that in 10 cases the capsular rent continues ulnarly proximal to the triquetrum causing rupture of the ulnocarpal ligaments. All the above cases belonged to the PLFD group, (8 cases of the PLFD+S and 2 cases of the PLFD–S group). From the mechanism of injury and the X-rays, a radial displacement of the wrist was proven, we thus considered them as cases of reverse perilunar instability (Fig. 4.33a–g). The presence of rupture of the ulnocarpal ligaments in perilunate injuries, has been mentioned before

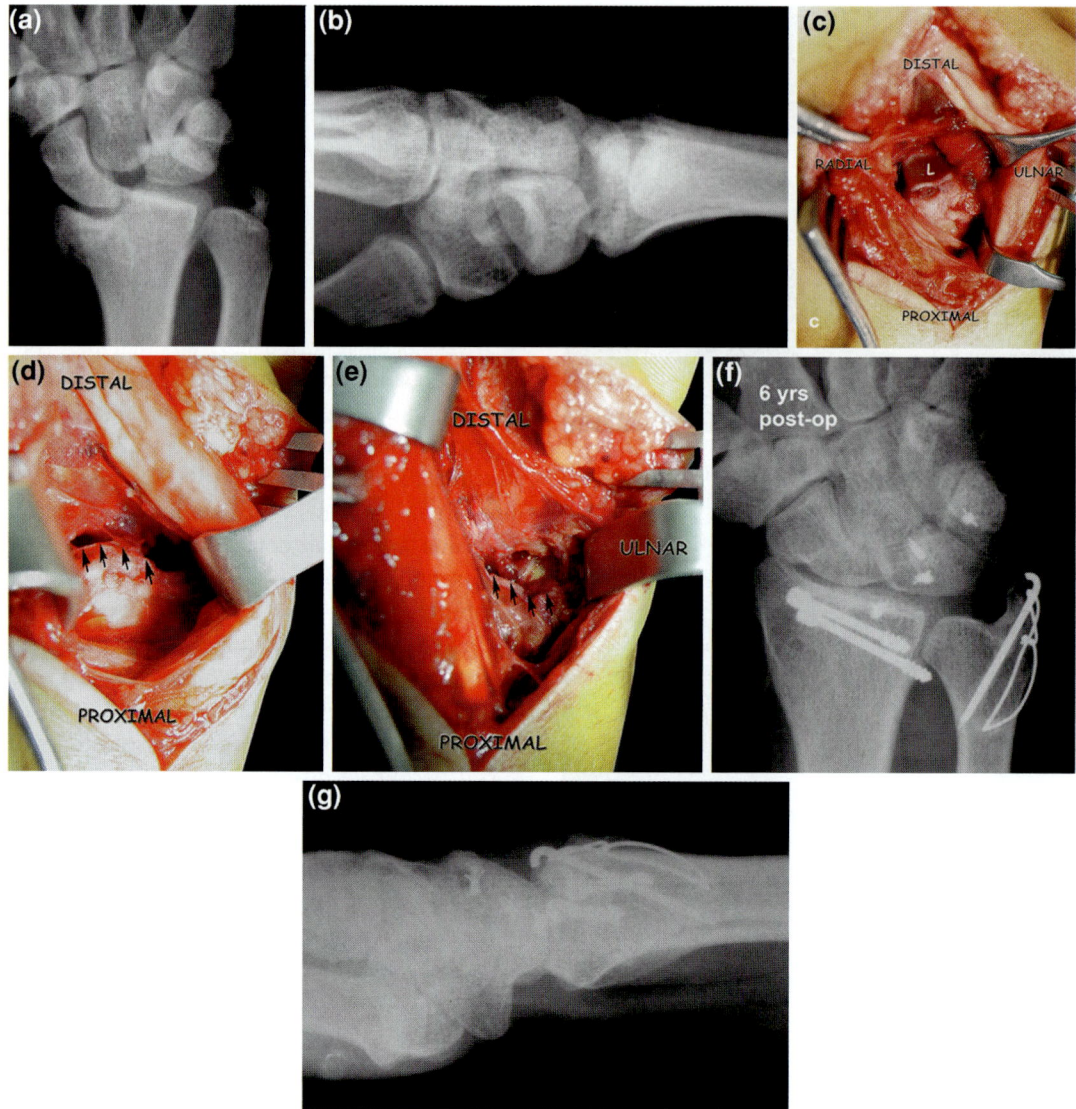

Fig. 4.33 A case of trans-styloid dorsal perilunate dislocation with the wrist radially displaced (**a**, **b**); The volar approach reveals the dislocated lunate (**c**); After reduction, *arrows* indicate the ruptured capsuloligamentous structures at the space of Poirier and LT joint (**d**); The rupture continues ulnarly to disrupt the ulnocarpal ligaments (*arrows*) (**e**); and The final X-rays 6 years postoperatively (**f**, **g**). With permission from [231]

[6, 84, 86]. However, the importance of recognizing the rupture of the ulnocarpal ligaments and the necessity for restoration of this rupture will be discussed later in this chapter.

The presence of skin abrasions, contusions, or ecchymosis at the hypothenar area and a radially deformed wrist, may indicate such a reversed perilunar instability type of injury (Fig. 4.34a, b).

4.5   Mechanism of Injuries

The exact mechanism of injury is not entirely clear, because the position of the hand and wrist at the moment of injury is seldom recalled by the patient. Seemingly similar mechanisms (hyperextension) generate different types of injuries

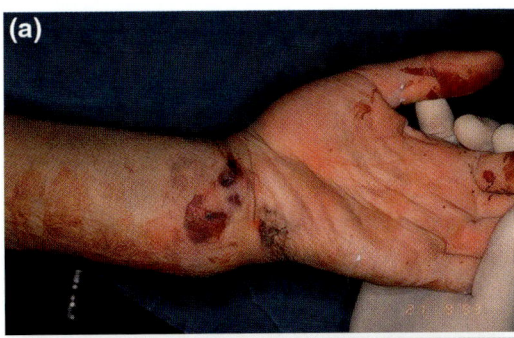

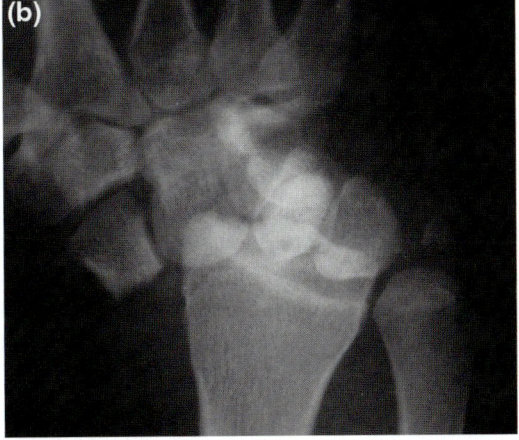

Fig. 4.34 Skin abrasions at the hypothenar area (**a**) and radial displacement of the wrist in the PA view (**b**), are indicative findings of a reversed perilunar instability type of injury. With permission from [231]

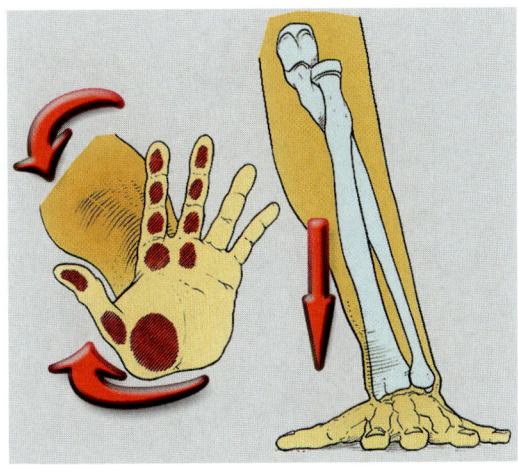

Fig. 4.35 Application of force at the thenar area produces a three-dimensional mechanism of injury: hyperextension, midcarpal supination, and ulnar deviation. With permission from [231]

(distal radius or scaphoid fractures, perilunate injuries) because the injury that will occur depends on a number of factors: (a) magnitude, direction, and site of torque application, (b) wrist position at the time of impact, (c) bone quality, (d) condition of the different ligaments, and (e) muscle protection reactivity [5, 58]. Some authors believe that the rate of loading determines the pattern of injury, with slower loading resulting in carpal fractures, and faster loading resulting in ligamentous injury [87]. The possibility of an indirect mechanism has also been mentioned where tensile forces are transmitted by ligaments, whereas compressive forces are transferred across the joint surfaces [5].

The amount of force required for these injuries to occur, most frequently results from motor vehicle accidents, sports injuries, and falls from substantial heights. However, no single mechanism, no matter how complex it is, is able to explain the entire spectrum of these injuries.

Based on fresh cadaver specimens, Mayfield [35] and Mayfield et al. [36] demonstrated these injuries to result from a three-dimensional mechanical concept consisting of a combination of extension, ulnar deviation, and intercarpal supination. The intercarpal supination is the rotational component of this injury, produced by loading the thenar of wrist cadavers with the forearm stabilized in pronation (equivalent to pronation of the forearm on the carpus as observed in actual clinical injuries). In that case, the axis of intercarpal supination passed through the triquetrum. The rotational component has been emphasized by Tanz since 1968 [88]. Nowadays, it is believed that axial and torsional forces are applied with the wrist in any combination of hyperextension, hyperflexion, and radial or ulnar deviation [5, 6, 26] (Fig. 4.35).

The described mechanism of injury has been implicated to explain the most common injuries, which are propagating from the radial to the ulnar side of the wrist. As mentioned before, the combination of dorsiflexion, radial deviation, and intercarpal pronation has been held responsible for injuries with reverse perilunar disruption (Fig. 4.36) (see Sect. 4.4).

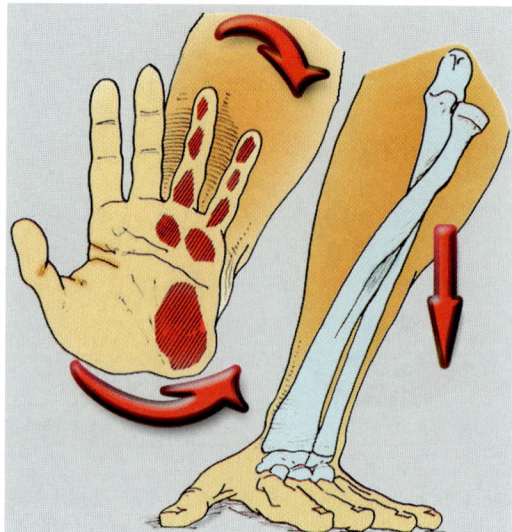

Fig. 4.36 Loading at the hypothenar area with the wrist in hyperextension could also produce midcarpal pronation and ulnar deviation, a mechanism which has been implicated to the development of reverse perilunar disruption. With permission from [231]

Special mechanisms have been described to explain perilunate injuries associated with fracture of the neck of the capitate (see Chap. 5) or fracture of the proximal pole of the scaphoid [89].

However, regardless of the mechanism of injury, which has academic interest, it is particularly important to determine the path that the disruption has followed in order to recognize, name, and treat the injury appropriately.

4.6 Diagnosis

4.6.1 Clinical Evaluation

A thorough investigation of the patient's history with special emphasis on the mechanism of injury is advisable. Due to the wide spectrum of injuries, we regularly face two extreme situations: at one end of the spectrum is a polytrauma patient, who is likely to have an obviously deformed wrist and at the other end is the patient with a painful wrist, who may not even recall a specific traumatic event [90]. Frequently, there is a striking paradox between the significance of the traumatic injury to the wrist and the paucity of clinical signs to suggest a serious injury [3, 91]. The patients complain of wrist pain and limited range of motion. Examination shows swelling and tenderness around the wrist and any attempt at a passive or active range of motion is painful. Crepitation may be appreciated in greater arc injuries during palpation. Inspection usually reveals a less obvious deformity of the wrist that is located slightly more distal than expected for a distal radial fracture (Fig. 4.37a, b). When present, skin abrasions, contusions, or ecchymosed areas may be helpful in determining the mechanism of injury.

The impressively high percentage of patients with missed diagnosis (even when they have been submitted to radiological control) has been

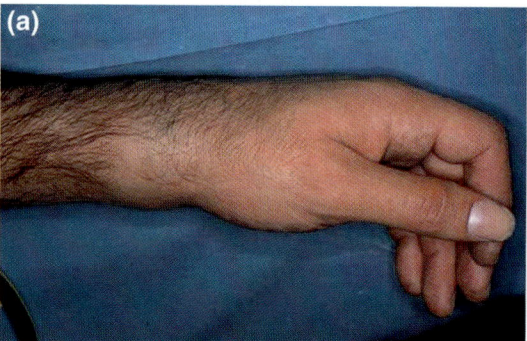
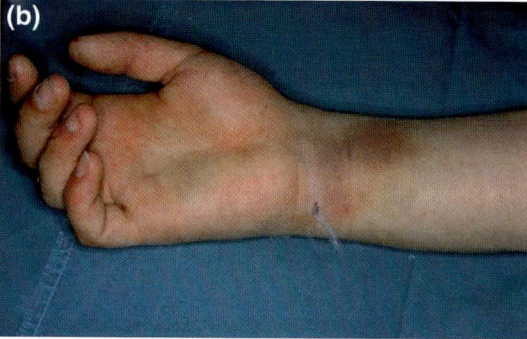

Fig. 4.37 **a**, **b** Frequently and despite the severity of the injury, the deformity of the wrist in perilunate injuries, is less obvious than in distal radius fractures. With permission from [231]

Table 4.2 Number of patients (percentage) with delay in operative treatment for each type of injury

	Operated on the same day	Operated between 2–7 days	Operated between 8–45 days	Operated after 45 days
PLFD+S	30 (57.6 %)	13 (25 %)	6 (11.5 %)	3 (5.7 %)
PLFD−S	3 (20 %)	5 (33.3 %)	5 (33.3 %)	2 (13.3 %)
PLD	9 (30 %)	5 (16.6 %)	12 (40 %)	4 (13.3 %)

Table 4.3 Number of patients (percentage) with delayed or missed diagnosis for each type of injury

	Diagnosed the same day	Diagnosed between 2–7 days	Diagnosed between 8–45 days	Diagnosed after 45 days
PLFD+S	41 (78.8 %)	5 (9.6 %)	4 (7.6 %)	2 (3.8 %)
PLFD−S	8 (53.3 %)	1 (6.6 %)	5 (33.3 %)	1 (6.6 %)
PLD	15 (50 %)	3 (10 %)	8 (26.6 %)	4 (13.3 %)

pointed out by many authors [5, 13, 92, 93]. The frequency with which this occurs in reported case series, varies from 25 to 43 % [5, 13, 94–96].

Misdiagnosis can be attributed to the severity of associated injuries, inadequate radiographs, inexperienced doctors, or underestimation because of spontaneous reduction. According to Herzberg et al. [13], 26 % of his patients were polytraumas. However, the lack of acquaintance with the radiologic images of an injured wrist is considered as probably the most important factor for the delayed or missed diagnosis. There were patients who were operated with fracture in their forearm, while the ipsilateral perilunate injury was missed or patients who were treated with injury of a finger, while at the same X-ray an obvious lunate dislocation was missed [97].

Herzberg et al. [13] supported that PLD and PLFD injuries are overlooked with the same frequency, while Garcia-Elias [5] stated that PLD injuries are more prone to be overlooked than PLFD, owing to the lack of an obvious pathology, such as a scaphoid fracture, which can rarely be left undiagnosed. The radiological diagnosis is difficult to escape if we follow Hill's [98] encouragement: "look for the lunate".

A vascular injury is not usual, while the vast majority are closed injuries. Open injuries represent less than 10 % [6, 13]. Median nerve compression is common and acute carpal tunnel syndrome is present in approximately 25 % of patients (range 16–46 %) [13, 16, 38, 42, 93, 99] therefore, a thorough neurologic examination of the median and ulnar nerves is important. During the palmar approach it is common to find the median nerve being compressed by the dislocated lunate or by the proximal carpal row, when the distal row is dorsally displaced. In most cases, recovery of the nerve function is expected after the reduction of the dislocation [93, 100].

In volar lunate dislocation fingers are flexed, while their active or passive extension causes severe pain [44].

Author's Personal Series (View)

By reviewing the medical records of our patients who were treated operatively (97 patients-98 cases), we found that the delay of the operative treatment does not coincide with the delay or missed diagnosis (Tables 4.2, 4.3). We found that timely diagnosis (same day as the accident) was done in 78.8, 53.3, and 50 % of PLFD+S, PLFD−S, and PLD cases, respectively. On the contrary, 21, 46.5, and 49.9 % of PLFD+S, PLFD−S, and PLD cases, respectively, were diagnosed with some delay. We concluded that lesser arc injuries (PLD) were more frequently missed in diagnosis because 39.9 % of the cases were diagnosed after the first week of the accident. It is also obvious, that if in an injured wrist there is no scaphoid or radial styloid fracture, any wrist derangement is very likely to escape.

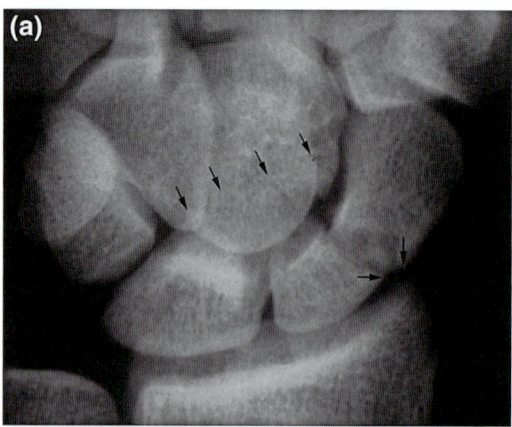

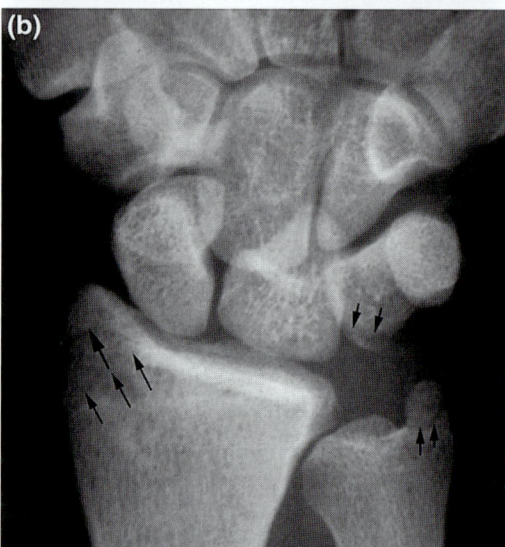

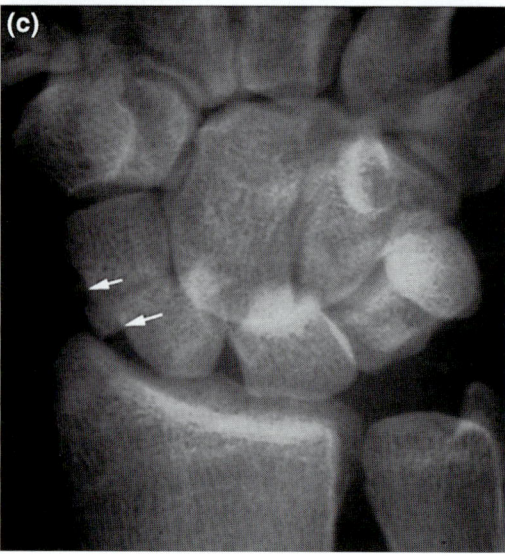

Fig. 4.38 Fractures indicative of perilunate injuries are: the fracture of the neck of the capitate (**a**), the fractures of the styloids (radial and ulnar) or the proximal triquetrum (**b**), and the displaced fracture of the scaphoid (**c**). With permission from [231]

4.6.2   Imaging Studies

Despite the fact that the radiographic evaluation is the cornerstone of diagnosis, it should be noted that approximately 20 % of perilunate injuries are misinterpreted on the initial radiographic evaluation [24]. Initial radiographs must include a neutral PA and a true L view.

The *PA radiological view* must be examined for disclosure of one or more of the following findings:

1. The existence of fractures indicative of disturbance of wrist architecture: fractures of radial and ulnar styloid, displaced or angulated fracture of the scaphoid, fracture of the lunate, or fractures of the bones of the distal carpal row. The detection of these fractures requires, prior to being recognized as individual, to first exclude the possibility of a perilunate injury (Fig. 4.38a–c).
2. The overriding of proximal and distal carpal row giving rise to the "crowded carpal sign" [101] (Fig. 4.39a, b).
3. Loss of carpal height and disruption of Gilula's arcs. Gilula [102] and Gilula et al. [103] defined three smooth carpal arcs that indicate intact carpal connections. The proximal (Arc I) and distal (Arc II) outlines of the proximal carpal row and the proximal outline (Arc III) of the distal carpal row, must be smooth and uninterrupted. If a discontinuity is detected, a grossly altered intercarpal relationship is indicated (Fig. 4.40a, b).
4. The relation and symmetry of the opposing articular surfaces. Loss of parallel alignment and overlapping or increased distance between adjacent bones must be assessed. We used in comparison the opposing articular surfaces of

Fig. 4.39 a, b Overlapping of the distal and proximal carpal rows in the PA view (*arrows*) is indicative of perilunate injury. With permission from [231]

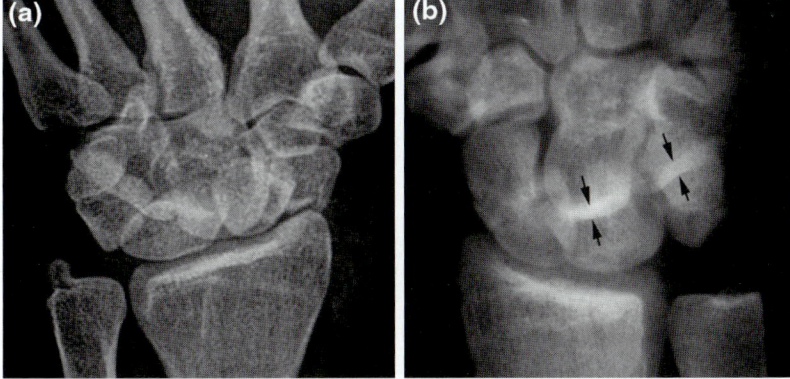

Fig. 4.40 Gilula's arcs in a normal wrist must be smooth and uninterrupted (a). *Arcs I* and *II* are disrupted in perilunate injuries (b). With permission from [231]

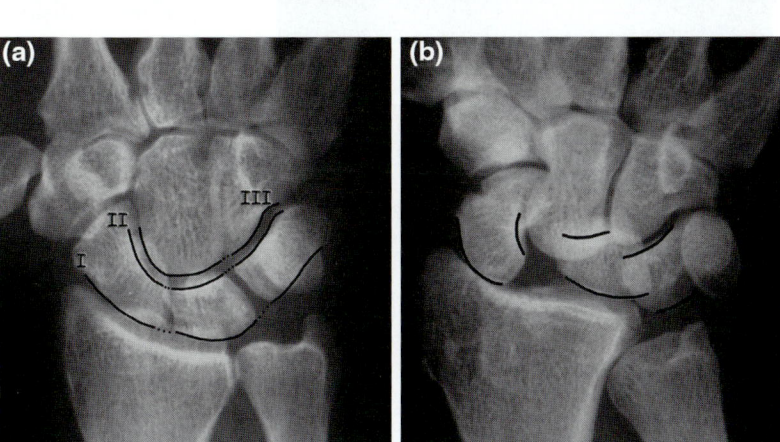

the distal carpal row that were usually normal (i.e., the capitohamate joint) (Fig. 4.41).

5. The shape of the carpal bones (especially of the scaphoid and lunate). A correctly aligned lunate appears trapezoidal on the PA view. If the lunate rotates dorsally or palmarly, its configuration changes to appear triangular or wedge-shaped [102]. The shape of the lunate is changed repeatedly during radial or ulnar deviation of the wrist, so it can easily lead to misunderstandings. In perilunate injuries, the lunate gets an abnormal or wedged shape as a result of its palmar rotation. The scaphoid shape and configuration should be inspected for evidence of abnormal posture. When the scaphoid is palmarly flexed, it appears foreshortened and is projected in cross section on the PA projection. This "ring sign" may indicate perilunate instability or can be a normal finding in a radially deviated wrist [104] (Fig. 4.42a–c).

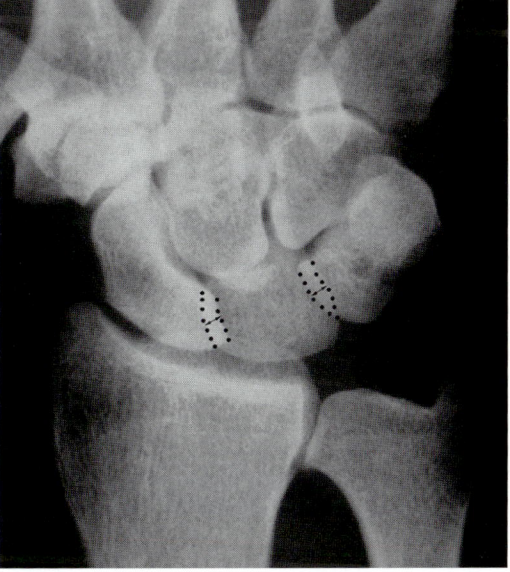

Fig. 4.41 Overlapping of the lunate with the adjacent scaphoid and triquetrum is indicative of perilunar instability. With permission from [231]

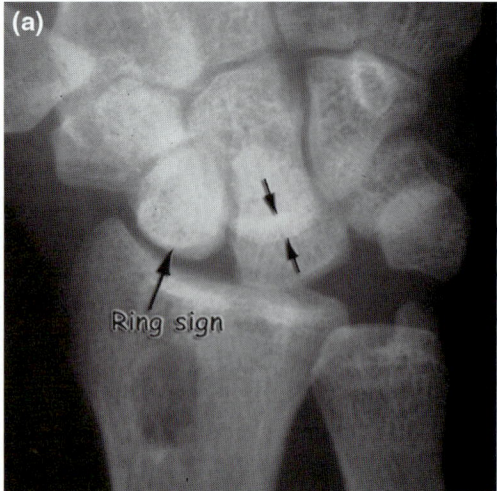

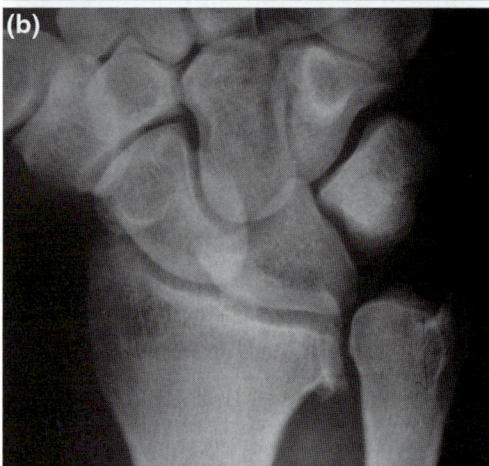

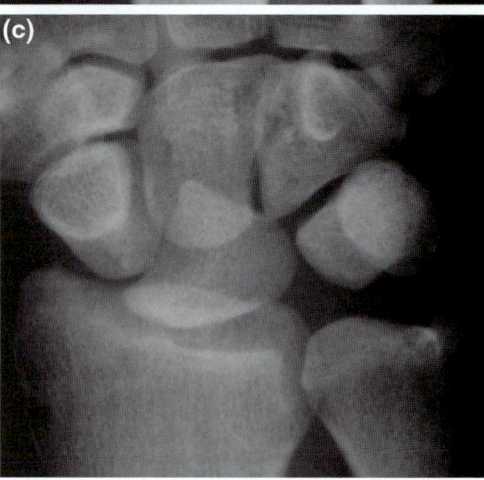

Fig. 4.42 Palmar flexed scaphoid produced the so-called "*ring sign*", while the lunate has a triangular shape overlapping the capitate (**a**). Abnormal shapes of the lunate (**b**, **c**). With permission from [231]

The *L radiological view*, must be truly lateral, with the wrist in neutral position. Since in this view the carpal bones are overlapped, there is a relative difficulty in interpreting, especially when the projection is oblique or when the wrist is radially or ulnarly deviated. In the L view, the following are confirmed:

1. The radius, lunate, and capitate axes must be in almost coaxial alignment and any deviation from this configuration needs further investigation. The normal coaxial alignment of the radius, lunate, and capitate is disrupted in perilunate dislocations. In dorsal perilunar dislocations, the distal concavity of the lunate no longer contains the proximal convexity of the capitate, the axis of which is dorsally displaced. In palmar lunate dislocations, the distal concavity of the lunate is facing palmarly (« spilled teacup sign») [105] and the axis of the radius and capitate are almost collinear (Fig. 4.43a–d). In rare palmar perilunate dislocations, the axis of the capitate is palmarly displaced, while the lunate still articulates with the radius. On the contrary, in dorsal lunate dislocations, the radius and capitate remain almost coaxial while the axis of the lunate is dorsally displaced (Fig. 4.44a, b).

2. The displacement of the head of the capitate in cases of greater arc injuries (Fig. 4.45).

3. The measurement of the angles between bone axes is not useful in fresh injuries. They are particularly useful to monitor the adequacy of reduction (closed or open), to observe if the initial reduction is maintained and also to evaluate the long-term outcome. The radiolunate, lunocapitate, and scapholunate are the angles we are mainly interested in.

Although there has been skepticism for the method [26], when uncertainty exists, a PA traction radiograph helps us describe with some accuracy the extent and clarify the path of injury. It also uncovers the full extent of the intraarticular damage that was not obvious in plain X-rays owing to bone overlapping (Fig. 4.46a–c).

Further investigation methods (tomography, cineradiography, bone scan, arthrogram, CT, and MRI) are usually not necessary in the acute

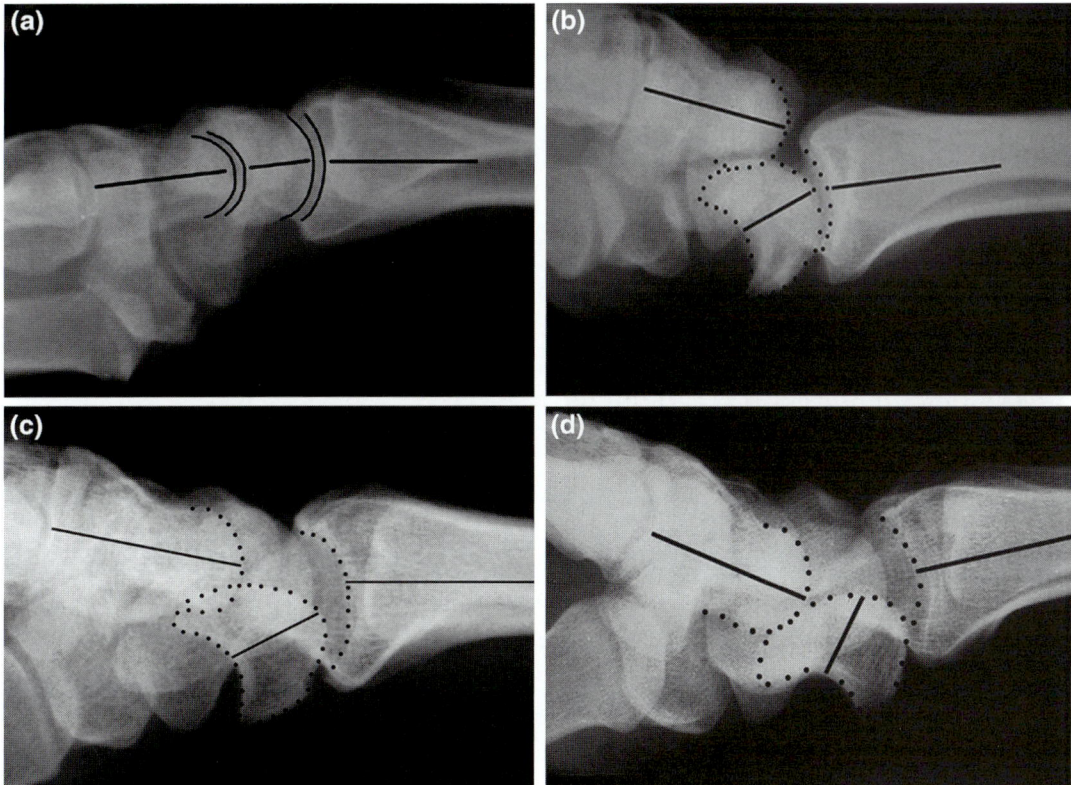

Fig. 4.43 In a normal wrist the radius, lunate, and capitate axes must be in almost coaxial alignment (**a**). Different stages of dorsal perilunar dislocation where the distal concavity of the lunate no longer contains the proximal convexity of the capitate (**b–d**). With permission from [231]

setting. These modalities may be useful in chronic or neglected cases.

4.7   Management

Because of the rarity and great diversity of these injuries, there is limited clinical experience for the assessment of the outcome of a particular therapeutic method. Most clinical studies referred to a small number of patients, with various types of injuries, treated in different modes, and at different periods of time. Only in recent years have appeared in the literature series of patients with specific type of injuries or specific treatment modalities [106–109], which makes it possible to draw conclusions regarding the treatment and prognosis [2, 18, 110].

The plan of treatment necessarily relies on the evaluation of the initial X-rays but no parallelism can be drawn between bone displacement and the magnitude of ligamentous injuries, since there is a possibility of partial or full spontaneous reduction. For this reason, the true extent of ligaments injury can only be assessed intraoperatively, while it is inappropriate to assume the ligament injury by the initial radiographs alone [24].

The time elapsed from injury is an important guiding factor to treatment options [111].

Early diagnosis and appropriate treatment, are prerequisites to prevent the development of instabilities, bone nonunion, and arthritis. Early treatment is definitely more effective than delayed treatment, which often requires salvage operations.

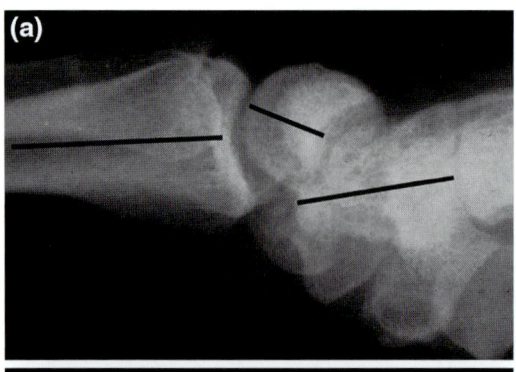

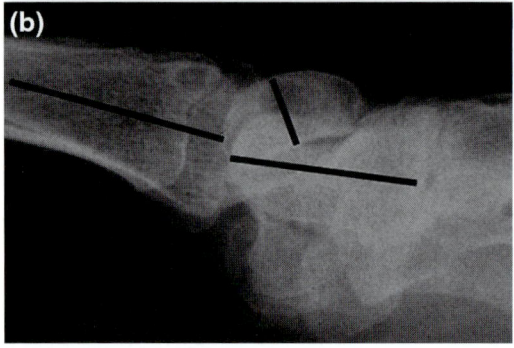

Fig. 4.44 In volar perilunate injuries, the lunate axis is displaced dorsal to the capitate axis (**a**), while in dorsal lunate dislocation the capitate is coaxial with the radius (**b**). With permission from [231]

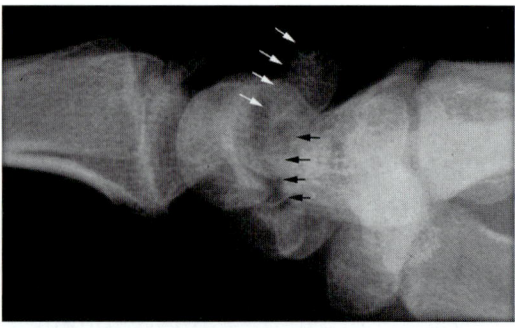

Fig. 4.45 In L view, the integrity of the head of the capitate is inspected. In this case, the head of the capitate was fractured, dorsally displaced, and rotated 180° (*arrows*). With permission from [231]

The lesser and greater arc injuries have a different philosophy to deal with. In lesser arc injuries, where ligamentous injuries predominate, the management principles are mainly directed in repairing and maintaining the ligamentous stability, while in greater arc injuries the management principles are mainly directed in the reduction, fixation, and union of the fractures. In the quite common combined injuries, we are interested in all of the above.

There is a trend for these injuries to be treated with open reduction and internal fixation because, although it is usually possible to grossly reduce the dislocation by closed manipulation, restoration of anatomic alignment of all injured structures cannot be achieved by closed means [112]. We endorse the view expressed by Moneim [46] according to whom: "if for some reason open reduction cannot be

carried out immediately, closed reduction should be carried out only to reduce the perilunate dislocation. It should be followed by open reduction and internal fixation as soon as the patient's condition allows".

Regardless of the way we choose to treat a perilunate injury, closed reduction must be made as soon as possible in all cases, unless we plan to treat operatively the patient, immediately after his/her admission to the hospital [112]. The reasons for the closed reduction to be done as soon as possible, are:

1. To relieve pressure on the median nerve and other soft tissue structures.
2. To diminish the time of increased tension of the capsule and therefore, of vascular deficit to the displaced bones [5].

In cases where early definitive surgical management is contraindicated (polytrauma or other medical conditions), we prefer to closely reduce the injury, splint the wrist, elevate the extremity to allow the edema to subside, and perform an open reduction during the first week postinjury.

Until the 1950s, most recommended methods for closed reduction of perilunar dislocations were based on Gunn's law (formulated in 1923 by Davis [113]), which states that "by positioning the dislocated joint in the position it was at the time of injury and then reversing the force, any dislocation should be easily reduced". In

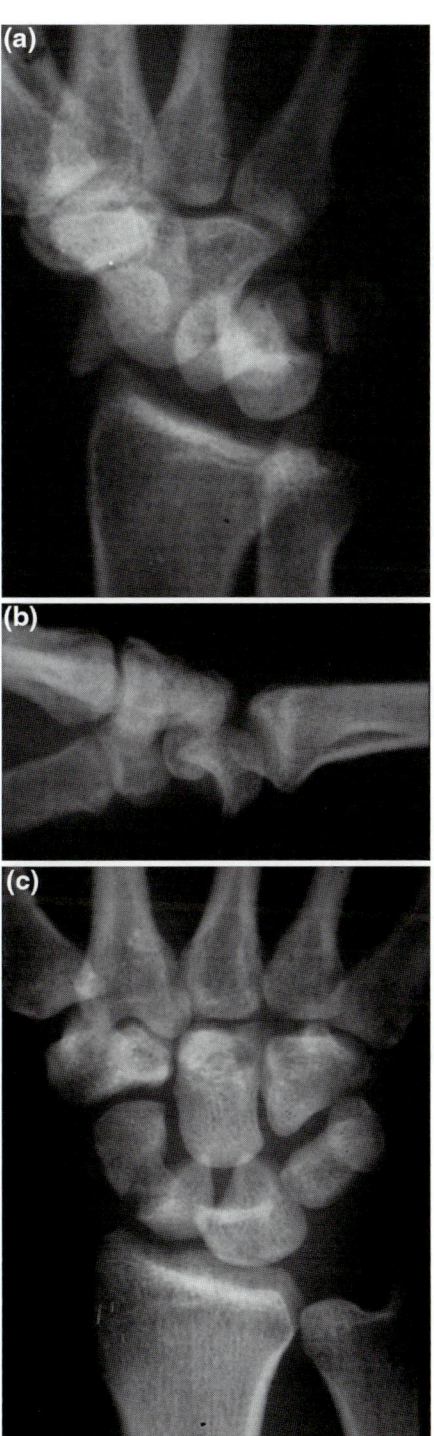

Fig. 4.46 Initial X-rays (**a**, **b**) may cause confusion on the definition of the type of injury, while the PA traction view easily clarifies its identity (**c**). With permission from [231]

other words, to reduce a dislocation, the mechanism of injury must be recreated. Initially, for the manipulation of reduction a broomstick was used as a lever, to press the lunate from the volar surface [113, 114]. Adams [115] stressed the harmful consequence that may result from hard objects used as a lever of reduction and recommended the use of thumb to press the lunate. Bohler [116] attributed irreducibility to muscle spasm and emphasized long (more than 20 min) application of continuous traction without manipulation, aimed at automatic reduction of the lunate. The method of continuous (skeletal) traction (up to 3 days) was applied in neglected cases, where the attempt for closed reduction had failed [117]. The most commonly used manipulation for closed reduction of perilunate dislocations are the guidelines proposed by Codman and Chase in 1905 [118] and by Tavernier in 1906, that were later modified by Watson-Jones [119]. The closed reduction must be atraumatic with complete muscle relaxation, either through general anesthesia or Bier's or axillary block. Forceful manipulation (as with local anesthesia) should be avoided because of the risk of further injury to ligaments or cartilage, while multiple attempts to reduce the lunate should be limited, as they may cause iatrogenic median nerve palsy [120].

Herzberg and Forissier [27], indeed, believe that closed reduction should not be attempted when the lunate is palmarly dislocated and rotated more than 90°, because closed reduction will inevitably fail and may even be harmful to the palmar radiolunate ligamentous remnants, if present.

The patient is placed supine and the elbow is flexed to 90°. A finger-trap suspension with 10–15 pounds of counterweight across the arm is used. A period of 5–10 min of uninterrupted traction is helpful to increase the joint spaces and makes the manipulations of reduction milder. At that time and during traction, PA and L radiographs are obtained, with the carpus distracted, to better evaluate the path of injury and the extent of the damage. The patient's wrist is extended while counter pressure is applied over the palmar

Fig. 4.47 a–d The steps taken for closed reduction of a dorsal perilunate injury (see text for details). With permission from [231]

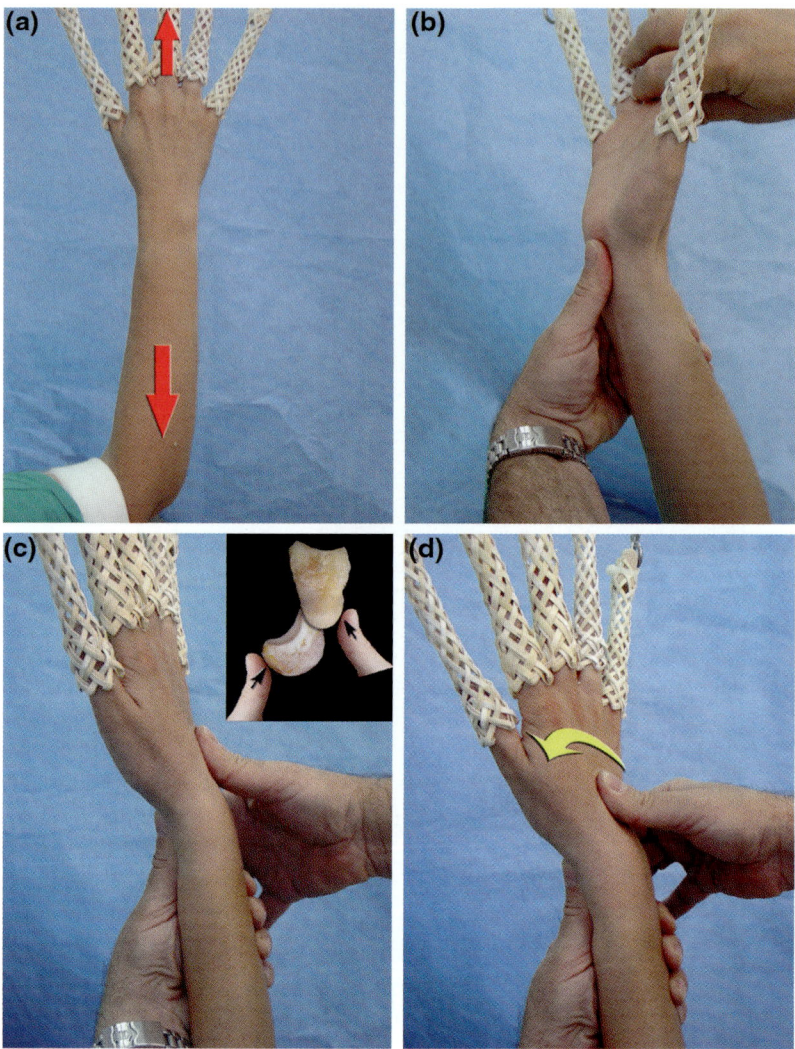

lunate with the surgeon's thumb. Gradual wrist flexion follows with direct pressure over the capitate until a snap occurs. This indicates that the proximal pole of the capitate has overcome the dorsal lip of the lunate and the dislocation is reduced. Pronation of the hand on the forearm may be required for this maneuver to succeed [2, 39, 44, 88] (Fig. 4.47a–d). The manipulation of closed reduction is the same, whether the injuries are of PLD or PLFD type.

Failure of closed reduction with gentle manipulations, necessitates open reduction in order to remove any obstacle, which is usually the interpolated capsule [24]. Of course, there are cases of irreducible perilunate injuries, usually referred to as greater arc injuries [121–123].

After a successful closed reduction we are faced with three options:

1. The closed reduction and cast immobilization will be the definitive treatment.
2. The closed reduction will be augmented with percutaneous pin fixation and cast immobilization.
3. A splint is applied and an open reduction is arranged when the conditions allow for it (the swelling subsides, the overall health of the patient improves, or when planning the referral to a specialized center).

4.7.1 Closed Reduction and Cast Immobilization as Definitive Treatment

In the past, many authors suggested that closed reduction should be the primary treatment for perilunate dislocations and fracture-dislocations and open reduction should be reserved for irreducible cases [94, 98, 124, 125]. The problem is that these injuries are inherently unstable, so that closed reduction and cast immobilization carry an unpredictable prognosis [15, 16, 25, 126]. Cooney et al. [17] noted that carpal instability was a problem after conservative treatment despite maintaining reduction in a cast for an average of 17 weeks. The reduction of the midcarpal joint by closed methods is not enough to ensure the maintenance of an anatomic alignment for the next 6 weeks. Because there is a serious potential for long-term complications (nonunion, instabilities, arthritis), we should be very reluctant to consider closed reduction and cast application as definitive treatment.

Adkison and Chapman [16] reviewed 55 patients with perilunate injuries who were all treated by closed reduction. They found that after anatomic reduction, 59 % of the wrists lost anatomic position during the first 6 weeks of treatment despite adequate external immobilization. The closed treatment alone was successful in achieving and maintaining an anatomic reduction in only 27 % of cases. The authors stated that failure of treatment is usually due to loss of the initial reduction during immobilization in a cast, as the carpus is inherently unstable in compression. Compression forces often cannot be controlled adequately with a cast alone.

Panting et al. [100] reported late displacement of an anatomic reduction and cast immobilization in 21 % of their patients.

Apergis et al. [127] performed a study, where 20 patients were treated by open reduction internal fixation (ORIF) and 8 patients by closed reduction and casting. All patients treated by casting had poor to fair results, while 65 % of ORIF patients had good and excellent results. The authors also concluded that these injuries are too unstable to be treated without fixation.

After reduction, if definitive closed treatment is contemplated, careful scrutiny of the pre- and post-reduction radiographs is necessary. The adequacy of reduction must be critically assessed and only perfect alignment accepted.

In greater arc injuries, difficulties to achieve anatomic reduction may be greater due to comminution of the fracture fragments or because of interference of ligamentous or capsular structures [121]. Even after a perfect reduction, the wrist could collapse in DISI deformity, where the proximal scaphoid and proximal carpal row rotate dorsally, while the distal scaphoid with the distal carpal row rotate volarly. Proper cast application requires a three-point support system with reduction pressure applied at specific areas both for lesser and greater arc injuries [5, 17, 24, 128]. Pressure is exerted dorsally over the capitate and the distal radius, while it is palmarly applied over the scaphoid tuberosity and pisiform. Pads are placed at the reduction points and careful cast molding is critical [7].

Concerning the *extent of immobilization* , despite the fact that some authors recommend the application of a long-arm cast [44], the maintenance of reduction does not seem to depend on the level of the cast applied [16]. However, in greater arc injuries, the immobilization must probably be more rigorous: a long-arm plaster that includes the thumb in opposition and the index and long fingers in an intrinsic-plus position [5, 44].

The recommended *position of immobilization* is not unanimously accepted. Despite the fact that occasionally all possible wrist positions of immobilization have been suggested (slight or full wrist flexion, neutral or slight dorsiflexion), which demonstrates that this method does not produce consistently reliable results, it seems that the prevailing view is with the wrist in neutral or slight palmar flexion [5, 15, 44, 105, 129]; for TS-PLFD injuries slight palmar flexion and radial deviation are recommended [5].

Regarding the *period of immobilization* , although in the past there was a tendency of immobilization for even less than a week [114, 115, 130], immobilization for 8–12 weeks, provided that the reduction is maintained anatomically, is most appropriate [23, 44, 111]. Possibly in greater arc injuries, the time is usually greater than the time for lesser arc injuries and can reach up to 17 weeks [17].

The unstable nature of these injuries requires the reduction to be weekly reassessed radiographically for at least the first 3 weeks, as gradual loss of reduction frequently occurs.

The *acceptance criteria of reduction* should be strict. Every residual malalignment of the bones, any dorsal or volar rotation of the intercalated proximal carpal row or any scapholunate dissociation, require operative intervention. We would not accept a lunocapitate angle greater than 15°, a scapholunate angle greater than 60°, or scapholunate dissociation greater than 4 mm. Scaphoid fractures with postreduction displacement greater than 1 mm or lateral intrascaphoid

angulation greater than 45° (normal values 15°–35°), should not be accepted [131–134].

Bibliographic data suggest that closed reduction and cast immobilization are often accompanied by

(a) A high incidence of scaphoid nonunion, reaching 50–75 % [16, 17, 135].

(b) Complications of ligamentous origin (SL dissociation, LT dissociation, rotatory subluxation of scaphoid, ulnar translocation) (Fig. 4.48a, b). Besides, it is known that ligamentous instability predisposes to scaphoid nonunion [136, 137].

(c) High incidence of post-traumatic arthritis [3].

(d) Potential perturbation of the kinematic behavior of the proximal carpal row, compared with patients treated with open reduction for the same type of injury [93] (Fig. 4.49a1–a3, b1–b3).

4.7.2   Closed Reduction and Percutaneous Fixation

If the reduction achieved by closed manipulation is completely anatomic and no further surgery is considered, we can try to maintain the reduction achieved using percutaneous Kirschner wires (K-wires). In addition, by retaining the bones in their anatomical position with K-wires, the healing capability of the intrinsic ligaments is enhanced [5]. However, the possibility of obtaining anatomic reduction with the closed method is strongly disputed and the method is indicated only in cases, where open reduction is contraindicated (polytrauma patients who may not be able to tolerate surgery) [40, 163]. The percutaneous fixation should be done fluoroscopically [106] or when possible, under arthroscopic direct vision [107, 138–141].

The percutaneous fixation with K-wires is made with the wrist reduced but still suspended by finger trap, with the traction released. The placement of the K-wires conforms to a specific technique, the stages of which are described below [5, 111, 138] (Fig. 4.50a–c):

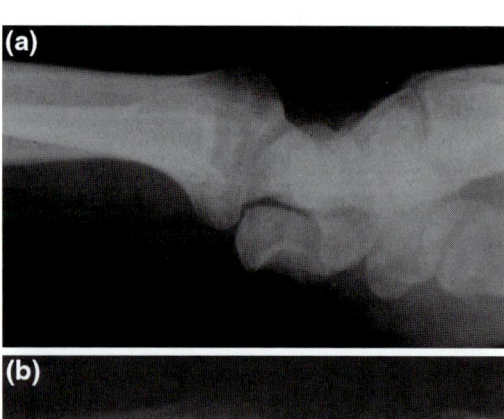
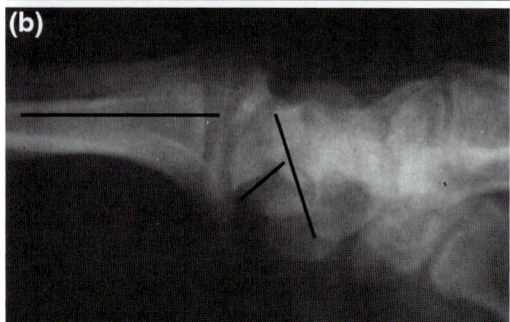

Fig. 4.48 Late presentation of a volar lunate dislocation (**a**), treated with closed reduction: DISI deformity and rotary subluxation of scaphoid (**b**)

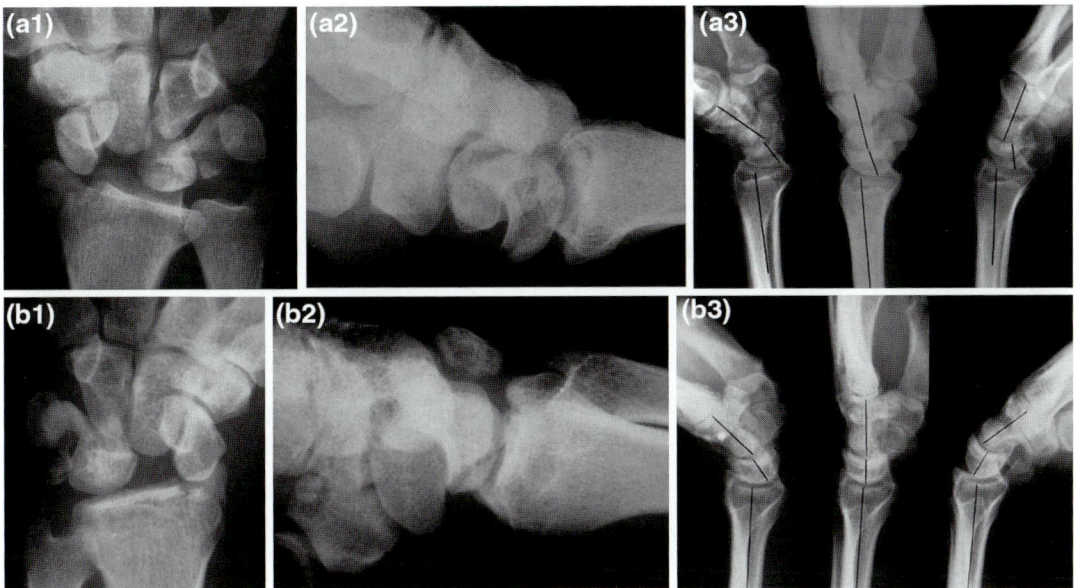

Fig. 4.49 Comparison of the L X-ray views through dorsiflexion, neutral, and palmarflexion of two patients with identical injuries (trans-styloid trans-triquetral dorsal perilunate), who were treated: the first patient with closed reduction (**a1–a3**) and the second patient with open reduction, ligamentous suturing, and osseous fixation (**b1–b3**). It is noted that the lunate of the patient treated with closed reduction, remains in dorsiflexion throughout the range of motion. Conversely the lunate of the second patient follows accordingly the range of wrist motion

1. In cases of scapholunate dissociation (perilunate or lunate dislocations), the procedure starts by inserting from the dorsum 2 K-wires at right angles, one into the lunate and the other into the scaphoid, which are used as "joysticks" to hold them in the reduced position by the assistant. The manipulation reduction of the scapholunate complex without using joysticks is difficult, since we are dealing with what Mayfield et al. [36] called: ***paradox of closed reduction***.[1]

---

[1] Both Mayfield et al. [36] in experimental studies and Taleisnik [44] in the clinical practice observed the so-called ***paradox of closed reduction***, namely, when the wrist is palmarflexed in order to relax the torn palmar radiocarpal ligaments and facilitate their approximation and healing, the scaphoid is placed in the undesirable, unstable palmarflexed position of presubluxaton. If the scaphoid is reduced with the wrist in dorsiflexion, a gap is produced between the torn palmar ligaments, and their healing is either prevented or delayed.

Ruby and Cassidy [15], prefer to stabilize first the capitolunate relationship. While exerting a volar translation force on the capitate, a single smooth K-wire is driven proximally from the capitate into the lunate.

2. The lunate is then retained in a neutral lateral position by a percutaneous pin placed through the radial aspect of the radial metaphysis across the radiolunate joint.

3. Two more K-wires are inserted from the medial aspect of the wrist across the LT joint to stabilize the ulnar side of the perilunate injury.

4. Fixation of the SL joint with two more pins that are transversely inserted from the anatomic snuffbox.

5. At this point, midcarpal joint mobility and congruity are inspected under fluoroscopy. If there is a tendency for capitate subluxation, a further K-wire is passed across the scaphoid to stabilize the scaphocapitate joint.

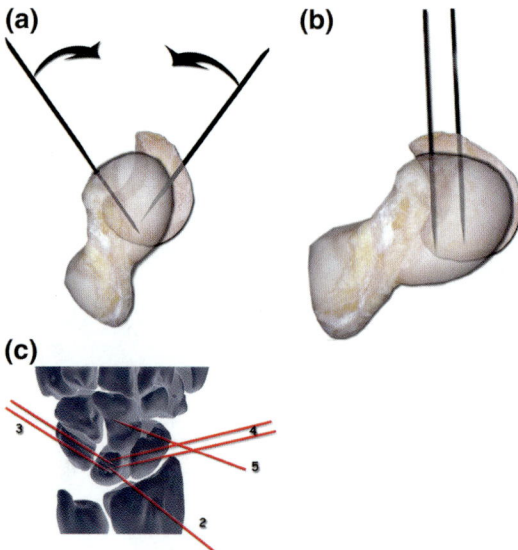

Fig. 4.50 Schematic depiction of the K-wires, by order of insertion, in cases of closed reduction and percutaneous fixation (**a–c**) (see text for details). With permission from [231]

In all cases, a subcutaneous neurovascular injury should be prevented by means of small skin incisions, followed by blunt dissection to identify and protect structures such as the radial artery and the superficial branches of the radial or ulnar nerves [142]. A drill guide may be helpful to introduce K-wires with safety.

The K-wires are left protruding through the skin, bent at right angles, or cut just under the skin to facilitate later removal. A padded splint is applied immediately after the final radiographs have been obtained. This is converted to a below elbow plaster cast, after swelling has subsided. Alternatively, an external fixator could be used, which permits cast-free after-treatment and neutralizes the applied loads, while maintaining normal carpal alignment during ligament healing [143].

Although percutaneous pinning under fluoroscopic guidance, can minimize the surgical trauma, the main disadvantage of this technique is that the assessment of an accurate reduction of the intercarpal alignment is always insufficient, when depending on a radiological aid [144].

The percutaneous fixation method is applied mainly for lesser arc injuries. Despite the fact that cases with percutaneous fixation of the scaphoid with K-wires [100, 126] or cannulated screws [106, 145, 146] have been reported in the literature, they usually referred to cases with isolated fracture of the scaphoid. Using this technique in complex perilunate injuries is a difficult task [111].

The cast or the external fixator and pins are removed at 8 weeks and therapy is started. However, most authors [7, 15, 142], recommend that after removal of the hardware, immobilization in a dorsal splint is continued for an additional 4 weeks, adding up to a total of 10–12 weeks.

4.7.3   Arthroscopic Reduction and Percutaneous Fixation

Arthroscopic reduction with percutaneous fixation, has been suggested by several authors as a useful alternative for the treatment of acute perilunate injuries [107, 140, 144, 147, 148]. As it is a minimally invasive surgical technique, it certainly decreases the extent of soft tissue dissection, preserving the blood supply to carpal bones, while the risk of joint stiffness resulting from capsular fibrosis is less than with open surgery.

Most cases reported in the literature involved exclusively TS-PLFD cases [107, 148] and only few series included PLD cases [144, 147].

It can be used for debridement, evaluation of damage, assessment of reduction and percutaneous fixation with K-wires of the reduced joints, percutaneous screw fixation for scaphoid fractures and even percutaneous bone grafting [107].

Main limitations are: (a) The method is only indicated for acute injuries and is currently limited to relatively simple cases, (b) The relatively high risk of extravasation due to the massive disruption of capsular structures, which is always present in perilunate injuries, can cause problems such as compartment syndrome

[40, 107], (c) Direct repair of the torn capsule or ligaments is not possible by this method [107, 144, 147]. Proponents of the method claim that the capsular structures can heal adequately with a good vascularity when they are properly approximated and protected for some period, and that open repair of interosseous ligaments is not necessary [144, 147].

Arthroscopic reduction and percutaneous fixation in perilunate injuries, is certainly a useful ancillary method although it is a technically demanding procedure. In the hands of experienced wrist arthroscopists, it is a promising method that may be considered in selected cases.

4.7.4 Open Reduction

Open reduction, which is considered today the method of choice, is performed either immediately after the injury or delayed 5–7 days to allow for the swelling to decrease. If delayed open reduction is selected, closed reduction of the dislocation must be preceded [24]. However, for anatomic reduction and appropriate fixation of the injured structures, there is a time limit as to when it can be done successfully.

The prevalence of open over closed reduction as definitive treatment with respect to long-term results, is based on the fact that we have more chances to achieve and maintain the anatomical reduction in the open rather than in the closed method [5, 17, 24, 86]. Additional reasons in favor of open reduction are that the existing extensive ligamentous lesions both dorsally and volarly, render these injuries unstable by definition, while the frequent presence of chondral lesions, especially from the head of the capitate (Fig. 4.51a–c) and comminution of scaphoid fracture, necessitate joint irrigation and removal or reattachment of the free osteochondral fragments [5, 10, 15, 16] (Fig. 4.52). During open reduction, there is a tendency for direct ligamentous repair in an attempt to improve long-term stability. Several studies have shown the superiority of this method, but it is not clear whether this is due to a greater accuracy of

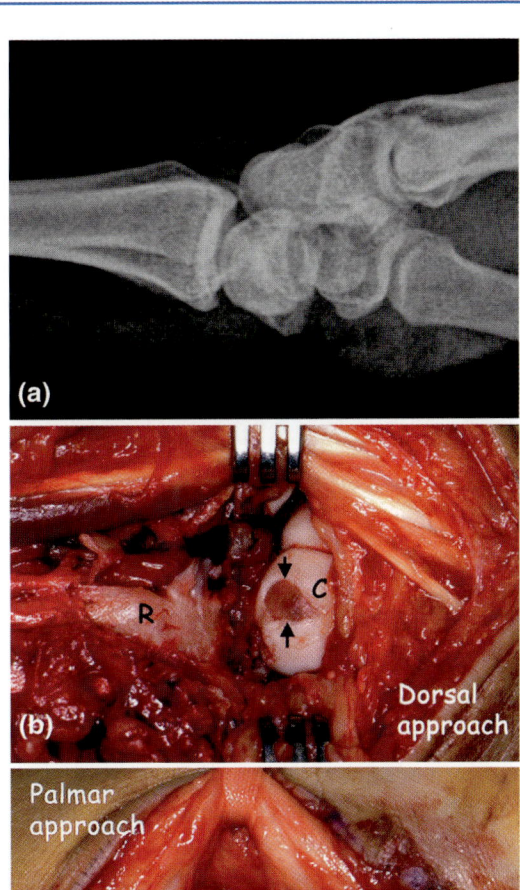

Fig. 4.51 A case of dorsal PLD (**a**) with an extensive chondral defect of the head of the capitate (*arrows*) (**b**). The chondral fragment was found with the palmar approach lying deep in the carpal tunnel and adjacent to the midcarpal rent (*wavy arrow*), through which it migrated from the dorsal to the palmar surface (**c**) (*R* Radius, *C* Capitate). With permission from [231]

reduction or due to the repair of the ligaments [10]. It continues to be unclear, which intercarpal or radiocarpal ligaments require direct repair and which heal by restoration of the osseous relationships [39].

Since perilunate and lunate dislocations are different stages of the same injury, their treatment is practically the same. Certainly, there is a

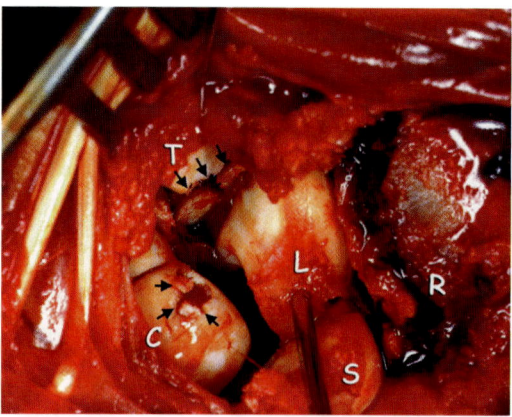

Fig. 4.52 The dorsal approach frequently reveals comminuted fracture or osteochondral fragments (*arrows*) necessitating joint irrigation. (*R* Radius, *C* Capitate, *T* Triquetrum, *L* Lunate, *and S* Scaphoid). With permission from [231]

large number of combined lesser and greater arc injuries published as case reports, but their treatment follows the same basic principles that will be described below.

Such rare cases of perilunate fracture-dislocations, are: Trans-scaphoid, trans-capitate, trans-triquetral, dorsal perilunate, fracture-dislocation [51, 52, 149]; trans-scaphoid dorsal perilunate fracture-dislocation with dorsal [150] or volar [151] dislocation of the proximal scaphoid pole; trans-triquetral, dorsal [45, 85, 152], or palmar [153] perilunate dislocation; trans-scaphoid, trans-triquetral, dorsal perilunate, fracture-dislocation [49, 154], or palmar lunate dislocation [48, 155]; trans-styloid, trans-scaphoid, trans-triquetral dorsal perilunate fracture-dislocation [156]; trans-styloid, trans-triquetral dorsal perilunate fracture-dislocation with fracture of the ulnar border of the distal radius [157]; trans-styloid, trans-scaphoid, trans-lunate dorsal perilunate fracture-dislocation [54, 56, 57];

dorsal perilunate dislocation with distal radius fracture [158]; palmar lunate dislocation with type Salter–Harris III distal radius fracture [159]; trans-triquetral (with nonunion scaphoid) dorsal perilunate fracture-dislocation [131]; trans-styloid, trans-scaphoid, trans-lunate, trans-triquetral fracture (reduced) [58]; trans-scaphoid, trans-lunate, trans-triquetral fracture (reduced) [61]; trans-scaphoid, trans-lunate fracture (reduced) [63]; trans-scaphoid, trans-capitate, trans-triquetral fracture (reduced) [50]; and trans-lunate, trans-triquetral (reduced) [60].

Rare cases of perilunate or lunate dislocations are: Peri-triquetral dorsal perilunate dislocation [41]; periscaphoid and lunate dorsal perilunate dislocation [74]; peri-scaphoid and lunate palmar lunate dislocation [64, 66, 69–71]; periscaphoid and lunate palmar lunate dislocation with complete scaphoid extrusion [67]; perilunate, peritriquetral palmar lunate dislocation [68]; and dorsal perilunate and dorsal radiocarpal dislocation [160].

We examine the issue of open reduction of these complex injuries, in three steps: (**a**) *The approach*, (**b**) *The assessment of injuries* (dorsally and palmarly), and (**c**) *The reconstruction* (dorsally and palmarly). When necessary, a differentiation is made depending on whether the injury is of dislocation or fracture-dislocation type.

Ninety seven patients (98 wrists) were operated at our institution for perilunate injuries. Table 4.4 indicates the operative approaches we used, according to the type of injury.

4.7.4.1 The Approach

Despite the overall consensus that open reduction and internal fixation is the treatment of choice for these complex injuries, the best

Table 4.4 The operative approaches used, according to the type of injury

PLD	N°	PLFD+S	N°	PLFD−S	N°
Combined (Dorsal, Palmar)	28	Combined (Dorsal, palmar)	35	Combined (Dorsal, Palmar)	11
Dorsal	2	Dorsal	15	Dorsal	3
Palmar	1	Triple (Dorsal, Palmar, Ulnar)	2	Triple (Dorsal, Palmar, Ulnar)	1

surgical approach is less clear and remains controversial. Surgical approaches that have been used are the dorsal, volar, and combined dorsal-volar techniques. The fear had always been that combined approach would lead to lunate and scaphoid avascular necrosis due to interference with their blood supply, but this has so far remained a theoretical rather than a real complication [10]. In addition, the choice of the most suitable approach is influenced by the fact that it has not yet been established, which intercarpal or radiocarpal ligaments require direct repair and which heal just by restoring the osseous relationships [86].

Proponents of the combined dorsal and volar approaches feel that they provide the benefits of improved exposure, better assessment of injured structures, ease of reduction, access to distal scaphoid fractures, the ability to repair volar ligaments, and carpal tunnel decompression [38, 112].

Proponents of the isolated dorsal approach [15, 16, 23, 46, 86, 125, 161–164] believe that suture repair of the volar ligaments is not absolutely necessary, as the volar capsule will heal when anatomic reduction is achieved after dorsal fixation. In addition, a second volar incision in a swollen wrist may impart further swelling, wound problems, carpal devascularization, and a slower recovery of digital flexion and grip strength [18, 38, 86]. They would use an additional volar approach, if a carpal tunnel release were to be performed or if a volarly dislocated lunate required open reduction. Herzberg [2] suggested that a single dorsal approach may be used when the rotation of the proximal scaphoid-lunate unit is less than 90° with respect to the radius. However, when the dislocated unit is rotated more than 90°, a volar carpal tunnel approach should be used first, because attempts at closed reduction are likely to fail due to volar capsule interposition and these attempts may moreover be harmful to the remaining ligamentous connections between the radius and lunate (Fig. 4.53).

Proponents of isolated palmar approach [86, 98, 116, 165–167], mainly refer to trans-caphoid perilunate fracture-dislocation injuries and they

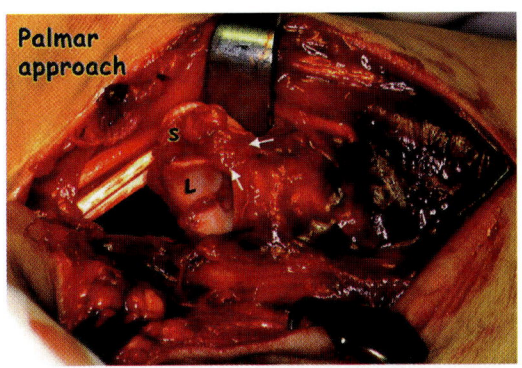

Fig. 4.53 In a case of trans-scaphoid volar lunate dislocation, the lunate (*L*) with the proximal scaphoid fragment (*S*) were volarly dislocated. In this case, the RSL ligament (*arrows*) seems to be intact. Any attempt for vigorous closed reduction could jeopardize its integrity. With permission from [231]

recommend to use a Russe approach to free the scaphoid fracture from interposed soft tissue, apply bone graft if indicated, and repair the anterior capsular rent.

Since 1973, when Dobyns and Swanson [168] first advocated combining dorsal and palmar approaches for these injuries, this option has gained wide recognition [3, 5, 8, 9, 14, 22, 24, 43, 90, 91, 120, 138, 164, 169, 170].

The main idea is that the volar approach allows the release of the carpal tunnel, suturing of the capsular rent at the level of the midcarpal joint and repairing the important volar ligaments. The dorsal approach allows us to control the adequacy of reduction, to repair the interosseous ligaments of the proximal carpal row, to stabilize the joints, and to reduce and fixate the fractures of carpal bones. It should be noted that the volar approach is not necessary in order to reduce the dislocation, but to repair the important palmar ligaments. Only in rare cases is the volar approach indispensable for the reduction of the dislocation, e.g., complete dislocation of the lunate (Stage IV) [3] or in chronic cases.

With the patient supine on the operating table, a general or regional anesthetic is administered. A tourniquet is placed on the arm to afford good visibility of the neurovascular and ligamentous structures.

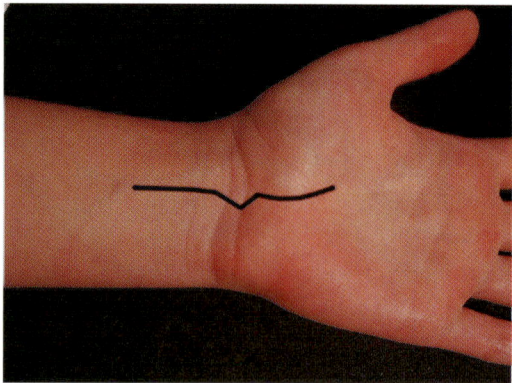

Fig. 4.54 The extended carpal tunnel approach

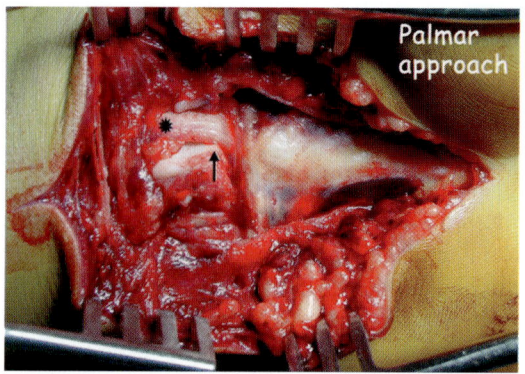

Fig. 4.56 A case in which the volarly dislocated and rotated by 90° lunate, compresses with its dorsal horn (*arrow*) the median nerve (*asterisk*). Nerve dysfunction is obvious. With permission from [231]

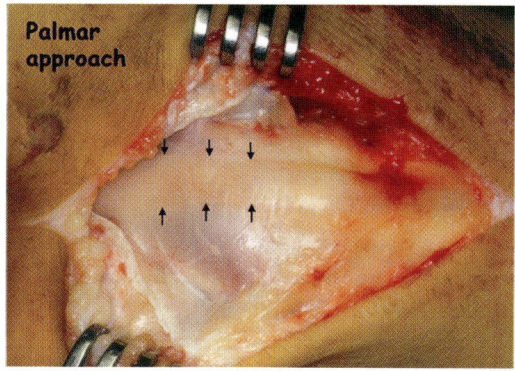

Fig. 4.55 In dorsal perilunate or volar lunate dislocations frequently the median nerve is lying immediately under the transverse ligament, somewhat flattened by the underlying dislocated bone (*arrows*). With permission from [231]

Regardless of the type of injury (PLD or PLFD type), both dorsal and palmar approaches are the same. Usually, we prefer to start with the palmar and then to proceed with the dorsal approach.

The Palmar Approach

An extended carpal tunnel incision is used, starting 3–4 cm proximal to the wrist crease, in line with the palmaris longus tendon. The incision is curved ulnarly at the proximal wrist crease to avoid injuring the palmar sensory branch of the median nerve, then parallel to the longitudinal thenar crease and ends at the distal region of the transverse carpal ligament in the midpalm (Fig. 4.54). The transverse carpal ligament and the antebrachial fascia are incised longitudinally. In every case, great care must be taken when dividing the transverse carpal ligament, so as not to injure the median nerve that is located more superficial than normal, compressed by the underlying lunate (in lunate dislocation) or proximal carpal row (in perilunate dislocation) (Fig. 4.55). At that stage, the median nerve should be carefully inspected for hematomas that suggest direct trauma to the nerve (Fig. 4.56). The palmar wrist capsule is exposed by manipulating the contents of the carpal canal. We usually retract the median nerve and the FPL tendon radially, and the rest of the flexor tendons, ulnarly (Fig. 4.57). In order to evaluate and reconstruct the ulnar capsuloligamentous structures, all flexor tendons and the median nerve are radially retracted. With the volar approach, great care must be taken not to disrupt the proximal ligamentous attachments of the lunate, since probably these are now the only vascular supplier (Fig. 4.58).

In PLFD+S type of injuries, instead of a carpal tunnel incision, a distally extended Henry exposure has been recommended by some authors [5, 135], as used for grafting scaphoid nonunions, while Inoue et al. [14] used an approach that combines Herbert's approach with a carpal tunnel release with an incision of "Y" fashion. Szabo and Newland [86], in cases of

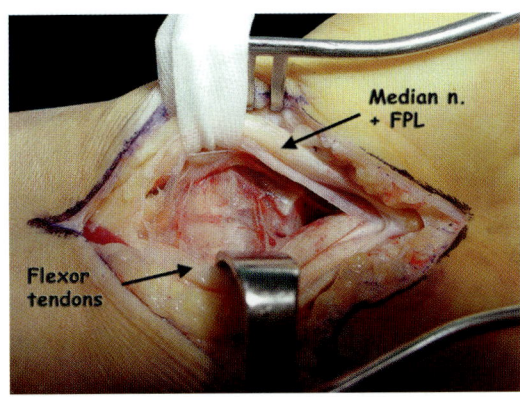

Fig. 4.57 Deep palmar approach by retracting the median nerve and the *FPL tendon* radially and the mass of *flexor tendons* ulnarly. With permission from [231]

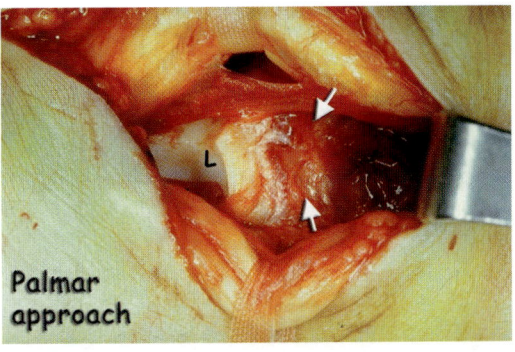

Fig. 4.58 Usually, in a volarly dislocated lunate its proximal ligamentous attachments (SRL ligament) remain intact and should be preserved. With permission from [231]

trans-scaphoid PLFD and if the carpal tunnel needs to be released, recommends an "S" type incision which necessitates identification of the palmar cutaneous branch of the median nerve. Herzberg [6] suggested a combined palmar approach: a radial incision for internal fixation of the scaphoid and a midline carpal tunnel approach to repair palmar carpal ligaments.

The Dorsal Approach

The dorsal approach consists of an 8 cm longitudinal midline incision or in line with the Lister's tubercle. The incision is carried down to the extensor retinaculum, raising skin flaps radially and ulnarly. The retinaculum is divided in line with the third dorsal compartment and the extensor pollicis longus (EPL) tendon is retracted radially. Dividing this compartment, attention is required not to injure the superficial radial nerve, the branches of which are crossing the third compartment radially. The second and fourth dorsal compartments are mobilized by subperiosteal dissection, without exposing the encompassing tendons, until the dorsal wrist capsule becomes visible (Fig. 4.59a–c).

At that stage, we need to think if the terminal branch of the posterior interosseous nerve, which is identified on the radial floor of the fourth compartment, should be resected for pain reduction [40], or if the nerve resection alters wrist proprioception reflexes [171]. Recent

publications are trying to resolve this issue [172–175].

The capsule could be distended and filled with blood, it may have already been disrupted in various ways or it could be intact. If the dorsal capsule is intact, we prefer to perform a ligament splitting capsulotomy as originally described by Berger and Bishop [176]. In this technique, the dorsal capsular incision is started ulnar to Lister's tubercle, splitting the dorsal radiocarpal ligament longitudinally to the triquetrum. The capsular incision is then continued in the radial direction, splitting the dorsal intercarpal ligament and making a radially based V-shaped flap. Further exposure can be achieved by extending the proximal limb of the capsulotomy along the dorsal rim of the distal radius (Fig. 4.60). The last step, inevitably results in a complete denervation of the dorsal wrist capsule. Alternatively, a dorsal nerve-sparing approach has been described [175].

If the dorsal capsule is torn, the arthrotomy can be extended, either longitudinally to create and elevate a radial and an ulnar capsular flap to expose the scapholunate, capitolunate, and lunotriquetral articulations, or incorporating the original capsular injury with a ligament-sparing dorsal capsulotomy.

Transverse arthrotomies [7], an inverted "T" –shaped capsulotomy [9] or a "Z" fashion capsulotomy [2] have also been in some instances described.

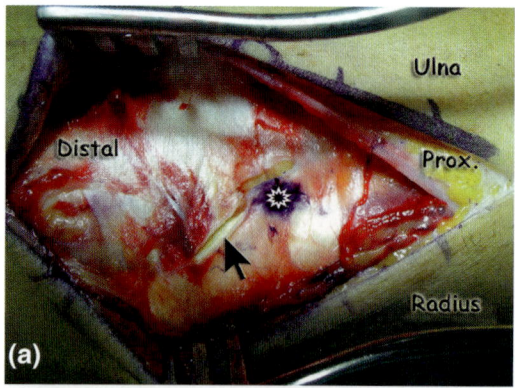

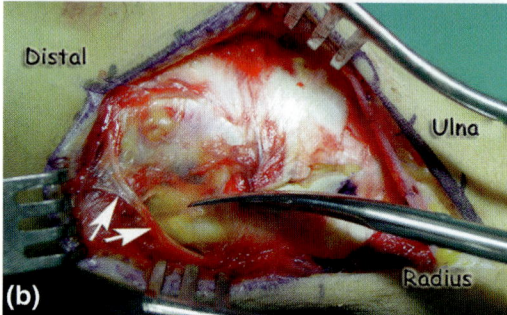

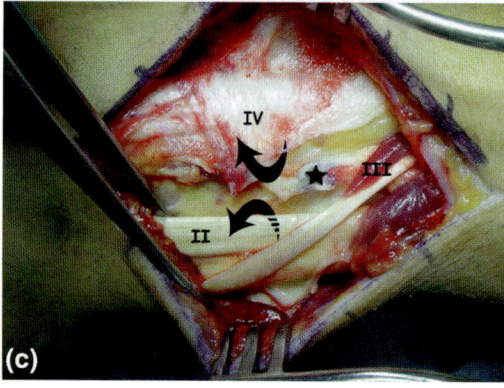

Fig. 4.59 Stepwise dorsal approach: Division of the third compartment (*arrow*), Lister's tubercle (*asterisk*) (**a**); the superficial radial nerve (*arrows*) is in danger when dividing the third compartment (**b**); and mobilization of the second and fourth dorsal compartments (**c**). With permission from [231]

4.7.5   The Assessment of the Injury

When we use combined approaches, it is useful to record the integrity of specific anatomic structures, following a prescribed order. The injury is first examined palmarly, then dorsally, and subsequently definitive repair is planned.

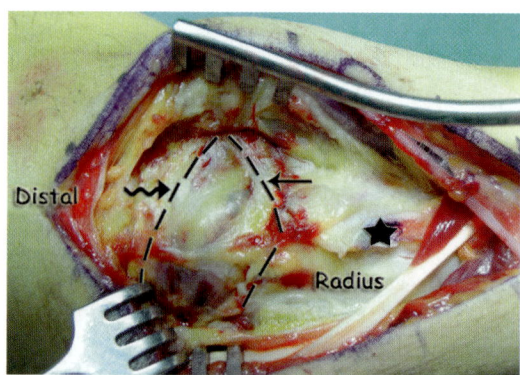

Fig. 4.60 The ligament splitting capsulotomy [176]. Splitting the DIC ligament (*wavy arrow*) and the DRC ligament (*straight arrow*). Lister's tubercle (*asterisk*). With permission from [231]

4.7.5.1 Palmar Findings

Lesser arc Injuries

With the nerve and flexor tendons retracted, the volar capsule is inspected. In unreduced dislocations, the distal articular surface of the lunate is immediately apparent protruding through the disrupted volar wrist capsule and rotated palmarward in different degrees. If closed reduction is preceded, a transverse rent of capsuloligamentous structures is consistently found. This rent is located at the level of the midcarpal joint, it has even or rugged torn edges and occurs in both perilunate and lunate dislocations (Fig. 4.61a, b). The rent is transverse or arc-shaped with its convex side facing distally. Its length is variable and comprises radial, distal or central and ulnar parts. The radial part usually involves the sulcus between the RSC and long RL ligaments. The integrity of the RSC ligament is a matter of controversy. We, as others [21, 40], believe that most often the RSC ligament is intact (Fig. 4.62a–c) and only rarely is it found ruptured or avulsed from radius (Fig. 4.63). Others believe that rupture of the RSC ligament is a frequent intraoperative [5, 6, 8, 26], or arthroscopic finding [144, 147]. Since the RSC and long RL are intraarticular ligaments covered with the joint capsule, the control of their integrity necessitates the removal of the superimposed synovial layer. In every case, the

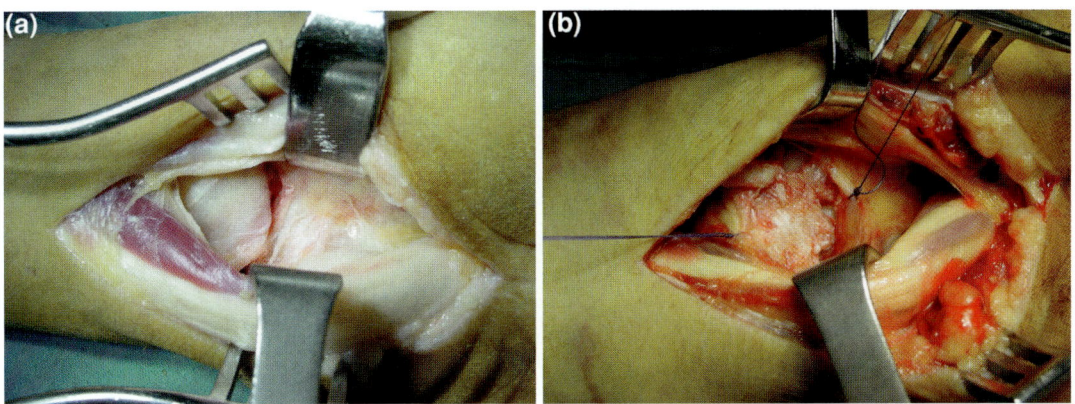

Fig. 4.61 The midcarpal rent could have even (**a**) or rugged (**b**) torn edges. With permission from [231]

integrity of the RSC ligament must be recorded and treated accordingly. The distal or central part of the rent involves the capsule of the lunocapitate joint (space of Poirier), while the ulnar part is located at the lunotriquetral region, rupturing the palmar lunotriquetral, and the continuation of the long RL ligament to the triquetrum (Fig. 4.62c). In some cases, the volar LT ligament can be avulsed with osseous articular fragment from the volar surface of the triquetrum. This was found in 5 out of 26 (19 %) of our acute or delayed cases treated before the 45th day.

The rupture of the SL and LT ligaments is given, in both perilunate and lunate dislocations, while the long and short RL ligaments are usually intact (Fig. 4.58), with the exception of cases with complete dislocation of the lunate, which is free of any ligamentous attachments (stage IV) (Fig. 4.64).

Greater Arc Injuries

The capsuloligamentous injuries are similar to those already described in lesser arc injuries, except that in some cases (mostly of greater arc), the ulnar part of the capsular rent continues proximal and ulnar to the triquetrum, affecting the ulnocarpal ligaments, the integrity of which must be verified (Fig. 4.33e in the Sect. 4.4.2). This was observed in 10 out of 97 cases (10.3 %) of perilunate injuries that were operatively treated by the author; all 10 cases were greater arc injuries.

Often through the capsular rent, the proximal scaphoid stays linked to the protruding lunate with the scapholunate ligament, if the latter maintains its integrity (Fig. 4.65). A fragment of the fractured triquetrum can also be linked to the dislocated lunate (Fig. 4.66). However, there are cases in the literature, where through this capsular rent, the lunate with the proximal scaphoid [73, 177, 178], or with the proximal capitate [179] are palmarly displaced even up to the distal forearm [162, 180]. At this stage, we have the opportunity to control the integrity of the dislocated lunate. It is not unusual to find fractures of the body [42, 63] or the horns of the lunate. The fracture of the palmar lunate horn is probably equivalent with rupture of the long RL ligament and needs to be addressed (Fig. 4.67).

4.7.5.2 Dorsal Findings

Lesser Arc Injuries

Rupture of the dorsal capsuloligamentous structures is not a usual finding. Rarely, the dorsal capsule and especially its radial part can be avulsed from the dorsal radial rim. Some authors [21, 37, 38, 42] support that in Mayfield's staged perilunar instability, lunate dislocation (Stage VI) presupposes rupture of the dorsal radiocarpal ligament. This involves the attachment of the ligament to the dorsal horn of

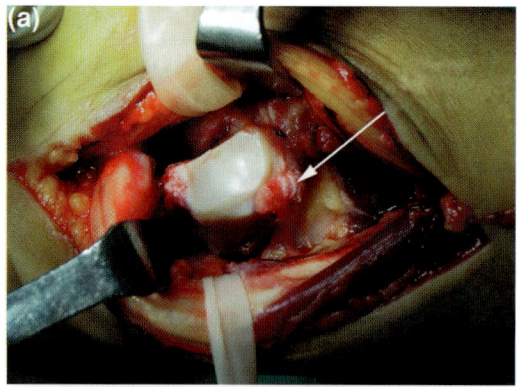

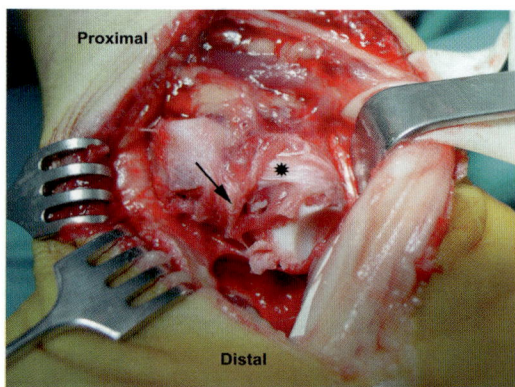

Fig. 4.63 *The arrow* indicates the ruptured RSC ligament in a volar lunate dislocation, while *the asterisk* indicates the intact LRL ligament

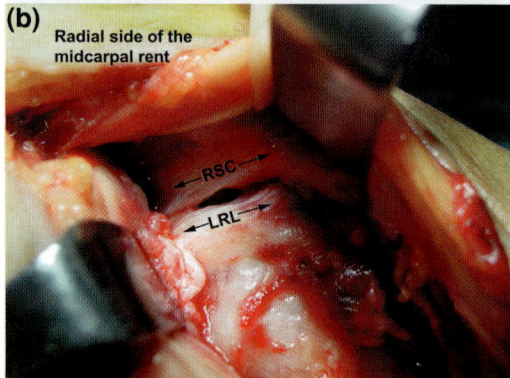

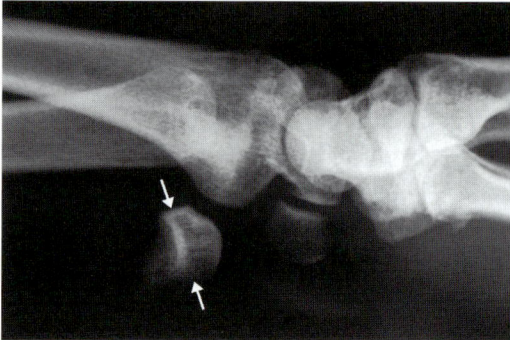

Fig. 4.64 Complete dislocation of the lunate (Stage IV) (*arrows*) predisposes to complete rupture of its ligamentous attachments

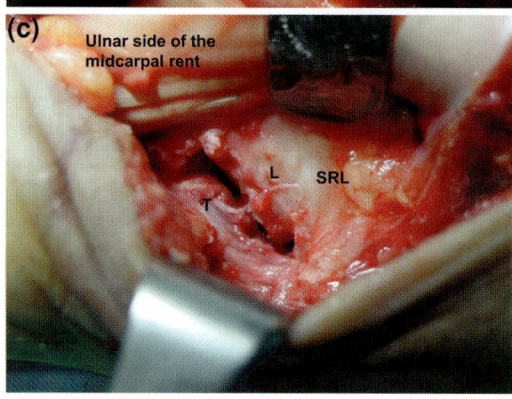

Fig. 4.62 In a volar lunate dislocation the arrow indicates the remnants of the LT ligament (**a**); Postreduction, both LRL and RSC ligaments are intact (**b**); and Rupture of the volar LT ligament (**c**). (*SRL* Short radiolunate ligament, *L* Lunate, *T* Triquetrum) [231]

the lunate, but the main ligament which is attached to the triquetrum, is usually intact.

After capsule elevation, the head of the capitate and the proximal pole of the scaphoid, which is dorsally subluxated, become visible. The lunate is covered partially or completely by

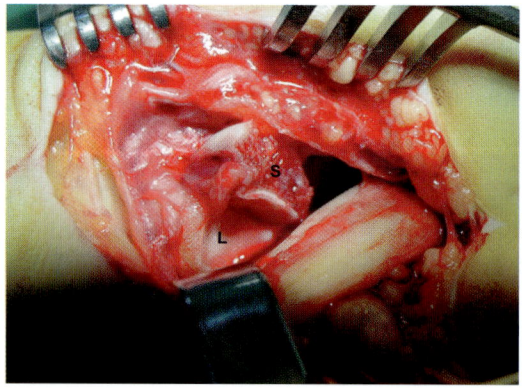

Fig. 4.65 The volarly dislocated lunate attached with an intact SL ligament to the proximal fragment of the scaphoid. (*S* Scaphoid, *L* Lunate)

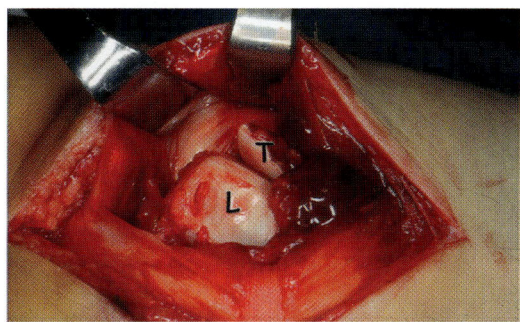

Fig. 4.66 The volarly dislocated lunate attached with an intact proximal LT ligament to the proximal fragment of the triquetrum. (*L* Lunate, *T* Triquetrum). With permission from [231]

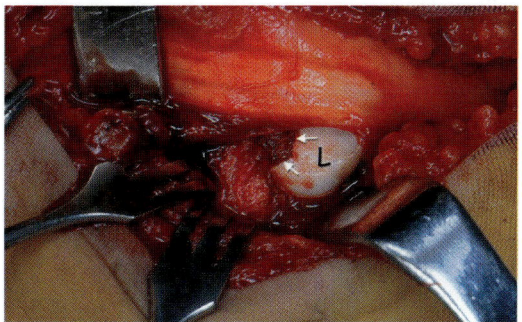

Fig. 4.67 A volarly dislocated lunate with fractured palmar horn (*arrows*), exerting pressure on the median nerve. (*L* Lunate). With permission from [231]

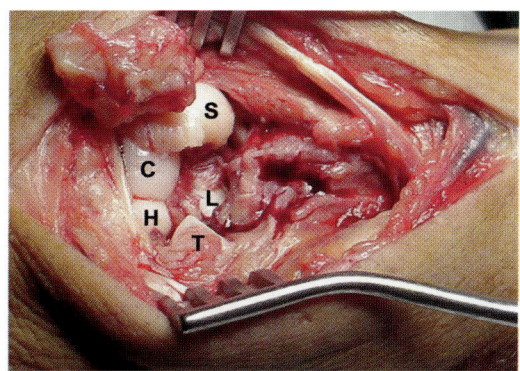

Fig. 4.68 With dorsal approach, after capsulotomy, the unreduced lunate is found embedded and partially covered by the capitate head. (*S* Scaphoid, *L* Lunate, *T* Triquetrum, *H* Hamate, *C* Capitate)

the head of the capitate (Fig. 4.68). After the carpal bones are exposed, cartilage damage is assessed. It is important to inspect all the carpal bones for damage, since chondral defects will be prognostic in long-term recovery [40]. The head of the capitate is a common area where cartilage defects of varying size are identified. It is usually indicative of the violence applied to the head of the capitate from the dorsal lip impaction of the lunate during dislocation. The presence of free osteochondral fragments needs to be addressed either by excision or reattachment. In addition, by inspecting the head of the capitate for cartilage erosion or chondral defects, we could roughly predict the development of midcarpal arthritis [6, 40].

The literature suggests that the SL interosseous ligament usually detaches from the scaphoid and remains connected to the lunate [1, 7, 22,

37, 38, 40, 111, 140], while others suggest that it is most often avulsed from the lunate [21, 43]. In fact, the SL ligament shows a much wider range of failures. Specifically, from 26 acute PLD cases treated operatively, we found the SL ligament: avulsed from the scaphoid (5 cases) or from the lunate (15 cases), ruptured in its midsubstance (1 case), and with peculiar types of disruption (5 cases). The latter types of disruption usually include cases where the dorsal SL ligament was avulsed from the lunate, while the proximal SL ligament was avulsed from the scaphoid (Fig. 4.69a–d). The good news is that in the vast majority of cases, the SL ligament is avulsed from its attachments (with or without bony fragment), rather than ruptured in its midsubstance.

Normally, the dorsal intercarpal ligament is intact, but its proximal part, i.e., the dorsal scaphotriquetral ligament, is often avulsed together with the dorsal SL ligament (Fig. 4.70a, b).

The lunotriquetral ligament is either torn or avulsed, with the same rate from the lunate or the triquetrum, with or without an osseous fragment. Some authors believe that the lunotriquetral ligament is avulsed more often from the triquetrum [21, 43] and others from the lunate [108], but frequently, there is no dorsal lunotriquetral ligament remaining for direct repair [7, 9].

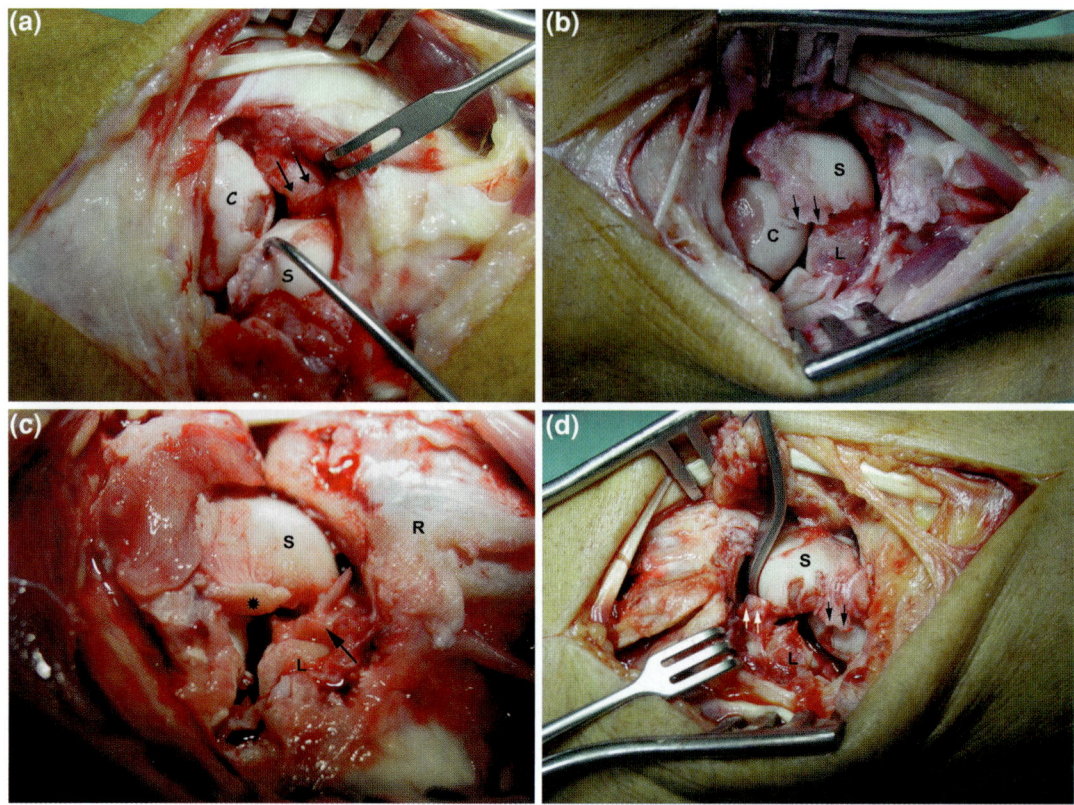

Fig. 4.69 Different types of SL ligament ruptures: The dorsal SL ligament (*arrows*) is detached from the scaphoid (**a**) or the lunate (**b**). The dorsal SL ligament appears detached from the lunate with an osseous fragment (*asterisk*), while the proximal portion of the ligament is detached from the scaphoid (*arrow*) (**c**). Same type of rupture without an osseous fragment (*arrows*) (**d**) (*S* Scaphoid, *C* Capitate, *L* Lunate, *R* Radius)

Greater Arc Injuries

Depending on the mechanism and the violence applied, an irregular rupture could be found, not only of the capsule but also of the dorsal retinaculum. Greater arc, in contrast with lesser arc injuries, show a high frequency of injuries of the dorsal capsuloligamentous structures manifested as: avulsion of the dorsal capsule from the radius with the DRC ligament intact, rupture of both capsule and DRC ligament, or avulsion fracture fragments from the dorsal radial rim (Fig. 4.71a–c). Excluding chronic cases, we found 26 cases (52 %) from 50 PLFD+S and 8 cases (61 %) from 13 PLFD−S, with injuries of these dorsal structures. The dorsal radiocarpal ligament can rupture anywhere in its course (avulsed from radius, ruptured in its midsubstance, or avulsed

with an osseous fragment from the dorsal triquetrum).

After capsule elevation, the head of the capitate and the fractured distal scaphoid become visible. The proximal scaphoid remains linked with the lunate through the "intact" scapholunate ligament.

In the past, there was the perception that scapholunate dissociation and scaphoid fracture are mutually exclusive, because the energy causing the injury will either tear the scapholunate ligament or fracture the scaphoid [16, 23, 26, 40, 100, 178, 181]. Even nowadays it has been suggested that, when the capitate displaces, the scaphoid must either fracture or rotate [86]. Mayfield [35] and Mayfield et al. [36] found that almost all TS-PLFD had some degree of

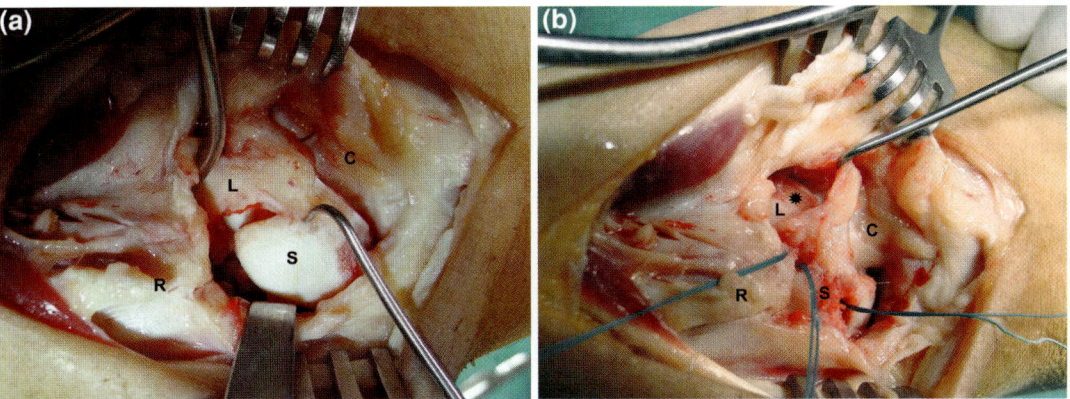

Fig. 4.70 Besides the rupture of the proximal SL ligament, the dorsal scaphotriquetral ligament appears to be intact (**a**), but it is actually avulsed from the dorsal horn of the lunate (*asterisk*) (**b**)

scapholunate ligament failure, ranging from small palmar tear to complete disruption. Concomitant scaphoid fracture and scapholunate dissociation, were confirmed in many clinical cases reported later [6, 89, 104, 138, 147, 150, 182–185] (Fig. 4.72), while Herzberg et al. [13] found this combination in 3.8 % of their patients and considered it as a factor of poorer prognosis. In some cases, the scapholunate ligament has a partial tear of its volar and proximal part, confirming the perception that the rupture of the ligament has started from the volar side [35]. In addition, the macroscopically intact scapholunate ligament does not necessarily ensure its biomechanical integrity. The coexistence of these two injuries renders the scapholunate complex particularly unstable, increasing the incidence of scaphoid nonunion [136, 182, 186]. In rare cases, the proximal scaphoid is dorsally displaced protruding through the dorsal capsule [89] or even more rarely rotated by 180° [122, 150] (Fig. 4.73a–c). In our series, 9 out of 50 cases (18 %) with acute or delayed injuries, exhibited concurrent scaphoid fracture and scapholunate dissociation. Seven of the above cases had complete rupture, while two of them had ruptured the volar and proximal part of the ligament.

The scaphoid fractures are usually located in its middle third and are frequently comminuted. According to Herzberg et al. [13], from 83

dorsal TS-PLFD, the scaphoid fractures were located in the middle third in 95 % (transverse in 72 %, comminuted in 22 %, and with a large intermediate fragment in 6 %) and in only 5 % they were located in the proximal third. In our series, from 51 TS-PLFD, 47 scaphoid fractures (92 %) were located at its waist. Sixteen of them were transverse (34 %) and 31 (65.9 %) were comminuted. Two fractures (3.9 %) were located at its proximal third and 2 fractures (3.9 %) were comminuted involving its distal third (Fig. 4.74a, b).

Fractures of the radial styloid are usually associated with rupture of the scapholunate ligament, regarded as TS-PLFD variance [3] (Fig. 4.49a1, b1). However, the combination of fractures of the radial styloid and the scaphoid is not unusual. The concomitant fractures of the radial styloid and the scaphoid associated with rupture of the scapholunate ligament, is a really rare injury (Fig. 4.75).

A relatively frequent variation of a greater arc type of injury is the scaphocapitate syndrome, which implies a perilunar dislocation with fractures of the scaphoid and the capitate, the latter being displaced with the proximal pole rotating by up to 180° (The scaphocapitate syndrome is analyzed in a separate chapter).

The fracture of the triquetrum may concern its body, an avulsion fracture fragment from its proximal surface or a volar articular fragment

Fig. 4.71 Different types of injury of the dorsal capsuloligamentous structures in greater arc injuries: avulsion of the dorsal capsule from the radius (*arrows*) with the DRC ligament intact (**a**); rupture of the DRC ligament (*arrows*) (**b**); avulsion fracture fragments from the dorsal radial rim (*arrows*) (**c**)

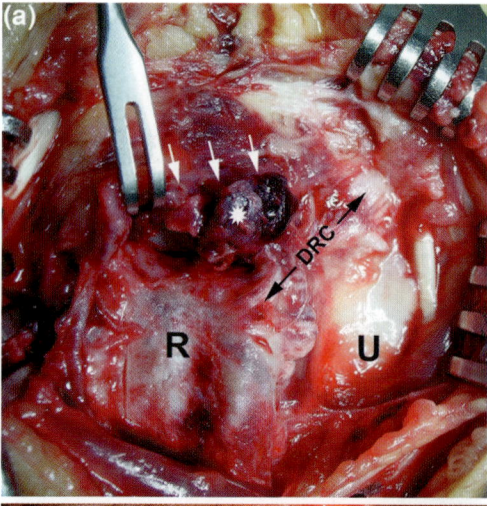

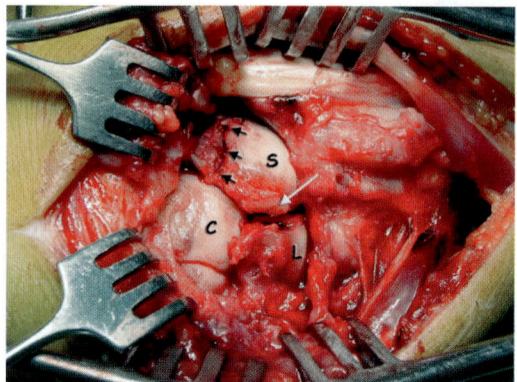

Fig. 4.72 The concomitant fracture of the scaphoid and SL ligament rupture in trans-scaphoid perilunate injuries, were found in 18 % of our patients. With permission from [231]

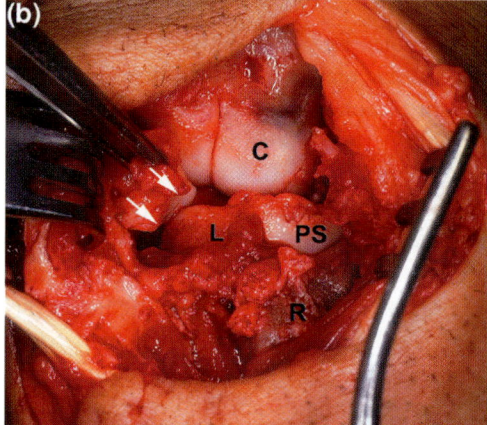

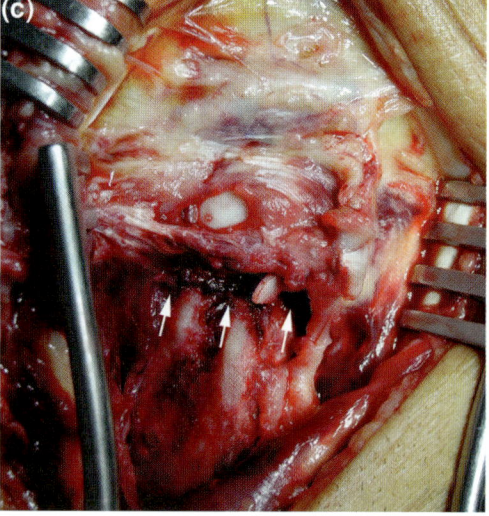

avulsed with the volar LT ligament, which remains linked with the lunate, while the main body is dislocated with the distal carpal row (Fig. 4.76). In some cases, an osseous fragment is identified at the dorsal surface of the triquetrum, either as an avulsion fracture from ligamentous attachments or after a chiseling action of the ulnar styloid process on the dorsum of the triquetrum [187] (Fig. 4.77a, b). Garcia-Elias et al. [95] supported that 1 out of 4 patients, instead of dislocation of the LT joint, presented with fracture of the body of the triquetrum or avulsion fracture from its proximal pole.

Inspection of the integrity of the capitate-hamate joint is recommended, since from 67 greater arc injuries treated operatively, we found 3 cases with capitate-hamate dissociation, which were not radiographically visible. This finding probably implies a complex mechanism of injury comprising an anterior-posterior crush type force [10] (Fig. 4.78).

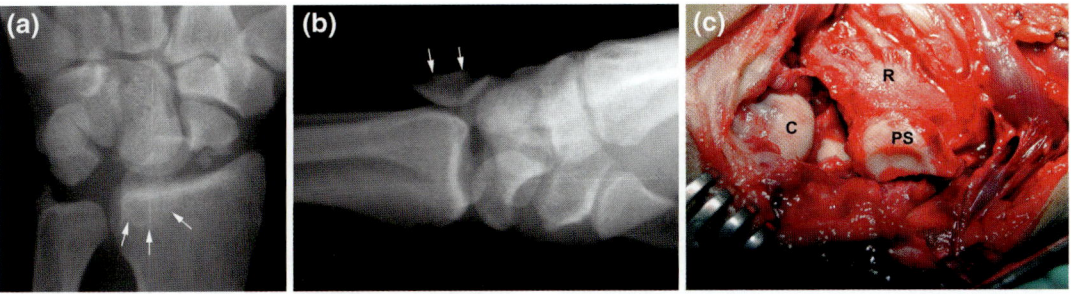

Fig. 4.73 A case with trans-scaphoid perilunate dislocation with the proximal pole of the scaphoid displaced dorsally (*arrows*) (**a**, **b**); it was lying on the dorsal surface of the radius and was detached from the lunate (**c**); (*PS* Proximal pole of the scaphoid, *R* Radius, *C* Capitate)

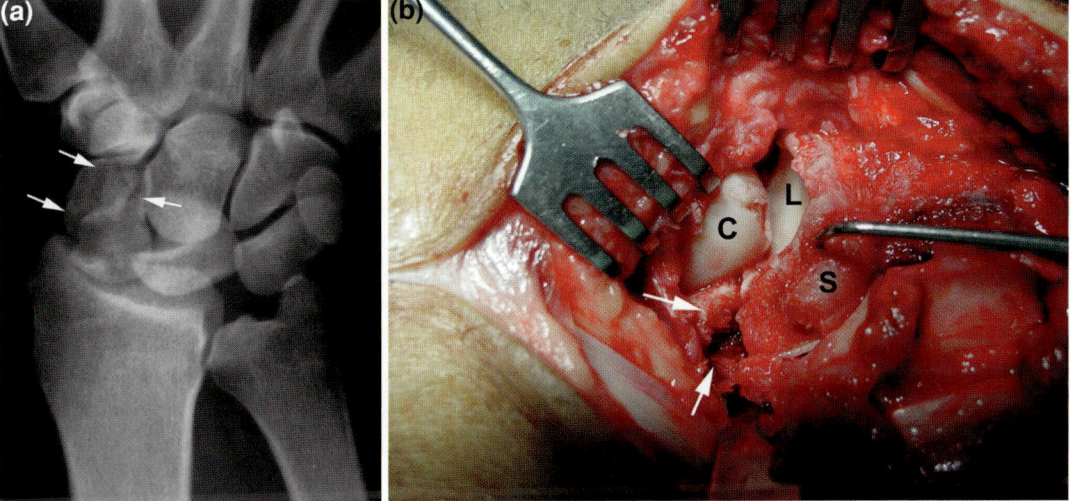

Fig. 4.74 A trans-scaphoid perilunate dislocation with comminution distal to the scaphoid waist (*arrows*) (**a**); an extensive osteochondral defect is detected at the capitate head (**b**) (*C* Capitate, *L* Lunate, *S* Proximal scaphoid)

Regardless of the type of injury (probably more frequently with greater arc injuries), the fracture of the ulnar styloid, is quite a common finding and it must be evaluated in relation to the integrity of the ulnocarpal ligaments and the stability of the DRU joint.

4.7.6 The Reconstruction

An important part of any open reduction is removing bone, cartilage, and soft tissue debris, by thoroughly irrigating the joint [9, 21].

4.7.6.1 Lesser Arc Injuries

Palmar Repair

In unreduced PLD cases, the lunate is reduced under direct vision, by manually pushing it in a dorsal direction while longitudinal traction on the hand is applied. With the lunate reduced, the constant finding of the transverse rent in the volar capsule is easily visualized. Suturing of the palmar rent precedes any dorsal reconstruction to prevent redislocation during the remainder of the operative procedure. Nonabsorbable suture (3-0) is used to repair this rent in the

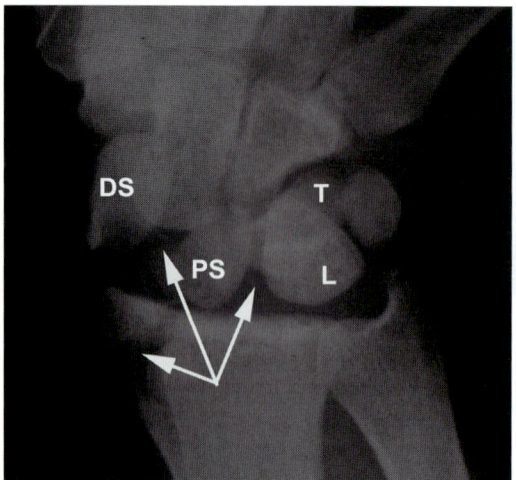

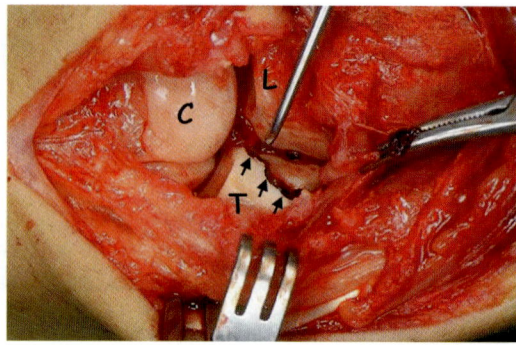

Fig. 4.76 Fracture of the radiovolar surface of the triquetrum (*arrows*) after the reduction of the dislocation (*L* Lunate, *C* Capitate, *T* Triquetrum). With permission from [231]

Fig. 4.75 A trans-styloid, trans-scaphoid dorsal perilunate dislocation associated with rupture of the SL ligament (*arrows*) (*DS* Distal scaphoid, *PS* Proximal scaphoid, *T* Triquetrum, *L* Lunate)

capsule. Care must be taken to place the sutures deep enough to include the deep ligamentous structures in the repair, since they are covered with a synovial layer that renders them indiscernible. It is usual practice to suture the whole length of the capsular rent, including the space of Poirier. However, we agree with Garcia-Elias [5] who stated that suturing should not include the space of Poirier (which is by nature a free space), since by closing this anatomically defined space with sutures, a palmar midcarpal stiffness may follow. Thus, our concern is focused on the radial and ulnar limb of the rent (Fig. 4.79a, b).

Suturing of the radial limb usually involves the sulcus between the RSC and long RL ligaments, while in cases where the RSC ligament is found disrupted or avulsed from the radius, it is also repaired using nonabsorbable sutures or with bone anchor to the radius. At present, the palmar SL ligament cannot be repaired, as it is covered by the intact long RL ligament. However, this seems to be of no concern, since the dorsal SL ligament is repaired and the SL joint is stabilized with K-wires; probably in the future, repairing the palmar SL ligament will become a matter of interest.

Attention is then turned to the ulnar limb of the rent, which is one of the main reasons for the palmar approach. It is essential to suture the palmar LT ligament, which is the strongest and most important part of the LT ligament. In cases where the volar LT ligament is avulsed with osseous articular fragment from the volar surface of the triquetrum, repair could be performed by inserting a bone anchor to the triquetrum. In rare, for lesser arc injury, cases where the capsular rent continues ulnarly to include the ulnocarpal ligaments, their suturing is equally important.

Once the volar rent has been repaired, attention is drawn dorsally, while the palmar wound is closed only at the skin level and at the end of the procedure.

Dorsal Repair

As during assessment of injuries, similarly during reconstruction, it is advisable to follow a specific sequence of steps. Different surgeons show a preference to a different sequence of reconstruction [111]. We, however, recommend the following order for dorsal repair:

As a preliminary step, it is often helpful to place 1.6 mm K-wires transversely into the scaphoid and the triquetrum using an inside-out technique, while the lunate is still free of ligamentous support. These K-wires are advanced until they reach the articular surfaces of the bones adjacent to the lunate, exiting radially and

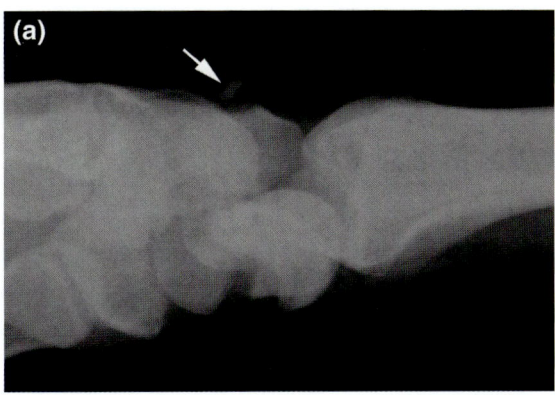
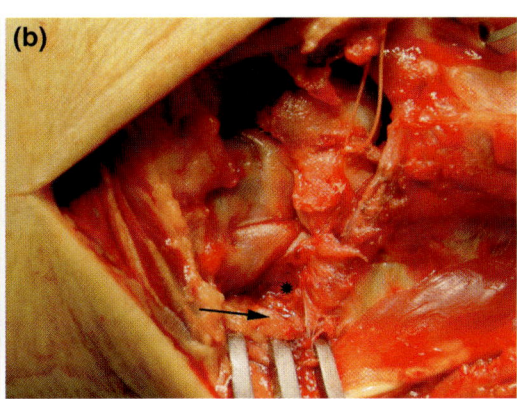

Fig. 4.77 A trans-scaphoid dorsal perilunate dislocation associated with an avulsion fracture fragment from the dorsal triquetrum (*arrow*) (**a**); the avulsed fragment originates from an area in which the DRC and DIC ligaments are attached (*asterisk*) (**b**)

ulnarly [37], and will be used later to stabilize the SL and LT joints.

Preparation of SL ligament repair. Before reducing the scapholunate interosseous interval, it is desirable to first place the sutures for repair depending on the type of SL injury. Direct repair of the ligament is preferred, provided that the ligament is of sufficient quality. This ligament is usually avulsed off bone, either the scaphoid or the lunate and is only rarely ruptured at its midsubstance. The bony bed is prepared by removing any interposed soft tissue. Creating a

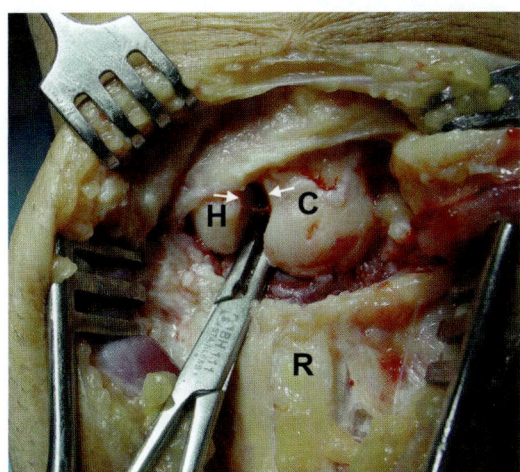

Fig. 4.78 In 4.4 % of our patients with greater arc injuries, a capito-hamate dissociation (*arrows*) was found (*H* Hamate, *C* Capitate, *R* Radius)

bleeding surface is not necessary in acute cases. One or two suture anchors are placed into the bed and used to repair the dorsal portion of the ligament later on. Any osteochondral fragment that may still be attached to the ligament is preserved and incorporated into the repair for better suture retention and healing potential [8]. Alternatively [188], drill holes are placed in the scaphoid pole or the lunate, exiting along the radial ridge of the scaphoid or the dorsal pole of the lunate. In this technique, the sutures are passed though the SLIL and then through the scaphoid or the lunate, to reapproximate and suture the SLIL later on. The sutures are not secured and tightened, until after scapholunate reduction and pinning have been performed. Skoff et al. [189] compared the classic Bunnell technique with that of bone anchors and found that both are equally strong with loads up to 40 N. However, the transosseous sutures technique is more demanding technically, lengthens the operative time, and there is always the risk of bone fracture (Fig. 4.80a–f). Conversely, bone anchors are easily applied and reduce the operative time, although there is concern over their fatigue strength (Fig. 4.70b).

Reduction of the SL joint. We prefer the joystick method by placing one 1.6 mm K-wire into the lunate and another one into the proximal scaphoid in a dorsal to palmar direction. The K-wires are advanced until they reach the palmar

Fig. 4.79 The midcarpal rent (**a**) probably needs to be sutured only to its radial and ulnar limb, in order to avoid postoperative stiffness

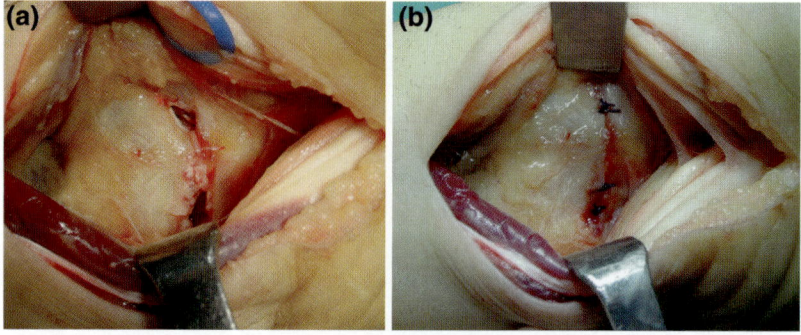

Fig. 4.80 A case of dorsal perilunate dislocation (**a**, **b**); the SL ligament was repaired with transosseous sutures (**c**, **d**) and stabilized using K-wires (**e**, **f**) (*S* Scaphoid, *L* Lunate). With permission from [231]

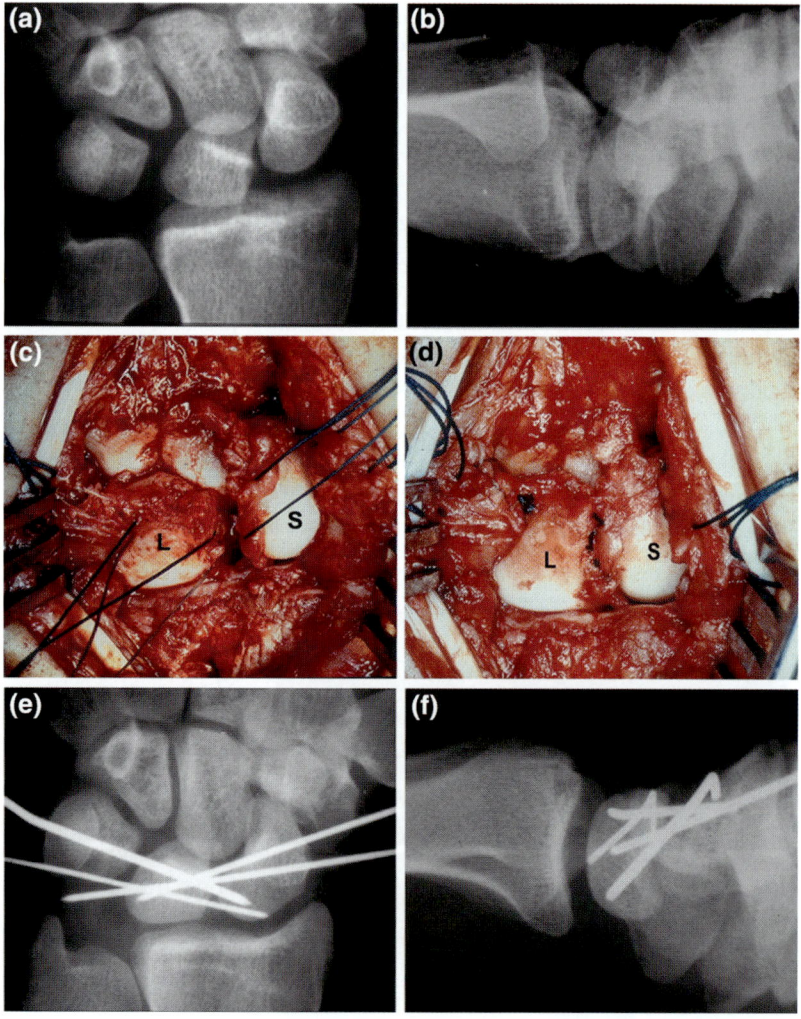

cortex of the bones, so they can be used as levers to reduce the scapholunate joint. The K-wires are introduced divergently in a way that after becoming parallel, they reduce the palmar flexion of the scaphoid and the dorsiflexion of the lunate. The compression of the SL joint is

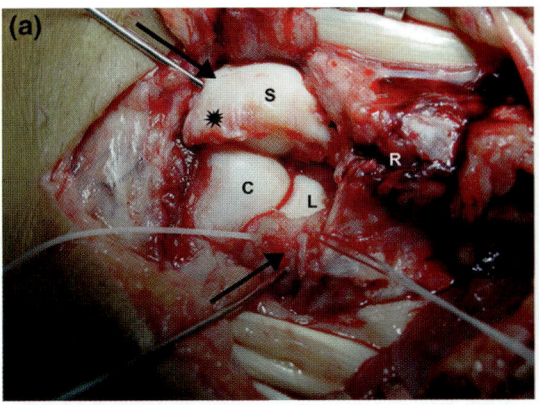
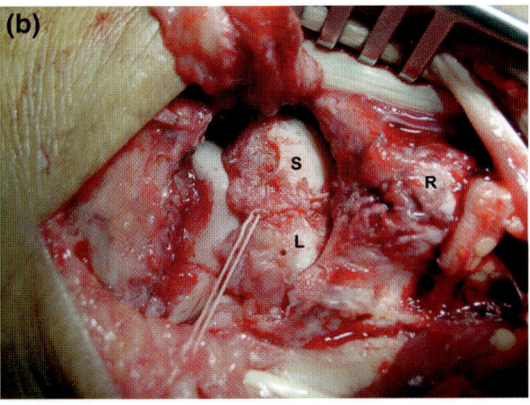
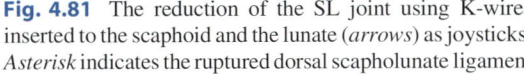

Fig. 4.81 The reduction of the SL joint using K-wires inserted to the scaphoid and the lunate (*arrows*) as joysticks. *Asterisk* indicates the ruptured dorsal scapholunate ligament (**a**). Its reconstruction was accomplished using two bone anchors inserted to the lunate (**b**) (*S* Scaphoid, *L* Lunate, *C* Capitate, *R* Radius)

accomplished by using a strong plier, which compresses both K-wires at their insertions to the bone, while at the same time an assistant is keeping apart the top of the wires (Fig. 4.81a, b). At that stage, it is important to control the proximal contour of the SL joint for proximal–distal displacement, by using a blunt Freer elevator to support the radioscapholunate joint. Alternatively, a towel clip can be used to compress the two bones together [40, 161].

Pinning of the SL interval is usually accomplished with two K-wires placed through the anatomic snuffbox, from the scaphoid to the lunate bone or by using the inside-out technique described earlier. An additional K-wire is advanced from the scaphoid waist region into the body of the capitate to prevent scaphoid flexion (Fig. 4.82a–d).

The *scapholunate ligament repair* is completed by tying the previously placed sutures through the bone anchors or the drill holes. The endings of the sutures are kept in order to be used later to repair the proximal part of the DIC ligament and the capsule.

Preparation of LT ligament repair. Frequently, there is no sufficient dorsal lunotriquetral ligament remaining for direct repair and we do not consider it an issue, since its biomechanically important palmar part has been

repaired. However, in cases of avulsion of LT ligament from bone, with or without an osseous fragment, it is advisable to repair it with a bone anchor, which we usually use either way, to repair the dorsal capsuloligamentous structures. However, to repair [108] or not [106, 190] the dorsal LT ligament is a matter of controversy.

Reduction of the LT joint. The triquetrum will typically assume an extended position and needs to be flexed relative to the lunate. The reduction is accomplished by using the joystick method and is judged by visualizing the distal contour of the lunate and triquetrum at the midcarpal joint. Two K-wires are inserted percutaneously from the ulnar side across the lunotriquetral joint, from the triquetrum into the lunate or by advancing into the lunate the K-wires that had been placed with the inside-out technique. Sometimes it is more convenient to introduce the K-wires in reverse, from lunate to triquetrum after palmarflexion of the wrist (Fig. 4.83a–i).

The adequacy of reduction of the proximal carpal row is best assessed by visualizing the midcarpal joint, after applying traction to the hand. There should be no step-off or rotation between the distal contours of the proximal carpal bones. Their flat dorsal surfaces should be smoothly aligned [161], while any exposed articular surface indicates incomplete reduction [7].

Fig. 4.82 A dorsal perilunate dislocation (**a, b**) where after ligamentous reconstruction, the LT and SL joints were stabilized using K-wires. An additional K-wire was inserted to the capitate to prevent scaphoid rotation. At the end of the procedure, an external fixator was applied (**c, d**)

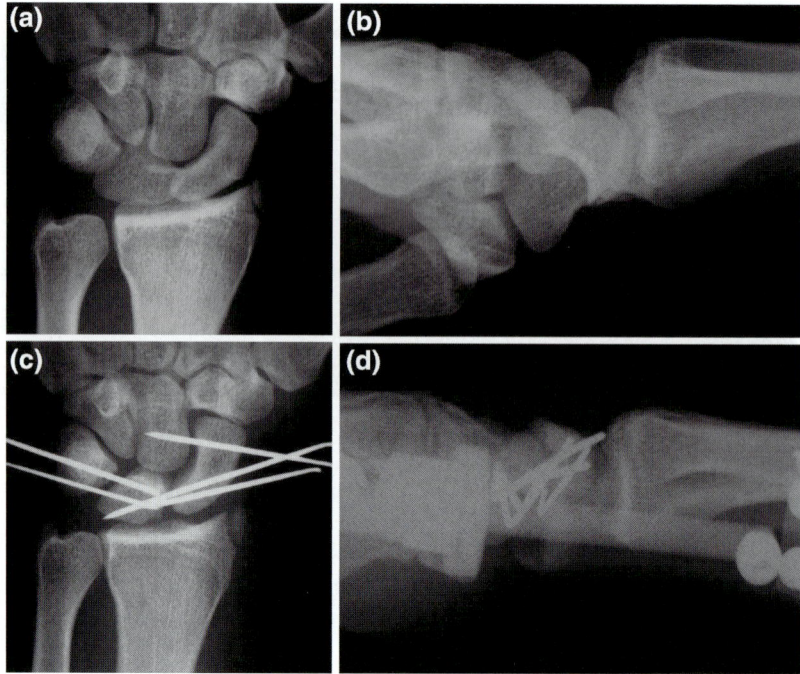

Repair of the DRC ligament. The repair technique depends on the type of ligament injury. If the DRC ligament has avulsed from the distal radius or the triquetrum, it is repaired with suture anchor(s) placed along the dorsal lip of the radius or the dorsal surface of the triquetrum. Midsubstance tears are repaired, using nonabsorbable sutures.

Repair of the dorsal capsuloligamentous structures. Repairing of these structures depends on the type of capsular approach. With longitudinal arthrotomy, the dorsal capsule should be repaired anatomically whenever possible. If a ligament splitting capsulotomy has been used, the radially based flap is brought down, suturing its apex to the triquetrum. Equally important is to reattach the proximal part of the DIC ligament, using the sutures of the previously inserted anchors to the scaphoid or the lunate [191] (Fig. 4.84a–g). The borders of the flap are sutured next, followed by retinacular repair in an effort to relocate the EPL to its original position. Finally, the palmar and dorsal wounds are closed only at the skin level.

Fluoroscopy or X-rays are used to confirm reduction and adequate placement of K-wires, which may be left percutaneous or buried beneath the skin. At the end of the procedure, we usually stabilize the wrist with an external fixator, mainly as a stress-shield, as it reduces strain on fractured bones and torn/stretched ligaments during healing [47, 192, 193] and also, to block the axial load of the cartilage on the injured proximal carpal row and maintain normal carpal alignment during the initial stages of ligament healing [143]. The external fixator and the trans-articular K-wires are removed 6 weeks postoperatively.

Several authors prefer to start the reconstruction by rebuilding the dislocated wrist around the lunate [1]. This is accomplished by securing the relationship of the lunate to the lunate fossa of the radius by inserting a K-wire temporarily, between the radial metaphysis and the reduced lunate [9, 21, 43, 86, 194]. Others, prefer to use this technique when there are difficulties in restoring carpal alignment despite the joystick method [7, 8], while some [15, 22], prefer to transfix the lunate to the capitate with a

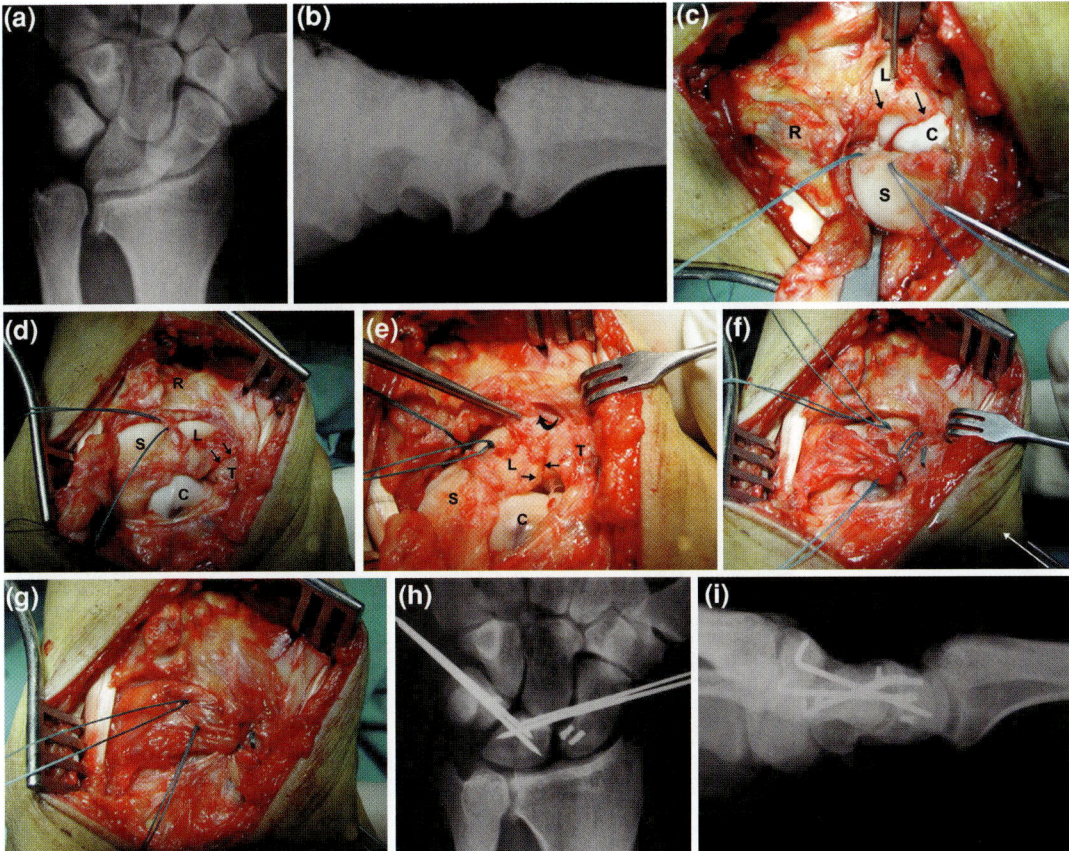

Fig. 4.83 A dorsal perilunate dislocation (Stage II) (**a**, **b**); the SL ligament was detached from the scaphoid (*arrows*) (**c**); after repairing the SL ligament using bone anchors and stabilizing the SL complex with K-wires, the dorsal LT ligament was detached from the triquetrum (*arrows*) (**d**); the dorsal LT ligament was inverted (*curved arrow*) while a step-off between lunate and triquetrum is illustrated (*double arrows*) (**e**); using a bone anchor inserted to the triquetrum, reconstruction of the dorsal LT and the DIC ligament was accomplished, while the LT joint was stabilized using a K-wire (*arrow*) (**f**, **g**); postoperative x-rays (**h**, **i**). With permission from [231]

K-wire, followed by the reduction and transfixion of the scaphoid to the lunocapitate complex.

Much perturbation exists in the literature when, after anatomical reduction and pinning of the SL joint, the dorsal SLIL is torn in such a way that it cannot be securely repaired. When encountered with this situation, we believe that it is of the outmost importance to fix the proximal DIC ligament and the dorsal capsule to the remnants of the dorsal SLIL, in order to reinforce the sutured ligament and provide a collagen substance to the repaired ligament [3]. In addition it has been suggested that direct suturing of the ligaments themselves is not always necessary, provided that there is no other tissue interposition [2, 47] and that even suboptimal ligamentous suturing may lead to an acceptable functional result, on the premise that free osteochondral fragments have been removed and the scapholunate joint has been anatomically reduced [138]. Various types of capsulodesis [1, 8, 21, 22, 40, 86, 195] or tenodesis [196–198] have also been proposed in such circumstances, but we never had to use them in acute cases.

A number of authors [2, 106, 110, 138], has been using K-wires to bridge the radiocarpal and/or midcarpal joints in order to ensure the axial alignment of the lunate. With the exception of the K-wire used to stabilize the scaphocapitate joint and rarely the triquetrohamate joint, we

Fig. 4.84 A dorsal perilunate dislocation (**a, b**); the dorsal portion of the SL ligament was detached from the lunate and its proximal portion from the scaphoid (*arrows*) (**c**); two bone anchors inserted to the scaphoid and lunate, were used for reconstruction (**d**); after reattachment of the dorsal capsular flap, sutures from the bone anchor immobilized the DIC ligament (*arrows*) (**e**); postoperative X-rays (**f, g**). With permission from [231]

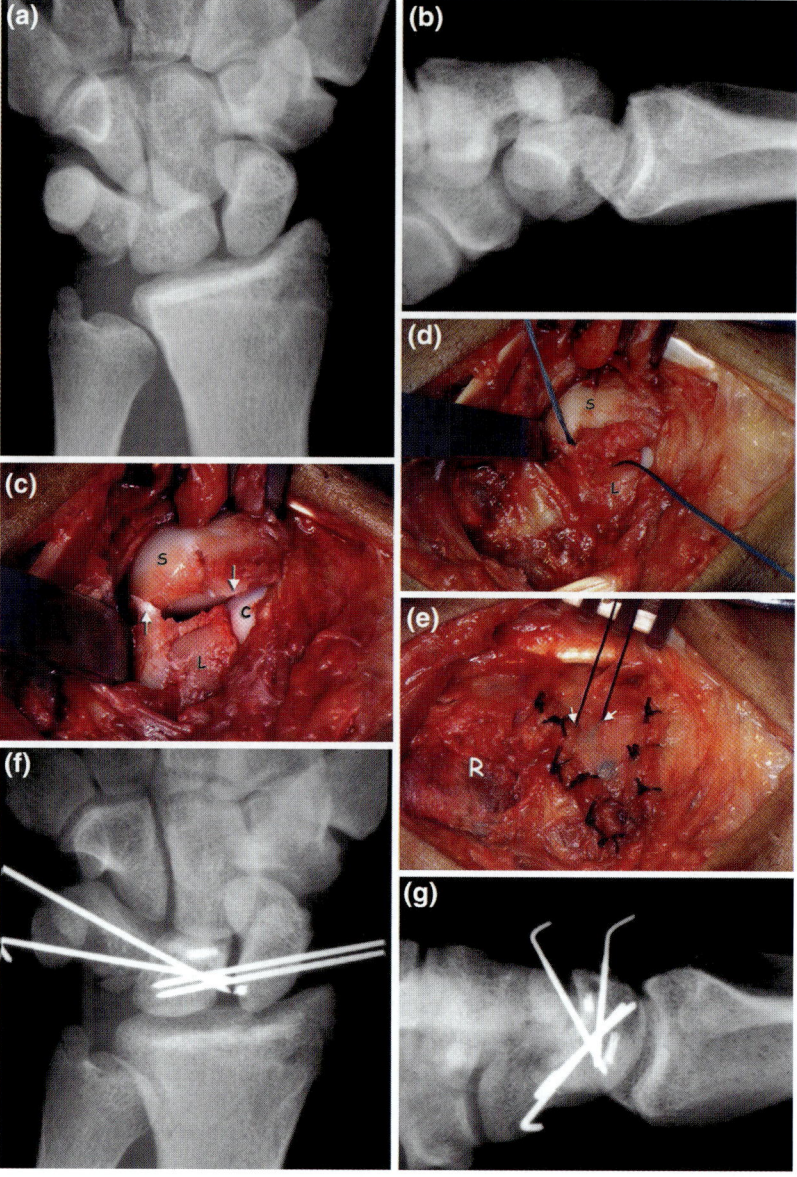

usually avoid bridging radiocarpal or midcarpal joints with K-wires, when we are dealing with injuries treated in the acute phase. The avoidance of bridging K-wires is due to the increased risk of pin loosening, chondrolysis, and broken hardware [8].

Many surgeons feel that the most critical issue in lesser arc injury is the repair of the SLIL. K-wires were traditionally used to protect the SLIL repair. However, concerns over pin tract infection and inability to provide adequate compression, have led some to advocate more rigid fixation of the scapholunate joint [7, 38]. Temporary headed or headless screws fixation [109, 161] or intraosseous cerclage [99, 140] between the scaphoid and lunate, have been described as methods for providing stronger fixation to preserve alignment during the critical period of ligamentous healing. Advantages of these techniques include subdermal location, decreased infection risk, increased stability, and the ability to apply compression. Furthermore,

Fig. 4.85 Excision of the lunate in a case with volar lunate dislocation (**a**), resulted in wrist collapse. Four months postoperatively, the scaphoid is palmarly flexed (*curved arrow*), the triquetrum translates distally and medially along the helicoidally shaped articular surface of the hamate (*straight arrow*) and the capitate migrates proximally (**b**). With permission from [231]

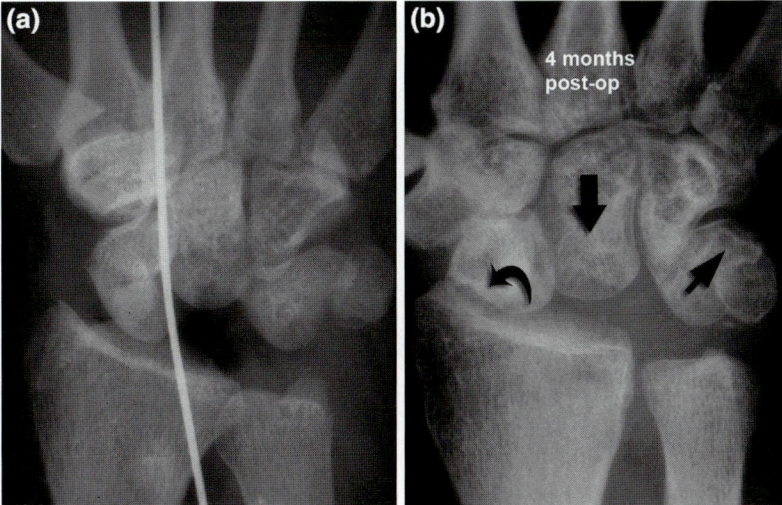

theoretically these patients may be started at an earlier ROM protocol [120]. Potential drawbacks include the need for a secondary surgical procedure usually at 5–6 months [40] to remove the implants, which are often broken with return of ROM [140]. However, in a comparison study of the two methods of fixation (temporary screws vs K-wires) on 18 patients (nine wrists in each group), the results were comparable in radiographic or clinical outcomes [109].

Excision of the lunate is not accepted in any acute case (Fig. 4.85a, b).

4.7.6.2 Greater Arc Injuries

Palmar Repair

Repairing of the transverse palmar rent is performed as has been previously described for lesser arc injuries. As already mentioned, rupture of the ulnocarpal ligaments is more frequent in greater arc injuries and we believe their reconstruction with nonabsorbable sutures is of paramount importance. Probably one of the reasons for the high frequency of ulnocarpal translation in perilunate injuries, as mentioned by Song et.al [199], is the unrecognized and unrepaired ruptures of the ulnocarpal and DRC ligaments. A number of authors [1, 6, 22], have occasionally fixed the midwaist fractures of the

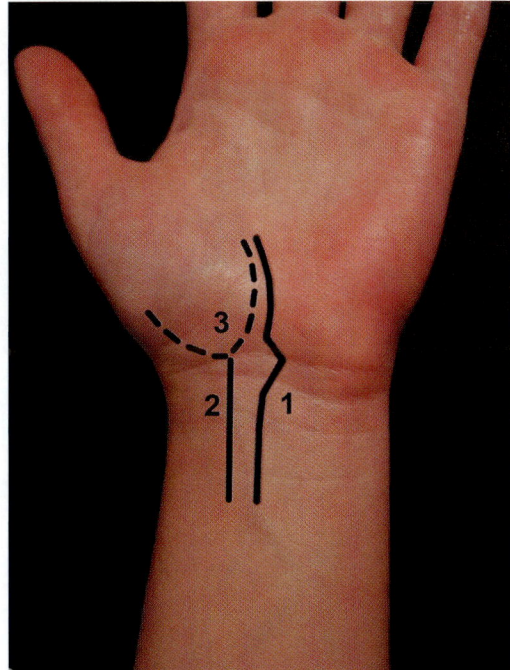

Fig. 4.86 The extended carpal tunnel approach (*1*), the Henry's approach (*2*), and the modification of the palmar approach (*3*) [14]

scaphoid with a cannulated screw, by advancing it from distal to proximal, using a modification of the palmar approach [5, 14, 200] (Fig. 4.86). However, we believe that additional capsular incision (with division of RSC and even STT

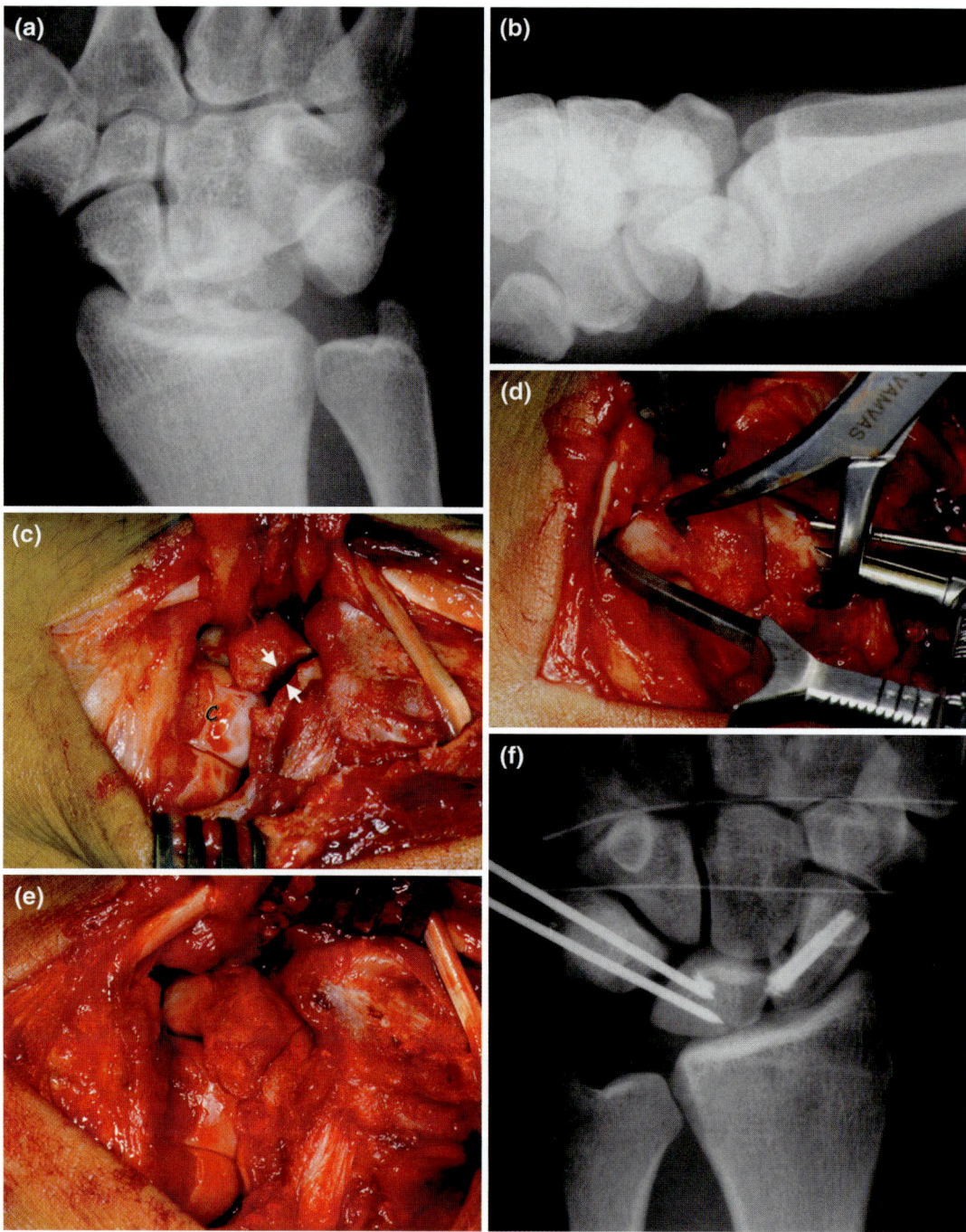

Fig. 4.87 A trans-scaphoid dorsal perilunate dislocation (**a**, **b**); after the reduction of the dislocation, the dorsal approach reveals the fractured scaphoid (*arrows*) (**c**); compression with a towel clip, temporary fixation with a K-wire, and cannulated screw application using the jig (**d**); anatomical reduction and fixation of the scaphoid (**e**); postoperative x-rays (**f**, **g**); 3 years postop the development of midcarpal joint stenosis is noted (*arrows*) (**h**). With permission from [231]

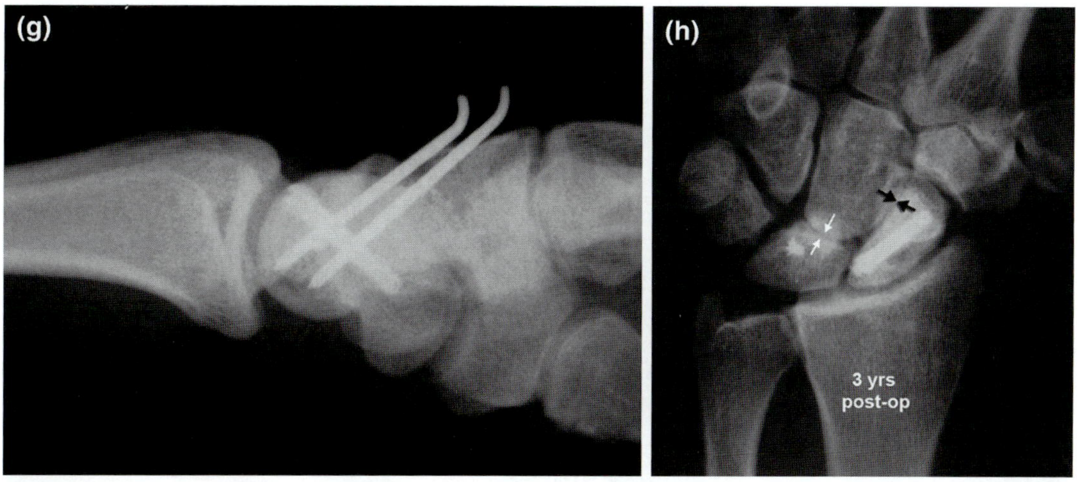

Fig. 4.87 (continued)

ligaments), which is necessary to insert the cannulated screw, could destabilize further an already unstable wrist. Consequently, we have not used a palmar incision to internally fix the fractures of the proximal pole or the waist of the scaphoid. The distal pole fractures possibly constitute an exception and are better treated with K-wires, using the palmar approach.

Dorsal Repair

In addition to the dorsal capsuloligamentous repair that has already been described in lesser arc injuries, the main fracture that must be dealt with, is the scaphoid fracture. The combined fractures of the scaphoid and capitate are analyzed in Chap. 5. Anatomic reduction and compressive fixation of the scaphoid fracture are necessary. Use of K-wires or screw fixation is equally acceptable and is based on surgeon preference. If there is no comminution, the scaphoid fracture fragments are anatomically reduced and provisionally stabilized with an eccentrically placed K-wire. Next, a guide wire is inserted along the long axis of the scaphoid on both the anteroposterior and L views [43, 201]. A cannulated screw is inserted anterogradely (from the dorsal edge of the proximal pole aiming the palmar-distal scaphoid tuberosity) [5, 14, 17, 200, 202] (Figs. 4.87a–h, 4.88a–i).

The presence of comminution favors the fixation of the scaphoid with K-wires rather than a compressive screw. The scaphoid is reduced (often with the use of 2 K-wires as joysticks), compressed (with the use of a towel clip), and stabilized with 2 K-wires, which are inserted from proximal to distal direction, exiting through the base of thenar. Alternatively, the K-wires are placed through the fracture surface to the distal fragment, before the reduction; after the fragments are anatomically reduced, the K-wires are advanced proximally to engage the proximal pole of the scaphoid (Fig. 4.89a–g). The comminution of the scaphoid fracture usually involves its dorsoradial surface and in this case autologous bone grafting from the distal radius could be used. When concomitant scaphoid fracture and SLIL injury are present, both injuries should be treated surgically. However, cross-fixation of the scaphoid to the lunate is recommended in any case, since the macroscopically intact SLIL does not necessarily ensure its biomechanical integrity (Fig. 4.90a–l).

Treatment of the LT interval follows. The triquetrum is reduced to the lunate, compressed, and pinned percutaneously with 2 K-wires. Any fracture of these bones must be identified, reduced, and fixed using any convenient method (K-wires, mini-screws, and bone anchor).

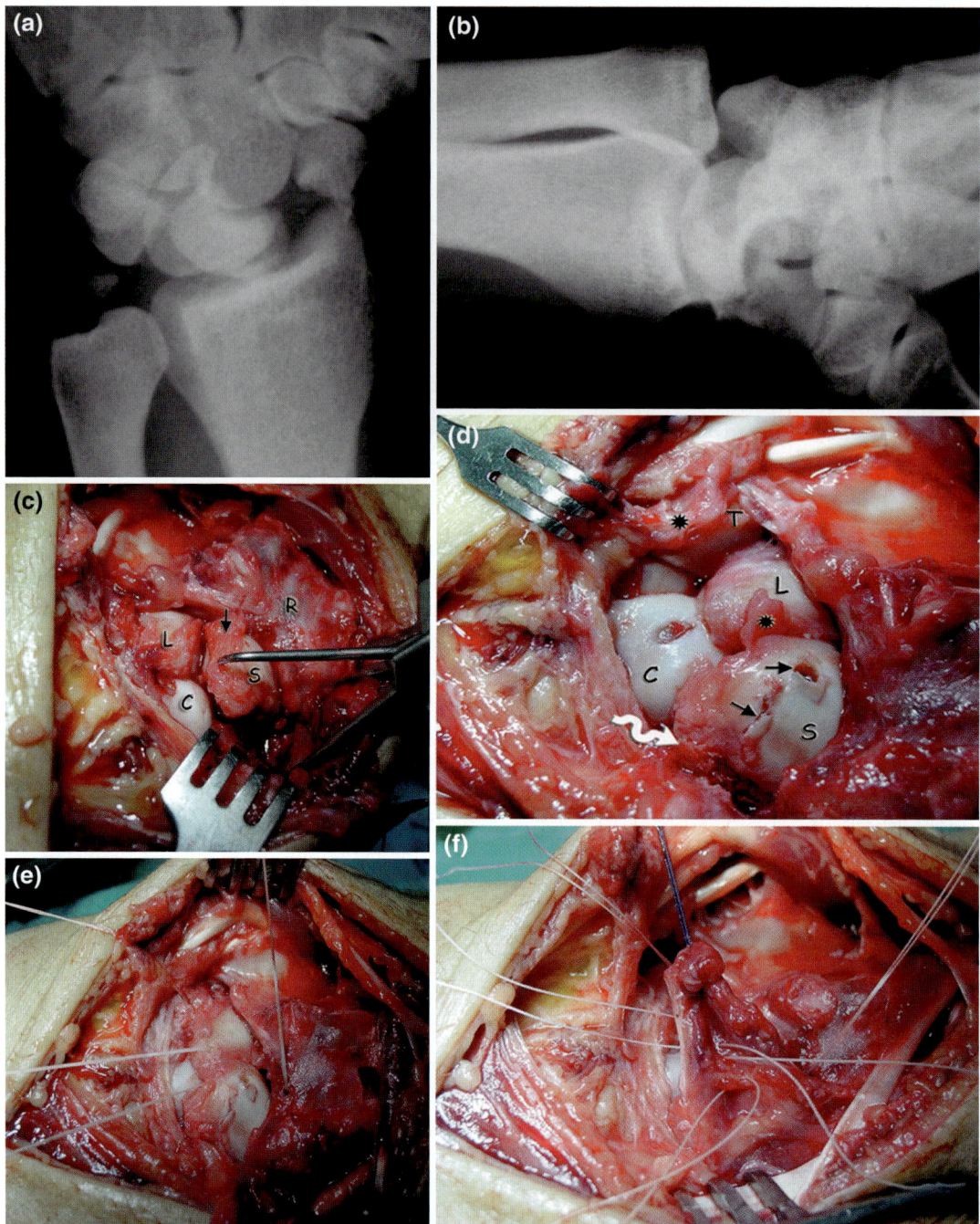

Fig. 4.88 A case with trans-scaphoid dorsal perilunate dislocation with displaced ulnar styloid fracture (**a**, **b**); It was treated with combined approach. The dorsal approach revealed avulsion of the SL ligament from the lunate (*arrow*) and a comminuted fracture of the scaphoid waist (**c**); Reduction and fixation of the scaphoid using a cannulated screw and autologous bone grafting from distal radius (*wavy arrow*). *Double arrows* indicate iatrogenic chondral injury produced during the insertion of the cannulated screw. The SL and LT ligaments were avulsed from the lunate (*asterisks*) (**d**); Capsuloligamentous reconstruction using absorbable bone anchors (**e**, **f**); postoperative (**g**) and final X-rays 6 months postinjury (**h**, **i**). With permission from [231]

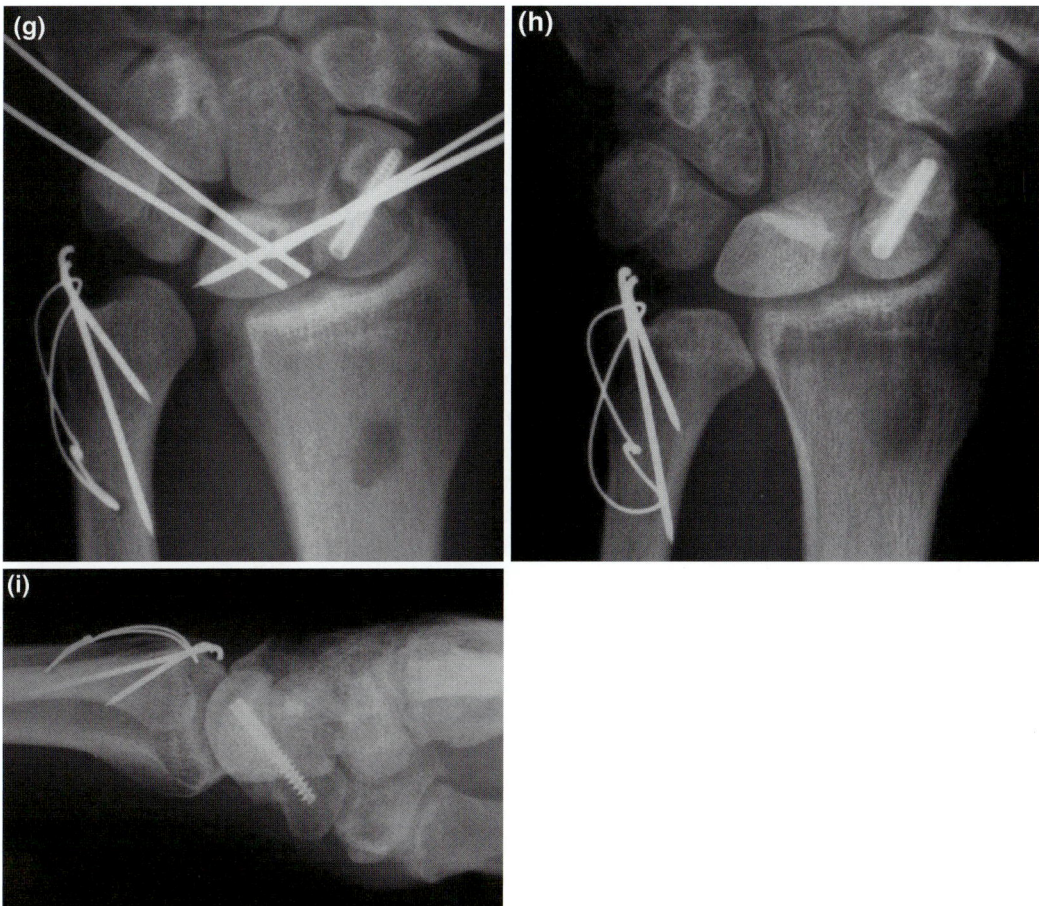

Fig. 4.88 (continued)

Fractures of the radial styloid and dorsal radial rim should be managed with a method depending on the size or comminution of the fracture. Headless screws, K-wires, bone anchors, and even low-profile plates could be used. Excision of fragments or part of the radial styloid is not an option [5, 161], since it could destabilize the radiocarpal joint (Fig. 4.91a–i).

It has been stated [3, 6] that in trans-radial styloid PLFD, it is not necessary to perform a palmar incision because the main palmar ligaments should be intact and displaced with the radial styloid. Nevertheless, in 12 out of 15 of our patients treated with combined approach, apart from the wide rupture of the palmar capsule, we found 2 cases with rupture of the ulnocarpal ligaments and 3 cases with fractured palmar lunate horn (Teisen type 1) [203], that required palmar reconstruction (Fig. 4.92a–e).

Cases with displaced fractures of the base of the ulnar styloid are approached through a separate longitudinal incision placed just palmar to the sixth dorsal compartment. A tension band technique is usually sufficient for stabilization of the ulnar styloid (Figs. 4.33f, 4.88g).

As in cases of lesser arc injuries, we usually stabilize the wrist, at the end of the procedure, with an external fixator maintaining the wrist in slight dorsiflexion, which is removed together with the trans-articular K-wires 6 weeks postoperatively. Alternatively, a short-arm splint could be used until stitches removal, which is then converted to short-arm cast for an average of 6 weeks.

Gunal et al. [204] contrary to the conventional methods, applied for a 10 weeks period a mini-external fixator between trapezium and lunate in two cases of TS-PLFD. One of them was treated with closed and the other with open reduction. As opposed to prevalent belief, they neither performed any ligamentous repair nor did they immobilize the wrist. Instead, they encouraged the patients to use their wrists freely, starting the day after operation. After 3.5 years follow-up, the clinical and radiological outcome was excellent.

4.8 Results

Evaluation of these injuries (treatment guidelines, long-term results) is difficult, since the literature does not always address a homogeneous group of patients. They were usually treated in different ways, at different chronic stages, and had different rehabilitation protocols applied. Below are some factors which are differentiating the result and are thus not comparable:

- Open or closed injuries?
- Which type of treatment (Closed, arthroscopically, or open reduction)?
- Diversity of surgical methods of reconstruction (K-wires or screws, repairing the ligaments or not).
- PLD or PLFD injuries?
- PLFD with fractured or intact scaphoid?
- Stage of displacement?
- Dorsal or volar perilunate injuries?
- Early or late management?
- Single (volar or dorsal) or combined approach?
- Duration and type of immobilization?
- Mid-term or long-term evaluation of the results?

Frequently, the literature reports refer to patients with different types of injuries and treatments [93, 100, 110, 170, 190], hence it is hard for the results to be credible. However, there are reports which, by referring to homogeneous groups of patients, allow drawing safer conclusions. As an example, there are reports concerning only patients with PLFD+S, who were treated operatively within 7–15 days post injury with either open reduction [18, 27, 108, 164, 167] or percutaneous fixation [106]. Others referred only to patients with acute PLD without scaphoid fracture [163, 205], to patients with chronic perilunate injuries (both PLD and PLFD) [206, 207], or to patients with chronic PLD [208].

Several authors [3, 209] have defended the superiority of open reduction and internal fixation over closed reduction and cast immobilization, concerning the functional result, while it is generally accepted that open injuries and delayed treatment are the most unfavorable factors affecting the long-term result.

It has been supported that greater arc have poorer prognosis than lesser arc injuries [100, 210]. Conversely, it has also been stated that the results of treatment for trans-scaphoid fracture-dislocations are generally better than for perilunate dislocations, because the fracture can heal to restore normal wrist kinematics, whereas in perilunate injuries the SLIL repair never results in normal function [181]. To complete the circle of conflicting reports, it has been argued that there are no significant differences between PLD and PLFD groups [13, 37, 169, 190] and that the only significant difference between these 2 groups is in the revised carpal height ratio, which in the PLD group had a larger value compared to the PLFD group [169].

The correlation between poor clinical result and radiological instability findings has been emphasized in patients with perilunate injuries (increased scapholunate interval and DISI alignment of the wrist) [2, 93, 210].

Despite optimal management, most patients experience loss of grip strength and motion and also develop radiographic signs of arthritis. However, these clinical measurements and radiographic changes do not correlate with patient satisfaction or their ability to return to work [13, 100, 110, 161].

Fig. 4.89 A trans-scaphoid volar dislocation of the lunate (Stage IV) to which an osseous fragment from the triquetrum (*arrow*) is attached through intact volar lunotriquetral ligament (**a**, **b**); dorsal approach reveals the fracture of the triquetrum (*arrows*), while absorbable bone anchors were introduced into the lunate for the reconstruction of the SL and LT ligaments (**c**); fixation of the fractured scaphoid and stabilization of the SL and LT joints with K-wires, while an external fixator was applied at the end to neutralize the applied loads (**d**, **e**); final X-rays 2 years postinjury (**f**, **g**). With permission from [231]

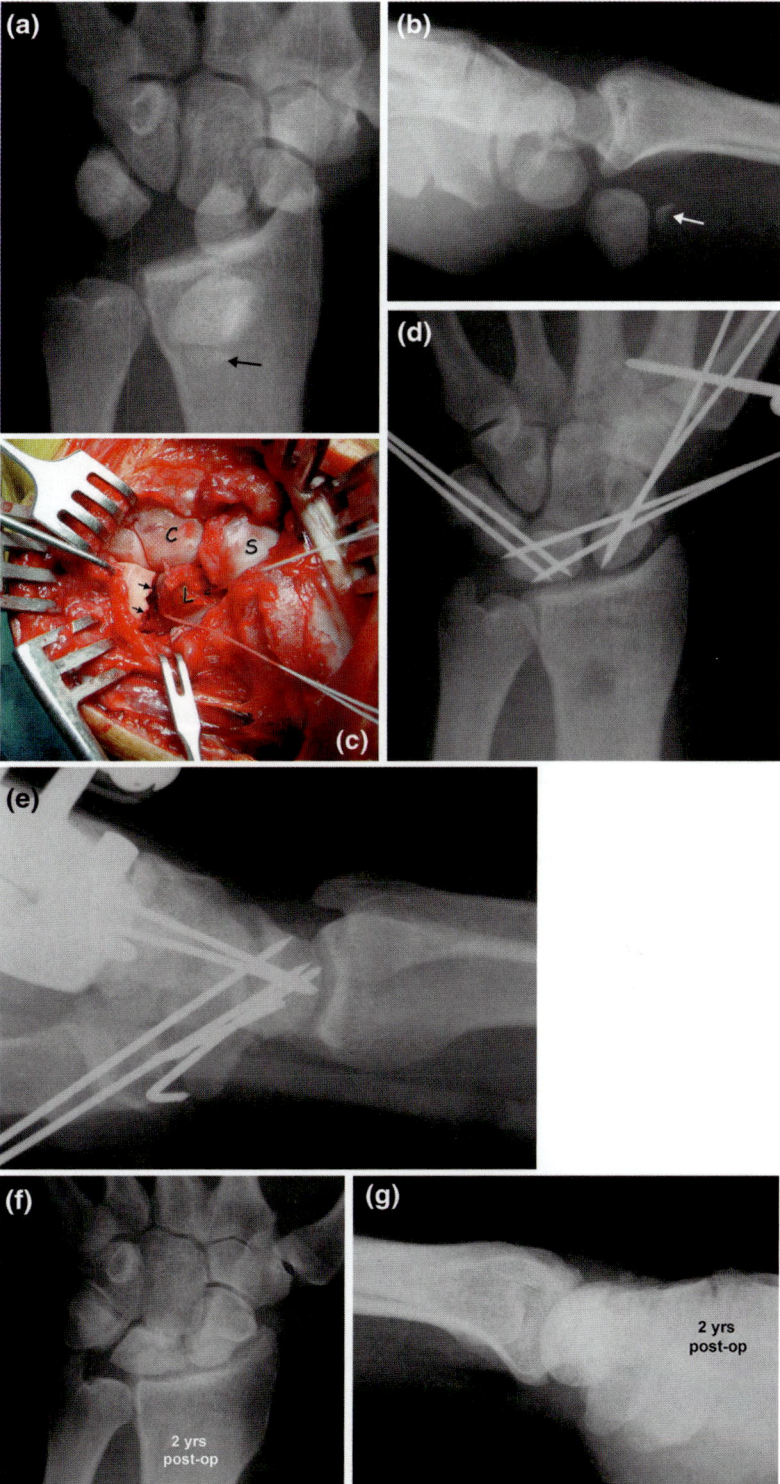

Fig. 4.90 Male 28-years old, with trans-scaphoid dorsal perilunate dislocation (**a**, **b**); He was treated with open reduction using only dorsal approach. The SL ligament macroscopically seems to be intact (*arrows*) (**c**); The scaphoid and the LT joint were stabilized using K-wires (**d**, **e**); 2 months later, there were no signs of scaphoid union the proximal pole of which showed signs of avascular necrosis, while the SL joint was widened (**f**); 5 months postoperatively, a SNAC wrist appearance was obvious (**g**); 16 months postinjury and after arthroscopic evaluation of the articular cartilage of the radioscaphoid joint, a scapholunocapitate fusion combined with lateral closing distal radial osteotomy for load redistribution was decided (**h**, **i**); 11 years postinjury, the X-ray and ROM were satisfactory (**j**–**l**), while the patient was symptoms free. With permission from [231]

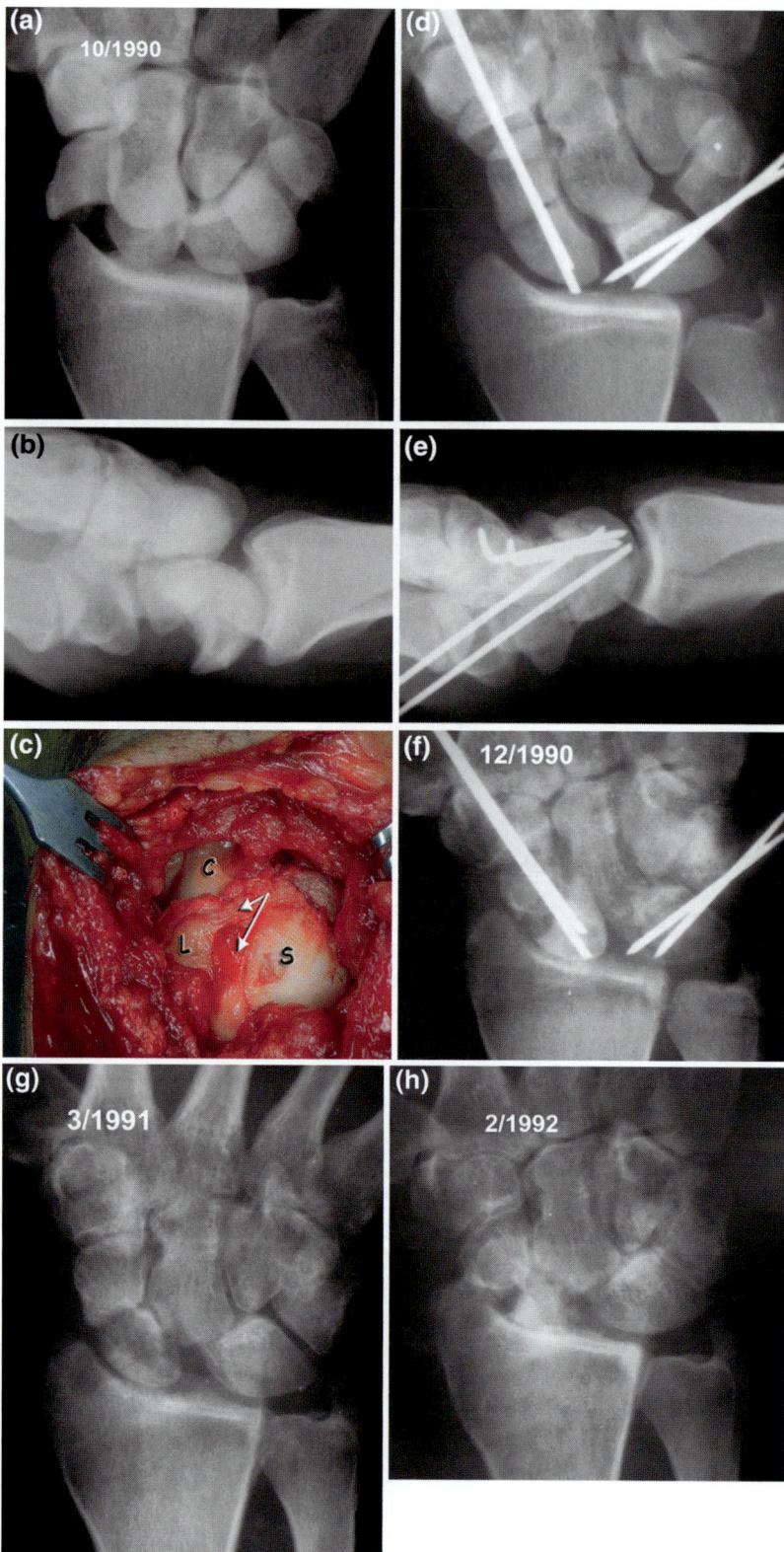

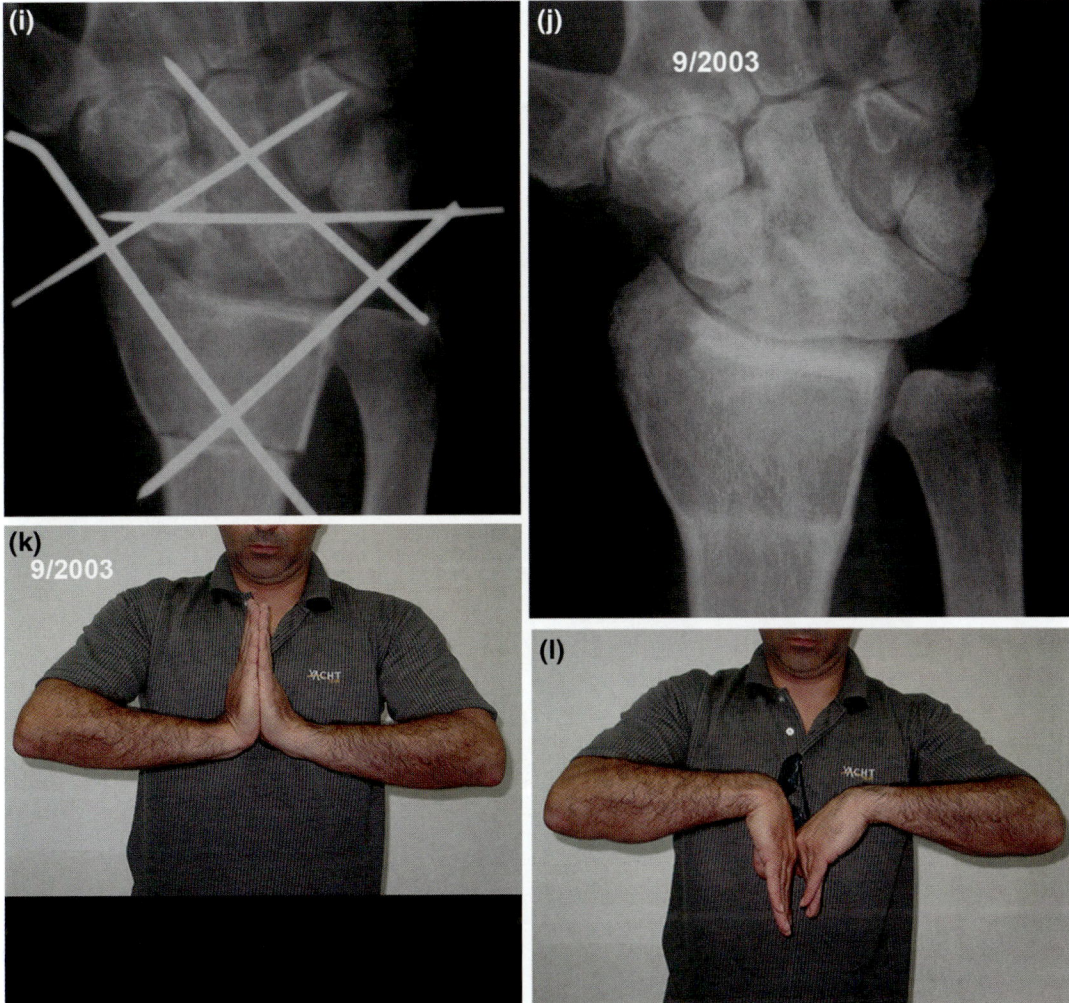

Fig. 4.90   (continued)

Hildebrand et al. [169] studied 22 patients (23 wrists) with some homogeneity: acute dorsal PLD or PLFD were treated in a similar fashion with combined operative approaches, fixation within the proximal carpal row, and postoperative immobilization for an average of 10 weeks. Results were estimated after mean follow-up of 37 months. Clinical examination revealed that flexion–extension, radioulnar deviation, and grip strength were 57, 58, and 73 %, respectively, in relation to the contralateral wrist. Radiographic measures showed an increase in the SL angle, a decrease in the revised carpal height ratio (which is contributed mainly to the loss of articular cartilage in the midcarpal joint), and development of arthritis in approximately 50 % of the cases. The Mayo wrist score was 66 and 73 % of the patients returned to full regular duties. The authors being worried over the results, which in spite of favorable conditions were suboptimal, pose the question whether operative or postoperative methods need to be modified; for instance, if earlier controlled motion can actually allow for improved ligament healing.

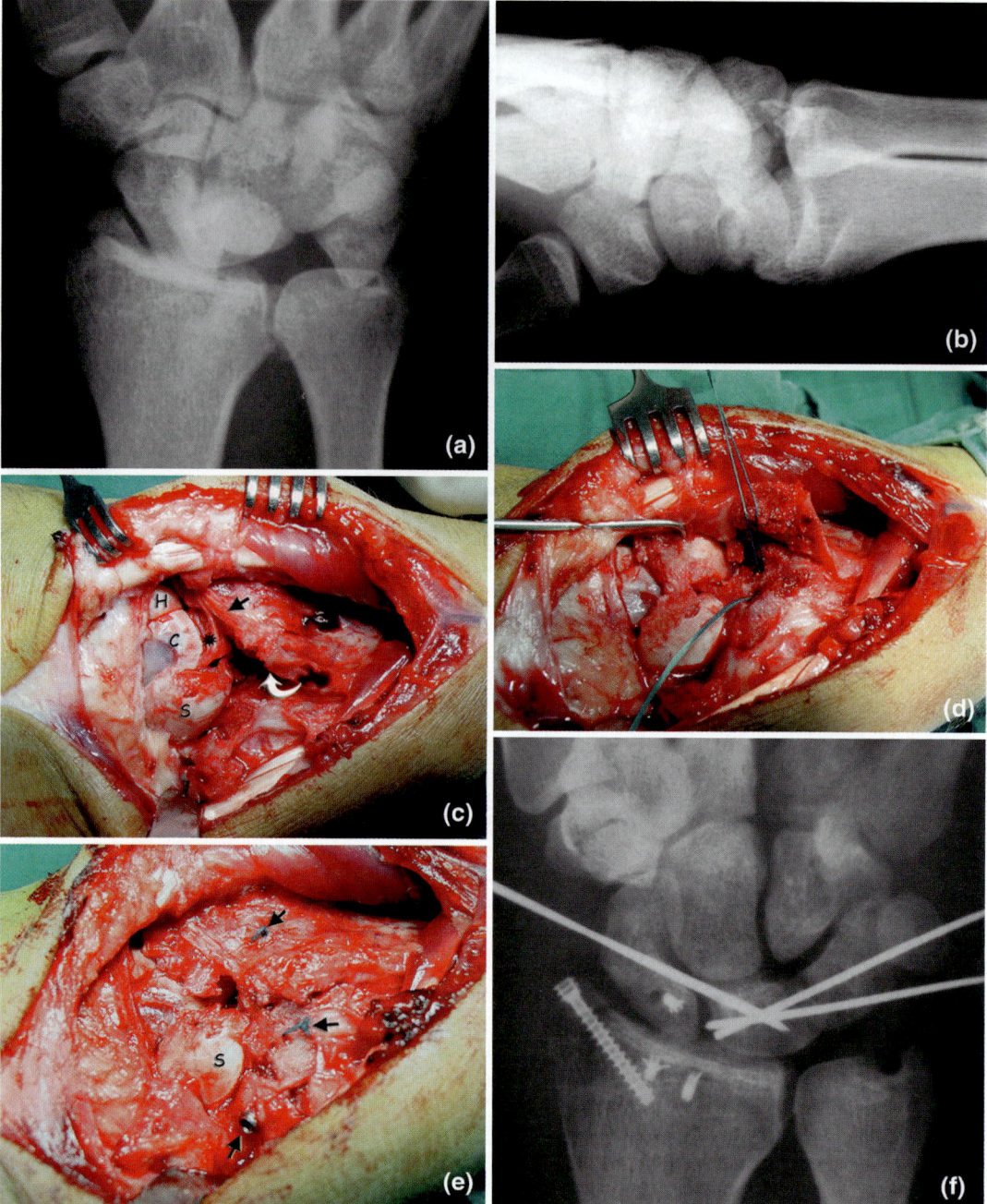

Fig. 4.91 A trans-styloid dorsal perilunate dislocation (**a**, **b**), was treated with open reduction with combined approaches; The dorsal approach revealed also a fracture of the dorsal radial rim (*curved arrow*), with the DRC ligament incorporated to the fracture fragment (*black arrow*), while the SL ligament was avulsed from the scaphoid (*asterisk*) (**c**); the reconstruction is accomplished using bone anchors and a cannulated screw for the radial styloid (*arrows*) (**d**, **e**); postoperative X-rays (**f**, **g**) and final X-rays 1 year later (**h**, **i**). With permission from [231]

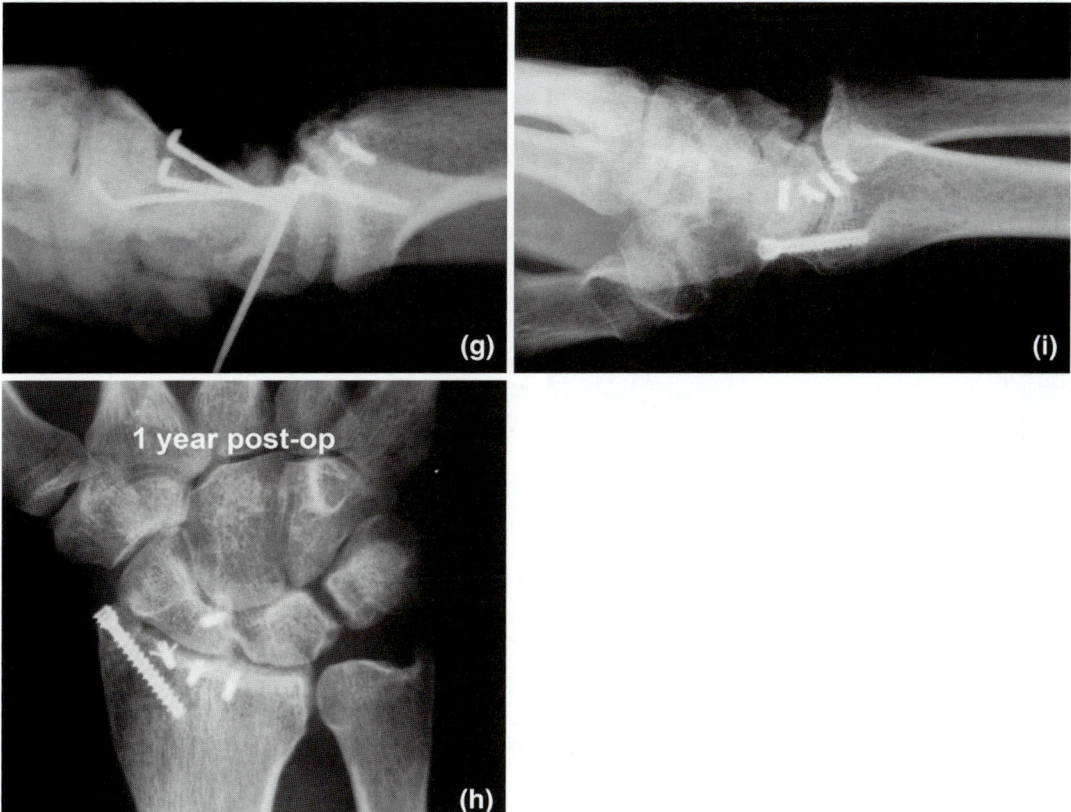

Fig. 4.91 (continued)

Komurcu et al. [211] compared six patients with PLFD treated acutely, with six patients whose treatment was delayed by an average of 26 days (range, 10–40 days). At an average follow-up of 45 months, patients in the early treatment group had better wrist ROM (129.5° vs. 95.5° flexion–extension arc), grip strength (34.0 vs. 26.3 kg), and clinical scores (89.2 vs. 72.5), while two of six patients in the delayed treatment group had radiographic evidence of midcarpal arthritis at final follow-up, compared to none in the early treatment group.

Inoue and Imaeda [167] studied 28 cases with TS-PLFD, which were divided into two groups depending on the postoperatively cast immobilization time (4 weeks and longer than 5 weeks of immobilization). They found that the postoperative cast immobilization time, seems to influence limitations in the range of wrist motion.

Inoue and Kuwahata [163], in a group of patients with perilunate dislocations without scaphoid fracture, found that patients who had scapholunate ligamentous repair and those who did not, had comparable clinical results. In the former group, however, the scapholunate relationship was maintained more consistently.

Minami and Kaneda [92] weighed the value of suturing the scapholunate ligament, by comparatively studying 32 patients with perilunate dislocations. Twelve of those patients had the scapholunate ligament sutured, whereas the remaining 20 did not. After a mean follow-up of 5 years, they concluded that the reconstruction of the SL ligament has better clinical and radiological results, compared to the patients who did not receive ligament reconstruction and that its suturing averts the development of wrist instability.

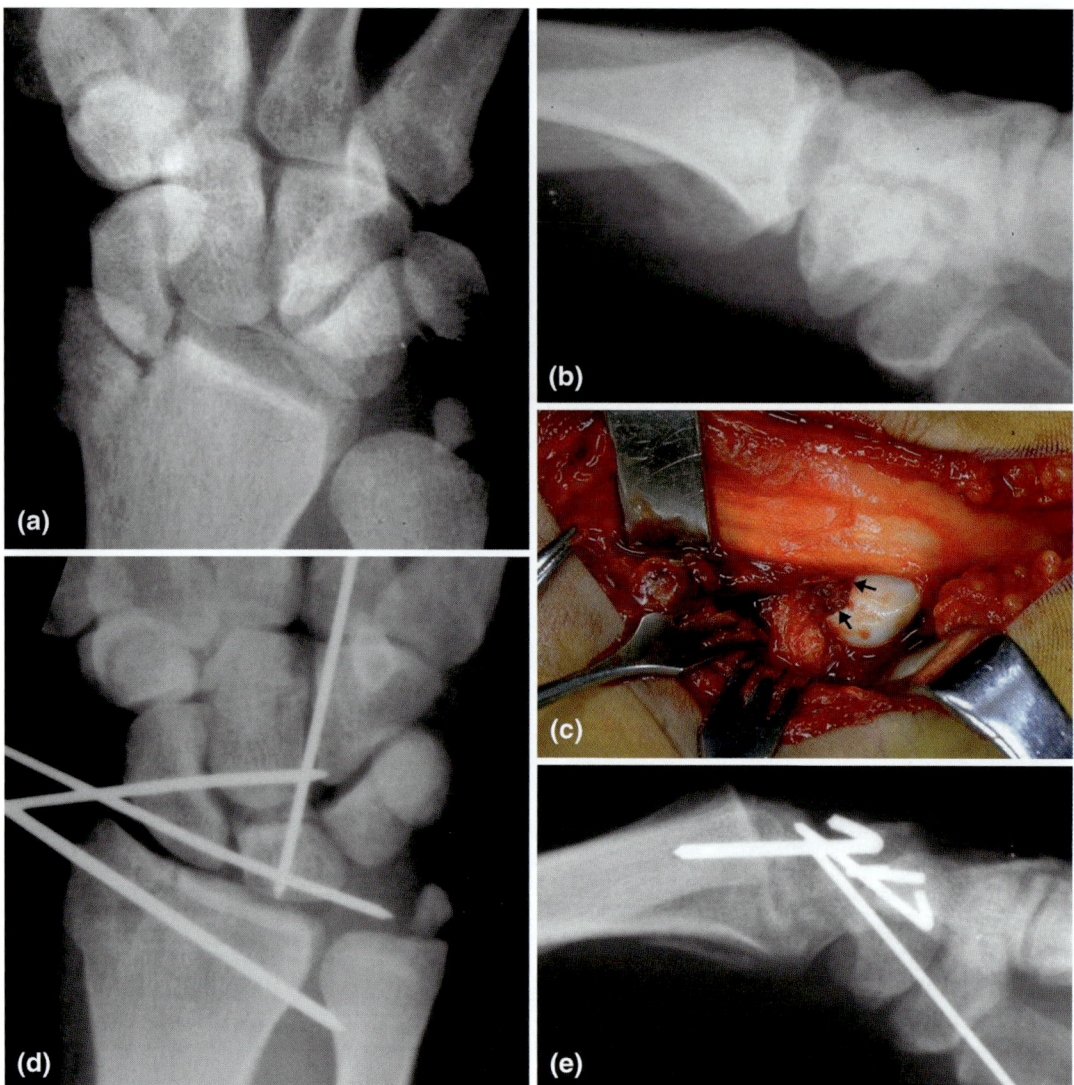

Fig. 4.92 A trans-styloid dorsal perilunate dislocation (**a**, **b**); the volar approach revealed a fracture of the palmar lunate horn (*arrows*) (**c**); which was held with a K-wire. Postoperative x-rays (**d**, **e**). With permission from [231]

Kremer et al. [190], in a study with 39 patients (9 PLD and 30 PLFD) found better outcome scores, in patients with partial denervation from anterior and posterior interosseous nerve resection, with normal SL angles, in white-collar workers, and in patients for whom a single dorsal or volar approach was sufficient for reduction.

Significant differences were also noted in the percentage of patients who returned to their previous employment following a perilunate injury. This percentage fluctuated between 45 [170] and 100 % [212].

As suggested by Garcia-Elias [5], patients with perilunate injuries required a long period of rehabilitation, which on average went up to 6 months, while they eventually gained 70 % range of motion and 75 % grip strength in comparison to their contralateral wrist. On the other hand, only one in three heavy manual workers returned to their previous employment. Dobyns

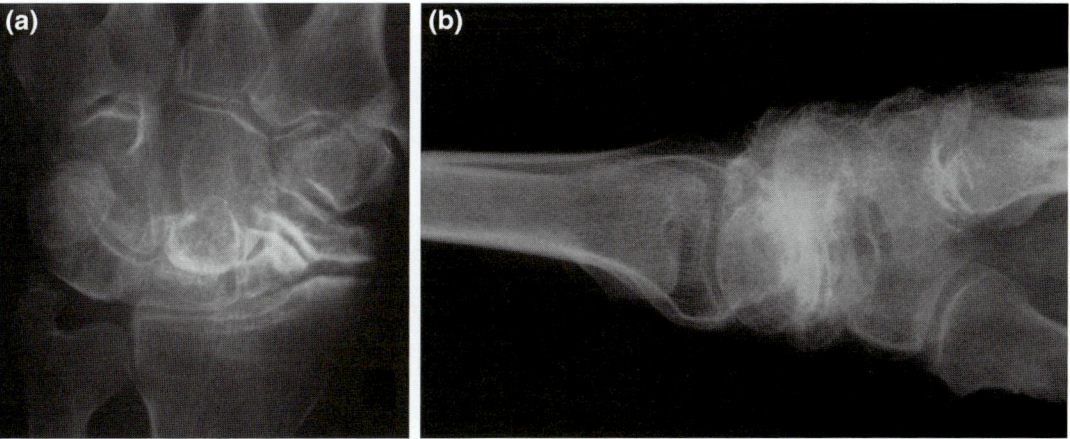

Fig. 4.93 a, b Undiagnosed case of trans-scaphoid dorsal perilunate dislocation with a remote history of injury. With permission from [231]

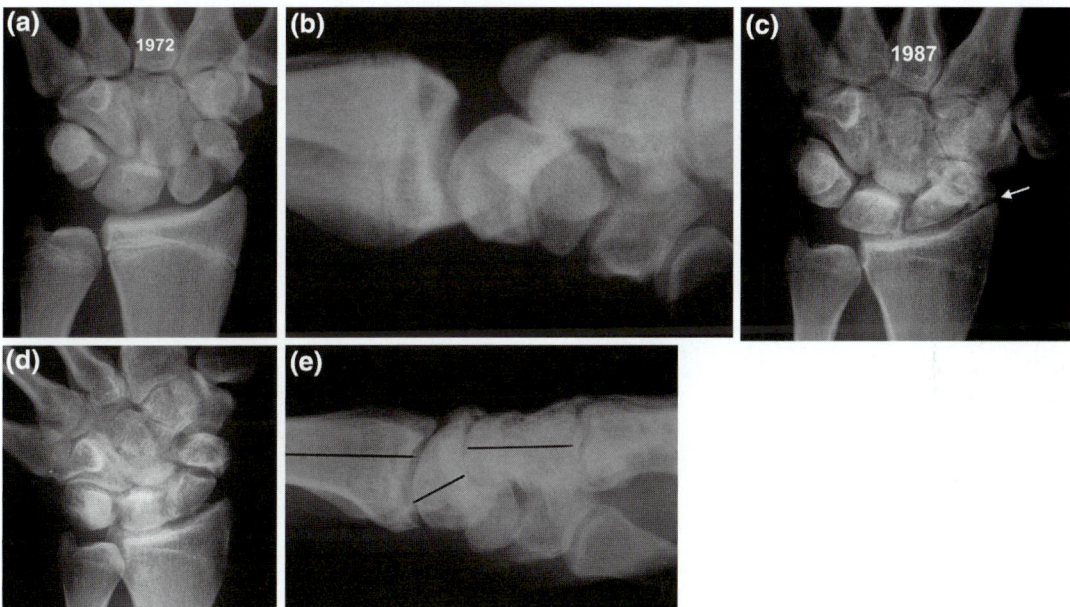

Fig. 4.94 A trans-scaphoid dorsal perilunate dislocation which was treated with closed reduction and cast application (**a, b**); 15 years later, a SNAC wrist with DISI malalignment was apparent. With permission from [231]

and Linscheid [104] supported that, following the conventional methods of ligament reconstruction, grip strength and range of motion were restored by 2/3 of the normal, while Ruby and Cassidy [15] stated that most patients will approximately regain 50 % normal range of motion. Kozin [111] mentioned that in the long-term the percentage of range motion reduction was 50 % and that of grip strength was 60 %. Additionally, Webber et al. [91] reported the requirement of several months for rehabilitation and regaining of range of motion and grip strength, although almost all patients were expected to exhibit some restriction in their range of motion. Heavy manual workers usually required 1 year to return to their previous employment.

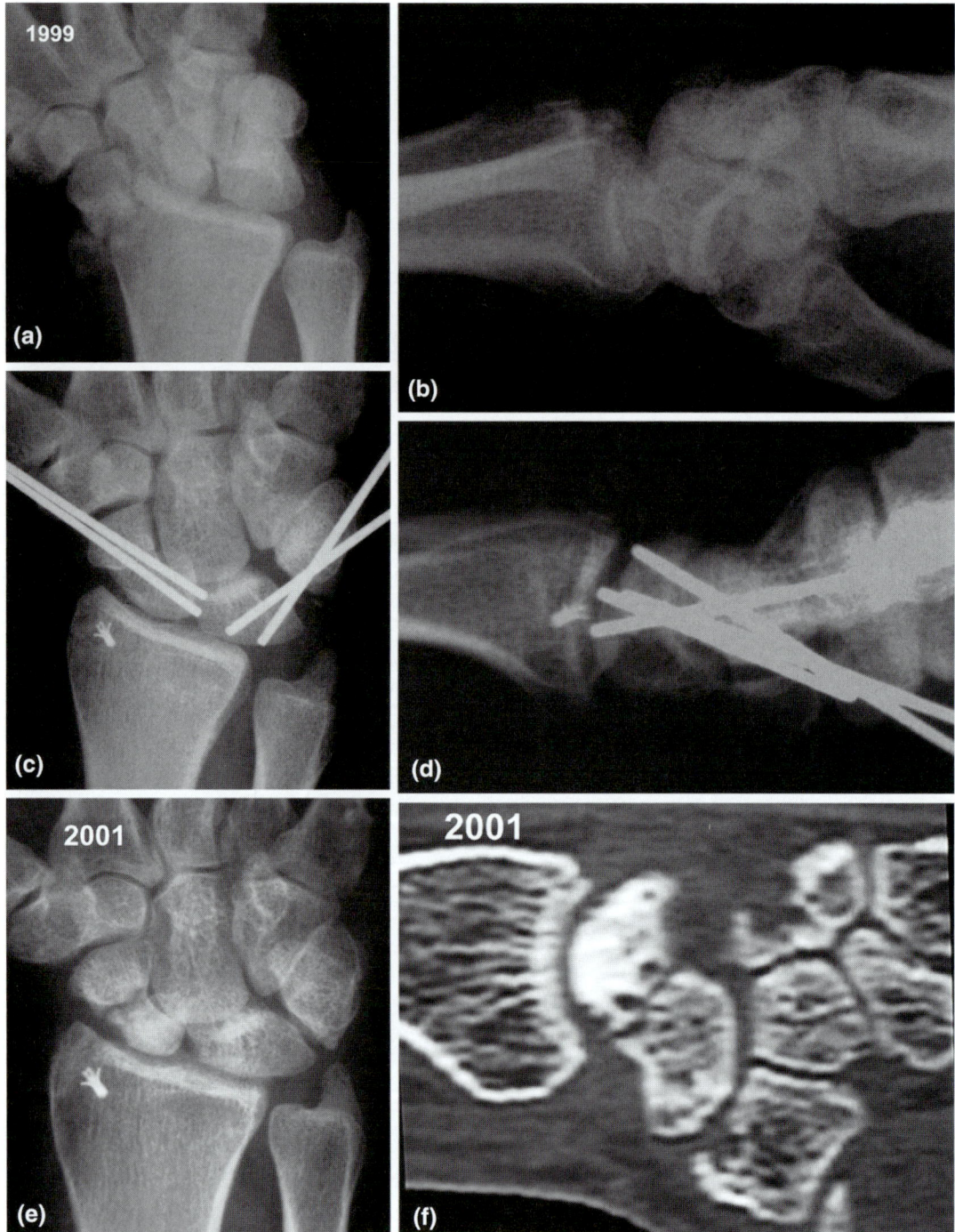

Fig. 4.95 An operatively treated trans-styloid, trans-scaphoid dorsal perilunate dislocation (**a–d**); 2 years later, the scaphoid failed to unite and its proximal pole showed signs of avascular necrosis (**e–g**); 7 years later, the patient refused any further treatment since he was symptoms free in spite of scaphoid nonunion (**h–j**)

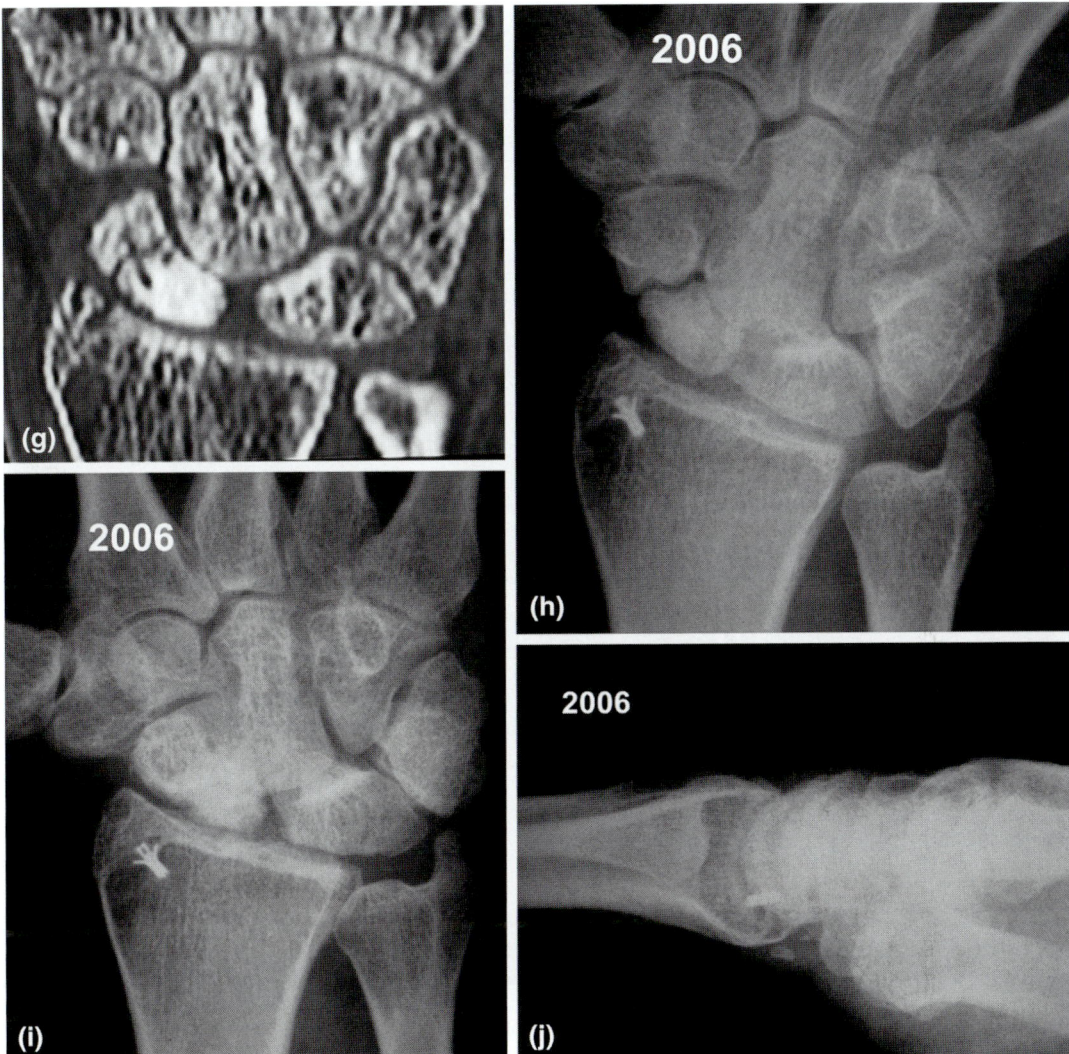

Fig. 4.95 (continued)

The overall good results referred after minimally invasive surgical methods with arthroscopic reduction and percutaneous fixation, still remain to be verified after a longer follow-up and a greater number of patients [107, 147].

Mayo wrist score [17], Krimmer wrist score [213], DASH questionnaire [214], PRWE score [215], and Herzberg's clinical and radiological outcome scores [13] have all been used to evaluate the outcome of patients with perilunate injuries.

4.9   Complications

Complications of these injuries are common and usually related to the original trauma.

Failure of diagnosis . Patients who have perilunate injuries often go undiagnosed. The frequency of missed diagnosis, as has already been written, varies from 25 to 43 % [5, 13, 94–96]. Delayed diagnosis constitutes the most serious early complication, since belated

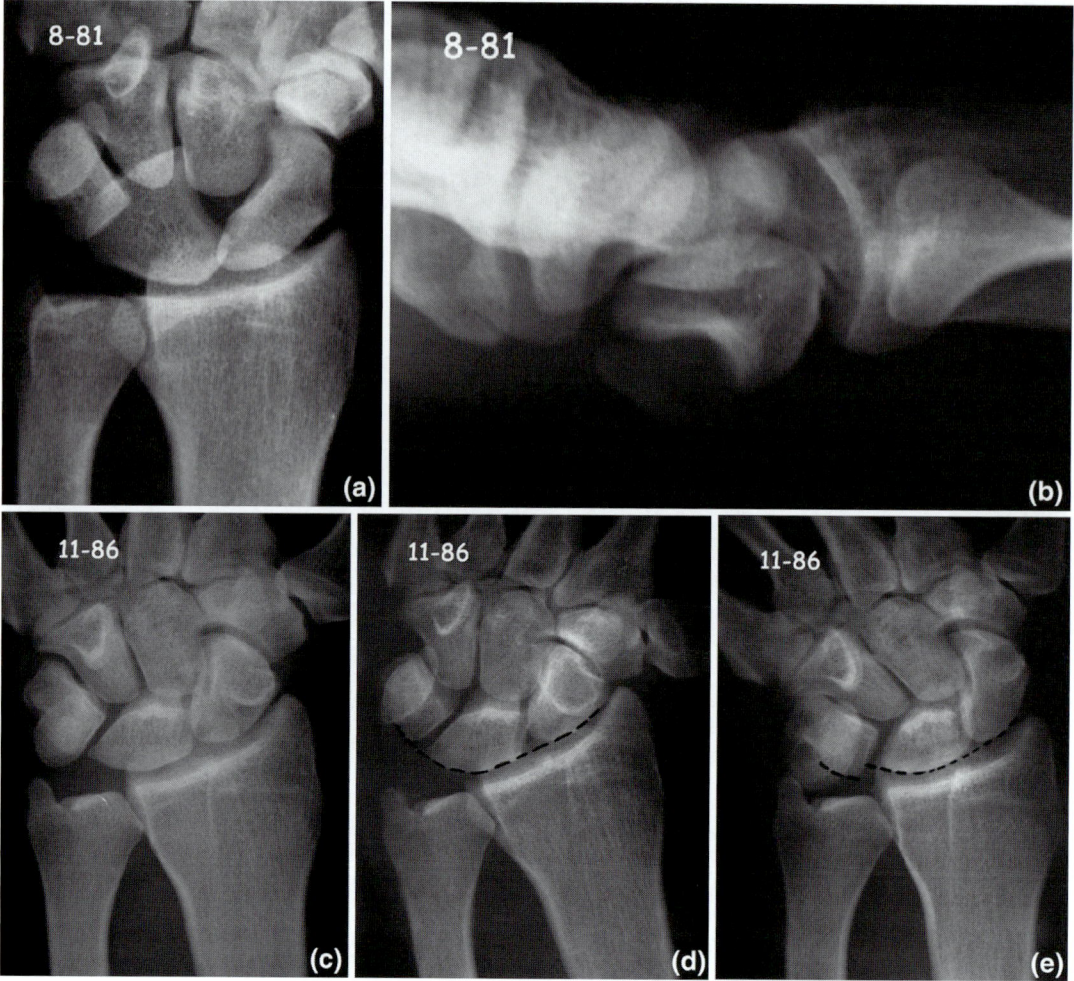

Fig. 4.96 A conservatively treated dorsal perilunate dislocation (stage III) (**a**, **b**); 5 years later, he presented with signs of LT instability with disruption of Gilula's arc during ulnar deviation (**c–e**). With permission from [231]

treatment is more difficult with unpredictable results [2, 25, 111]. In general, with injuries less than 2-months old, patients have good outcomes after open reduction and internal fixation. On the contrary, a salvage operation is frequently necessary for patients who are treated after 2 months [37] (Fig. 4.93a, b).

Median nerve neuropathy. Is a usual finding in acute injuries and an acute carpal tunnel syndrome is present in approximately 25 % of patients (range, 16–46 %) [13, 16, 38, 42, 93, 99]. Initial evaluation frequently reveals paresthesia in the median nerve distribution, because of the pressure exerted to the nerve by the

dislocated lunate or the palmar lunate horn in cases of perilunate dislocations, where the distal carpal row is dorsally displaced. Rarely, an extensive hematoma contributes to the nerve pressure. Reduction of the dislocation usually results in good prognosis [111, 164]. Delayed treatment may lead to persistent median neuropathy [120], while late presentation of median nerve paresthesias may result in carpal tunnel release, with a volarly dislocated lunate being undiagnosed. Rarely has ulnar nerve paresis been reported, resulting from pressure exerted by the dislocated lunate [216].

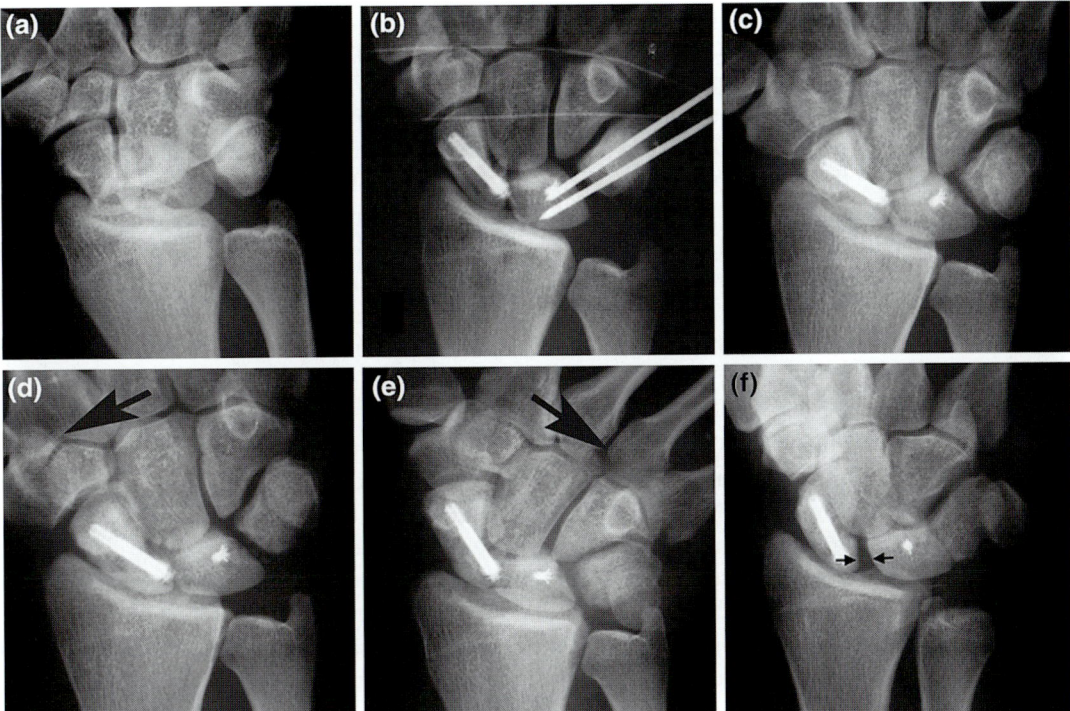

Fig. 4.97 A trans-scaphoid dorsal perilunate dislocation (**a**); it was treated with open reduction and internal fixation (**b**); postoperatively, the scapholunate distance seems to be normal in neutral position (**c**) and during radial (**d**) and ulnar deviation (**e**); the SL distance widens in AP fist view (**f**)

Vascular derangement of carpal bones.
A vascular necrosis of the scaphoid, lunate, or proximal capitate constitute potential complications regardless of the severity of the injury. This complication may occur after significant displacement of the bones, which implies denudation from ligamentous attachments, leading to necrosis and fragmentation [155, 179, 180]. Conversely, there have been reports where, despite the considerable displacement of the lunate along with the proximal scaphoid pole, early management resulted in a good functional outcome without vascular changes of the displaced bones [177]. Vascular changes of the scaphoid usually refer to its proximal pole, are followed by greater arc injuries and are basically transient [164]. Avascular necrosis of the lunate is extremely uncommon, since its vascularity is maintained by the short radiolunate ligament. However, transient ischemia of the lunate is frequently observed and lasts for months. The lunate appears radiodense compared to the surrounding osteopenic carpal bones during immobilization, but progressively vascularity is restored [5, 7, 24, 100, 217]. Lunate fragmentation and collapse have rarely been reported [217, 218]. White and Omer [219] studied 24 cases of perilunate injuries (PLD and PLFD); in 3 patients (12.5 %) they observed transient vascular compromise of the lunate that was restored. Panting et al. [100] reported that 12 out of 61 patients (19.6 %) with lunate dislocation (with or without scaphoid fracture) presented vascular changes and 3 of them finally developed avascular necrosis and collapse. They further supported that early reduction has less influence on vascularity than does the violence of injury and that vascular changes (although frequently transient) are more common in greater arc injuries.

Scaphoid nonunion. Incomplete fracture reduction, delayed operative treatment, and suboptimal fixation of the scaphoid fracture, increase the incidence of nonunion and of vascular changes of the scaphoid [202]. Green [220] had demonstrated the association between reduced bone vascularity and compromised callus formation in scaphoid nonunion. Scaphoid nonunion in nonoperatively treated patients is extremely high [127], while in the surgically treated patients the union rate of the scaphoid ranges between 75 and 100 % [2, 106, 108–110, 148, 170, 190, 211] (Figs. 4.94a–e, 4.95a–j).

Wrist instability. (CID or CIND) is a frequent complication when perilunate injuries are treated with closed reduction and cast immobilization [3, 96], but also in cases of insufficient repair after open reduction [24]. Failure to repair the volar LT ligament and the DRC ligament are responsible for long-term development of VISI alignment of the wrist [202]. Ulnar translation of the wrist has been reported by several authors [7, 10, 190, 199, 221]. According to Song et al. [199], ulnar translation is often overlooked and frequently associated with operatively treated perilunate injuries. They recognized that ulnar translation may be of varying degrees and may not always be significant. They proposed that pinning the lunate to the radius reduces the risk of ulnar translation of the wrist. Wollstein et al. [222] using Gilula and Weeks' [223] method of measuring lunate uncovering, concluded that neutral PA or radial deviation radiographs should be used and compared with the normal values (40 and 49 %, respectively) when assessing ulnocarpal translation. We believe that unrecognized and unrepaired ruptures of the ulnocarpal and DRC ligaments are mainly responsible for ulnar translocation. Wrist instability is hard to manage when treated belatedly; frequently, salvage operations must be recruited (partial fusions, proximal row carpectomy, wrist arthrodesis) (Fig. 4.96a–e). Many authors consider the SL interval and the SL angle as factors indicative of instability. In our series, an interesting and frequent finding even in TS-PLFD cases was the widening of the SL joint in the AP fist view; while in PA view during radial and ulnar deviation, it seemed to be normal. This is probably due to the unrepaired palmar SL ligament (Fig. 4.97a–f).

Chondrolysis and arthritis. According to the literature, perilunate injuries are associated with an incidence of posttraumatic arthritis, ranging between 50 and 56 %, after 3–6 years postinjury [13, 17, 23, 109, 111, 169, 190]. Forli et al. [110] postulated that degenerative changes are likely to increase with time, since they found 67 % of arthritic changes after a follow-up of 13 years, while functional outcome may be independent of these changes.

Although arthritis develops more frequently following closed reduction compared to open reduction [3], it is quite common even in cases treated with open reduction, joint irrigation, and optimal reconstruction. It makes sense for the arthritis to develop mainly at the midcarpal joint, since the lunocapitate joint is the one subjected to the greatest force, as is indicated by the increased frequency of osteochondral defects at the head of the capitate. Degenerative changes could also be observed at the radiocarpal level. However, early development of midcarpal arthritis in certain cases is quite impressive, despite the adequate treatment performed. This complication is considered by many as chondrolysis resulting in osteoarthritis [24]. Early arthritis is quite different to the late degenerative arthritis developed due to articular incongruity. It is manifested in the form of stenosis or obliteration of the adjacent articular surfaces, with or without the formation of subchondral cysts, and in a period of less than 6 months postinjury (Fig. 4.98a–c).

The rapid development of degenerative changes is related to:

(a) *The destruction of the articular cartilage at the initial injury*. Borrelli et al. [224] reported that a significant and possibly nonreversible damage of the articular cartilage, leading to the development of osteoarthritis, was observed after a single high-energy impact load on the cartilage. Frequent chondral defects at the head of the capitate are indicative of the force applied on the articular cartilage at the time of

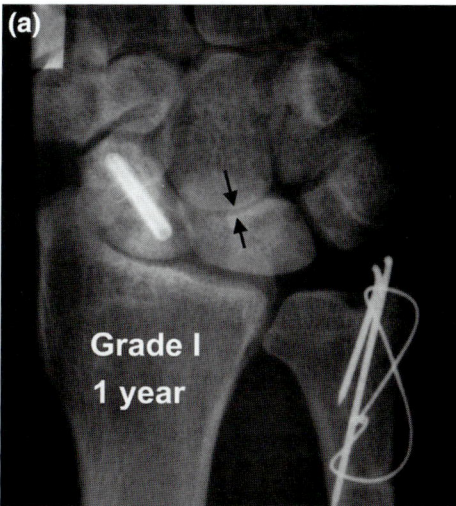

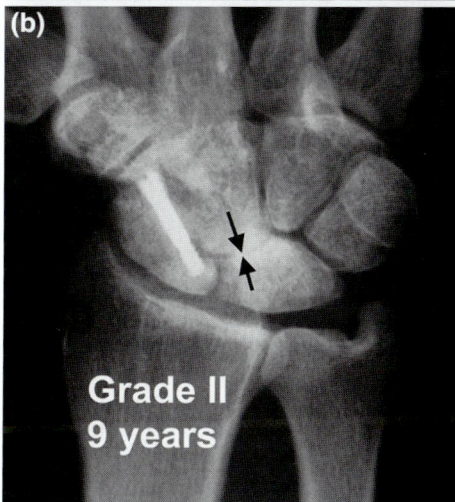

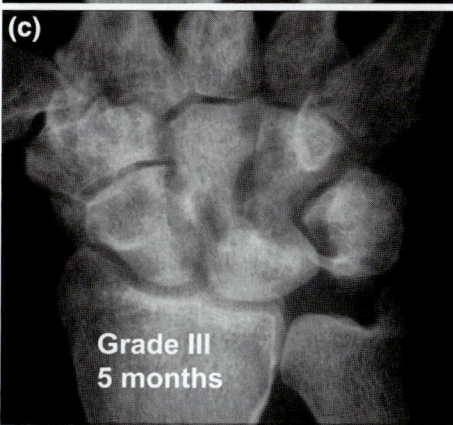

Fig. 4.98 Chondrolysis or midcarpal arthritis are of different degrees and developed at various chronic stages (a–c)

injury. In addition, repeated passage of K-wires through the joint surfaces and forced vigorous reduction maneuvers have been considered as iatrogenic injury of the cartilage [86].

(b) *The disruption of the blood supply of the midcarpal joint*, either from injury itself or the surgical approach. Simank et al. [225] experimentally produced cartilage injury with vessels ligation, as early as 6 weeks of ischemia. The cartilage destruction was maximal after an ischemic period of 24 weeks. It is known [226] that dorsally, the largest and most consistent is the intercarpal arch, which provides the major blood supply to the distal carpal row and contributes to the vascularity of the lunate and triquetrum. Coursing over the neck of the capitate, the intercarpal arch is at risk through the dorsal exposure.

Considering that the above are effective, we may not have many choices over the initial cartilage damage, we can, however, remove the chondral debris with sufficient irrigation of the joint and most significantly avoid extending the deep dorsal approach beyond the neck of the capitate.

In our series, we followed-up 67 patients (68 wrists) for 3.8 years on average (12–176 months). The distribution was: 45 greater arc and 23 lesser arc injuries. There were 41 acute, 18 delayed, and 7 chronic cases. Arthritis of all grades [227] was found in 50 % of greater arc and in 41.1 % of lesser arc injuries. However, advanced grades of arthritis (Grade II and III) were found in 14.2 % of greater and 17.6 % of lesser arc injuries.

Pin tract infection. Pins that are cut beneath the skin lessen the risk of infection, but if the pins are left outside the skin, the patients are advised to clean the site of insertion every day with an antiseptic solution. If pin tract infection occurs and it is diagnosed early, a short course of antibiotics is usually effective. If diagnosis is delayed, there is a potential risk for septic arthritis and osteomyelitis, in which case the pin(s) has/have to be prematurely removed and a 3–6 week course of antibiotics is required. Early removal of the pin may compromise ligamentous repair [8, 86].

Wrist stiffness. The majority of patients with perilunate injuries will exhibit wrist stiffness to a smaller or greater degree, which may reach 50 % of the normal range of motion [15, 111]. Szabo and Newland [86] stated that some loss of motion is unavoidable, since ligaments heal with scar, which has different mechanical properties from the original ligaments. Prevention of stiffness may require improvements in fixation that allow early motion, while maintaining carpal relationships. In relatively simple cases, fixation within proximal carpal row and stabilization of the radiocarpal joint (probably with a mini-external fixator between scaphoid and distal radius) will allow to start early an oblique plane of motion from radial extension to ulnar flexion, termed the "dart throwers" motion, in which midcarpal motion is maximized while radiocarpal motion is limited.

Ruptured tendons. Are usually observed in chronic and neglected cases [228, 229].

References

1. Murray PM (2003) Dislocations of the wrist: carpal instability complex. J Am Soc Surg Hand 3(2):88–99
2. Herzberg G (2002) Acute perilunate dislocations and fracture-dislocations. In: EFORT (ed) Surgical techniques in orthopaedics and traumatology, vol 5. 55-370-E-10. Elsevier
3. Herzberg G, Cooney WP (1998) Perilunate fracture dislocations. In: Cooney WP, Linscheid RL, Dobyns JH (eds) The wrist: diagnosis and operative treatment, vol 1. Mayo Clinic, Mosby, pp 651–683
4. Sauder DJ, Athwal GS, Faber KJ et al (2007) Perilunate Injuries. Orthop Clin North Am 38:279–288
5. Garcia-Elias M (2004) Perilunar injuries including fracture dislocations. In: Berger R, Weiss AP (eds) Hand surgery, vol 1. Lippincott Williams & Wilkins, ch 27, pp 511–523
6. Herzberg G (2010) Perilunate fracture dislocations. In: Cooney W (ed) The wrist. Diagnosis and operative treatment, 2nd edn. Lippincott Williams & Wilkins, ch 24, pp 550–578
7. Kozin SH (2010) Perilunate dislocations. In: Cooney W (ed) The wrist: Diagnosis and operative treatment. Lippincott Williams & Wilkins, pp 532–549
8. Najarian R, Nourbakhsh A, Capo J et al (2011) Perilunate injuries. Hand 6:1–7
9. Blazar PE, Murray P (2001) Treatment of perilunate dislocations by combined dorsal and palmar approaches. Techn Hand Upper Extrem Surg 5:2–7
10. Melsom DS, Leslie IJ (2007) Carpal dislocations. Curr Orthop 21:288–297
11. Carmichael KD, Bell C (2005) Volar perilunate trans-scaphoid fracture-dislocation in a skeletally immature patient. Orthopedics 28(1):69–70
12. Massicot R, Uzel AP, Ceolin JL et al (2005) Dorsal trans-scaphoid perilunate dislocation in a 9-year-old child. Eur J Pediatr Surg 15(2):140–143
13. Herzberg G, Comtet JJ, Linscheid RL et al (1993) Perilunate dislocations and fracture dislocations: a multicenter study. J Hand Surg [Am] 18:768–779
14. Inoue G, Tanaka Y, Nakamura RE (1990) Treatment of trans-scaphoid perilunate dislocations by internal fixation with the Herbert screw. J Hand Surg [Br] 15:449–454
15. Ruby LK, Cassidy C (2003) Fractures and dislocations of the carpus. In: Browner BD, Jupiter JB, Levine AM, Trafton PG (eds) Skeletal trauma: basic science, management, and reconstruction. Saunders, pp 1267–1314
16. Adkison JW, Chapman MW (1982) Treatment of acute lunate and perilunate dislocations. Clin Orthop 164:199–207
17. Cooney WP, Bussey R, Dobyns JH et al (1987) Difficult wrist fractures: perilunate fracture-dislocations of the wrist. Clin Orthop 214:136–147
18. Herzberg G (2000) Acute dorsal trans-scaphoid perilunate dislocations: open reduction and internal fixation. Techn Hand Upper Extrem Surg 4:2–13
19. Kerr CD, Gunderson RJ (1995) Concomitant perilunate dislocation of the wrist with posterior radial head subluxation: case report. J Trauma 38:941–943
20. Lahoti OP, Callanan I, Reidy DP et al (1995) Elbow fractures with carpal injuries. J Hand Surg [Br] 20:620–622
21. Grabow RJ, Catalano L III (2006) Carpal dislocations. Hand Clin 22:485–500
22. Idler RS (2001) Carpal dislocations and instability. In: Watson HK, Weinzweig J (eds) The wrist. Lippincott Williams & Wilkins, pp 203–229
23. Green DP, O'Brien ET (1980) Classification and management of carpal dislocations. Clin Orthop 149:55–72
24. Kozin SH, Murphy MS, Cooney WP (1998) Perilunate dislocations. In: Cooney WP, Linscheid RL, Dobyns JH (eds) The wrist: diagnosis and operative treatment, vol 1. Mayo Clinic, Mosby, pp 632–650
25. Vo DP, Mohler LR, Trumble TE (2002) Lunate and perilunate dislocations. In: Trumble T (ed) Carpal

fracture-dislocations. American Academy of Orthopaedic Surgeons, pp 27–35

26. Johnson RP (1980) The acutely injured wrist and its residuals. Clin Orthop 149:33–44

27. Herzberg G, Forissier D (2002) Acute dorsal trans-scaphoid perilunate fracture-dislocations: medium-term results. J Hand Surg [Br] 27:498–502

28. Witvoet J, Allieu Y (1973) Lesions traumatiques fraiches. Rev Chi Orthop 59(1):98–125

29. Smith DK, Murray PM (1996) Avulsion fractures of the volar aspect of triquetral bone of the wrist: a subtle sign of carpal ligament injury. Am J Roentgenol 166(3):609–614

30. Hawken RMA, Fullilove SM (2007) Delayed post-traumatic midcarpal dislocation. J Hand Surg [Eur] 32(5):554–555

31. Shaw JC, Wilson FC (1970) Radial perilunar dislocation: report of a case. J Bone Joint Surg Am 52:556–558

32. Graham TJ (2003) The inferior arc injury: an addition to the family of complex carpal fracture-dislocation patterns. Am J Orthop 32(9):10–19

33. Lowdon IM, Simpson AH, Burge P (1984) Recurrent dorsal trans-scaphoid perilunate dislocation. J Hand Surg [Br] 9:307–310

34. Scharizer E (1995) Scaphoid pseudarthrosis and capitate fracture. Handchir Mikrochir Plast Chir 27:38–42

35. Mayfield JK (1980) Mechanism of carpal injuries. Clin Orthop 149:45–54

36. Mayfield JK, Johnson RP, Kilcoyne RK (1980) Carpal dislocations: pathomechanics and progressive perilunar instability. J Hand Surg [Am] 5:226–241

37. Sauder DJ, Athwal GS, Faber KJ et al (2010) Perilunate injuries. Hand Clin 26:145–154

38. Stanbury SJ, Elfar JC (2011) Perilunate dislocation and perilunate fracture-dislocation. J Am Acad Orthop Surg 19:554–562

39. Kennedy SA, Allan CH (2012) Mayfield et al. Classification: carpal dislocations and progressive perilunar instability. Clin Orthop 470(4):1243–1245

40. Kardashian G, Christoforou DC, Lee SK (2011) Perilunate dislocations. Bull Hosp Jt Dis 69(1):87–96

41. Bollen SR (1988) Peri-triquetral-lunate dislocation associated with ulnar nerve palsy. J Hand Surg [Br] 13(4):456–457

42. Bain GI, McLean JM, Turner PC et al (2008) Translunate fracture with associated perilunate injury: 3 case reports with introduction of the translunate arc concept. J Hand Surg [Am] 33(10):1770–177006

43. Schimizzi A, Catalano L (2010) Carpal dislocations. In: Slutsky D (ed) Principal and practice of wrist surgery. Saunders, ch 43, pp 465–472

44. Taleisnik J (1985) The wrist. Churchill Livingstone, New York

45. Leung YF, Ip SPS, Wong A et al (2007) Trans-triquetral dorsal perilunate fracture dislocation. J Hand Surg [Eur] 32(6):647–648

46. Moneim MS (1988) Management of greater arc carpal fractures. Hand Clin 4(3):457–468

47. Kohut G, Smith A, Giudicio M et al (1996) Greater arc injuries of the wrist treated by internal and external fixation - six cases with mid-term follow-up. Hand Surg 1(2):159–166

48. Harrington P, Quinlan WB (1999) Palmar lunate trans-scaphoid, trans-triquetral fracture-dislocation. J Hand Surg [Br] 24:493–496

49. Soejima O, Iida H, Naito M (2003) Transscaphoid-transtriquetral perilunate fracture dislocation: report of a case and review of the literature. Arch Orthop Trauma Surg 123:305–307

50. Sabat D, Dabas V, Suri T et al (2010) Transscaphoid, Transcapitate, Transhamate fracture of the wrist. J Hand Surg [Am] 35(7):1093–1096

51. Sandoval E, Cecilia D, Garcia-Paredero E (2008) Surgical treatment of trans-scaphoid, transcapitate, transtriquetral, Perilunate fracture-dislocation with open reduction, internal fixation and lunotriquetral ligament repair. J Hand Surg [Eur] 33(3):377–379

52. Weseley MS, Barenfield PA (1972) Trans-scaphoid, trans-capitate, trans-triquetral perilunate fracture dislocation of the wrist: a case report. J Bone Joint Surg Am 54:1073–1078

53. Graham TJ, Condit DP, Culver JE (1995) Patterns of injury associated with radial styloid fractures. In: The proceedings of VI international federation for societies for surgery of the hand, Edited by V.S.G.H.et.al. Vastamaki M. Bologna: Monduzzi Editore

54. Noble J, Lamb DW (1979) Translunate scapho-radial fracture: a case report. Hand 11(1):47–49

55. Ruitgers R, Kortmann J (1988) A case of translunate luxation of the carpus. Acta Orthop Scand 59(4):461–463

56. Toft P, Bertheussen K, Otkjaer S (1985) Translunate, transmetacarpal, scapho-radial fracture with perilunate dislocation; a case report. J Hand Surg [Br] 10(3):382–384

57. Weissenborn W, Sabri W (1988) Complex dislocation fracture of the wrist: transscaphoid-translunar-transstyloid dislocation fracture. Handchir Mikrochir Plast Chir 20:107–110

58. Amaravati RS, Saji MJ, Rajagopal HP (2005) Greater arc injury of the wrist with fractured lunate bone: a case report. J Orthop Surg 13(3):310–313

59. Briseno M, Yao J (2012) Lunate fractures in the face of a perilunate injury: an uncommon and easily missed injury pattern. J Hand Surg [Am] 37:63–67

60. Van Leeuwen DH, Buijze GA, Ring D (2012) Ulnar to radial dorsal fracture-dislocations of the wrist: a report of 2 cases. J Hand Surg [Am] 37:500–502

61. Christodoulou L, Palou CH, Chamberlain ST (1999) Proximal row transcarpal fracture from a punching injury. J Hand Surg [Br] 24(6):744–746

62. Conway WF, Gilula LA, Manske PR et al (1989) Translunate, palmar perilunate fracture-subluxation of the wrist. J Hand Surg [Am] 14:635–639

63. Takase K, Yamamoto K (2006) Unusual combined scaphoid and lunate fracture of the wrist: a case report. J Hand Surg [Am] 31:414–417

64. Brown R, Muddu B (1981) Scaphoid and lunate dislocation a report on a case. Hand 13(3):303–307

65. Capo JT, Armbruster EJ, Hashem J (2010) Proximal carpal row dislocation: a case report. Hand 5(4):444–448

66. Chalidis BE, Dimitriou CG (2010) Palmar dislocation of the scapholunate bone-ligament-bone complex. J Hand Surg [Br] 35(4):322–324

67. Domeshek LF, Harenberg PS, Rineer CA et al (2010) Total scapholunate dislocation with complete scaphoid extrusion: case report. J Hand Surg [Am] 35(1):69–71

68. Fowler JL (1988) Dislocation of the triquetrum and lunate: brief report. J Bone Joint Surg Br 70(4):665

69. Healey DC, Giachino A, Conway AF (2002) Periscaphoid perilunate dislocation of the wrist: a case report. J Bone Joint Surg Am 84:1201–1204

70. Komura S, Yokoi T, Suzuki Y (2011) Palmar-divergent dislocation of the scaphoid and the lunate. J Orthop Traumatol 12:65–68

71. Lee B-J, Kim S–S, Lee S-R et al (2010) Palmar scaphoid dislocation associated with dorsal perilunate dislocation: case report. J Hand Surg 35(5):726–731

72. Lundkvist L, Larsen CF, Juul SM (1991) Dislocation of the lunate, triquetral, and hamate bones: case report. Scand J Plast Reconstr Surg Hand Surg 25:83–85

73. Sarrafian SK, Breihan JH (1990) Palmar dislocation of scaphoid and lunate as a unit. J Hand Surg [Am] 15:134–139

74. Yamabe E, Nakamura T, Matsumura T et al (2008) Palmar dislocation of the scaphoid with dorsal perilunate dislocation. J Hand Surg [Eur] 33(5):682–683

75. Reagan DS, Linscheid RL, Dobyns JH (1984) Lunotriquetral sprains. J Hand Surg [Am] 9:502–514

76. Saffar P (1984) Carpal luxation and residual instability. Ann Chir Main 3:349–352

77. Viegas SF, Patterson RM, Peterson PD et al (1990) Ulnar-sided perilunate instability: an anatomic and biomechanic study. J Hand Surg [Am] 15:268–278

78. Viegas SF (1998) Ulnar-sided wrist pain and instability. Am Acad Orthop Surg 25:215–218

79. Melone CP, Nathan R (1992) Traumatic disruption of the triangular fibrocartilage complex: patho-anatomy. Clin Orthop 275:65–73

80. Murray PM, Palmer CG, Shin AY (2012) The mechanism of Ulnar-sided perilunate instability of the wrist: a cadaveric study and 6 clinical cases. J Hand Surg [Am] 37:721–728

81. Horii E, Garcia-Elias M, An KN et al (1991) A kinematic study of luno-triquetral dissociations. J Hand Surg [Am] 16:355–362

82. Ritt MJ, Linscheid RL, Cooney WP III et al (1998) The lunotriquetral joint: kinematic effects of sequential ligament sectioning, ligament repair, and arthrodesis. J Hand Surg [Am] 23:432–445

83. Moritomo H, Murase T, Arimitsu S et al (2008) Change in the length of the ulnocarpal ligaments during radiocarpal motion: possible impact on triangular fibrocartilage complex foveal tears. J Hand Surg [Am] 33:1278–1286

84. Chin A, Garcia-Elias M (2008) Combined reverse perilunate and axial-ulnar dislocation of the wrist: a case report. J Hand Surg [Br] 33:672–676

85. Nunn D (1986) Trans-triquetral mid-carpal dislocation. J Hand Surg [Br] 11:432–433

86. Szabo R, Newland C (2010) Ligamentous repair for acute lunate and perilunate dislocations. In: Gelberman R (ed) The wrist: master techniques in orthopaedic surgery, 3rd edn. Lippincott Williams & Wilkins, ch 22, pp 243–262

87. Mayfield JK, Gilula LA, Totty WG (1992) Carpal fracture-dislocations. In: Gilula LA (ed) Traumatized hand and wrist: radiographic and anatomic correlation. Saunders WB, Philadelphia PA

88. Tanz SS (1968) Rotation effect in lunar and perilunar dislocations. Clin Orthop 57:147–152

89. Viegas SF, Hoffmann FJ (1988) Palmar lunate dislocation with a dorsal scaphoid fracture variant. J Hand Surg [Am] 13:440–443

90. Green DP (1988) Carpal dislocations and instabilities. In: Green DP (ed) Operative hand surgery, 2nd edn. Churchill Livingstone, New York, pp 875–938

91. Webber JB, Bashner B, Fye M (1991) Acute lunate and perilunate dislocation. Orthopedics 14:630–632

92. Minami A, Kaneda K (1993) Repair and/or reconstruction of scapholunate interosseous ligament in lunate and perilunate dislocations. J Hand Surg [Am] 18:1099–1106

93. Minami A, Ogino T, Ohshio I et al (1986) Correlation between clinical results and carpal instability in patients after reduction of lunate and perilunate dislocations. J Hand Surg [Br] 11:213–220

94. Campbell RD, Lance EM, Yeoh CB (1964) Lunate and perilunar dislocation. J Bone Joint Surg Br 46(1):55–72

95. Garcia-Elias M, Irisarri C, Henriquez A et al (1986) Perilunar dislocation of the carpus: a diagnosis still often missed. Ann Chir Main 5:281–287

96. Saffar P (1994) Dislocations of the carpal bones. Rev Prat 44(18):2442–2445

97. Juhl M, Saether J (1987) Simultaneous dislocation of the interphalangeal joint of the thumb and the carpal lunate. J Trauma 27:581–582

98. Hill NA (1970) Fractures and dislocations of the carpus. Orthop Clin North Am 1:275

99. Trumble T, Verheyden J (2004) Treatment of isolated perilunate and lunate dislocations with combined dorsal and volar approach and intraosseous cerclage wire. J Hand Surg [Am] 29:412–417

100. Panting AL, Lamb DW, Noble J et al (1984) Dislocations of the lunate with and without fracture of the scaphoid. J Bone Joint Surg Br 66:391–395

101. Klein A, Webb LX (1987) The crowded carpal sign in volar perilunar dislocation. J Trauma 27:82–84

102. Gilula LA (1979) Carpal injuries: analytic approach and case exercises. Am J Roentgenol 133:503–517

103. Gilula LA, Destouet JM, Weeks PM et al (1984) Roentgenographic diagnosis of the painful wrist. Clin Orthop 187:52–64

104. Dobyns JH, Linscheid RL (1984) Fractures and dislocations of the wrist. In: Rockwood CA, Green DP (eds) Fractures in adults. JB Lippincott, Philadelphia, pp 411–510

105. Green DP, O'Brien ET (1978) Open reduction of carpal dislocations: indications and operative techniques. J Hand Surg [Am] 3:250–265

106. Chou Y-C, Hsu Y-H, Cheng C-Y et al (2012) Percutaneous screw and axial kirschner wire fixation for acute transscaphoid perilunate fracture dislocation. J Hand Surg [Am] 37:715–720

107. Jeon I-H, Kim H-J, Min W-K et al (2010) Arthroscopically assisted percutaneous fixation for trans-scaphoid perilunate fracture dislocation. J Hand Surg [Eur] 35(8):664–668

108. Knoll VD, Allan C, Trumble TE (2005) Trans-scaphoid perilunate fracture dislocations: results of screw fixation of the scaphoid and lunotriquetral repair with a dorsal approach. J Hand Surg [Am] 30(6):1145–1152

109. Souer JS, Rutgers M, Andermahr J et al (2007) Perilunate fracture–dislocations of the wrist: comparison of temporary screw versus K-wire fixation. J Hand Surg [Am] 32(3):318–325

110. Forli A, Courvoisier A, Wimsey S et al (2010) Perilunate dislocations and transscaphoid perilunate fracture–dislocations: a retrospective study with minimum ten-year follow-up. J Hand Surg [Am] 35:62–68

111. Kozin SH (1998) Perilunate injuries: diagnosis and treatment. J Am Acad Orthop Surg 6:114–120

112. Jones D, Kakar S (2012) Perilunate dislocations and fracture dislocations. J Hand Surg [Am] 37:2168–2174

113. Davis GG (1923) Treatment of dislocated semilunar carpal bones. Surg Gynecol Obstet 37:225–229

114. Conwell HE (1925) Closed reduction of acute dislocation of the semilunar carpal bone. Ann Surg 92:289

115. Adams JD (1925) Displacement of the semilunar carpal bone: an analysis of twelve cases. J Bone Joint Surg Am 7:665–681

116. Bohler L (1956) The treatment of fractures, 5th edn. Grune & Stratton, New York, pp 826–854

117. Stevenson DL (1940) Dislocations of the carpal lunate. Br Med J 1:129

118. Codman EA, Chase HM (1905) The diagnosis and treatment of fracture of the carpal scaphoid and dislocation of the semilunar bone, with a report of thirty cases: part II. Ann Surg 41:863

119. Watson–Jones R (1943) Fractures and joint injuries, 3rd edn. Churchill Livingstone, pp 568–577

120. Yao J, Jagadish A (2010) Carpus: Perilunate and greater arc injuries. In: Slutsky DJ (ed) Principles and practice of wrist surgery. Saunders, ch 44, pp 473–486

121. Jasmine MS, Packer JW, Edwards GS (1988) Irreducible trans-scaphoid perilunate dislocation. J Hand Surg [Am] 13:212–215

122. O'Carroll PF, Gallagher JE (1983) Irreducible trans-scaphoid perilunate dislocation. Ir J Med Sci 152:424–427

123. Weiss C, Lasik RS, Spinner M (1970) Irreducible trans-scaphoid perilunate dislocation: a case report. J Bone Joint Surg Am 52:565–568

124. Aitken AP, Nalebuff EA (1960) Volar transnavicular perilunar dislocation of the carpus. J Bone Joint Surg Am 42:1051–1057

125. Campbell RD, Thompson TC, Lance EM et al (1965) Indications for open reduction of lunate and perilunate dislocations of the carpal bones. J Bone Joint Surg Am 47(5):915–937

126. Sowa DT, Hotchkiss RN, Weiland AJ (1995) Symptomatic proximal translation of the radius following radial head resection. Clin Orthop 317:106–113

127. Apergis E, Maris J, Theodoratos G et al (1997) Perilunate dislocations and fracture-dislocations: closed and early open reduction compared in 28 cases. Acta Orthop Scand Suppl 68:55–59

128. Cooney WP III, Linscheid RL, Dobyns JH (1991) Fractures and dislocations of the wrist. In: Rockwood CA, Green DP, Bucholz RW (eds) Fractures in Adults, vol 1, 3rd edn. JB Lippincott, New York, pp 563–678

129. Webber JB, Bashner B, Fye M (1991) Answer please: acute volar lunate dislocation. Orthopedics 14(5):625–630–632

130. Cave EF (1941) Retrolunar dislocation of the capitate with fracture or subluxation of the navicular bone. J Bone Joint Surg Am 23:830–840

131. Alt V, Sicre G (2004) Dorsal transscaphoid-transtriquetral perilunate dislocation in pseudarthrosis of the scaphoid. Clin Orhop 426:135–137

132. Amadio PC, Berquist TH, Smith DK et al (1989) Scaphoid malunion. J Hand Surg [Am] 14:679–687

133. Fernandez DL, Eggli S (2001) Scaphoid nonunion and malunion: how to correct deformity. Hand Clin 17:631–646

134. Pachucki A, Prendinger G (1988) Perilunar dislocations and dislocation fractures–evaluation of treatment results using the newest data on carpal instability. Handchir Mikrochir Plast Chir 20:27–32

135. Cooney WP, Dobyns JH (1980) Fracture of the scaphoid: a rational approach to management. Clin Orthop 149:90–97

136. Monsivais JJ (1986) The role of carpal instability in scaphoid nonunion: casual or causal? J Hand Surg [Br] 11:201–206

137. Sennwald G (1987) The wrist: anatomical and pathophysiological approach to diagnosis and treatment. Springer, Berlin

138. Garcia-Elias M (1999) Carpal instabilities and dislocations. In: Green DP, Hotchkiss RN, Pederson WC (eds) Green's operative hand surgery, 4th edn, vol 1. Churchill Livingstone, New York, ch 28, pp 865–928

139. Ruch DS, Poehling GG (1996) Arthroscopic management of partial scapholunate and lunotriquetral injuries of the wrist. J Hand Surg [Am] 21:412–417

140. Weil W, Slade JF, Trumble TE (2006) Open and arthroscopic treatment of perilunate injuries. Clin Orthop 445:120–132

141. Whipple TL (1995) Acute scaphoid fracture fixation. In: Vastamaki M (ed) Current trends in hand surgery. Elsevier, Amsterdam, pp 75–78

142. Garcia-Elias M (2011) Carpal instability. In: Wolfe S, Hotchkiss RN, Pederson WC, Kozin SH (eds) Green's operative hand surgery, 6th edn. Elsevier Churchill Livingstone, ch 15, pp 465–522

143. Fernandez DL, Mader K (2000) The treatment of complex carpal dislocations by external fixation. Injury 31:92–101

144. Park MJ, Ahn JH (2005) Arthroscopically assisted reduction and percutaneous fixation of dorsal perilunate dislocations and fracture-dislocations. Arthroscopy 21(9):1153

145. Bond CD, Shin AY (2000) Percutaneous cannulated screw fixation of acute scaphoid fractures. Techn Hand Upper Extrem Surg 4:81–87

146. Haddad FS, Goddard NJ (2000) Acutrak percutaneous scaphoid fixation. Techn Hand Upper Extrem Surg 4:78–80

147. Kim JP, Lee JS, Park MJ (2012) Arthroscopic reduction and percutaneous fixation of perilunate dislocations and fracture-dislocations. Arthroscopy 28(2):196–203

148. Wong TC, Ip FK (2008) Minimally invasive management of trans-scaphoid perilunate fracture-dislocations. Hand Surg 13:159–165

149. Leung Y-F, Ip SPS, Wong A et al (2006) Transscaphoid transcapitate transtriquetral perilunate fracture–dislocation: a case report. J Hand Surg [Am] 31:608–610

150. Inoue G, Miura T (1991) Transcaphoid perilunate dislocation with a dorsal dislocated proximal scaphoid fragment: report of 2 cases. Acta Orthop Scand 62(4):394–396

151. Roger DJ, Williamson SC, Whipple R (1994) Ejection of the proximal scaphoid in a trans-scaphoid perilunate fracture dislocation: a case report. Clin Orthop 302:151–155

152. Mittal RL, Sharma RK (1991) Unusual wrist injuries in India. Int Orthop 15(1):45–48

153. Skelly WJ, Nahigian SH, Hidvegi EB (1991) Palmar lunate transtriquetral fracture dislocation. J Hand Surg [Am] 16:536–539

154. Kloss BT, Patierno SR, Sullivan AM (2010) Transcaphoid perilunate dislocation. Int J Emerg Med 3:501–502

155. Stevanovic M, Schnall SB, Filler BC (1996) Trans-scaphoid, transtriquetral, volar lunate fracture-dislocation of the wrist: a case report. J Bone Joint Surg Am 78:1907–1910

156. Schranz PJ, Fagg PS (1991) Trans-radial styloid, trans-scaphoid, trans-triquetral perilunate dislocation. J R Army Med Corps 137:146–148

157. Yamaguchi H, Takahara M (1994) Transradial styloid, transtriquetral perilunate dislocation of the carpus with an associated fracture of the ulnar border of the distal radius. J Orthop Trauma 8:434–436

158. Bell MJ (1983) Perilunar dislocation of the carpus and an associated Colle's fracture. Hand 15:262–266

159. Sharma H, Azzopardi T, Sibinski M et al (2007) Volar lunate dislocation associated with a Salter-Harris type III fracture of the distal radial epiphysis in an 8 year-old child. J Hand Surg [Eur] 32(1):77–79

160. Klein A, Bohret S (1986) Dorsal dislocation of the radiocarpal joint with associated dorsal perilunar dislocation. J Can Assoc Radiol 37(3):201–202

161. Budoff JE (2008) Treatment of acute lunate and perilunate dislocations. J Hand Surg [Am] 33:1424–1432

162. Digiovanni B, Shaffer J (1995) Treatment of perilunate and transscaphoid perilunate dislocations of the wrist. Am J Orthop 24:818–826

163. Inoue G, Kuwahata Y (1997) Management of acute perilunate dislocations without fracture of the scaphoid. J Hand Surg [Br] 22:647–652

164. Moneim MS, Hofammann KE, Omer GE (1984) Transscaphoid perilunate fracture-dislocation: result of open reduction and pin fixation. Clin Orthop 190:227–235

165. Fikry T, Lamine A, Harfaoui A et al (1993) Carpal perilunar dislocation: clinical study (apropos of 39 cases). Acta Orthop Belg 59:293–300

166. Hee HT, Wong HP, Low YP (1999) Transscaphoid perilunate fracture/dislocations—results of surgical treatment. Ann Acad Med Singap 28:791–794

167. Inoue G, Imaeda T (1997) Management of trans-scaphoid perilunate dislocations. Arch Orthop Trauma Surg 116:338–340

168. Dobyns JH, Swanson GE (1973) A 19 year-old with multiple fractures. Minn Med 56:143–149

169. Hildebrand KA, Ross DC, Patterson SD et al (2000) Dorsal perilunate dislocations and fracture-dislocations: questionnaire, clinical, and radiographic evaluation. J Hand Surg [Am] 25:1069–1079

170. Sotereanos DG, Mitsionis GJ, Giannakopoulos PN et al (1997) Perilunate dislocation and fracture dislocation: a critical analysis of the volar-dorsal approach. J Hand Surg [Am] 22:49–56

171. Hagert E, Persson JKE (2010) Desensitizing the posterior interosseous nerve alters wrist proprioceptive reflexes. J Hand Surg [Am] 35:1059–1066

172. Dellon AL (2010) Commentary:desensitizing the posterior interosseous nerve alters wrist proprioceptive reflexes: it is ok to lose your nerve. J Hand Surg [Am] 35(7):1067–1069

173. Hagert E, Persson JK, Werner M et al (2009) Evidence of wrist proprioceptive reflexes elicited after stimulation of the scapholunate Interosseous ligament. J Hand Surg [Am] 34:642–651

174. Hagert E (2010) Proprioception of the wrist joint: a review of current concepts and possible implications on the rehabilitation of the wrist. J Hand Ther 23:2–16

175. Hagert E, Ferreres A, Garcia-Elias M (2010) Nerve-sparing dorsal and volar approaches to the radiocarpal joint. J Hand Surg [Am] 35:1070–1074

176. Berger RA, Bishop A (1997) A fiber splitting capsulotomy technique for dorsal exposure of the wrist. Techn Hand Upper Extrem Surg 1:2–10

177. Ekerot L (1995) Palmar dislocation of the trans-scaphoid-lunate unit. J Hand Surg [Br] 20:557–560

178. Stern PJ (1984) Trans-scaphoid-lunate dislocation: a report of two cases. J Hand Surg [Am] 9:370–373

179. Pandit R (1998) Proximal and palmar dislocation of the lunate and proximal scaphoid as a unit in a case of Scaphocapitate syndrome: a 32-month follow-up. J Hand Surg [Br] 23:266–268

180. Mamon JF, Tan A, Pyati P et al (1991) Unusual volar dislocation of the lunate into the distal forearm: case report. J Trauma 31:1316–1318

181. Trumble TE (2002) Carpal fracture-dislocations: monograph series. Am Acad Orthop Surg

182. Braithwaite IJ, Jones WA (1992) Scapho-lunate dissociation occurring with scaphoid fracture. J Hand Surg [Br] 17:286–288

183. Sakada T, Miyazawa T, Ninomiya S et al (1994) Anterior dislocation of the proximal fragment of a scaphoid fracture: a case report. J Hand Surg [Am] 19:1042–1044

184. Schakel M (1986) Trans-scaphoid palmar lunate dislocation with concurrent scapholunate ligament disruption. J Hand Surg [Am] 11:653

185. Vender MI (1989) Acute scaphoid fracture with scapholunate gap. J Hand Surg [Am] 14:1004–1007

186. Cheng CY, Hsu KY, Tseng IC et al (2004) Concurrent scaphoid fracture with scapholunate ligament rupture. Acta Orthop Belg 70:485–491

187. Garcia-Elias M (1987) Dorsal fractures of the triquetrum—avulsion or compression fractures? J Hand Surg [Am] 12:266–268

188. Lavernia CJ, Cohen MS, Taleisnik J (1992) Treatment of scapholunate dissociation by ligamentous repair and capsulodesis. J Hand Surg [Am] 17(2):354–359

189. Skoff HD, Hecker AT, Hayes WC et al (1995) Bone suture anchors in hand surgery. J Hand Surg [Br] 20:245–248

190. Kremer T, Wendt M, Riedel K et al (2010) Open reduction for perilunate injuries–clinical outcome and patient satisfaction. J Hand Surg [Am] 35:1599–1606

191. Viegas SF, Dasilva MF (2000) Surgical repair for scapholunate dissociation. Techn Hand Upper Extrem Surg 4:148–153

192. Fernandez DL (1993) Technique and results of external fixation of complex carpal injuries. Hand Clin 9:625–637

193. Fernandez DL, Ghillani R (1987) External fixation of complex carpal dislocations: a preliminary report. J Hand Surg [Am] 12:335–347

194. Tomaino MM (2004) Preliminary lunate reduction and pinning facilitates restoration of carpal height when treating perilunate dislocation, scaphoid fracture and nonunion, and scapholunate dissociation. Am J Orthop 33(3):153–154

195. Blatt G (1987) Capsulodesis in reconstructive hand surgery: volar capsulodesis following excision of the distal ulna. Hand Clin 3:81

196. Van Den Abbeele KLS, Loh YC, Stanley JK et al (1998) Early results of a modified Brunelli procedure for scapholunate instability. J Hand Surg [Br] 23:258–261

197. Almquist EE, Bach AW, Sack JT et al (1991) Four-bone ligament reconstruction for treatment of chronic complete scapholunate separation. J Hand Surg [Am] 16:322–327

198. Linscheid RL, Dobyns JH (1992) Treatment of scapholunate dissociation: rotatory subluxation of the scaphoid. Hand Clin 8:645–652

199. Song D, Goodman S, Gilula LA et al (2009) Ulnocarpal translation in perilunate dislocations. J Hand Surg [Eur] 34(3):388–390

200. Viegas SF, Bean JW, Schram RA (1987) Transscaphoid fracture-dislocation treated with open reduction and Herbert screw internal fixation. J Hand Surg [Am] 12:992–999

201. Menapace KA, Larabee L, Arnoczky SP et al (2001) Anatomic placement of the Herbert-Whipple

screw in scaphoid fractures: a cadaver study. J Hand Surg [Am] 26:883–892

202. Trumble TE (2002) Transscaphoid perilunate dislocations. In: Trumble T (ed) Carpal fracture-dislocations, Monograph series. American Academy of Orthopaedic Surgeons, pp 49–57

203. Teisen H, Hjarbaek J (1988) Classification of fresh fractures of the lunate. J Hand Surg [Br] 13(4):458–462

204. Gunal I, Oztuna V, Hazer B (1998) Trapeziolunate external fixation for transscaphoid perilunate dislocations of the wrist: report of 2 cases. J Hand Surg [Am] 23:158–161

205. Raab DJ, Fischer DA, Quick DC (1994) Lunate and perilunate dislocations in professional football players: a five-year retrospective analysis. Am J Sports Med 22:841–845

206. Inoue G, Shionoya K (1999) Late treatment of unreduced perilunate dislocations. J Hand Surg [Br] 24:221–225

207. Siegert JJ, Frassica FJ, Amadio PC (1988) Treatment of chronic perilunate dislocations. J Hand Surg [Am] 13:206–212

208. Rettig ME, Raskin KB (1999) Long- term assessment of proximal row carpectomy for chronc perilunate dislocation. J Hand Surg [Am] 24:1231–1236

209. Lacour C, De Peretti F, Barraud O et al (1993) Perilunar dislocations of the carpus: value of surgical treatment. Rev Chir Orthop Reparatrice Appar Mot 79:114–123

210. Altissimi M, Mancini GB, Azzarà A (1987) Perilunate dislocations of the carpus: a long-term review. Ital J Orthop Traumatol 13(4):491–500

211. Komurcu M, Kurklu M, Ozturan KE et al (2008) Early and delayed treatment of dorsal transscaphoid perilunate fracture-dislocations. J Orthop Trauma 22:535–540

212. Schaller P, Grűnert J (1998) Spatergebnisse nach operativer Behandlung von perilunaren Luxationen und Luxationsfrakturen. Handchir Mikrochir Plast Chir 30:298–302

213. Krimmer H, Wiemer P, Kalb K (2000) Comparative outcome assessment of the wrist joint—mediocarpal partial arthrodesis and total arthrodesis [in German]. Handchir Mikrochir Plast Chir 32:369–374

214. Hudak PL, Amadio PC, Bombardier C (1996) Development of an upper extremity outcome measure: the DASH (disabilities of the arm, shoulder and hand) [corrected]. The upper extremity collaborative group (UECG). Am J Ind Med 29:602–608

215. MacDermid JC, Turgeon T, Richards RS et al (1998) Patient rating of wrist pain and disability: a reliable and valid measurement tool. J Orthop Trauma 12:577–586

216. Yamada K, Sekiya S, Oka S et al (1995) Lunate dislocation with ulnar nerve paresis. J Hand Surg [Br] 20:206–209

217. Gellman H, Schwartz SD, Botte MJ et al (1988) Late treatment of a dorsal transscaphoid, transtriquetral perilunate wrist dislocation with avascular changes of the lunate. Clin Orthop 237:196–203

218. Mueller JJ (1984) Avascular necrosis and collapse of the lunate following a volar perilunate dislocation: a case report and review of this complication in dislocations of the wrist. Orthopedics 7:1009–1014

219. White RE, Omer GE (1984) Transient vascular compromise of the lunate after fracture-dislocation or dislocation of the carpus. J Hand Surg [Am] 9:181–184

220. Green DP (1985) The effect of avascular necrosis on Russe bone grafting for scaphoid nonunion. J Hand Surg [Am] 10:597–605

221. Markiewitz AD, Ruby LK, O'Brien ET (1997) Carpal fractures and dislocations. In: Lichtman DM, Alexander AH (eds) The wrist and its disorders, 2nd edn. Saunders, pp 189–233

222. Wollstein R, Wei C, Bilonick RA et al (2009) The radiographic measurement of ulnar translation. J Hand Surg [Br] 34:384–387

223. Gilula LA, Weeks PM (1978) Post-traumatic ligamentous instabilities of the wrist. Radiology 129:641–651

224. Borrelli J, Torzilli PA, Grigiene R et al (1997) Effect of impact load on articular cartilage: development of an intra-articular fracture model. J Orthop Trauma 11:319–326

225. Simank HG, Graf J, Fromm B et al (1992) What is the effect of para-articular fractures on hyaline joint cartilage? Experimental electron optic studies of the rabbit on post-traumatic subchondral vascularization disorders. Unfallchirurg 95(6):280–283

226. Gelberman RH, Gross MS (1986) The vascularity of the wrist: identification of arterial patterns at risk. Clin Orthop 202:40–49

227. Knirk JL, Jupiter JB (1986) Intra-articular fractures of the distal end of the radius in young adults. J Bone Joint Surg Am 68:647–659

228. Stern PJ (1981) Multiple flexor tendon ruptures following an old anterior dislocation of the lunate: a case report. J Hand Surg [Am] 63:489–490

229. Stevens KJ, Pathak G, Davis TR (1994) Volar dislocation of the lunate causing multiple flexor tendon ruptures: an unusual manifestation of pyrophosphate arthropathy. J Hand Surg [Br] 19:195–196

230. Mullan GB, Lloyd GJ (1980) Complete carpal disruption of the hand. Hand 12(1):39–42

231. Apergis E (2004) καταγματα-εξαρθρήματα του καρπου. Konstantaras Medical Books, Athens

Scaphocapitate Syndrome

5

5.1 Introduction

The term "scaphocapitate syndrome" refers to the combination of a fracture through the waist of the scaphoid and a fracture of the neck of the capitate, the head of which rotates by 90°–180° [1–3].

The first references about a "scaphocapitate syndrome" were made by Lorie [4] and Perves et al. in 1937 [5], who were the first to describe a trans-scaphoid trans-capitate perilunate fracture-dislocation. In the English literature the first reference was in 1940 from Nicholson [6]. However, the term "scaphocapitate syndrome" was introduced by Fenton [7] in 1956 who described two patients with a proximal capitate fracture that was rotated 180°, but neither of them was reported to have an associated perilunate dislocation. Since then, about 43 cases have been published, involving adults. In children only 4 cases have been published [8–11], the youngest being 11-years old [12] with simultaneous fractures of the scaphoid and capitate, but these fractures were undisplaced.

Kaulesar Sukul and Johannes [13] made a literature review of 13 cases of scaphocapitate syndrome from 1955 to 1987, while Milliez et al. [14] of 25 cases from 1937 to 1992.

5.2 Incidence

The frequency of the scaphocapitate syndrome is not clearly known. Rand et al. [15] reported that capitate fractures accounted for 1.3 % of all carpal fractures; 0.3 % were isolated capitate fractures, 0.6 % were of scaphocapitate syndrome type and 0.4 % were fractures of the capitate in association with PLFD type of injuries. Geissler and Slade [16] stated that fractures of the capitate account for 1–2 % of all carpal fractures.

In our series, from 67 greater arc injuries (52 PLFD+S and 15 PLFD-S) we found 10 fractures of the capitate (14.9 %), which were manifested in various ways (Table 5.1 and Fig. 5.1).

Herzberg et al. [17] reported that in the trans-scaphoid-PLFD group, the most frequent variant was the trans-scaphoid, trans-capitate type and constituted 8 % of all PLFD injuries.

Adler and Shaftan [18] stated that the reported incidence of this injury may be unduly low, owing to failure of diagnosis and that a higher index of suspicion would lead to the recognition and treatment of more such injuries.

5.3 Mechanism of Injury

Fenton [7] assumed that during a fall, with the hand in dorsiflexion and radial deviation, the pointed radial styloid process (the chisel) impinges on the waist of the scaphoid, which is supported by the sturdy capitate (the anvil). When the force is moderately strong, the scaphoid alone will fracture, but when the blow is particularly sharp and violent, the capitate will also fracture [19].

E. Apergis, *Fracture-Dislocations of the Wrist*,
DOI: 10.1007/978-88-470-5328-1_5, © Springer-Verlag Italia 2013

Table 5.1 Data of our series

Case	Delay	Type-nomenclature	Scaphoid #	Capitate #	F-U/result
1	Same day	Trans-scaphoid, Trans-capitate dorsal perilunate	Waist	Transverse proximal pole. Head dislocated dorsally, rotated 90°, facing dorsally	15 years/scaphoid and capitate union. No arthritis
2	Same day	Trans-scaphoid, Trans-capitate, Trans-triquetral dorsal perilunate	Waist	Transverse neck. Head dislocated dorsally, rotated 180°, facing distally	2 years/scaphoid and capitate union. No arthritis
3	Same day	Trans-scaphoid, Trans-capitate, dorsal perilunate (open injury)	Waist	Transverse neck. Head dislocated palmarly, rotated 90°, facing dorsally	15 years/scaphoid union, capitate nonunion. Midcarpal arthritis. Symptoms free
4	Same day	Trans-scaphoid, Trans-Capitate, palmar perilunate	Proximal pole	Displaced para-sagittal of the capitate head	Lost
5	Same day	Trans-scaphoid, Trans-capitate, Trans-lunate, peri-triquetral, palmar lunate dislocation	Waist	Transverse neck. Body and head dislocated palmarly, rotated 90° facing palmarly	1 year/scaphoid and capitate union. Excessive RC arthritis
6	1 week	Wrist reduced. Scaphocapitate syndrome ?	Waist nonunion	Transverse proximal pole. Head rotated 180° facing distally	1 year/scaphoid nonunion, capitate union. No arthritis
7	1 week	Wrist reduced. Scaphocapitate syndrome	Distal pole comminuted	Transverse neck. Head dislocated dorsally. Rotated 180° facing distally	6.3 years/scaphoid and capitate union. No arthritis
8	4.5 months	Wrist reduced. Scaphocapitate syndrome	Waist	Transverse proximal pole, rotated 180°, facing distally	1 year/scaphoid and capitate union. Signs of AVN
9	1 week	Wrist reduced. Scaphocapitate syndrome	Waist	Transverse neck. Modest head displacement	1 year/scaphoid and capitate union. No arthritis
10	3 months	Wrist reduced. Peri-scaphoid, Trans-capitate	Avulsed STT from trapezium	Transverse proximal pole. Modest head displacement	7 years/capitate union. Rapid development of AVN. SLC fusion

STT Scapho-Trapezium-Trapezoid, *AVN* Avascular necrosis, *SLC* Scapholunocapitate

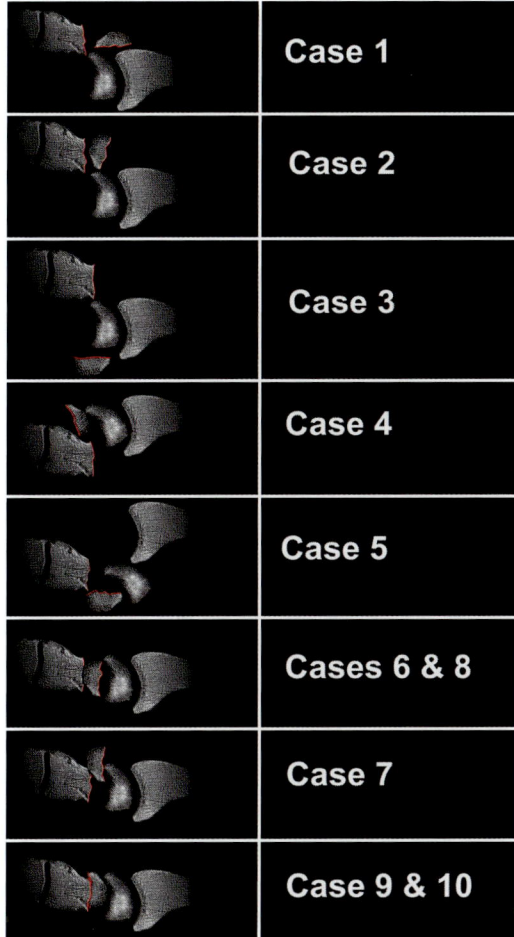

Fig. 5.1 Our cases with the corresponding drawings of the capitate fractures and their different types of displacement

Adler and Shaftan [18] in their review of 91 capitate fractures, suggested that indirect trauma was the most common mechanism of fractures of the capitate.

Although, a direct blow to the dorsum of the volar-flexed wrist has been implicated [3, 20], most authors [9, 20], agree with the mechanism proposed by Stein and Siegel [21] based on anatomical studies on cadaver wrists, according to which the patient falls on the outstretched hand and the wrist goes into marked dorsiflexion. The capitate fracture is caused by the impaction of the capitate neck to the dorsal lip of the radius, while the scaphoid fracture is caused by the tension created at the midcarpal joint level by the forced extension. We can reasonably assume that capitate fracture precedes chronically the scaphoid fracture. Rotation of the proximal fragment appears to occur secondarily, forced by the distal fragment, as this returns to neutral position [2, 22] (Figs. 5.2 and 5.3a–h).

However, none of the above-mentioned mechanisms seems to apply in several of the reported cases [3, 23].

5.4 Pathologic Anatomy of the Injury

According to the prevailing view, the scapho-capitate syndrome constitutes the final stage of a greater arc injury, starting from the radial side of

Fig. 5.2 Schematic depiction of the mechanism of injury: With the wrist in dorsiflexion the capitate fractures impacting to the dorsal lip of the radius (**a**); the scaphoid fractures after tension at the midcarpal joint level (**b**); the capitate head is forced to rotate by the distal fragment, as this returns to neutral position (**c**, **d**). With permission from [76]

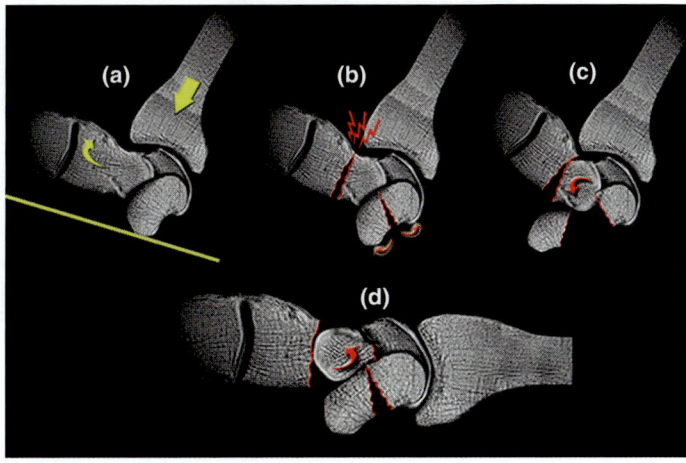

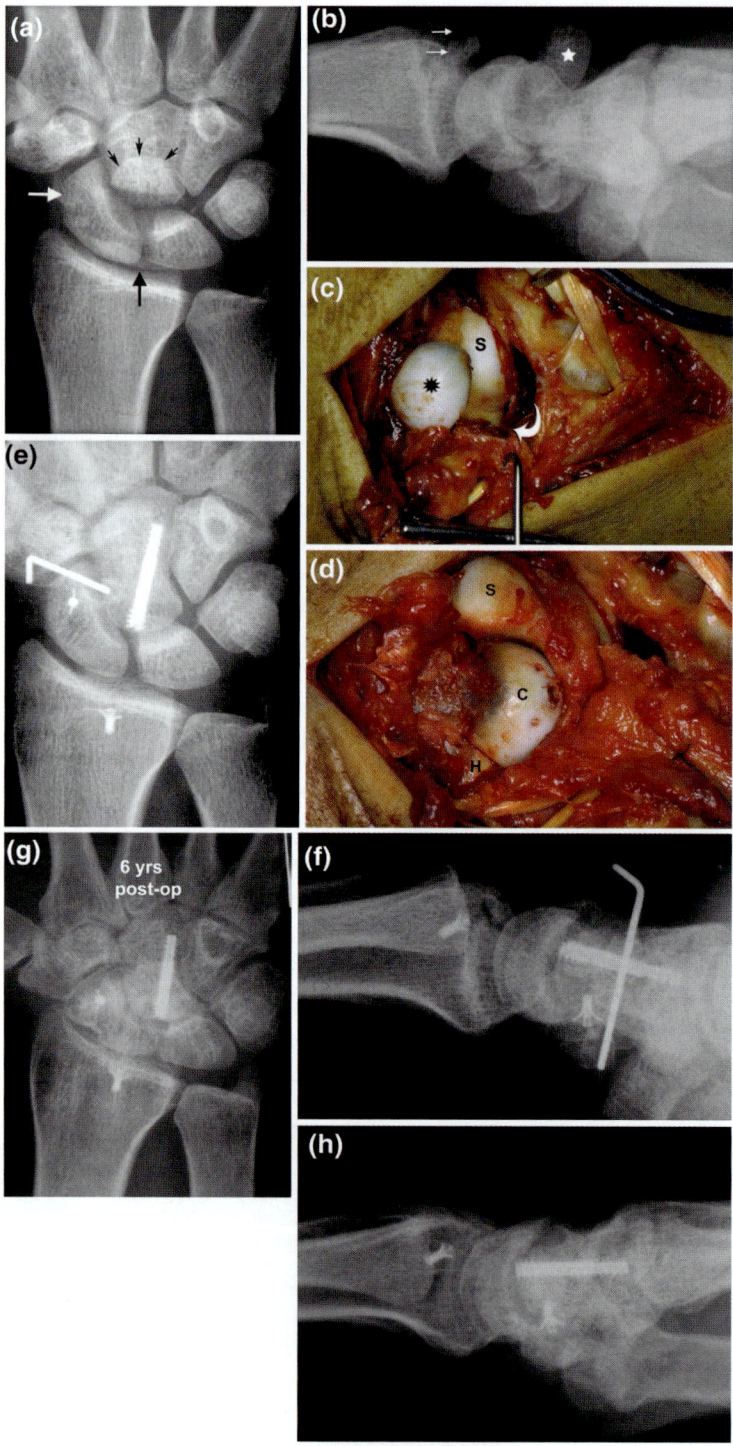

◀ Fig. 5.3 Case 7. Male, 27-years old. Preoperative PA view in which the proximal capitate fragment is rotated by 180° (*small arrows*), the fracture of the distal pole of the scaphoid (*white arrow*) and the fracture of the distal radial rim (*black arrow*) (**a**); in *L* view, the head of the capitate is dorsally displaced and rotated by 180° (*asterisk*), while white arrows indicate the fractured dorsal radial rim (**b**); appearance at surgery, dorsal approach; the head of the capitate (*asterisk*) and the displaced dorsal radial fragment (*curved arrow*) (*S* Scaphoid) (**c**); after reduction and fixation of the capitate head with a headless screw, while the scaphoid with the dorsal approach, looks intact (**d**); with a separate volar approach, the fractured distal scaphoid was reduced and fixated using a bone anchor and a K-wire while the dorsal radial rim was fixed with a bone anchor; postoperative X-rays (**e**, **f**); 6 years postoperatively (**g**, **h**). With permission from [76]

the wrist and progressing through osseous structures around the lunate [24]. The injury essentially constitutes a trans-scaphoid, trans-capitate perilunate injury, which appears with the wrist being dislocated or reduced, spontaneously [25] or with closed reduction after manipulation [9, 26–29]. The wrist can be reduced but the capitate head remains displaced, with its proximal pole rotated by 90°–180° [2, 9, 14, 26–33] (Fig. 5.4a, b), while a case of scapho-capitate syndrome has been described with the head of the capitate palmarly displaced deep to the median nerve, which was tended over it [34].

It has also been stated that the scaphocapitate syndrome represents an incomplete form of the perilunate pattern of injury [20].

Kaulesar Sukul and Johannes [13] distinguished two types of trans-scaphoid, trans-capitate fracture dislocation, one in which rotation of the capitate is limited or does not occur at all, and the other where there is a 180° rotation of the capitate fragment; this implies that a perilunate dislocation was originally present.

Vance et al. [3] stated that there are two common and three uncommon patterns of injury. The first two appeared with the same incidence: In the first one, transverse fractures of the scaphoid and capitate occurred without dislocation, while the inverted capitate fragment remained in articulation with the lunate. The other presentation was a dorsal perilunate dislocation. The three other uncommon patterns that have been noted are: volar perilunate dislocation of the wrist and proximal part of the capitate, the isolated volar dislocation of the proximal part of the capitate and the isolated dorsal dislocation of the proximal part of the capitate.

Rand et al. [15] maintained that the term "scaphocapitate fracture syndrome" adds confusion to the terminology and they suggested that this term must be abandoned in favor of considering this as a special case of "trans-scaphoid, trans-capitate, perilunar fracture dislocation".

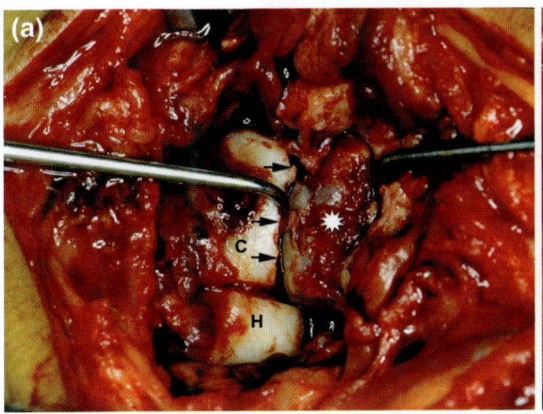 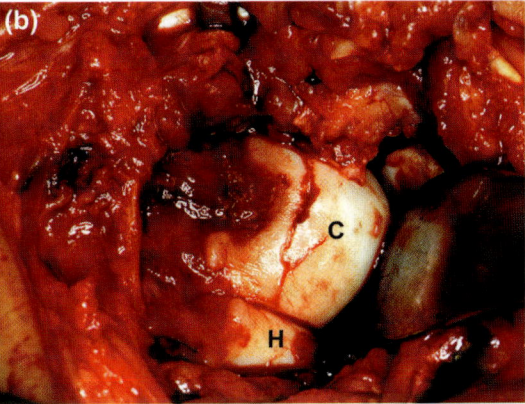

Fig. 5.4 The fractured surface of the neck of the capitate (*black arrows*) is in contact with the articular surface of its head (*asterisk*) (**a**); the appearance after reduction of the capitate head (**b**) (*H* Hamate, *C* Capitate). With permission from [76]

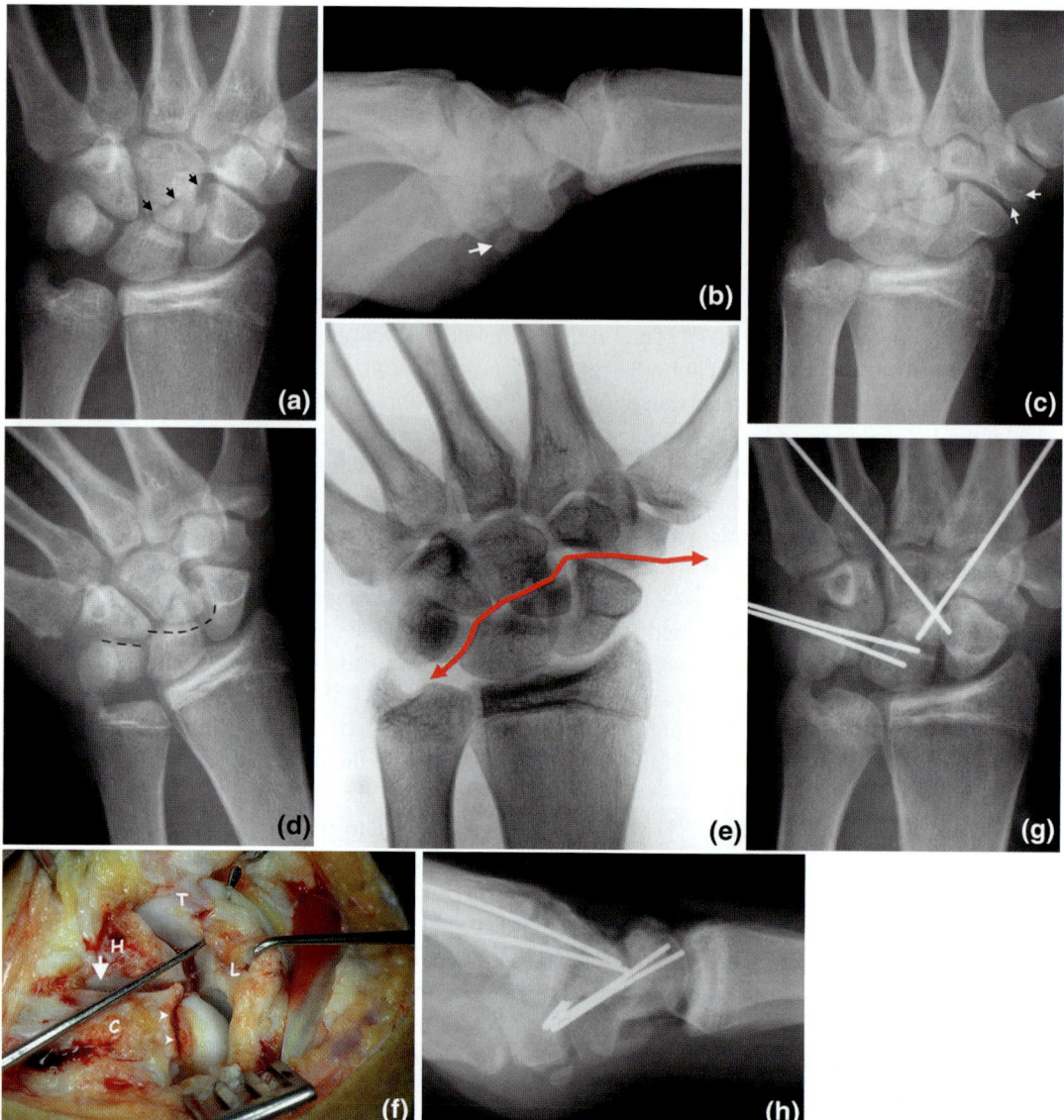

Fig. 5.5 Case 10. Male, 19-years old, with a 3-month old reported injury, treated with a splint for 2 weeks. The P-A view indicated an oblique fracture of the capitate (*arrows*) (**a**); the lateral and oblique views, showed an avulsed osseous fragment from the trapezium (probably the attachment of the STT ligament) (*white arrows*) (**b, c**); in ulnar deviation, disruption of Gilula's arc is apparent (**d**); the presumptive path of injury (**e**); appearance at surgery, dorsal approach. The fractured capitate (*white arrows*), a mild dissociation between capitate and hamate (*arrow*), while the probe shows the disruption of the LT ligament (*H* Hamate, *C* Capitate, *L* Lunate, *T* Triquetrum) (**f**); postoperative appearance (**g, h**); 6 months later the midcarpal joint had been obliterated, while the capitate showed signs of AVN (**i**); a midcarpal fusion was performed (**j**); the radiographic appearance and the ROM 7 years postoperatively (**k-n**). With permission from [76]

There is some confusion in the literature regarding the terminology and diversity in the appearance of these injuries [13, 15]. Any misunderstanding would be addressed, if we accepted that the term "scaphocapitate syndrome" should only be used in cases of a reduced wrist, with concomitant fractures of the scaphoid and the neck of the capitate, with its proximal pole rotated by 90°–180°.

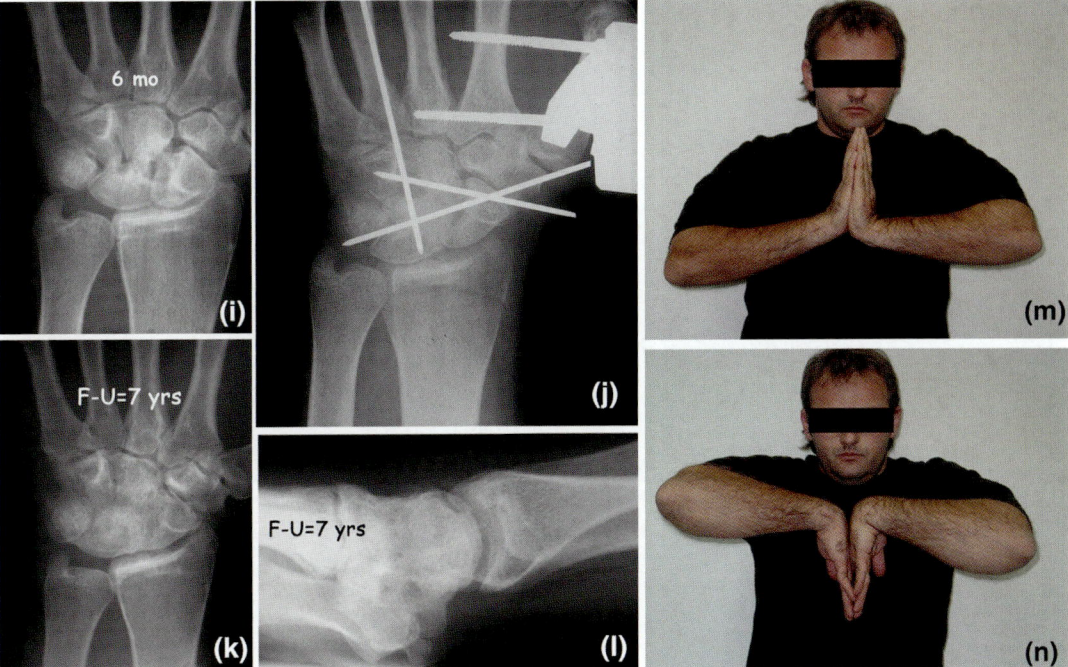

Fig. 5.5 (continued)

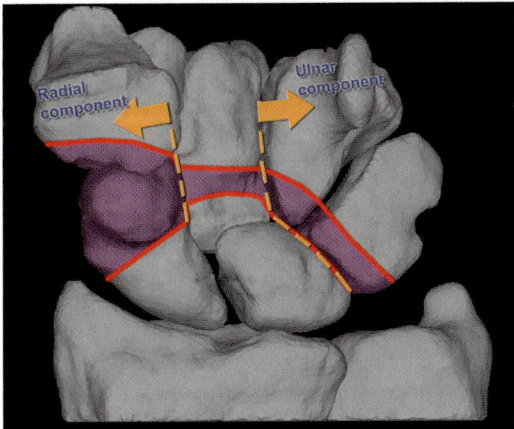

Fig. 5.6 Every displaced, angulated, or rotated fracture of the capitate constitutes a greater arc injury (confined to *shadowed area*), which is associated with a radial and an ulnar component. Both components could be related with injuries that are not detectable in X-rays, e.g., STT or LT ligament injury

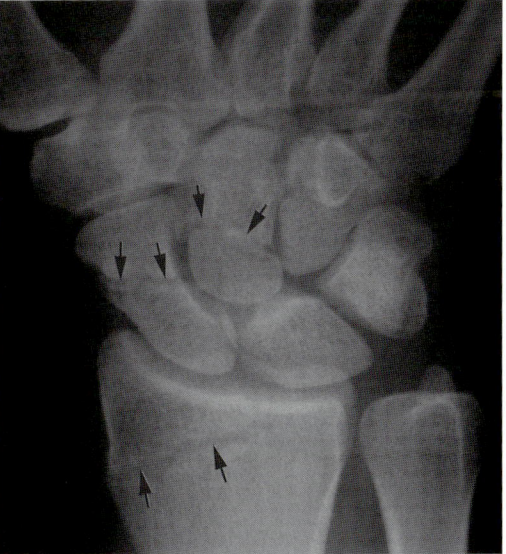

Fig. 5.7 The combined undisplaced or minimally displaced fractures of the radius, scaphoid, and capitate probably indicate the first stage of a progressively developing greater arc injury

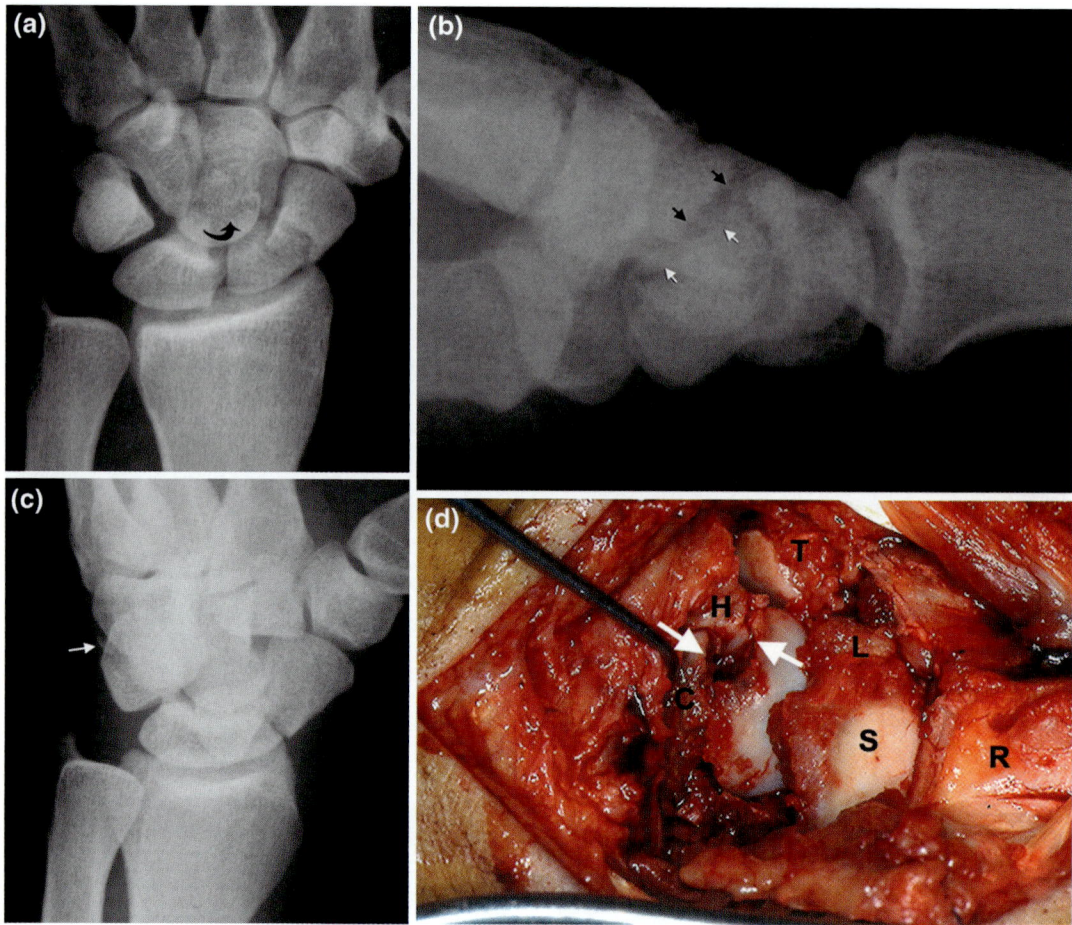

Fig. 5.8 Case 9. Male, 39-years old. He was referred as having a displaced fracture of the scaphoid. A fracture of the capitate neck with rotation and volar displacement of the capitate head were apparent (**a**, **b**); oblique view indicated an avulsion fragment from the dorsal surface of the hamate (**c**); appearance at surgery with dorsal approach; the displacement of the capitate fracture (*arrows*) (**d**); reduction and fixation of the capitate using a headless screw and temporary fixation with 2 K-wires (**e**); the reduced and fixated with a headless screw scaphoid using bone grafts; the tail of the hamate showed a compression fracture (*arrow*) (**f**); final X-rays 1 year postoperatively (**g**, **h**). With permission from [76]

Compared to the simple, isolated, and undisplaced fractures of the capitate, there are reports of isolated fractures of the capitate neck with palmar dislocation of the proximal pole [35, 36] or with the proximal pole rotated by 180°, without an apparent associated scaphoid fracture [22, 37, 38]. There are doubts however, as to whether these are really isolated fractures of the capitate. When one considers the central position of the capitate, surrounded by the other carpal bones and the base of the third metacarpal, it is difficult to accept that such displacement and rotation of the proximal capitate can occur in isolation.

Two of our cases had displaced fractures of the capitate neck, combined with injuries distal to the waist of the scaphoid. One of these was a comminuted fracture of the distal pole of the scaphoid, which was hardly shown on the X-rays (Fig. 5.3a–h) and the other was an avulsion fracture from the radiovolar surface of the trapezium (Fig. 5.5a–n), corresponding to the attachment of the STT ligament. Both injuries had an associated rupture of the LT ligament and both could easily be overlooked. A similar case with fracture of the capitate associated with STT and LT ligaments rupture, has already been reported [39].

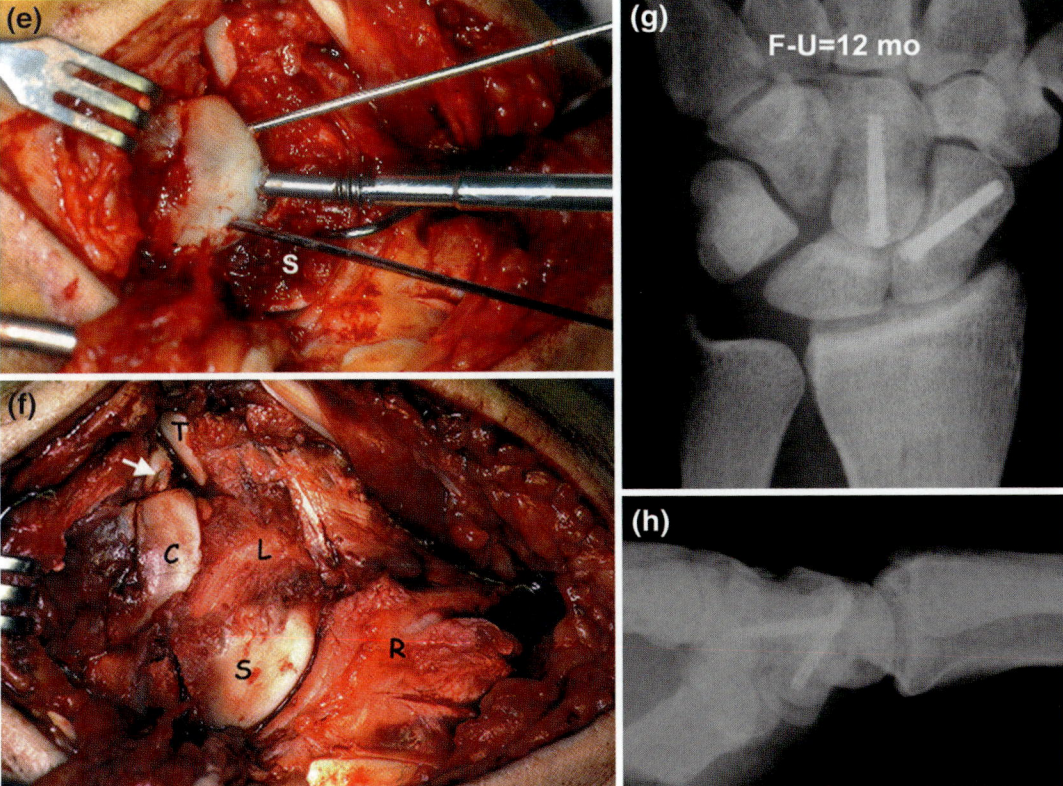

Fig. 5.8 (continued)

We consider that every displaced, angulated, and/or rotated fracture of the neck of the capitate indicates indeed a greater arc injury and that they are always associated with a radial and an ulnar component. The radial component could be located between the waist of the scaphoid and the trapezium-trapezoid bones (including rupture of the STT ligament, which is not detectable by X-rays). The ulnar component is usually a lunotriquetral ligament injury, but may be a fracture of either the triquetrum or the hamate bones (Fig. 5.6). Reported cases of combined fractures of the scaphoid and capitate neck with no or little displacement [12], probably represent the first stage of this progressively developing injury (Fig. 5.7).

Possibly, in cases of displaced fractures of the capitate neck with otherwise normal X-rays, a midcarpal arthrogram or arthroscopy is indicated to identify possible coexisting ligamentous injuries, indicating a path of injury, other than the path through the scaphoid.

The final delineation of the injury depends on two factors: (a) the direction of the force of the injury (usually radial to ulnar, although pure dorsopalmar application of force is possible) and (b) the magnitude of the applied force, which determines how many of the three columns of the wrist are injured.

Therefore, the term ''scaphocapitate syndrome'' constitutes only one subtype of a group of injuries and it may be better to use the term ''capitate syndrome'' instead of ''scaphocapitate syndrome''. The former can be defined as a displaced fracture through the neck of the capitate, with associated bony and/or ligamentous injuries on the radial and/or ulnar sides of the wrist [40].

5.5   Diagnosis

Diagnosis is based on careful radiographic evaluation but the true extent of injury can easily be missed. The injury may be labeled as an isolated fracture of the scaphoid or a typical trans-scaphoid perilunate fracture-dislocation, while the lesion to the capitate may be overlooked [20]. A posteroanterior traction radiograph (with the hand suspended in finger-traps) is useful, since the squared-off end of the proximal capitate is easily seen in this view [2]. This radiographic appearance has also been characterized as «cut-off-top-of-an-egg» [41] (Fig. 5.3a). Sometimes in questionable cases the diagnosis is made with the aid of computed tomography [42] or MRI [43, 44].

Delayed, deficient, or even complete lack of diagnosis of these injuries, are unfortunately quite common occurrences [14, 19, 45, 46]. In 1/3 out of 26 cases mentioned in the literature from 1937 until 1994, there was a delay in diagnosis of more than 15 days [14], some even 2 years later [46]. Boisgard et al. [47] reported that 8 out of 26 cases, evaded diagnosis during the initial assessment, in spite of the adequate radiological control performed.

The injury could be manifested with three basic radiographic patterns: (a) As incomplete injury with fractures of both the scaphoid and capitate, which are undisplaced or with minimal displacement (Figs. 5.7, 5.8a–h), (b) As a classic scaphocapitate syndrome, with fractures through the waist of the scaphoid and the capitate neck, with the wrist reduced and the head of the capitate displaced or rotated in varying degrees (Fig. 5.9a–k) and (c) As a trans-scaphoid, trans-capitate perilunar fracture dislocation (Fig. 5.10a–h).

The capitate fracture is usually located to its proximal or middle third and rarely to its distal third [15]. Geissler and Slade [16] recognized four major patterns of fractures in the capitate. These include: transverse fracture of the proximal pole of the capitate, transverse fracture of the body of the capitate, verticofrontal fracture and a parasagittal fracture pattern.

Associated fractures with this type of injury have also been described: fractured triquetrum [48–50], lunate [14] and radial styloid [21, 51], while more frequently reported, is an associated fracture of the distal radius [3, 9, 15, 18, 21, 52, 53].

Patients with preexisting nonunion of the scaphoid are vulnerable to dorsiflexion injuries, since the protective role of the scaphoid is omitted and the force is applied directly to the neck of the capitate from the dorsal radial rim [54] (Fig. 19 in chapter of acute PLI).

5.6   Management

Early reports recommended the excision of the head of the capitate and its replacement with an anchovy-type fascial graft, since avascular necrosis and nonunion were considered inevitable [6, 7, 21, 55].

Conservative treatment may lead to good results in undisplaced concomitant fractures of the scaphoid and capitate [12]. Jones [25] reported an excellent result in a patient treated only with immobilization, while the capitate was allowed to heal with its proximal portion rotated by 180°. Adler and Shaftan [18] reported that one of their patients, who sustained a trans-scaphoid, trans-capitate, dorsal perilunate fracture-dislocation with the head of the capitate rotated by 180°, was treated with closed reduction. After 5 months of immobilization he had a painless wrist with full flexion–extension arc and good strength, although he developed osteonecrosis of both proximal scaphoid and capitate.

It is understood that if closed reduction is attempted, any displacement of the capitate or scaphoid fractures is an indication for open reduction, but generally the result after conservative treatment is far from satisfactory [56].

Most authors [9, 12, 22, 23, 47, 57–60] agree that regardless of the radiographic appearance of the injury, open reduction and internal fixation is the treatment of choice. In cases of trans-scaphoid, trans-capitate PLFD, the combined approach is recommended, while in pure scaph-ocapitate syndrome the dorsal approach is usually sufficient. The capitate fragment is usually devoid of any soft tissues and is reduced relatively easy to the neck with manual pressure, by applying traction to the hand. K-wires or headless screws may be placed from the proximal to the distal side and have been equally successful for the fixation of the scaphoid and capitate. Reduction and fixation of the capitate must precede that of the scaphoid, otherwise the reduction of the latter is extremely difficult [3, 59] (Fig. 5.11a–h).

Transient avascular changes of the proximal capitate are usually seen, but the union of the fracture generally remains unaffected [20], while the possible objection that operative intervention might lead to necrosis seems unjustified [13]. Kohut et al. [61] reported that in three out of six patients with trans-scaphoid, trans-capitate PLFD, the first dorsal intermetacarpal artery and vein were implanted into the fractured proximal pole of the capitate to assist revascularization; other than that, all of them were treated during the first 12 days from injury. The fractured capitate united in all six cases and in one case the density of the proximal pole of the capitate increased temporarily.

When the capitate fracture is comminuted or if the treatment is applied belatedly, primary bone grafting is indicated [49, 59].

In cases of symptomatic osteonecrosis of the capitate head or severe damage of the articular cartilage, the excision of the fragment and a partial fusion (LC or SLC) with autologous bone grafting are indicated.

For injuries diagnosed late, i.e., after 2 months, the management depends on the patients' symptoms. As long as the scaphoid fracture has already or is about to unite, probably the best solution is patient monitoring, since some of them remain asymptomatic or with well tolerated symptoms for many years, despite the malposition of the capitate head. On the contrary, symptomatic patients with bone malalignment probably require some type of midcarpal fusion [20, 46].

We treated ten patients with capitate fracture (two cases with isolated fracture of the capitate were excluded). Five cases were considered as scaphocapitate syndrome and were treated with an average delay of 6 weeks (range, 1–18 weeks), while five cases belonged to the PLFD type of injuries and were treated the same day of the injury. They were all treated with open reduction and internal fixation. One patient was uncontactable for follow-up. The average follow-up of the remaining patients was 4.8 years (range, 1–15 years). Eight out of nine scaphoid fractures and nine out of ten capitate fractures were united successfully. Three out of ten cases developed signs of arthritis (two at the midcarpal and one at the radiocarpal level) and two patients developed signs of avascular necrosis, while one of them was subjected to scapholunocapitate fusion (Table 5.1).

5.7 Complications

Nonunion, osteonecrosis and the development of arthritis in the long-term, are potential complications regardless of the applied method of treatment [12, 15, 20]. Early open, anatomical reduction, and stable fixation are prerequisites to minimize the above complications.

The capitate is at particular risk for avascular necrosis, because its proximal pole is entirely intra-articular and also has peculiar vascularity. According to experimental studies [43, 47, 62–64], the capitate receives its vascularity from dorsal and palmar sources. In the majority of specimens (67 %) the dorsal vessels supply the major part of the capitate. In 33 % of specimens, the vascularity to the capitate head originates entirely from the palmar surface. Regardless of pattern, the proximal pole is supplied in a retrograde fashion in all specimens and is dependent on distal–to-proximal flow across the capitate waist analogous to the blood supply of the proximal scaphoid. The more proximal the fracture of the capitate is, the greater is the risk of aseptic necrosis [63]. Milliez et al. [65] classified

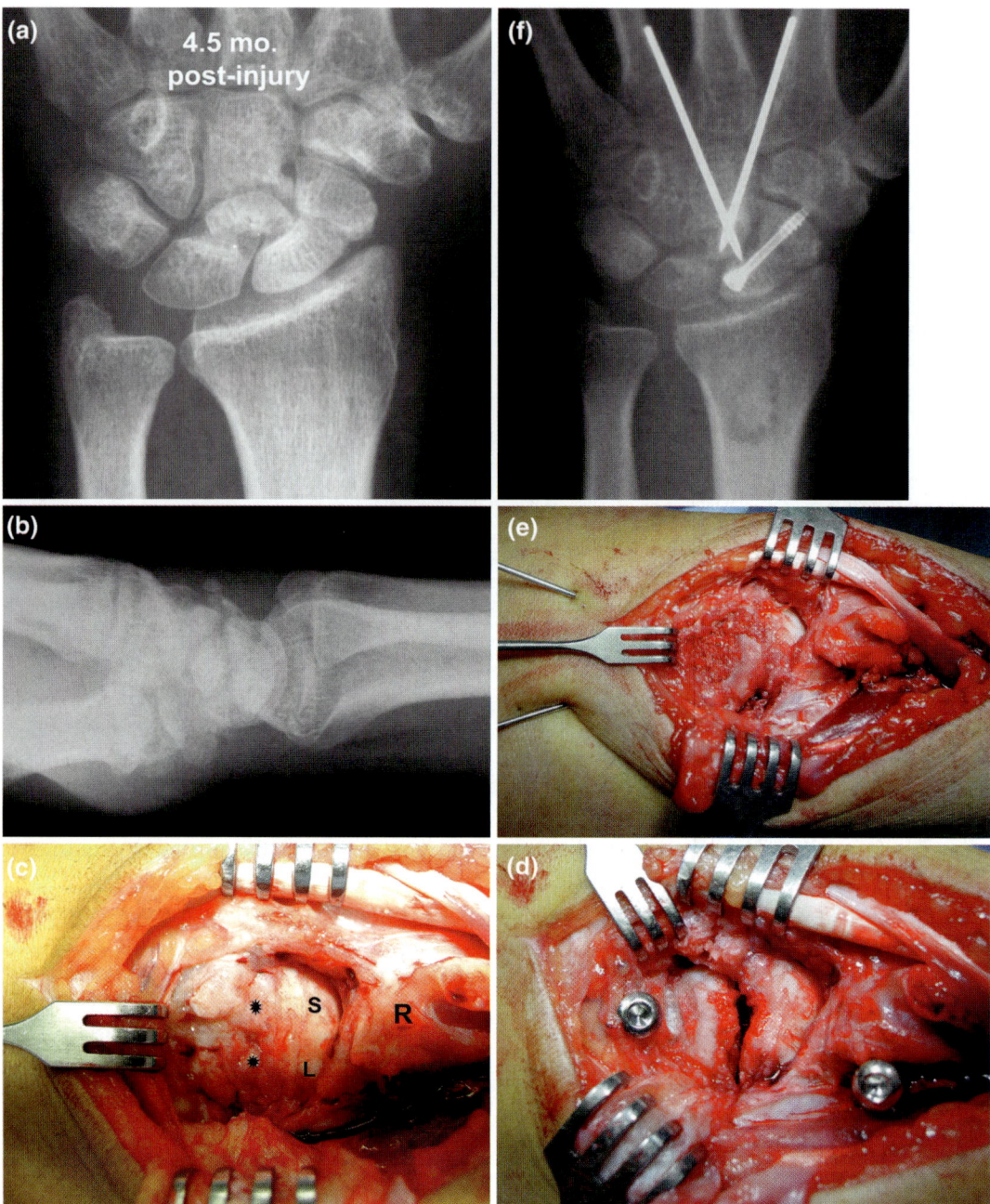

Fig. 5.9 Case 8. Male, 24-years old, with a 4.5 month-old reported injury. He was treated for a fractured scaphoid with a below-elbow cast for 3 months. The fracture and rotation of the capitate head were apparent in the X-rays (**a**, **b**); with the dorsal approach abundant scar tissue was located to the dorsal surface of the capitate (*asterisks*) (**c**); removal of the scar tissue and relocation of the capitate head which was proved to be particularly friable, using 2 screws and a lamina spreader for reduction (**d**); the capitate was reduced, the bone was grafted and fixated with 2 K-wires, while the scaphoid was fixated with a cannulated screw (**e**); postoperative X-rays (**f**, **g**); radiographic appearance and ROM after 12 months (**h–k**)

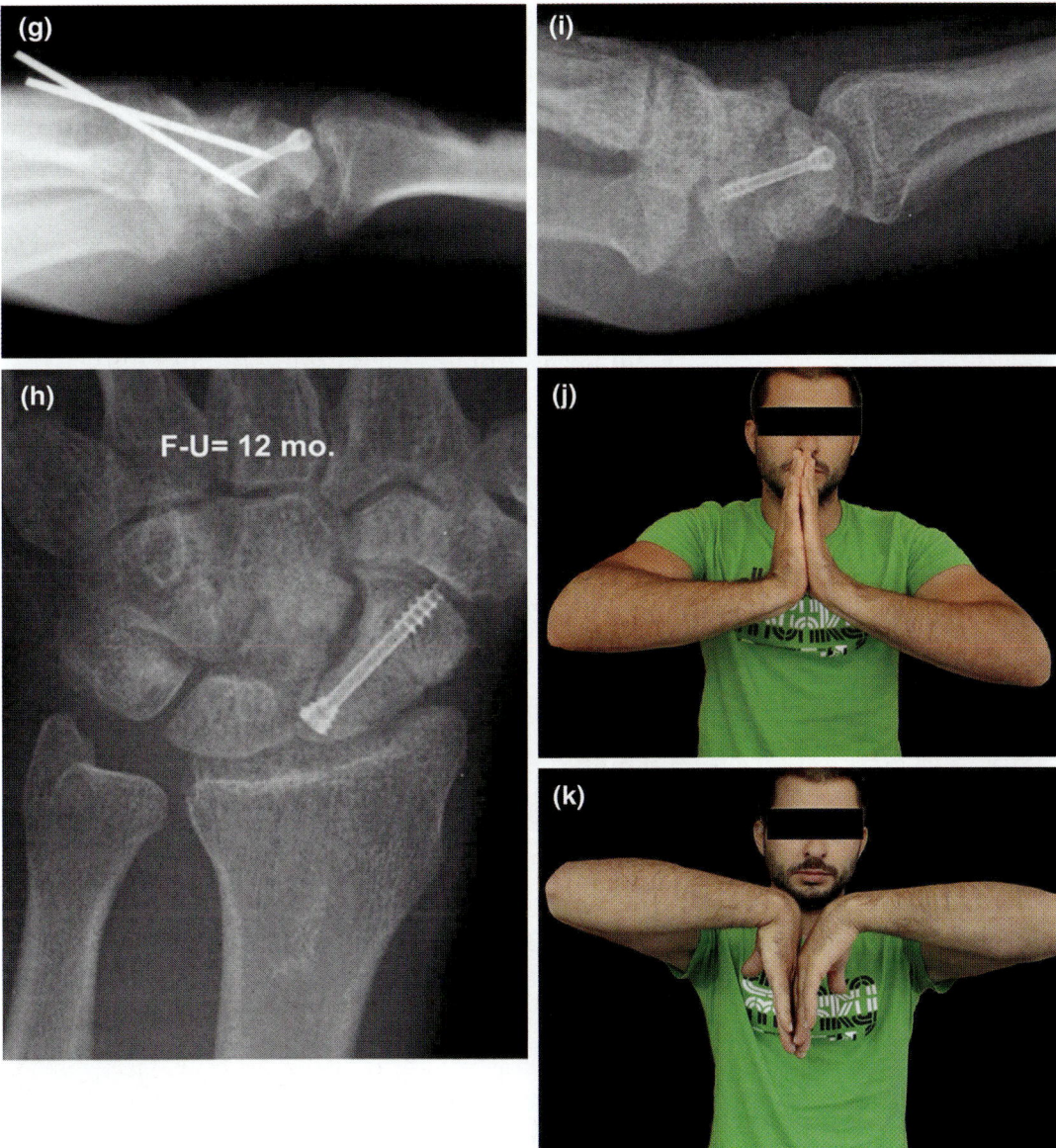

Fig. 5.9 (continued)

the avascular necrosis of the capitate into three types. In type I (which is the most common) the necrosis involves only the proximal pole, in Type II it involves the distal portion of the capitate, while in type III it involves the entire capitate. Avascular necrosis has been reported infrequently in isolated capitate fractures but is more common in higher-energy fractures, particularly when the capitate is rotated [16, 66].

The true incidence of capitate nonunion in cases with scaphocapitate syndrome is not known, but it is known that the most substantial and under-recognized complication of isolated capitate fractures is that of nonunion, the

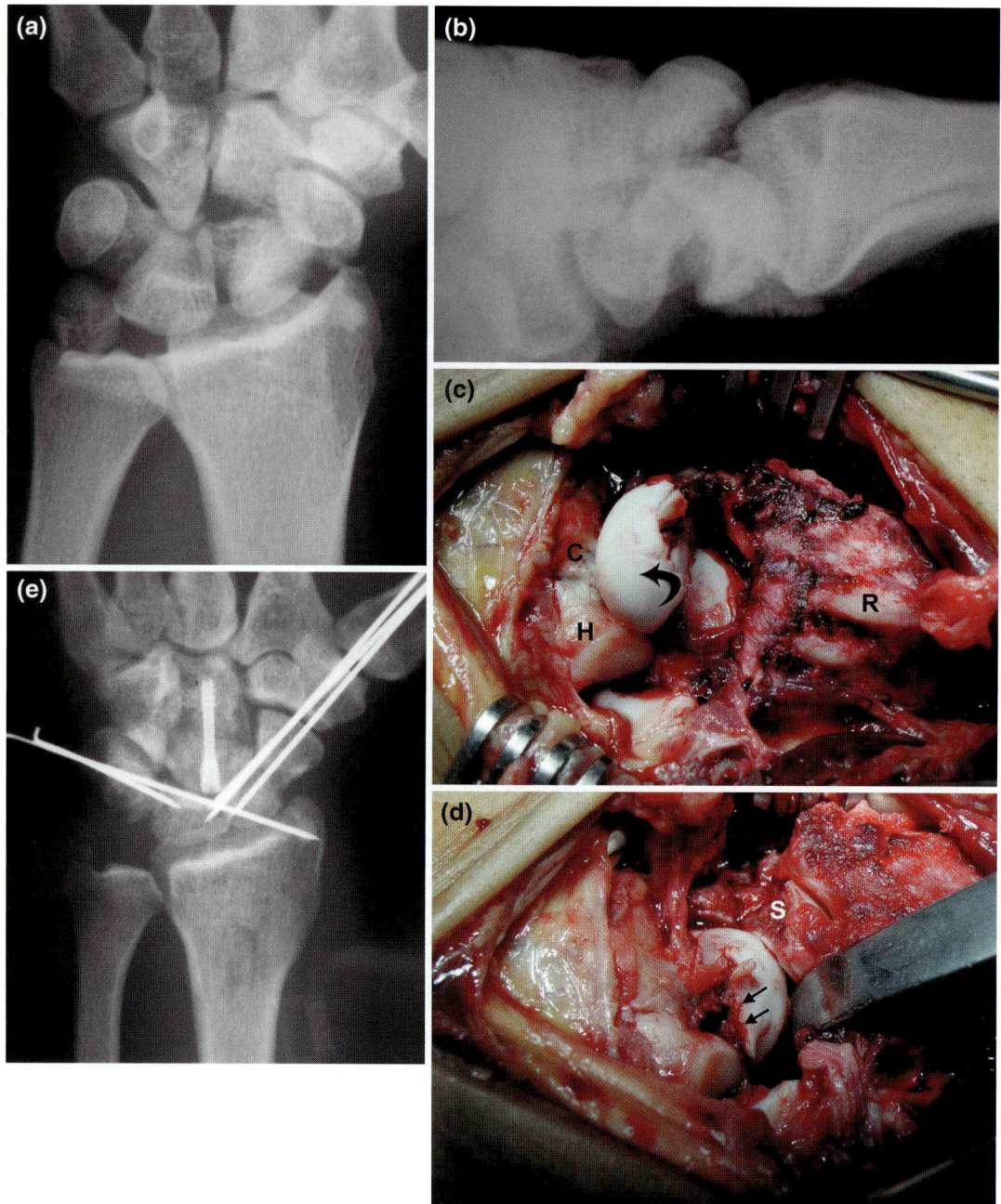

Fig. 5.10 Case 2. Male, 31-years old. Trans-scaphoid, trans-capitate, trans-triquetral dorsal perilunate fracture dislocation with the head of the capitate dorsally displaced, rotated by 180° and facing distally (**a**, **b**); with the dorsal approach, rotation of the capitate head was apparent (*curved arrow*) (*C* Capitate, *H* Hamate, *R* Radius) (**c**); double arrows indicate the comminution of the fractured capitate (*S* Scaphoid) (**d**); postoperative X-rays (**e**, **f**); final follow-up X-rays after 2 years (**g**, **h**)

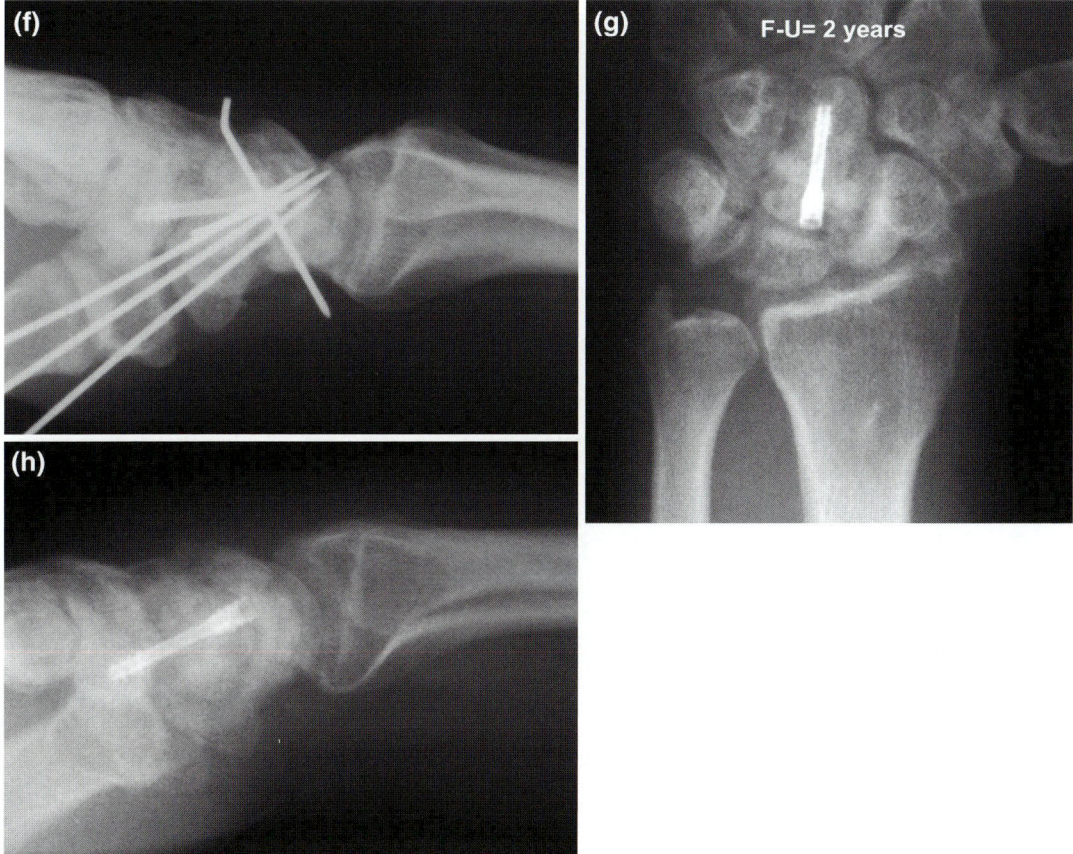

Fig. 5.10 (continued)

incidence of which ranges between 19.6 and 56 % [67, 68] (Fig. 5.12a–l).

Nonunion of the capitate may be related to both vascular and mechanical factors and is usually associated with absorption of the fracture surfaces and shortening of the capitate [15, 69–71]. This shortening induces carpal collapse and overloading to the scaphotrapezial-trapezoidal and triquetral hamate joints, on either side. In cases of capitate shortening, the fragments should be distracted to accept an intercalary graft, regain the lost length and restore carpal stability [15, 16, 70, 72].

Rand et al. [15], reported 13 cases of fractures, three of which were isolated and two of which progressed to nonunion after non-operative treatment. Freeman and Hay [69] introduced

a case with nonunion of the capitate presented with a painful snapping wrist, while Rayan [73] reported a case with occult wrist pain due to capitate nonunion. Both were cases with isolated injury to the capitate.

Kammermeier et al. [74] considered the uninjured palmar V ligament responsible for the development of capitate nonunion.

Rico et al. [75] presented a case with nonunion of an isolated fracture of the capitate, which was successfully treated with iliac bone graft and K-wires fixation. They stated that although isolated capitate fractures were less frequent, the incidence of pseudarthrosis was greater than in fractures of the capitate associated with other injuries. Reviewing the literature they found 10 cases of capitate nonunion.

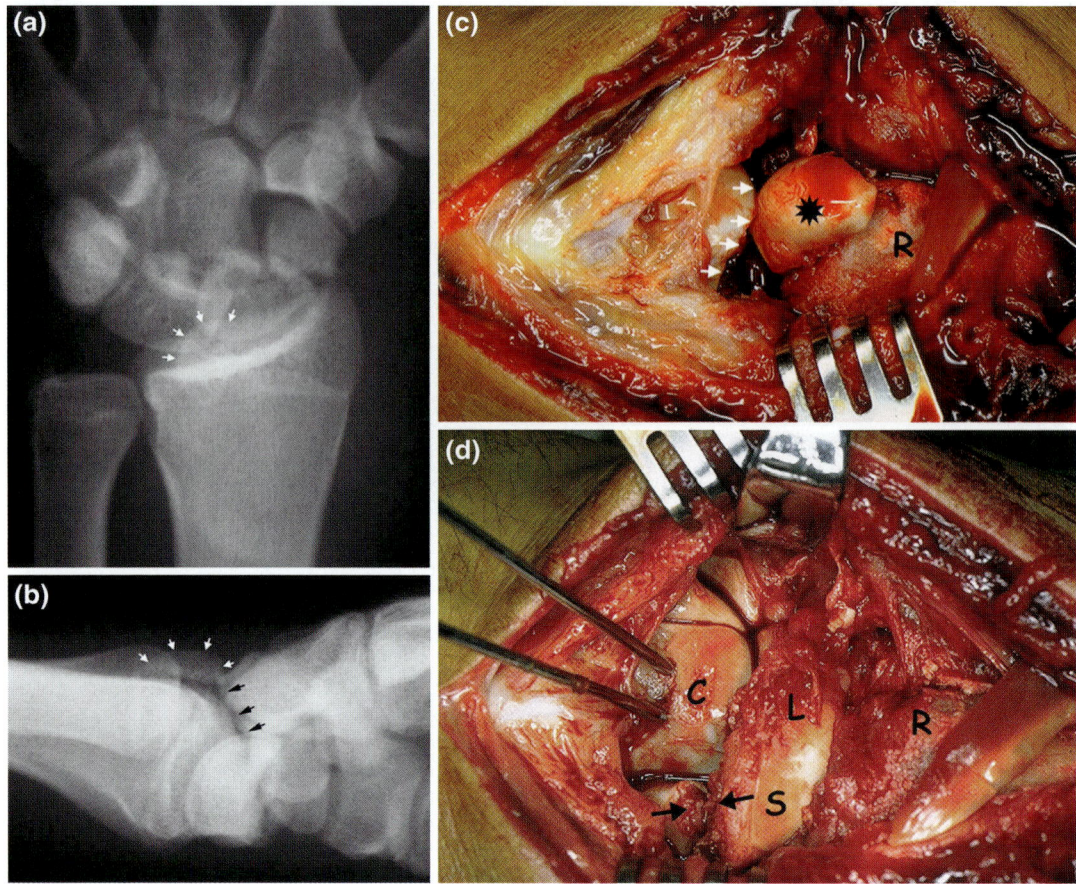

Fig. 5.11 Case 1. Male, 16-years old. Trans-scaphoid, trans-capitate dorsal perilunate fracture dislocation with the proximal head of the capitate located at the dorsal surface of the distal radius and rotated by 90° (**a**, **b**); fracture of the neck of the capitate (*white arrows*) and the head of the capitate (*asterisk*) located on the dorsal surface of the radius (**c**); reduction and fixation with 2 K-wires of the capitate while comminution of the dorsal scaphoid was obvious (*arrows*) (*C* Capitate, *S* Scaphoid, *L* Lunate, *R* Radius) (**d**); postoperative X-rays (**e**, **f**); 15 years postoperatively (**g**, **h**). With permission from [76]

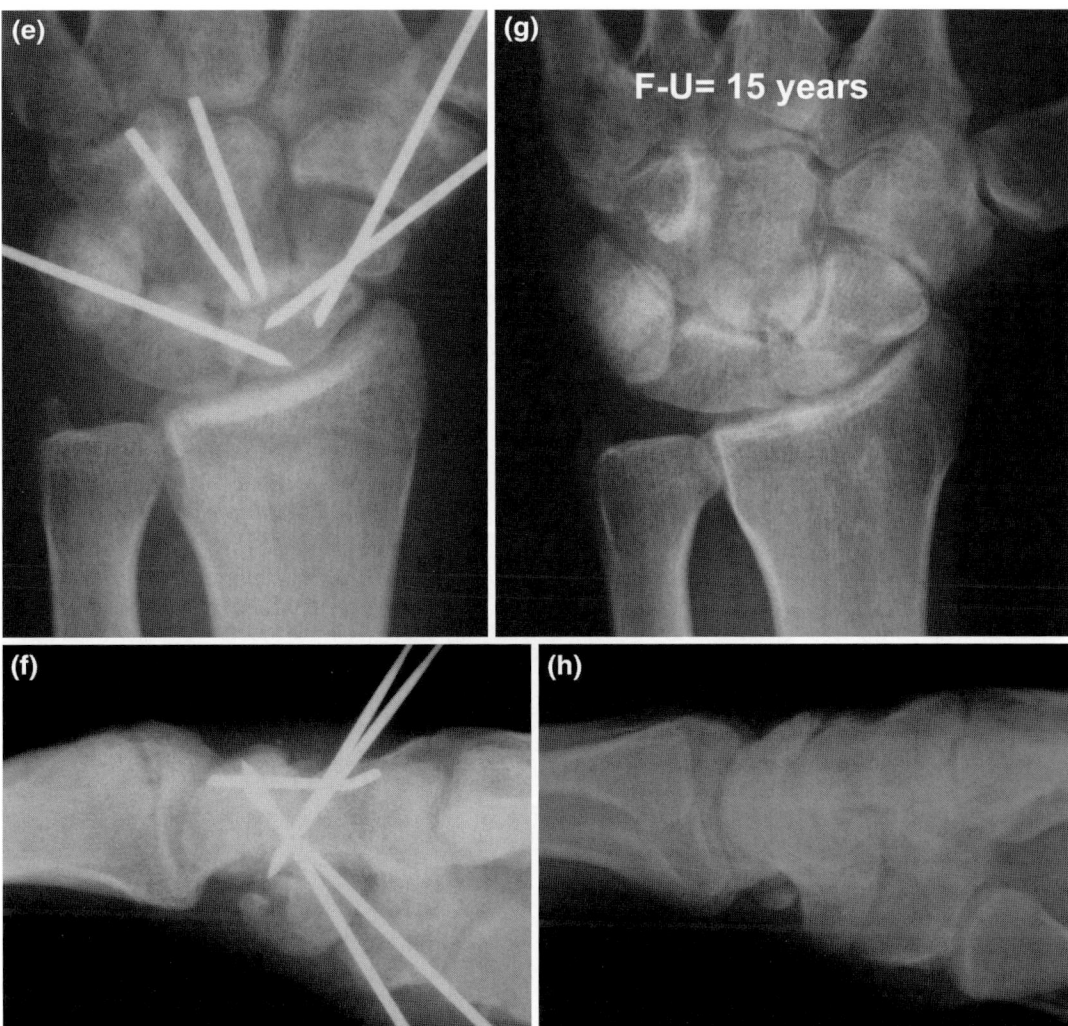

Fig. 5.11 (continued)

Fig. 5.12 Case 3. Male, 33-years old, polytrauma patient. Wrist bones were ejected through the volar wound without neurovascular injury (*S* Scaphoid, *L* Lunate, *C* capitate) (**a**, **b**); initial radiographs (**c**, **d**); reduction and fixation with combined approach (**e**, **f**); 2 years later a nonunion of the capitate was apparent (**g**); the patient refused the suggested operation since he had only mild discomfort. The radiological and clinical course vindicated the patient, as 15 years later he remains symptoms free with only minor restriction of ROM (**h–l**). With permission from [76]

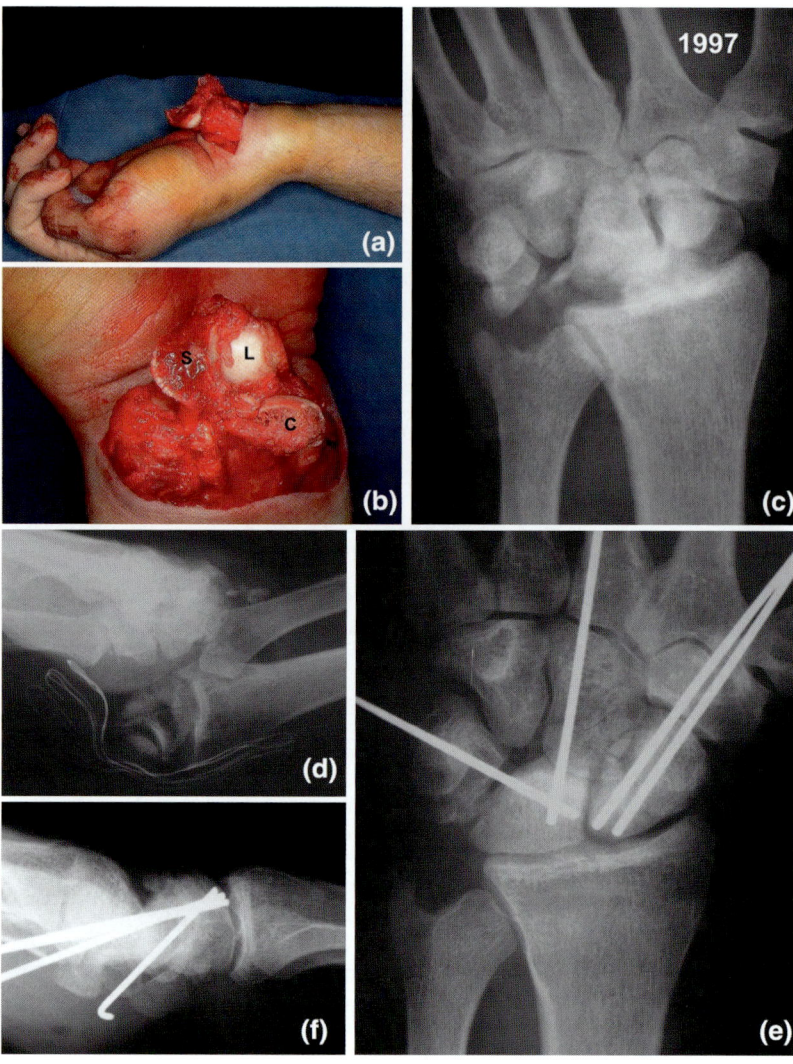

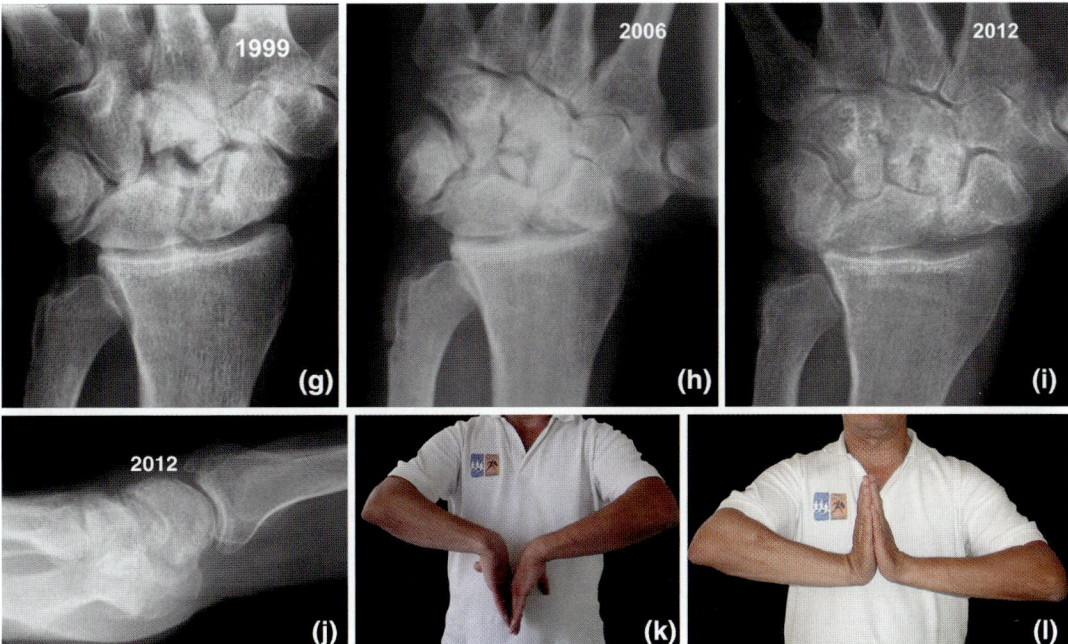

Fig. 5.12 (continued)

Rand et al. [15] reported that the incidence of post-traumatic arthritis in patients with scapho-capitate syndrome reached 66 %.

Marsh and Lampros [48] demonstrated that the proximal capitate fragment may undergo necrosis if left unreduced, a view also supported by others [59].

Kohut et al. [61] treated six patients with greater arc injuries and capitate fractures, with open reduction and K-wires fixation. After a follow-up of 6.4 years all wrists showed mild or moderate (one patient) arthritic changes. Only one patient was entirely free of pain, whereas the others experienced some discomfort or pain at various activity levels.

References

1. Cooney WP (1998) Isolated carpal fractures. In: Cooney WP, Linscheid RL, Dobyns JH (eds) The wrist, diagnosis and operative treatment, vol 1. Mosby, pp 474

2. Garcia-Elias M (1999) Carpal instabilities and dislocations. In: Green DP, Hotchkiss RN, Pederson WC (eds) Green's operative hand surgery, vol 1. Churchill Livingstone, New York, ch 28, pp 865–928

3. Vance RM, Gelberman RH, Evans EF (1980) Scaphocapitate fractures. Patterns of dislocation, mechanisms of injury, and preliminary results of treatment. J Bone Joint Surg Am 62:271–276

4. Lorie JP (1937) Un caso de fractura del escaphoides carpiano y del hueso grande. Cir Ortop Traumatol Habana 5:125–130

5. Perves J, Rigaud A, Badelon L (1937) Fracture par decapitation du grand os avec deplacement dorsal du corps de l'os simulant une dislocation carpienne. Rev Orthop 24:251–253

6. Nicholson CB (1940) Fracture dislocation of the os magnum. J R Nav Med Serv 26:289–291

7. Fenton RL (1956) The naviculo-capitate fracture syndrome. J Bone Joint Surg Am 38:681–684

8. Compson JP (1992) Trans-carpal injuries associated with distal radial fractures in children: a series of three cases. J Hand Surg [Br] 17:311–314

9. Mazur K, Stevanovic M, Schnall SB et al (1997) Scaphocapitate syndrome in a child associated with a distal radius and ulna fracture. J Orthop Trauma 11:230–232

10. Sawant M, Miller J (2000) Scaphocapitate syndrome in an adolescent. J Hand Surg [Am] 25(6):1096–1099

11. Wulff RN, Schmidt TL (1998) Carpal fractures in children. J Pediatr Orthop 18:462–465
12. Anderson WJ (1987) Simultaneous fracture of the scaphoid and capitate in a child. J Hand Surg [Am] 12:271
13. Kaulesar Sukul DM, Johannes EJ (1992) Transscapho-transcapitate fracture dislocation of the carpus. J Hand Surg [Am] 17:348–353
14. Milliez PY, Dallaserra M, Thomine JM (1993) An unusual variety of scapho-capitate syndrome. J Hand Surg [Br] 18:53–58
15. Rand JA, Linscheid RL, Dobyns JH (1982) Capitate fractures: a long-term follow-up. Clin Orthop 165:209–216
16. Geissler WB, Slade JF (2011) Fractures of the carpal bones. In: Wolfe SW, Hotchkiss RN, Pederson WC, Kozin SH (eds) Green's operative hand surgery, 6th edn. Elsevier Churchill Livingstone, ch 18, pp 639–707
17. Herzberg G, Comtet JJ, Linscheid RL et al (1993) Perilunate dislocations and fracture dislocations: a multicenter study. J Hand Surg [Am] 18:768–779
18. Adler JB, Shaftan OW (1962) Fractures of the capitate. J Bone Joint Surg Am 44:1537–1547
19. Schliemann B, Langer M, Kösters C (2011) Successful delayed surgical treatment of a scaphocapitate fracture. Arch Orthop Trauma Surg 131:1555–1559
20. Amadio PC, Taleisnik J (1999) Scaphocapitate syndrome. In: Green DP (ed) Operative hand surgery. Churchill Livingstone, New York, p 851
21. Stein F, Siegel MW (1969) Naviculocapitate fracture syndrome; a case report. J Bone Joint Surg Am 51:391–395
22. Dee W, Winckler S, Brug E (1994) Fracture and dislocation fracture of the os capitatum. Review of the literature and case report. Unfallchirurg 97:478–484
23. Meyers MH, Wells R, Harvey JP (1971) Naviculo-capitate fracture syndrome. J Bone Joint Surg Am 53:1383–1386
24. Johnson RP (1980) The acutely injured wrist and its residuals. Clin Orthop 149:33–44
25. Jones GB (1955) An unusual fracture-dislocation of the carpus. J Bone Joint Surg Br 37:146–147
26. Brekkan A, Karlsson J, Thorsteinsson T (1983) Case report 252. Scapho-capitate fracture of the right wrist with dislocation and rotation to 180 degrees of the proximal fragment of the capitate. Skeletal Radiol 10:193–291
27. Pandit R (1998) Proximal and palmar dislocation of the lunate and proximal scaphoid as a unit in a case of Scaphocapitate syndrome. A 32-month follow-up. J Hand Surg [Br] 23:266–268
28. Sandor L, Dosa G (1987) The scapho-capitate fracture syndrome (Fenton). Unfallchirurg 90:547–549
29. Zilch H (1986) The scapho-capitate fracture syndrome. Handchir Mikrochir Plast Chir 18:59–60
30. Mabee JR, Pritchard B (1997) An unusual transcapitate fracture of the wrist. Am J Emerg Med 15:584–586
31. Moneim MS (1988) Management of greater arc carpal fractures. Hand Clin 4:457–468
32. Resnik CS, Gelberman RH, Resnick D (1983) Transscaphoid, transcapitate, perilunate fracture dislocation (scaphocapitate syndrome). Skeletal Radiol 9:192–194
33. Schild H, Mueller HA, Klotter HJ (1983) Trans-scaphoid transcapitate dislocation fraction (naviculo-capitate fracture syndrome)–a rare wrist combined injury. Rontgenblatter 36:299–302
34. Mudgal C, Lovell M (1995) Scapho-capitate syndrome: distant fragment migration. Acta Orthop Belg 61:62–65
35. Guiral J, Gracia A, Diaz-Otero JM (1993) Isolated fracture of the capitate with a volar dislocated fragment. Acta Orthop Belg 59:406–408
36. Richards RR, Paitich CB, Bell RS (1990) Internal fixation of a capitate fracture with Herbert screws. J Hand Surg [Am] 15:885–887
37. Sabat D, Arora S, Dhal A (2011) Isolated capitate fracture with dorsal dislocation of proximal pole: a case report. Hand 6:333–336
38. Volk AG, Schnall SB, Merkle P et al (1995) Unusual capitate fracture: a case report. J Hand Surg [Am] 20:581–582
39. Chantelot C, Peltier B, Demondion X et al (1999) A trans STT, trans capitate perilunate dislocation of the carpus. A case report. Ann Chir Main Memb Super 18:61–65
40. Apergis E, Darmanis S, Kastanis G et al (2001) Does the term scaphocapitate syndrome need to be revised? A report of 6 cases. J Hand Surg [Br] 26:441–445
41. Ipsen T, Larsen CF (1985) A case of scapho-capitate fracture. Acta Orthop Scand 56:509–510
42. Robbins MM, Nemade AB, Chen TB et al (2008) Scapho-capitate syndrome variant: 180 degree rotation of the proximal capitate fragment without identifiable scaphoid fracture. Radiology Case reports 3:3:1–5
43. Calandruccio JH, Duncan SF (1999) Isolated nondisplaced capitate waist fracture diagnosed by magnetic resonance imaging. J Hand Surg [Am] 24:856–859
44. Schick S, Trattnig S, Gabler C et al (1999) Occult fractures of the wrist joint: high resolution image magnification roentgen versus MRI. Rofo Fortschr Geb Rontgenstr Neuen Bildgeb Verfahr 170:16–21
45. Maser SA, Harding SP, Harhay JS (1992) Answer please. Scaphocapitate fracture syndrome. Orthopedics 15(1378):1384–1386

46. Steffens K, Luce S, Koob E (1969) Unusual course of scapho-capitate syndrome. Handchir Mikrochir Plast Chir 26:12–14

47. Boisgard S, Bremont JL, Guyonnet G et al (1996) Scapho-capitate fracture. Apropos of a case, review of the literature. Ann Chir Main Memb Super 15:181–188

48. Marsh AP, Lampros PJ (1959) The naviculo-capitate fracture syndrome. Am J Roentgenol 82:255–256

49. Weseley MS, Barenfield PA (1972) Trans-scaphoid, trans-capitate, trans-triquetral perilunate fracture dislocation of the wrist: a case report. J Bone Joint Surg Am 54:1073–1078

50. Hohenbleicher R (1976) Das "naviculo-capitate fracture" syndrome. Unfallheilkunde 79:281–283

51. Pfeiffer KM (1978) Perilunar, transscaphoid, transcapital, transstyloid fracture-dislocation of the wrist. Operative reconstruction. Handchir 10:39–40

52. Fenton RL, Rosen H (1950) Fracture of the capitate bone: report of two cases. Bull Hosp Jt Dis 11:134

53. Hsu TL, Hsu SK, Chen HM et al (2011) Simultaneous fractures of the distal radius and capitate. Curr Orthop Pract 22(1):E5–E6

54. Scharizer E (1995) Scaphoid pseudarthrosis and capitate fracture. Handchir Mikrochir Plast Chir 27:38–42

55. Kimmel RB, O'Brien ET (1982) Surgical treatment of avascular necrosis of the proximal pole of the capitate: case report. J Hand Surg [Am] 7:284–286

56. Andreasi A, Coppo M, Danda F (1986) Trans-scapho-capitate perilunar dislocation of the carpus. Ital J Orthop Traumatol 12:461–466

57. Arbter D, Piatek S, Wichlas F et al (2009) The scaphocapitate fracture syndrome (Fenton). Handchir Mikrochir Plast Chir 41(3):171–174

58. Herzberg G (2010) Perilunate fracture dislocations. In: Cooney W (ed) The wrist. Diagnosis and operative treatment, 2nd edn. Lippincott Williams & Wilkins, ch 24, pp 550–578

59. Hofmeister EP, Shin AY (2002) Capitate and triquetrum fracture dislocations. In: Trumble T (ed) Carpal fractures-dislocations. American academy of orthopaedic surgeons, monograph series 21, pp 59–66

60. Peters A, Plesch J, Schacht U (1997) Scaphocapitate dislocation-fracture of the wrist joint in the setting of multiple injury. Chirurgie 68:1187–1189

61. Kohut G, Smith A, Giudici M et al (1996) Greater arc injuries of the wrist treated by internal and external fixation-six cases with mid-term follow-up. Hand Surg 1:159–166

62. Gelberman RH, Gross MS (1986) The vascularity of the wrist. Identification of arterial patterns at risk. Clin Orthop 202:40–49

63. Grend VR, Dell P, Glowczewskie F et al (1984) Intraosseous blood supply to the capitate and its correlation with aseptic necrosis. J Hand Surg [Am] 9:677–680

64. Panagis JS, Gelberman RH, Taleisnik J et al (1983) The arterial anatomy of the human carpus. Part II: the intraosseous vascularity. J Hand Surg [Am] 8(4):375–382

65. Milliez P, Kinh Kha H, Allieu T, Thomine J (1991) Osteonecrose aseptique essentielle du grand os. Int Orthop 15(2):85–94

66. Botte MJ, Pacelli LL, Gelberman RH (2004) Vascularity and osteonecrosis of the wrist. Orthop Clin North Am 35:405–421

67. Vigler M, Aviles A, Lee SK (2010) Other carpal fractures: lunate, triquetrum, capitate, hamate, hamate hook, trapezoid/trapezium. In: Slutsky D (ed) Principles and practice of wrist surgery. Saunders Elsevier, Philadelphia, ch 25, pp 289–300

68. Yoshihara M, Sakai A, Toba N et al (2002) Nonunion of the isolated capitate waist fracture. J Orthop Sci 7(5):578–580

69. Freeman BH, Hay EL (1985) Nonunion of the capitate: a case report. J Hand Surg [Am] 10:187–190

70. Heim U (1986) Pseudarthrosis of the capitate. Handchir Mikrochir Plast Chir 18:158–160

71. Minami M, Yamazaki J, Chisaka N et al (1987) Nonunion of the capitate. J Hand Surg [Am] 12:1089–1091

72. D'Hondt B, Safi A, Bruser P (1997) Pseudarthrosis of the capitate bone. Report of 2 cases. Handchir Mikrochir Plast Chir 29:27–31

73. Rayan GM (1994) Occult wrist pain due to capitate nonunion. South Med J 87:402–404

74. Kammermeier V, Schwarz M, Geishauser M et al (1991) Pseudarthrosis of the capitate bone with special reference to ligamentous stabilization. Handchir Mikrochir Plast Chir 23:265–269

75. Rico AA, Holguin PH, Martin JG (1999) Pseudarthrosis of the capitate. J Hand Surg [Br] 24:382–384

76. Apergis E (2004) καταγματα-εξαρθρήματα του καρπου. Konstantaras Medical Books, Athens

Palmar Perilunate Dislocations or Fracture-Dislocations

6

6.1 Introduction

The first case of palmar trans-scaphoid perilunate dislocation was probably published by Goulioud and Arcelin in 1908 [1].The palmar perilunate dislocations constitutes about 3 % of all perilunate injuries [2–4]. Witvoet and Allieu [5] in a retrospective study among 85 cases of perilunate injuries, found five palmar perilunate dislocations (6 %). Saunier and Chamay [6] in a review of the literature, reported only 12 cases of palmar perilunate dislocations, 50 % of which had an associated fracture of the scaphoid. Finally, in a multicenter study, Herzberg et al. [2] found that from 166 cases of perilunate injuries, 5 (3 %) were of palmar type.

Our knowledge about these injuries derives only from a few isolated cases that have been reported in the literature. The earliest report of a dorsal dislocation of the lunate proven by radiographic examination was published in 1906, by Thebault (quoted by Taleisnik [1]).

6.2 Mechanism of Injury

There is ambiguity in the literature regarding the mechanism of injury, since these injuries have not been experimentally reproduced and the patients can rarely recall the mechanism of injury.

The mechanisms that have been described so far are listed below:

- Forced hyperflexion after falling on the dorsum of the wrist [7–9], or hyperflexion with the wrist being trapped in machinery [10].
- Forced hyperflexion and supination of the wrist relative to the radius [3].
- Hyperflexion of the wrist associated with ulnar deviation [6, 11].
- Hyperflexion, ulnar deviation and pronation of the wrist [12].
- Wrist hyperflexion with a longitudinal loading force transmitted through the capitate [13].
- Axial force on a volarly flexed and radially deviated wrist, with the forearm in pronation [14].
- Fall on a hyperextended wrist with supination of the forearm and proximal row on the fixed hand and distal row [15, 16].
- The midcarpal displacement could be recreated by supination of the proximal segment on the extended distal segment, with the rotation occurring around the triquetrum. (Based on a postmortem study of a wrist with a volar perilunate dislocation of a patient who died 2 weeks later from associated injuries) [17].

From the above we assume that two main force components are implicated: (a) Hyperflexion (combined with palmar translation of metacarpals) which is often produced after a direct blow to the dorsum of the wrist and (b) The rotational component, where the distal carpal row and metacarpals are forced to pronation, while the proximal carpal row together with the forearm are forced to supination. This rotational dissociation is the same mechanism of injury

E. Apergis, *Fracture-Dislocations of the Wrist*,
DOI: 10.1007/978-88-470-5328-1_6, © Springer-Verlag Italia 2013

responsible for the palmar radiocarpal dislocations, except that the level of the disruption is
located at the radiocarpal rather than the midcarpal joint.

Pournaras and Kappas [18] suggested that a
predisposing anatomical factor may contribute to
this injury pattern since the contralateral healthy
wrist of the patient they presented with volar
perilunar dislocation, showed a VISI alignment
of the wrist. A preexisting abnormal radio-luno-
capitate alignment has also been mentioned by
Roman et al. [19]. Park and Steinberg [20] stated
that prior wrist injuries, may contribute to subtle
wrist instability, thus predisposing to an acute
volar perilunate dislocation while Niazi [16]
considered that laxity of the ligaments makes a
wrist susceptible to dislocations.

6.3 Pathologic Anatomy of the Injury

Like the more frequent dorsal perilunate dislocations these extremely rare injuries are produced after a progressively increasing
ligamentous injury in which the head of the
capitate is dislocated volar to the lunate. At a
more advanced stage, the lunate dislocates dorsally and the rest of the wrist returns to its original position. This constitutes the purely
ligamentous form of the injury [16, 21], where
the ligamentous attachments of the lunate to the
scaphoid initially and to the triquetrum subsequently, rupture, while at the final stage of this
perilunar instability, the SRL and the ulnolunate
ligaments rupture and the lunate dislocates dorsally. It seems that this perilunar instability
progresses with the axis of rotation located at the
triquetrum.

Following the above, we assume that the
progressive stages of this injury evolve as follows: Stage I: Fracture of the scaphoid or SL
dissociation; Stage II: The capitate head (i.e.,
distal carpal row) dislocates volarly with or
without the palmar fragment of a fractured
lunate; Stage III: LT dissociation; and Stage IV:
The lunate, deprived of soft tissues dislocates
dorsally.

As an example, the cases presented by Minami
et al. [22] and by Youssef and Deshmukh [4]
represented a Stage II injury, where the lunate and
triquetrum remained in their normal position with
the radius, while the scaphoid and distal carpal
row had migrated volarly.

In trans-scaphoid volar perilunate dislocations (like their dorsal equivalent) concomitant
scaphoid fracture and scapholunate dissociation
have been described in a case presented by
Nishiyama et al. [14].

Like their dorsal counterpart, the volar perilunate injuries exhibit a transverse disruption of
the volar carpal ligaments [8, 20, 23].

Often, the volar perilunate injuries are manifested as a fracture-dislocation injury, like their
corresponding dorsal variants are evidenced as
greater arc injuries. The most frequent concomitant fracture is that of the scaphoid, but of
particular interest is the next most common
fracture which is the fracture of the lunate.
Equally interesting is that the fracture of the
lunate is oriented at the frontal plane, usually
involves its central part and less frequently its
palmar pole. This means that the frequently
referred mechanism of palmar hyperflexion,
must be associated with a longitudinal loading
force transmitted through the capitate, where its
head impinges to the distal articular surface of
lunate separating it into two fragments. In that
case, the capitate and consequently the entire
distal carpal row, in association with the palmar
fragment of the lunate are palmarly subluxated
in different degrees, while the dorsal part of the
lunate is displaced dorsally. Probably, in cases
of volar perilunate fracture-dislocations with the
lunate fractured and the scaphoid intact, the
existence of a radial component of the injury,
e.g., rupture of STT ligaments must be
speculated.

According to the classification of Teisen and
Hjarbaek [24], the transverse fracture through
the body of the lunate constitutes a type V
fracture, which is highly unstable since the head
of the capitate maintains the two fragments
apart. Treated conservatively these fractures
usually end up with a nonunion as the case
mentioned by Ruijters and Kortmann [25].

In trans-scaphoid volar perilunate injury the fractured surface of the scaphoid lies on the frontal plane which means that during hyperflexion of the wrist, the scaphoid fractures after impaction to the volar rim of the radius. In such cases, the proximal scaphoid fragment remains with the lunate [26] (Fig. 6.1a–e).

Usually, the volar perilunate fracture-dislocation is associated with fracture of the scaphoid [2, 6, 7, 9, 10, 27, 28], the lunate [25, 29, 30], or both [11, 13, 31]. The impaction of the scaphoid to the radial styloid can cause fracture of the latter without fracture of the scaphoid [8, 12] or fractures of both the scaphoid and radial styloid [6, 32].

Irregular forms of volar perilunate injury, resembling greater arc injuries, have also been mentioned in the literature [11, 19, 23, 33], while Mueller [34] reported a case of volar perilunate dislocation leading to avascular necrosis and fragmentation of the lunate.

6.3.1   Dorsal Dislocation of the Lunate

The dorsal dislocation of the lunate represents the end stage of the volar perilunate dislocation (just as a volar lunate dislocation represents the end stage of the more common dorsal perilunate dislocation injury pattern) [20].

Bilos and Hui [8] reported two cases with dorsal dislocation of the lunate, both of which were treated with open reduction, ligaments suturing, and pin fixation, since after the initially closed reduction the dislocation recurred easily. After 12 and 15 months follow-up the results were good, despite the fact that in one of the patients, increased density of the lunate without collapse was noted at 1 year.

Schwartz et al. [35] reported a patient with a 2 months old dorsal lunate dislocation and carpal collapse, who presented pain, limited wrist motion, and inability to extend the long, ring and small finger metacarpophalangeal joints. Closed reduction was impossible and the patient was treated operatively with proximal row carpectomy and tendon reconstruction. The lunate was deprived of soft tissues and subsequent histologic examination showed complete avascular necrosis. Rupture of extensor tendons, which were trapped between the midcarpal joint preventing closed reduction of a volar perilunate dislocation, have also been mentioned by Minami et al. [22]. The authors were not aware if the tendons were torn or subsequently ruptured because of vascular compromise.

Bjerregaard and Holst-Nielsen [12], also report a case of dorsal dislocation of the lunate where through a transverse rent of the dorsal capsule the lunate was found beneath the fourth extensor compartment. The patient was treated 2 months postinjury with scapholunocapitate fusion.

One of two patients presented by Park and Steinberg [20] had dorsal lunate dislocation caused by an acute on chronic injury which was rupture of the lunotriquetral ligament. Probably the patient previously had a complex type of instability (CIC) due to insufficiency of both lunotriquetral and radiotriquetral ligaments that resulted in VISI alignment which was the predisposing factor to dislocate the lunate dorsally after the new trauma episode.

Markiewitz et al. [36] supported that dorsal dislocation of the lunate may be associated with rupture of the long and short radiolunate ligaments, which must be repaired through a palmar approach, since their deficiency may allow ulnar translation of the wrist.

Patients with dorsal lunate dislocation usually present with prominence of the lunate on the dorsum of the hand [4].

Certainly there are cases of neglected dorsal lunate dislocation which were accidentally found during a routine X-ray for another reason (Fig. 6.2a, b). In such cases the treatment is dictated by the symptoms [4].

6.4   Diagnosis

In acute cases physical findings consist of a swollen painful wrist and a silver fork deformity, which is more distal than in the fracture of the distal radius with volar displacement (Smith's fracture) [6]. Because of the rarity of this injury,

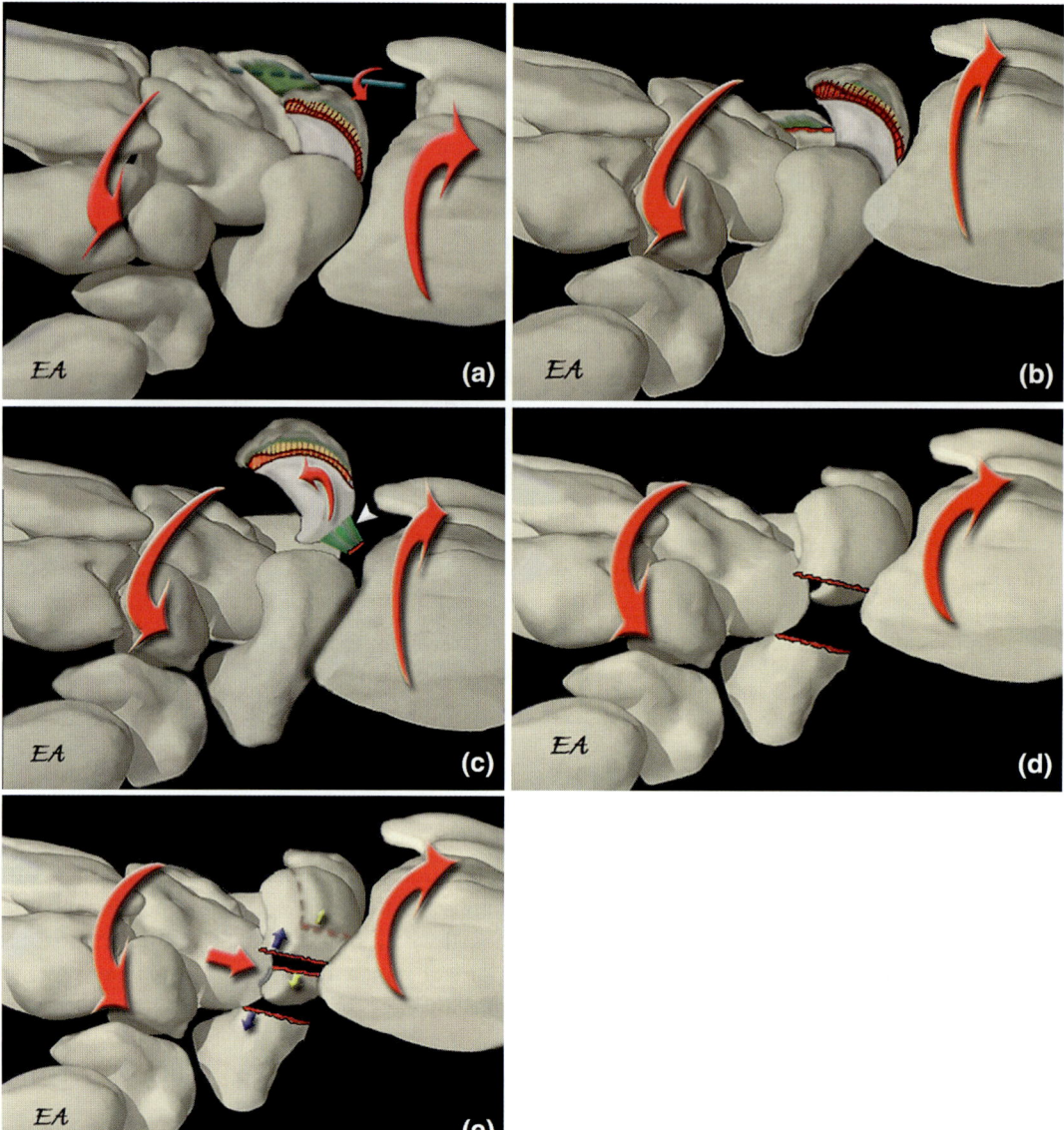

Fig. 6.1 Electronical depiction of the presumed mechanism of injury: The rotational dissociation of the wrist at the midcarpal level (*arrows*) could produce a palmar perilunate dislocation. The axis of rotation is located at the triquetrum, the metacarpals and distal carpal row are rotated in pronation, while the proximal carpal row together with the forearm are forced in supination. At an initial stage the SL ligament ruptures and all carpal bones apart from the LT complex, subluxate volarly (**a**); at a next stage, the LT ligament also ruptures and all carpal bones except the lunate, are volarly dislocated, while the head of the capitate forces the lunate to displace dorsally and at the same time rotate volarly (**b**); at a final stage, the wrist relocates to its normal position, while the lunate is ejected dorsally with simultaneous rupture of the short and long RL ligaments (*white arrow*) (**c**); in volar perilunate fracture-dislocations the most frequently involved fractures are those of the scaphoid and/or lunate, with their fractured surfaces oriented at the frontal plane. This finding correlates with a mechanism of hyperflexion injury, where the scaphoid fractures after impaction to the volar radial rim and the lunate after impaction from the head of the capitate (**d**, **e**). With permission from [42]

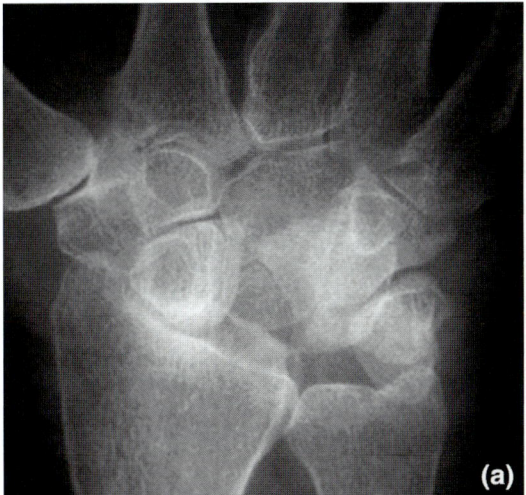

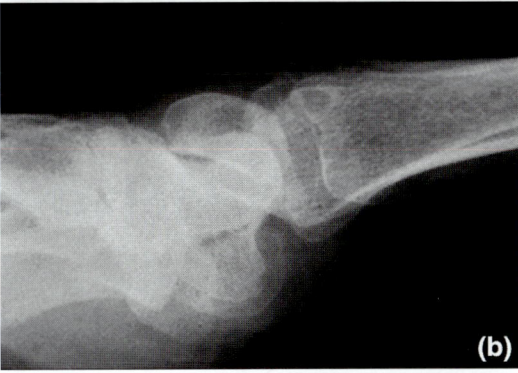

Fig. 6.2 **a**, **b** Female, 70-years old. A case of neglected dorsal lunate dislocation, which was found accidentally after a minor wrist injury. With permission from [42]

the proper diagnosis is likely to be missed. The two classic X-ray views are usually diagnostic. Because any coexisting fractures of the scaphoid or the lunate are oriented in the frontal plane, their recognition is difficult on the standard PA view. The diagnosis is most easily made on the lateral view [36, 37].

Klein and Webb [38] described the « crowded carpal sign» which is due to the overlapping of the proximal and distal carpal rows (however, it can also be found in the more frequent dorsal variant). Plain X-rays with the wrist distracted under anesthesia or a CT-scan in selected cases may add to diagnosis [23].

Fractures of the palmar pole of the lunate could be an ominous sign, hiding an incomplete or reduced volar perilunate dislocation [13, 39].

Numbness in the median nerve distribution has also been reported, early [22] or late in a missed volar perilunate dislocation [4].

6.5 Management

The rare volar perilunate injuries are exceedingly unstable injuries and should be managed like the more frequent dorsal perilunate dislocations, with open reduction using both palmar and dorsal approaches and internal fixation [3, 15, 37]. Closed reduction should be the initial step in management when open reduction is not possible immediately after injury.

Taleisnik [1] described the manipulation of closed reduction as follows: Under satisfactory anesthesia and muscle relaxation, a finger trap traction is applied and continued for several minutes before manipulation is tried. The reduction of the dorsally shifted lunate is attempted by direct pressure from the dorsum (the lunate is more readily palpable than in volar dislocations), while at the same time the hand is palmarflexed and rotated into supination around an imaginary pivot point passing through the triquetrum. The author claimed that volar perilunate dislocations are more difficult to reduce than the dorsal variety, and when reduced they are more likely to recur. He recommended that immobilization is more effective with the wrist in neutral or slight dorsiflexion. Green and O'Brien [17] also suggested that the manipulation of closed reduction could be accomplished with supination of the hand and distal row on the fixed forearm and proximal row.

Fernandes et al. [9] supported that closed reduction achieved in a case of trans-scaphoid volar perilunate fracture dislocation was very unstable except in position of extreme dorsiflexion, while Niazi [16] claimed that the closed reduction achieved of a perilunate dislocation, was found to be unstable in neutral or extension positions.

Although successful treatment has been reported with closed reduction alone [9, 16], in trans-scaphoid volar perilunate fracture-dislocations, closed reduction has been applied as initial

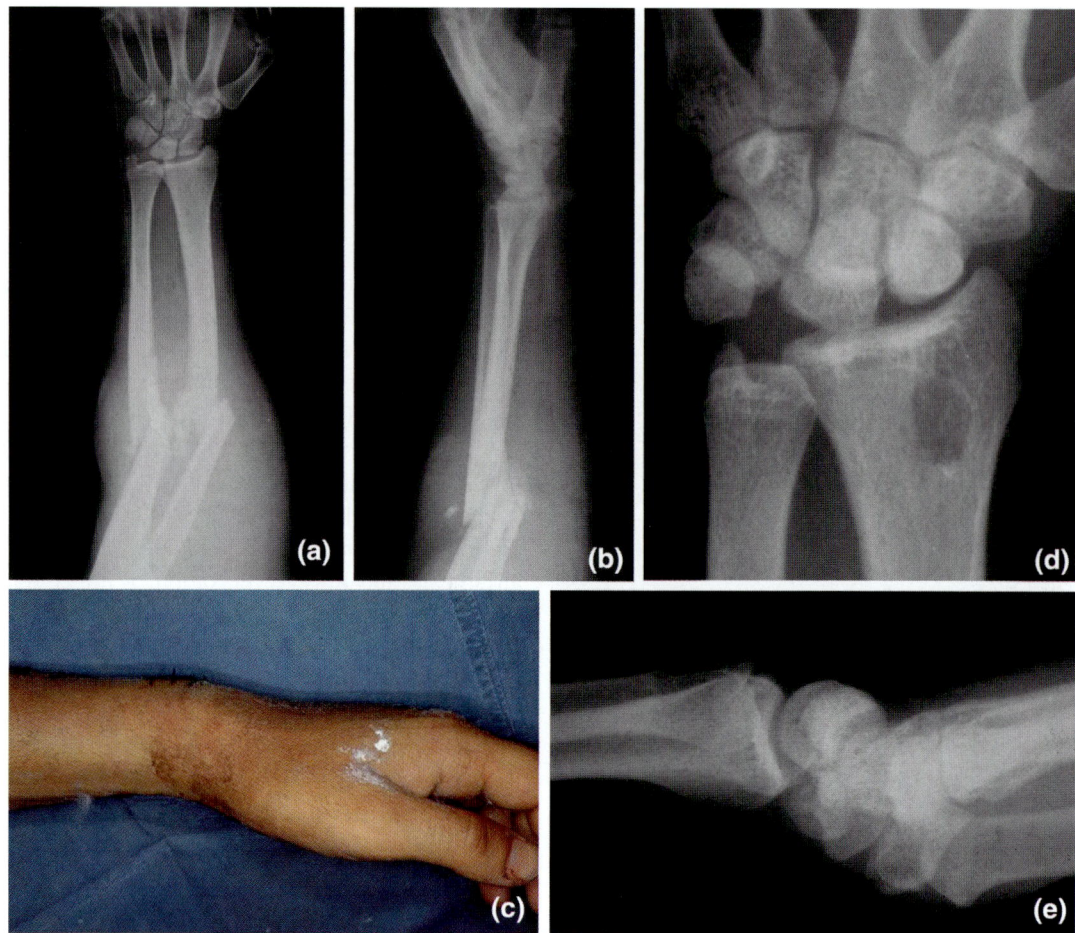

Fig. 6.3 Male, 28-years old. A polytrauma patient (fracture of *left* femur and left forearm, dislocation of the *right* elbow, ligamentous injuries at both knees). Same day, the fractures of the femur and forearm were operatively treated. Initial X-rays of the fractured forearm, where the wrist joint is also indicated (**a**, **b**); next day, changing the forearm wound, wrist deformity and crepitation were discovered (**c**); wrist X-rays revealed a trans-scaphoid volar perilunate fracture-dislocation (**d**, **e**); with a dorsal approach, except for the fractured scaphoid, an oblique fracture of the capitate head was found (*arrows*), while the SL and LT ligaments were intact (**f**, **g**); Postoperative X-rays (**h**, **i**); final appearance 3 months postinjury. (*R* Radius, *S* Scaphoid, *L* Lunate, *C* Capitate). (Comments: **a**) although careful evaluation of the initial forearm X-rays reveal the fractured scaphoid, obviously a spontaneous reduction concealed the magnitude of the injury, **b**) since the LT joint was intact, probably the case constitutes an incomplete type of injury). With permission from [42]

treatment, but it was soon followed by open reduction and fixation of the scaphoid due to the unstable character of the injury [6, 10, 13, 26, 32, 37].

Whenever closed reduction was the definitive treatment, it resulted in malunion [2, 9] or nonunion of the scaphoid. Conversely, open reduction and stable fixation of the fractured scaphoid usually rendered good results [2, 27, 28, 40], even in delayed treatment [14].

Several authors [6, 17, 23, 26, 32] prefer to internally fix the scaphoid through a volar incision, and percutaneously pinning the reduced joints. Others [36], prefer to use a dorsal approach for its versatility and better exposure (Fig. 6.3a–k).

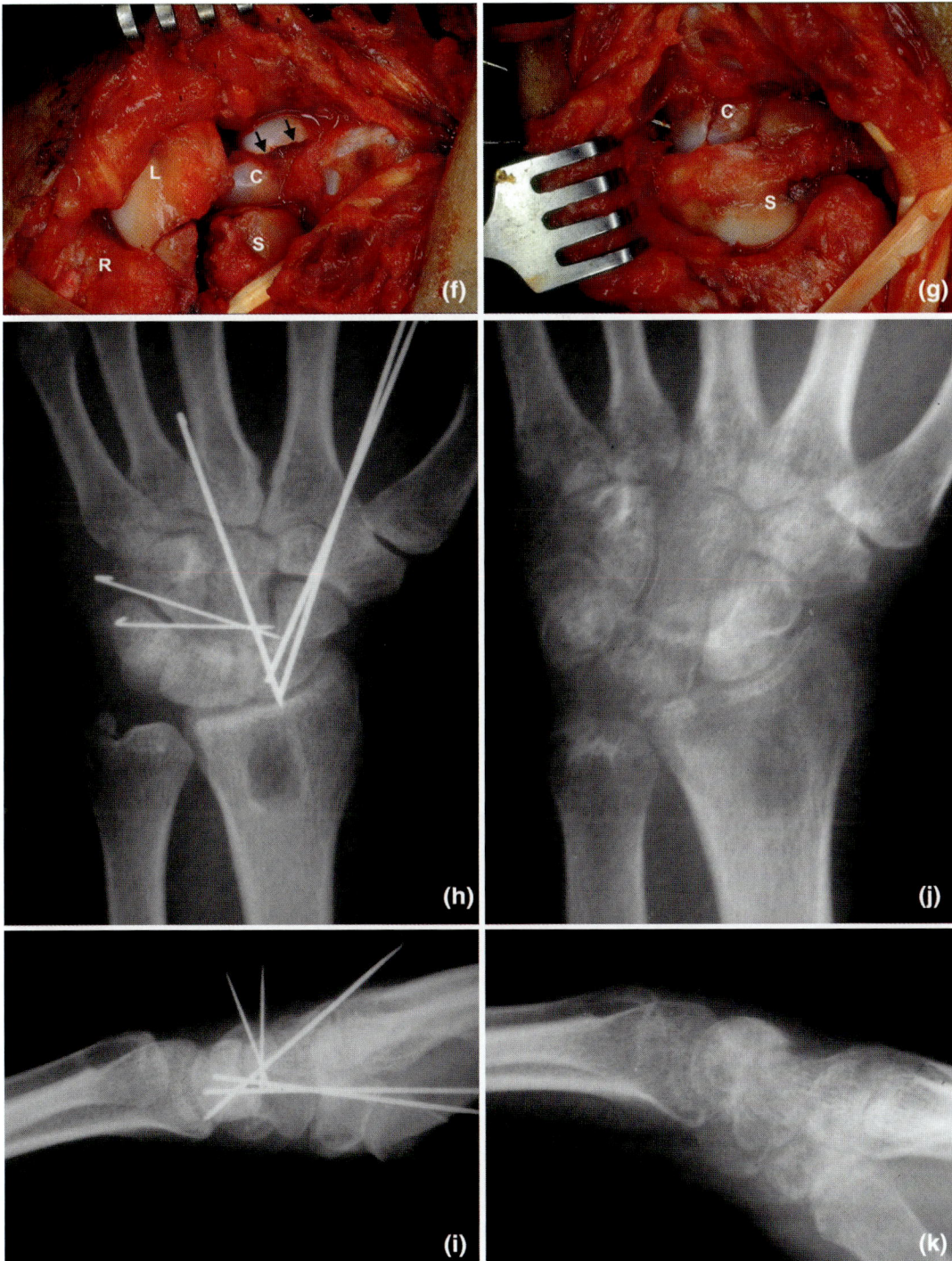

Fig. 6.3 (continued)

Green and O'Brien [17] in cases of volar perilunate dislocations, recommended closed reduction and percutaneous K-wires for 8 weeks, whereas any residual scaphoid subluxation should be corrected via a dorsal approach.

Similarly, in cases of lunate fracture stable fixation with a headless screw or K-wires is mandatory [13].

Various authors [6, 10, 18, 32, 36], have suggested that purely ligamentous volar perilunate dislocations when treated with closed reduction and cast immobilization are more likely to give satisfactory results than does the fracture dislocation counterpart.

Proximal row carpectomy has been applied in an acute trans-scaphoid, translunate volar perilunate fracture-dislocation, with the distal scaphoid pole free of any tissue attachment located just under the extensor retinaculum [11].

The outcome was considered significantly worse for those patients who underwent surgical treatment much later after the initial injury [4].

Post-traumatic instability of the wrist, avascular necrosis of the proximal pole of the scaphoid, and intracarpal osteoarthritis are possible complications when the progression of such an injury is not satisfactory [6, 41].

References

1. Taleisnik J (1985) The wrist. Churchill Livingstone, New York
2. Herzberg G, Comtet JJ, Linscheid RL et al (1993) Perilunate dislocations and fracture dislocations: a multicenter study. J Hand Surg [Am] 18:768–779
3. Garcia-Elias M (1999) Carpal instabilities and dislocations. In: Green DP (ed) Green's operative hand surgery (ch 28), Churchill Livingstone, New York, pp 865–928
4. Youssef B, Deshmukh SC (2008) Volar perilunate dislocation: a case report and review of the literature. Open Orthop J 2:57–58
5. Witvoet J, Allieu Y (1973) Lesions traumatiques fraiches. Rev Chi Orthop 59:98–125
6. Saunier J, Chamay A (1981) Volar perilunar dislocation of the wrist. Clin Orthop 157:139–142
7. Aitken AP, Nalebuff EA (1960) Volar transnavicular perilunar dislocation of the carpus. J Bone Joint Surg Am 42:1051–1057
8. Bilos ZJ, Hui PW (1981) Dorsal dislocation of the lunate with carpal collapse. Report of two cases. J Bone Joint Surg Am 63:1484–1486
9. Fernandes HJA, Koberle G, Ferreira GH et al (1983) Volar transscaphoid perilunar dislocation. Hand 15:276–280
10. Hayeems EB, Schemitsch EH (1996) Volar transscaphoid perilunate fracture dislocation: case report and review. J Trauma 40:1031–1033
11. Peshin C, Mahajan S, Singh H et al (2009) Volar transcaphoid perilunate dislocation; a case report. Internet J Orthop Surg 13:1. doi:10.5580/8bf
12. Bjerregaard P, Holst-Nielsen F (1988) Transstyloid dorsal luxation of the lunate. Case report. Scand J Plast Reconstr Surg Hand Surg 22:261–264
13. Conway WF, Gilula LA, Manske PR et al (1989) Translunate, palmar perilunate fracture-subluxation of the wrist. J Hand Surg [Am] 14(4):635–639
14. Nishiyama Y, Sato K, Nakamura T (2012) Radial and volar perilunate trans-scaphoid fracture dislocation: a case report. Hand Surg 17(1):93–97
15. Green DP (1988) Carpal dislocations and instabilities. In: Green DP (ed) Operative hand Surgery. Churchill Livingstone, New York, pp 875–938
16. Niazi TB (1996) Volar perilunate dislocation of the carpus: a case report and elucidation of its mechanism of occurrence. Injury 27:209–211
17. Green DP, O'Brien ET (1980) Classification and management of carpal dislocations. Clin Orthop 149:55–72
18. Pournaras J, Kappas A (1979) Volar peilunar dislocation. A case report. J Bone Joint Surg Am 61:625–626
19. Roman A, Sendino M, Salomon G et al (1994) A rare case of carpal dislocation. Ann Chir Main Memb Super 13(3):207–213
20. Park MJ, Steinberg DR (2012) Volar perilunate dislocations: possible association with prior wrist injuries. Hand 7:217–220
21. Marya SK, Khurana JS, Dave PK (1987) Volar perilunar dislocation of the carpus-a case report. Injury 18:357–358
22. Minami A, Ogino T, Hamada M (1989) Rupture of extensor tendons associated with a palmar perilunar dislocation. J Hand Surg [Am] 14(5):843–847
23. Masmejean EH, Romano SJ, Saffar PH (1998) Palmar perilunate fracture-dislocation of the carpus. J Hand Surg [Br] 23:264–265
24. Teisen H, Hjarbaek J (1988) Classification of fresh fractures of the lunate. J Hand Surg [Br] 13:458–462
25. Ruijters R, Kortmann J (1988) A case of translunate luxation of the carpus. Acta Orthop Scand 59:461–463
26. Kalra M, Menon J, Sharma B (2005) A rare case of volar trans-scaphoid perilunate dislocation. Injury Extra 36(9):405–406
27. Schwartz GB (1986) A volar transscaphoid perilunate fracture dislocation. Orthop Rev 15:170–173

28. Woodward AH, Neviaser RJ, Nisenfeld F (1975) Radial and volar perilunate transscaphoid fracture dislocation. South Med J 68:926–928

29. Mason GC, Bowman MW, Fu FH (1986) Translunate, perilunate fracture-dislocation of the wrist. A case report. Orthopedics 9:1001–1004

30. Vichard P, Tropet Y, Balmat P et al (1991) Reflections on 4 cases of ante-lunar carpal luxations. Ann Chir Main Memb Super 10:331–336

31. Noble J, Lamb DW (1979) Translunate scapho-radial fracture. Hand 11:47–49

32. Carmichael KD, Bell C (2005) Volar perilunate trans-scaphoid fracture-dislocation in a skeletally immature patient. Orthopedics 28(1):69–70

33. Wodecki P, Guigui P, Masmejean E (2002) Volar transcaphocapitate perilunate disclocation of the carpus: a new variety, a new approach. Chir Main 21:143–147

34. Mueller JJ (1984) Avascular necrosis and collapse of the lunate following a volar perilunate dislocation: a case report and review of this complication in dislocations of the wrist. Orthopedics 7:1009–1014

35. Schwartz MG, Green SM, Coville FA (1990) Dorsal dislocation of the lunate with multiple extensor tendon ruptures. J Hand Surg [Am] 15:132–133

36. Markiewitz AD, Ruby LK, O'Brien ET (1997) Carpal fractures and dislocations. In: Lichtman DM, Alexander AH (eds) The wrist and its disorders (ch 13), 2 edn. WB Saunders, Philadelphia, pp 189–233

37. Garcia-Elias M, Geissler W (2005) Carpal instability. In: Wolfe SW, Hotchkiss RN, Pederson WC, Kozin SH (eds) Green's operative hand surgery (ch 14), Elsevier Churchill Livingstone, London, pp 535–604

38. Klein A, Webb LX (1987) The crowded carpal sign in volar perilunar dislocation. J Trauma 27:82–84

39. Hawken R, Fullilove SM (2007) Delayed post-traumatic midcarpal dislocation. J Hand Surg [Eur] 32(5):554–555

40. Amar MF, Loudyi D, Chbani B et al (2009) Volar transscaphoid perilunate fracture dislocation. A case report. Chir Main 28(6):374–377

41. Kozin SH (1998) Perilunate injuries: diagnosis and treatment. J Am Acad Orthop Surg 6:114–120

42. Apergis E (2004) καταγματα-εξαρθρήματα του καρπου. Konstantaras Medical Books, Athens

Delayed and Chronic Perilunate Dislocations

7

7.1 Definition

The time limits used to characterize perilunate injuries into acute, delayed, and chronic, could neither be strict nor specific. However, time restrictions must be set for therapeutic and prognostic reasons and also for the purpose of understanding each other. Thus, Herzberg [1] suggested that *acute injuries* should be considered as those injuries diagnosed within the first week, *delayed* should be those diagnosed 7–45 days after the injury and *chronic* as those diagnosed after the 45th day.

7.2 Diagnosis

The percentage of patients with perilunate injuries escaping diagnosis fluctuates between 16 and 25 % [2–4]. The majority of patients with neglected perilunate injuries present with distinct wrist dysfunction. Wrist pain, paresthesia, or even anesthesia of the median nerve distribution, significant reduction of grip strength, and range of motion, were usually the clinical picture of patients [5–7]. At a later stage, they may present with arthritis of the radiocarpal or midcarpal joints with different degrees of functional deficit and articular remodeling [8]. Patients examined several years after the accident, present symptoms of either carpal tunnel syndrome or rupture due to attrition of the flexor tendons [6, 9, 10] (Fig. 7.1a–k).

However, the symptoms are not always as obvious. There are patients with isolated wrist injury, who underestimated its importance and requested medical assistance later, usually complaining for carpal tunnel symptoms [11] (Fig. 7.2a–n). There are also patients who had experienced in the past a high-energy injury involving the wrist, which was missed. The following years they experienced mild or even no symptoms at the wrist, to which they had adapted and the wrist injury was radiologically diagnosed by chance, much later.

7.3 Treatment Options

In any case, delay in diagnosis constitutes an important factor affecting the long-term result [2, 11]. Herzberg et al. [4] reported that patients treated after a delay of more than 45 days had significantly worse clinical outcomes. Inoue and Shionoya [6] reported that cases treated after 2 months post-injury, had unsatisfactory results compared to patients treated within the first 2 months (average clinical score was 58 and 82 points, respectively).

Howard and Dell [12] suggested that closed reduction may be attempted up to 2 weeks following injury, they considered the time period between the second–sixth week the "gray area", while after the 6th week they supported that open reduction with combined approach is necessary. The question remains, what further

E. Apergis, *Fracture-Dislocations of the Wrist*,
DOI: 10.1007/978-88-470-5328-1_7, © Springer-Verlag Italia 2013

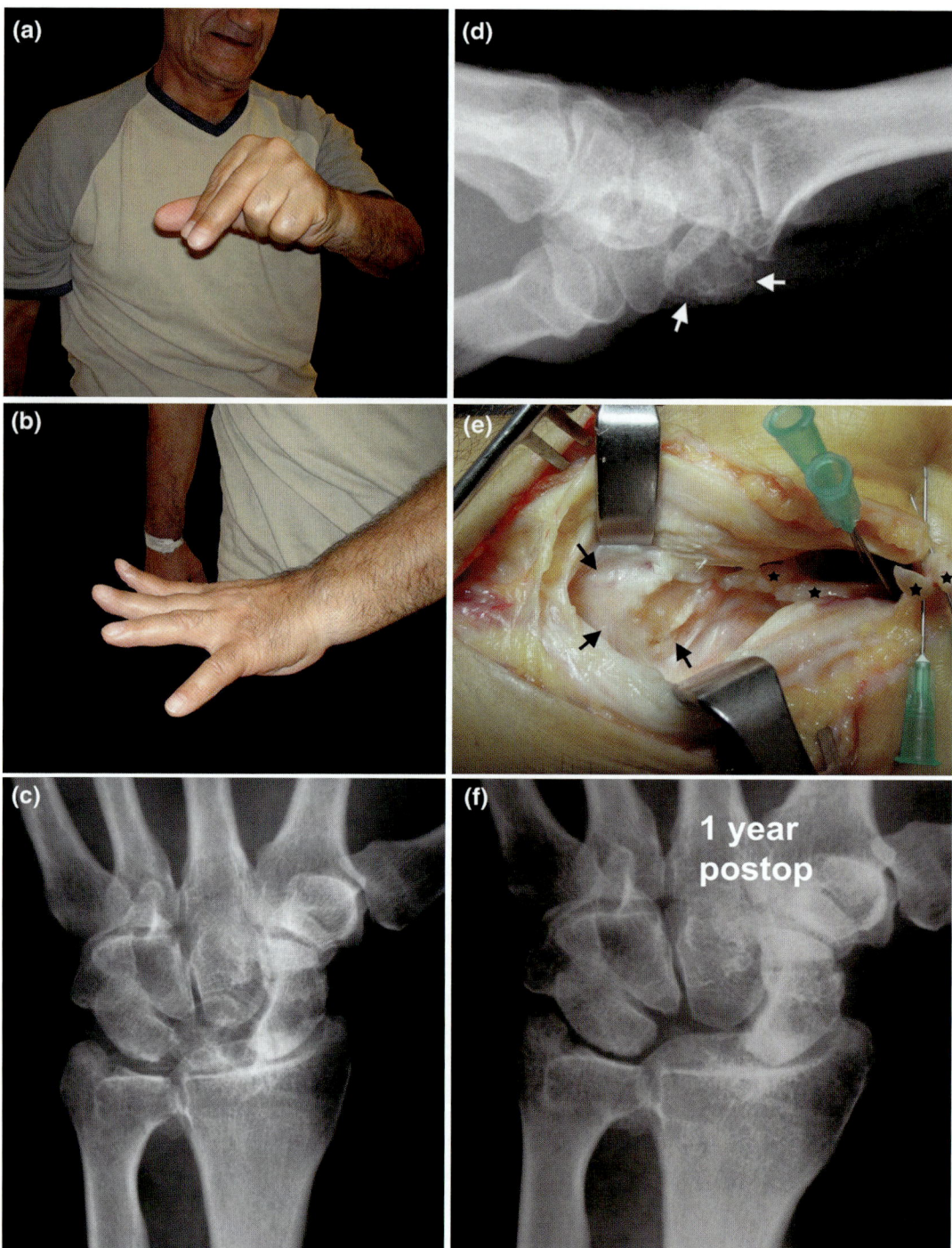

Fig. 7.1 Male, 63-years old. Reported finger hypesthesia at median nerve distribution and inability to flex the index and middle fingers (**a**, **b**), due to neglected palmar dislocation of the lunate, following a 20-year-old injury he vaguely remembered (**c–d**); excision of the lunate and reconstruction of the flexor tendons were performed. Palmar approach revealed the palmarly dislocated lunate (*arrows*) and attritional rupture of the deep and superficial flexors of the affected fingers (*asterisks*) (**e**); comparing the X-rays 1 and 4 years postoperatively, no carpal collapse was noticed (**f–h**); ROM 4 years postoperatively (**i–k**)

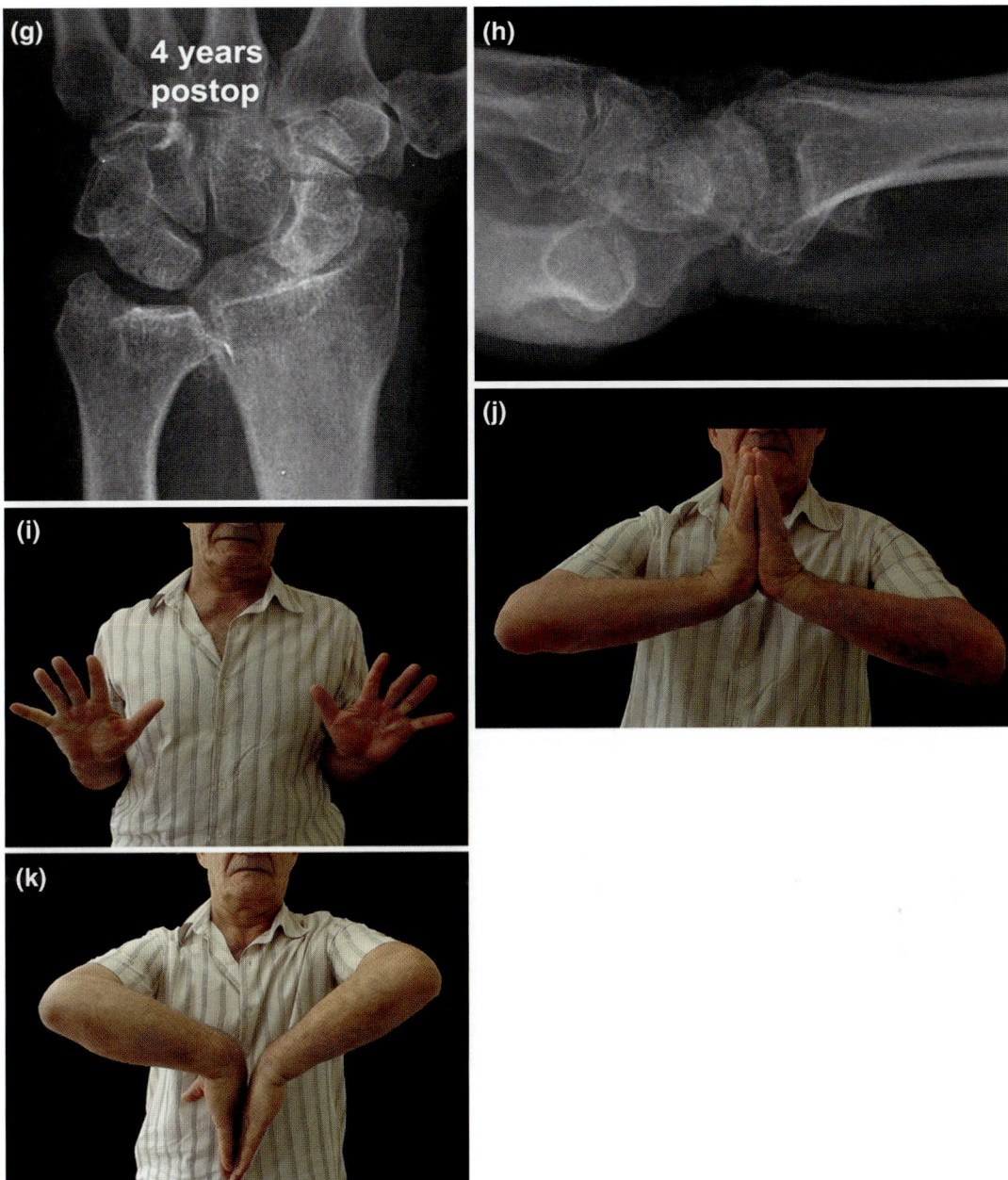

Fig. 7.1 (continued)

damage may be caused by our effort to perform close reduction to a month-old injury.

The upper time limit considered consistent with an acceptable result has been reported to be 6 weeks [13, 14], 8 weeks [6], 12 weeks [7, 15, 16], 18 weeks [17], and 5 months [5]. Others support the attempt of open reduction, regardless of the time that has intervened [12, 18, 19].

In literature, the most delayed open reductions attempted, were of a trans-scaphoid perilunate dislocation 8 months post-injury, where the condition of the cartilage of the lunate and

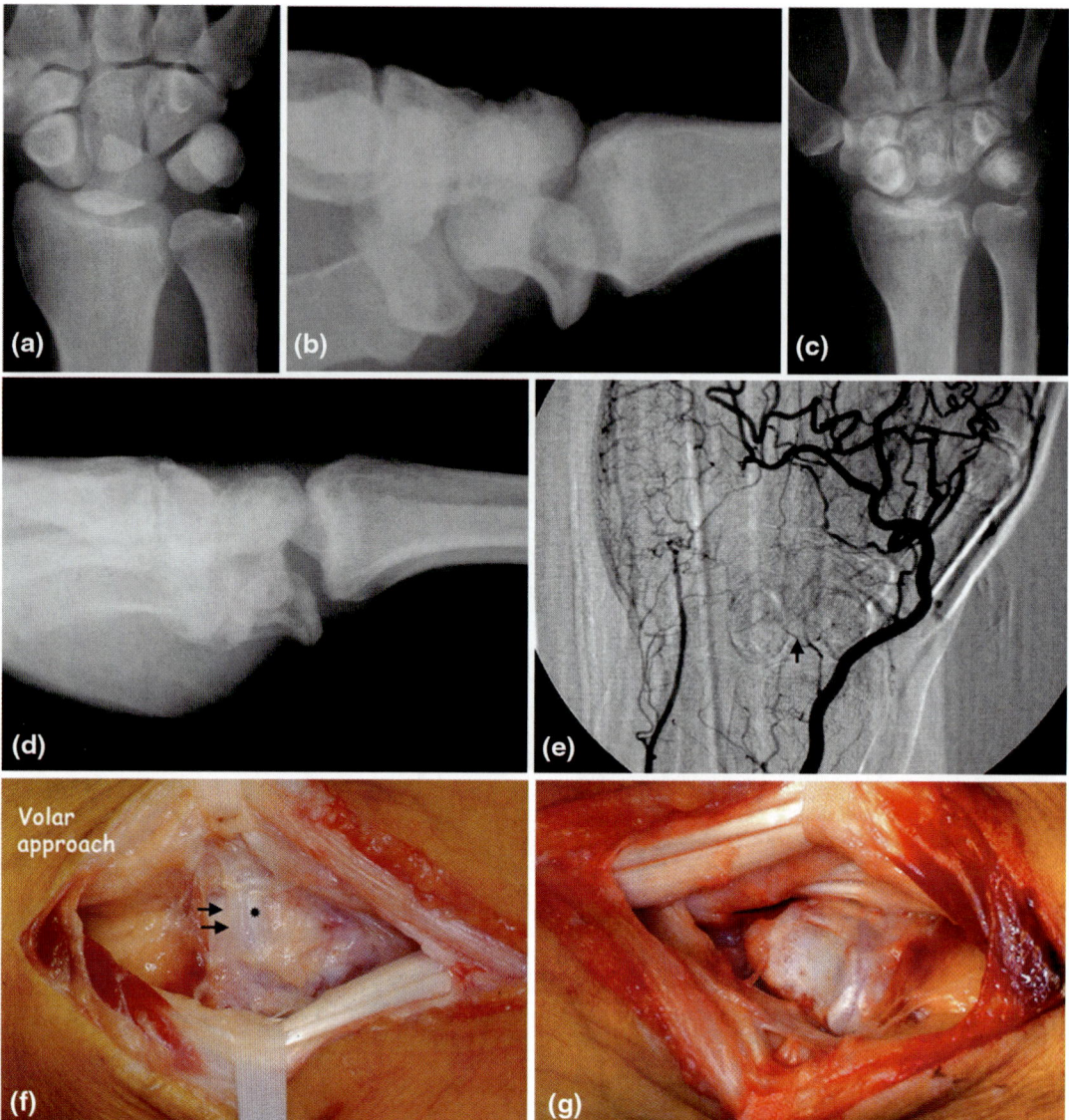

Fig. 7.2 Male, 52-years old, right-handed, with a 4-month old reported injury. It was initially considered a simple injury and a cast was applied. Fifteen days later he was subjected to carpal tunnel release due to numbness of the index and middle fingers. Three months later, pain and numbness continued, he therefore requested medical assistance and a palmar dislocation of the lunate was diagnosed. Initial X-rays (**a, b**); X-rays after 4 months indicated substantial osteopenia and the displacement of the lunate was upgraded from stage II to stage III (**c, d**); based on the arteriogram, vascularization of the lunate by a radial artery branch was presumed (**e**); palmar access exposed the palmar pole of the lunate (*asterisk*), while the distal articular surface was occupied by fibrous tissue (*arrows*) (**f**); its removal revealed cartilage denudation of the articular surface (**g**); dorsal access, following the raise of the capsular flap, revealed the presence of abundant scar tissue (*asterisk*) at the location of the lunate (**h**); following the removal of scar tissue, the lunate was reduced with difficulty and was particularly friable. Lunocapitate fusion with cancellous bone grafts from the distal radius was performed. Post-operative X-rays (**i, j**); the radiological result 3 years later, showing lunate fragmentation (**k, l**); the range of motion was satisfactory and the patient reported pain only after heavy manual work (**m, n**) (*S* Scaphoid, *C* Capitate, *H* Hamate, *T* Triquetrum, *R* Radius). With permission from [44]

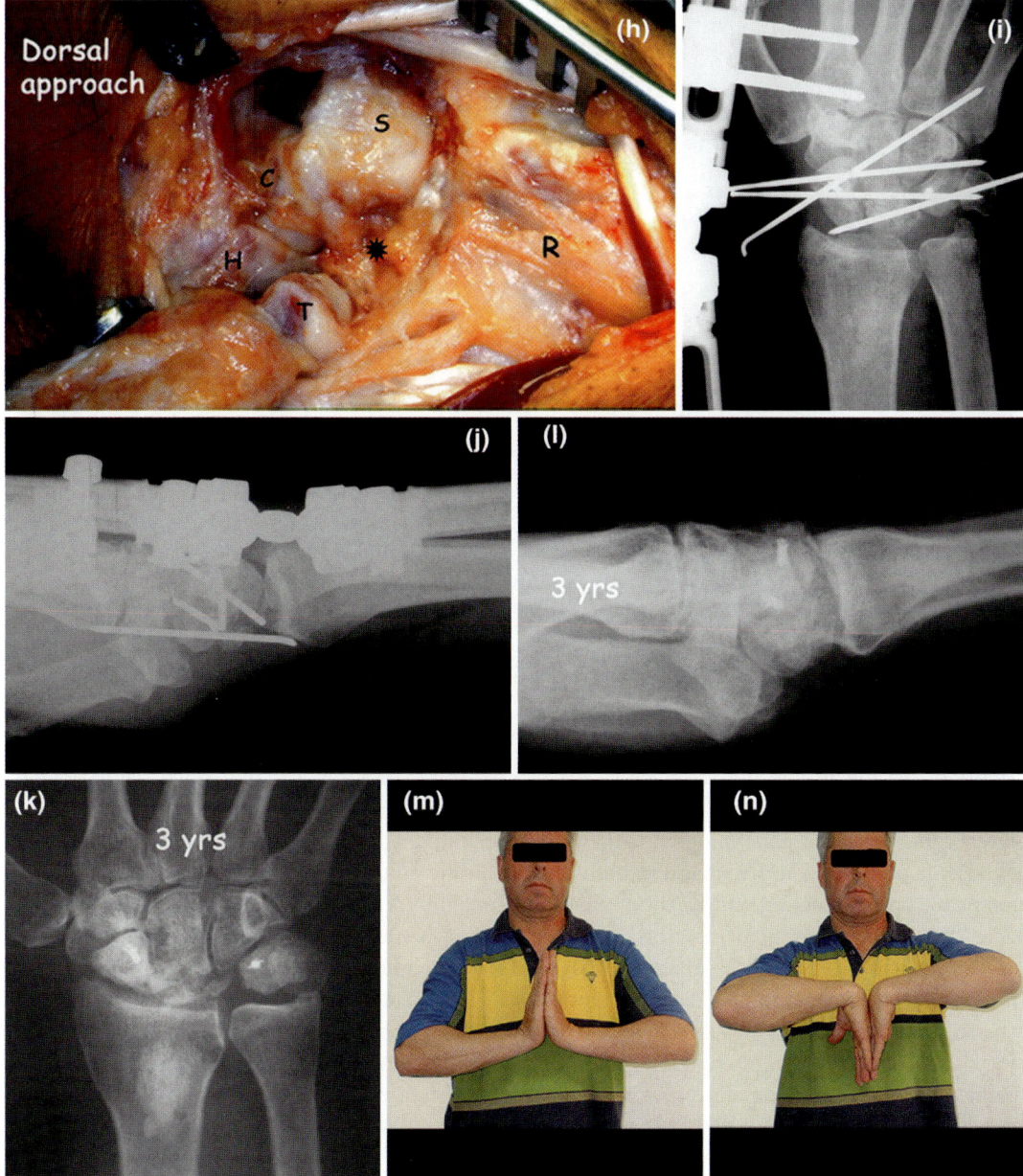

Fig. 7.2 (continued)

the scaphoid was found to be good and which presented with an excellent result after a 5 year follow-up [20]; also, a case with perilunate dislocation, treated with open reduction and internal fixation 35 weeks post injury, showed an excellent functional result after a follow-up of 19 months [7].

The treatment methods of chronic perilunate injuries vary in literature and involve open reduction and internal fixation [17], proximal

Table 7.1 Operative options depending on the condition of the articular cartilage of specific anatomical areas

Articular cartilage	Arthritis			Operative options
Head of capitate	No			Proximal row carpectomy
Distal lunate	No/Yes			
Radial fossae	No			
Head of capitate	Yes	No	No	Partial fusion
Distal lunate	No	Yes	No	
Radial fossae	No	No	Yes	
Head of capitate	Yes			Wrist fusion
Distal lunate	Yes			
Radial fossae	Yes			

row carpectomy [21–26], partial wrist fusions [11, 16, 27], wrist arthrodesis [28], and lunate excision [14, 29].

Siegert et al. [7] treated 15 patients with 16 chronic perilunate dislocations or fracture-dislocations with various methods and they noted that the level of improvement of patients who had wrist arthrodesis or proximal row carpectomy did not exceed that of ORIF. Unanimously, the results of isolated excision of a carpal bone (usually of the lunate) are not satisfactory [6, 7, 11, 15, 16, 23].

According to Inoue and Shionoya [6], when diagnosis is performed earlier than 2 months, an attempt for open reduction and fixation must be made. When however it is performed after 2 months post injury, the best results are achieved with proximal row carpectomy. Yao and Jagadish [30] and Jones and Kakar [31] advocated that any injury that has persisted for more than 4–6 weeks should not be primarily repaired and a salvage procedure should be performed, because contracture of the volar ligaments and irreversible carpal bone ischemia may preclude successful open reduction and ligament repair.

The longest period that a chronic perilunate injury must be treated with open reduction, is unknown. The word "must" instead of "may" is deliberately used, since any chronic dislocation can be reduced, regardless of the time that has intervened, but the result will not be a functional one. Hence the question that arises is: what is the time period that can intervene, in order for an open reduction to be attempted on a chronic perilunate dislocation, so that the result is functional in the long term?

It should also be considered, that none of the cases of neglected perilunate dislocations mentioned in the literature presents disruption in the vascularity of the lunate at the time of diagnosis, regardless of the time intervened. Disruption in vascularity develops only after attempting open reduction and is not usually transient, but leads to fragmentation of the bone (Fig. 7.2a–n). Transient vascular compromise was noted postoperatively, in three out of four patients with chronic lunate and perilunate dislocations presented by Takami et al. [17]. Three cases (out of 14) presented by Dhillon et al. [5] with neglected volar lunate dislocations with 21–22 weeks of delay, developed avascular necrosis of the lunate after open reduction. A similar case of chronic lunate dislocation, which was operatively treated after 6 months of delay, was presented by Weir [32]. After a follow-up of 1 year, X-ray showed complete collapse and fragmentation of the lunate. A reported exception is the case by Gellman et al. [13], where a trans-scaphoid dorsal perilunate dislocation, neglected for 3 months, presented avascular changes of the lunate preoperatively. However, after open reduction and internal fixation, the patient regained a full, pain-free wrist motion with complete resolution of the roentgenographic changes of the lunate after a follow-up of 4 years.

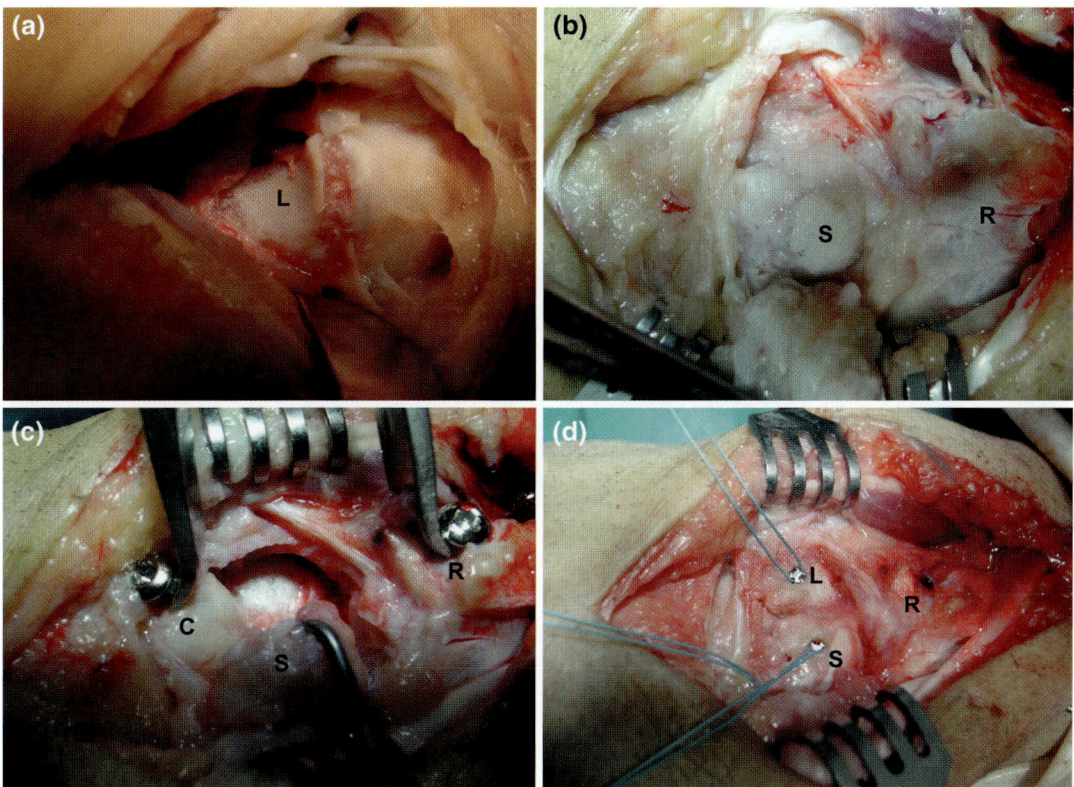

Fig. 7.3 A 4 months old lunate dislocation after volar approach (**a**); abundant scar tissue occupied the space previously located by the lunate (*dorsal approach*) (**b**); removal of the scar tissue and distraction of the joint with a lamina spreader using screws located at the radius and capitate (**c**); with the lunate reduced, insertion of bone anchors for capsuloligamentous reconstruction (**d**) (*L* Lunate, *S* Scaphoid, *C* Capitate, *R* Radius)

Hence, the atraumatic technique required for maintaining the precarious vascularity of dislocated bones, comes frequently in contrast with the manipulations required for the reduction of the chronically dislocated wrist.

Both patient-related and injury-related variables influence decision making [11]. As for the latter, mainly three factors must be taken into consideration during the reduction of a neglected perilunate dislocation:

1. The contraction of the capsuloligamentous structures and the development of scar tissue.
2. The condition of the articular cartilage (especially of the distal lunate) that has eroded during time.
3. The friability of the dislocated lunate, which has become osteopenic as it does not withstand physiologic loads for a long time.

Evidently, the severity of each of the above factors varies among patients and among injuries. The contraction of the capsuloligamentous structures can most likely be dealt with by applying gradual distraction to the wrist with an external fixator, through a one, or more commonly, two-stage operation [33–37]. The second operation after the application of the external fixator is usually performed 7–10 days after gradual application of distraction. As far as the other two factors are concerned though, our options are limited. However, these are the factors that will determine the surgical methods applied and which by order of preference are the following:

1. Open reduction, ligamentous reconstruction or substitution, and internal fixation.

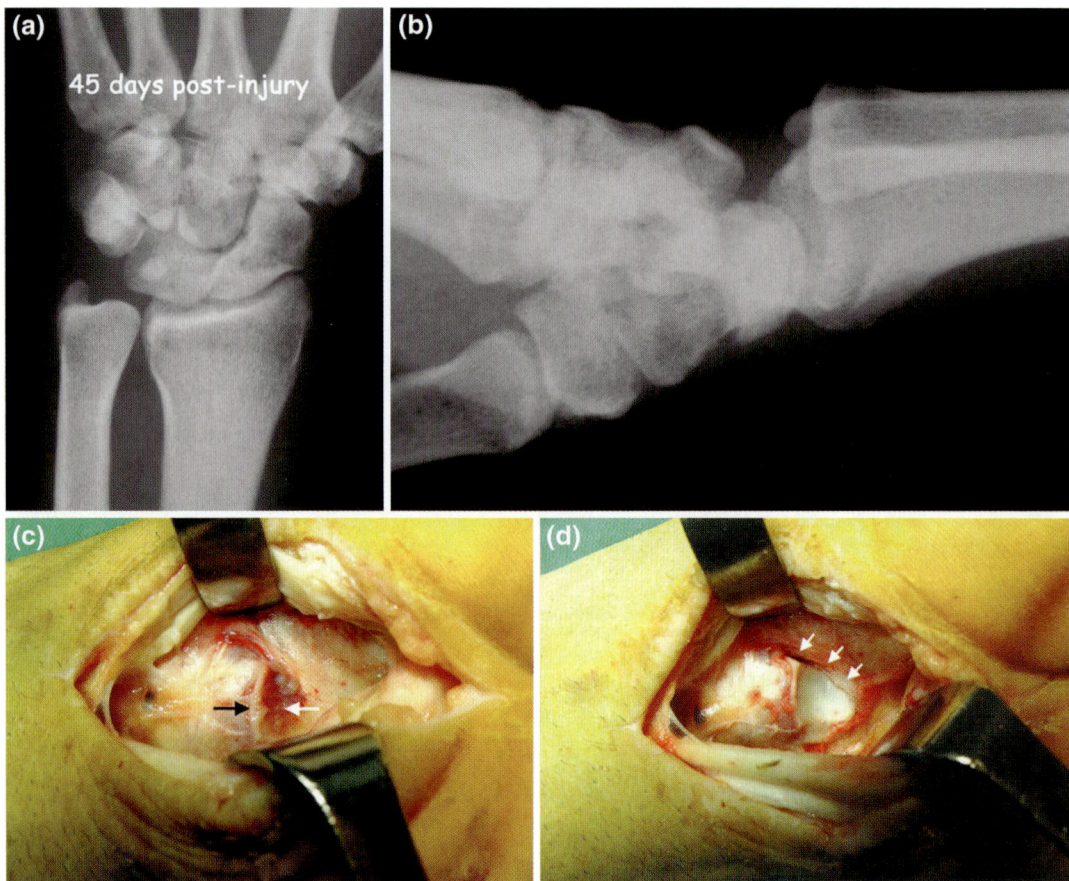

Fig. 7.4 Male, 27-years old, dorsal perilunate disloca-tion with a 6 weeks old injury, which escaped diagnosis (**a, b**); palmar access exposed scar tissue (*white arrow*) at the distal articular surface of the lunate (*black arrow*) (**c**); following the removal of the scar tissue the articular cartilage appeared to be in good condition (*white arrows* show the midcarpal rent) (**d**); dorsal access revealed the scar tissue proximal of the capitate (*asterisk*), which presented with a chondral defect (*arrow*) (**e**); after dislocation reduction, ligamentous reconstruction was performed using bone anchors (**f**); fixation was limited at the proximal carpal row and external fixation was applied (**g, h**); 3 months later, omission to place a transfixing pin, bridging the two rows, led to dorsal subluxation of the capitate head (**i, j**). With permission from [44]

2. Partial wrist fusion (scapholunocapitate or lunocapitate or four-corner fusion with sca-phoid excision [11, 16] or scaphocapitate with lunate excision [16, 27]).
3. Proximal row carpectomy and
4. Wrist fusion.

Which method will be chosen among the last three (2, 3 or 4), will depend upon the condition of the joint cartilage of the head of the capitate, the distal lunate, and the radial fossae (Table 7.1).

Consequently, how a neglected injury will be treated, does not depend as much upon the time limits set by the literature, but upon sur-geon's experience and the anatomical condi-tions encountered. In any case, successful delayed open reduction produces better func-tional results than any salvage operation [2, 7, 13, 17, 32, 38] and functional and radiological results are better in delayed than in chronic injuries [5, 39].

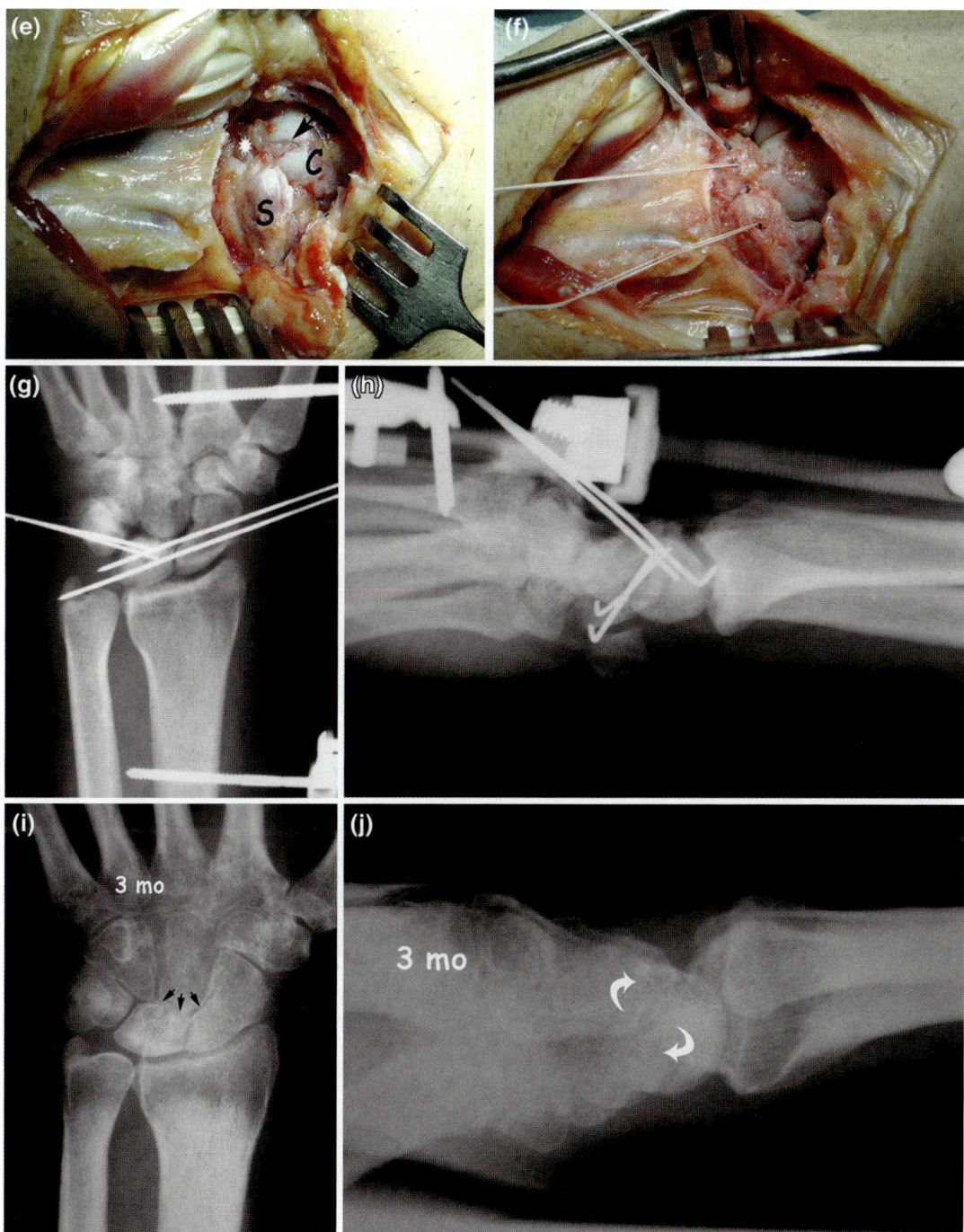

Fig. 7.4 (continued)

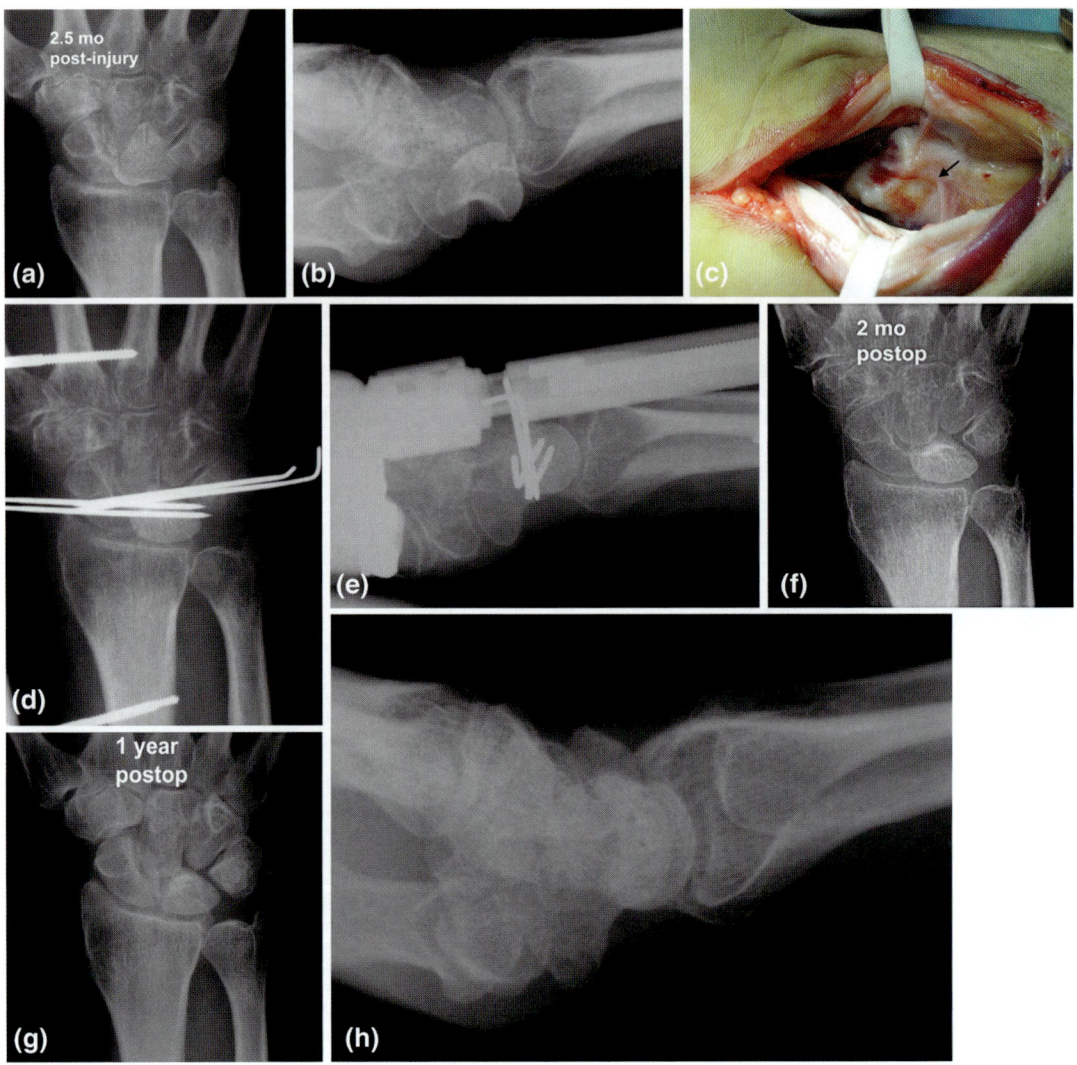

Fig. 7.5 Male, 58-years old, a 2.5 months old lunate dislocation (**a, b**); arrow shows the only vascular supply to the volarly dislocated lunate (**c**); postop X-rays (**d, e**); 2 months later, transient ischemia of the lunate was apparent (**f**); final X-rays 1 year postop (**g, h**)

It is properly supported [11, 39] that the decision on the type of operation, should be taken intraoperatively, according to the condition of the articular cartilage of the midcarpal and radiocarpal joints.

Kailu et al. [39] proposed to use the International Cartilage Repair Society grading system (ICRS) to grade the severity of the cartilage damage as follows: *ICRS 0 (normal):* Macroscopically normal cartilage without notable defects; *ICRS 1 (nearly normal):* The cartilage has superficial lesions (fibrillation, softening, fissures); *ICRS 2 (abnormal):* Defects that extend deeper but involve <50 % of the cartilage thickness; *ICRS 3(severely abnormal):* Lesions that extend through >50 % of the cartilage thickness but not through the subchondral bone plate; and *ICRS 4 (severely abnormal):* Cartilage defects that extend into the subchondral bone. The authors suggested that in delayed or chronic cases with low-grade cartilage damage (ICRS I and ICRS II), open reduction and internal fixation should be attempted, while in high-grade damage (ICRS III and ICRS IV), a salvage procedure should be considered.

The basic principles for reduction of neglected perilunate dislocations are identical with those for acute injuries. We believe that, up to 2 or 3 months post-injury, an open reduction and internal fixation should be attempted with the following essential steps:

1. Combined (dorsal and palmar) approach, as this diminishes the amount of force necessary for the reduction.
2. Removing of the scar tissue occupying the space opposite the lunate fossa (dorsally) and the distal articular surface of the lunate (palmarly).
3. Assessment of the articular cartilage i.e., distal lunate, head of the capitate.
4. Distraction of the joint, with an external fixator or other distraction device like lamina spreader (Fig. 7.3a–d)
5. Reduction of the dislocation, by using the most atraumatic technique possible and by maintaining the soft tissues of the proximal lunate intact. Using sharp or blunt instruments to help the reduction of the lunocapitate joint, as has been suggested [5, 16, 37], threatens the integrity of the friable lunate.
6. Fixation of the lunate with K wires with the adjacent bones. While transfixing pins (bridging rows or radius) are not necessary in acute injuries, they are essential in delayed cases in order to avoid recurrence of subluxation (Fig. 7.4a–j).
7. Retaining external fixator in slight distraction postoperatively to preserve the carpal height (Fig. 7.5a–h).

Capsular or ligamentous flaps (Blatt or DIC ligament flaps) may be needed to supplement the deficient SL interosseous ligament [15]. Reinforcement with tendon grafts of the SL ligament in neglected perilunate dislocations is most likely referred to in literature as a theoretical possibility, since only Howard and Dell [12] applied it in practice, emphasizing the technical difficulties of this method. Probably, the contraction of the capsuloligamentous structures and the scar tissue developed in cases older than 2–3 months, contribute to adequate stability and wrist stiffness, so that capsulodesis or tendon grafts are not necessary measures, a view also supported by Massoud and Naam [16] and Dhillon et al. [5]. If it's feasible, we insert one or two bone anchors to the proximal scaphoid or lunate to augment the remnants (if any) of the SL ligament with the proximal DIC ligament and the dorsal capsule.

In cases of neglected trans-scaphoid fracture-dislocations, where comminution, bone resorption or ischemic changes of the scaphoid may be encountered, simple bone grafts or vascularized bone grafts may be needed.

In the case of open reduction, as well as the case of partial fusion, chronic contracture of the capsuloligamentous structures, renders difficult the accurate alignment of the joint between the lunate and the capitate. If the lunocapitate joint is fixed with a K-wire (during open reduction) or fused (in partial fusion) with dorsal angulation, then dorsal impingement of the capitate to the dorsal radial rim will produce a painful restriction of dorsiflexion of the wrist.

Kailu et al. [39] supported that loss of the articular cartilage at the midcarpal joint, leads to the decrease of carpal height ratio postoperatively, which has adverse effects on wrist function. They are considered important to protect the articular cartilage postoperatively, especially in chronic cases in which the joint capsule is contracted and the articular cartilage is inevitably under compression after reduction. This was accomplished by using an external fixator in a neutralizing mode, to block the axial load on the cartilage of the proximal carpal row and to maintain normal carpal alignment during the initial stages of ligament healing. Concerning the distraction, Bathala and Murray [8] highlighted that when attempting to reduce a chronically dislocated carpus, the surgeon must take into account that shortening of the median nerve and the radial and ulnar arteries will have occurred.

For injuries dated more than 3 months, usually our options are confined to a salvage procedure (proximal row carpectomy, partial or total wrist fusion), depending on the condition of the articular cartilage of the head of the capitate, distal lunate, and of radial fossae.

Massoud and Naam [16] retrospectively reviewed 19 patients for chronic perilunate injuries with a mean delay of 29 weeks (range, 13–35), who were treated with open reduction and internal fixation. They divided the patients into two groups based on the type of injury: 13 patients with greater arc and 6 patients with lesser arc injuries and they attempted to compare the functional outcome. They found no significant differences between the two groups concerning pain (VAS), active ROM and grip strength. Statistically, significant difference was found concerning the Mayo wrist scoring system according to which, good to excellent result was achieved in 69 % of patients with greater arc injuries compared with 33 % of patients with lesser arc injuries. They concluded that patients with lesser arc injuries have a less successful outcome. In addition, they commented that the reduction of greater arc was technically easier than that of lesser arc injuries.

Rettig and Raskin [40] treated with proximal row carpectomy 12 patients with stage III and IV perilunate dislocations, which had remained undiagnosed for a period of 8 weeks until 6 months. In seven of the patients, they discovered small cartilaginous defects at the head of the capitate. After a follow-up of 40 months on average, the patients demonstrated significant pain relief, functional range of motion, and satisfactory grip strength (arc of flexion–extension 80o and grip strength 80 % of the contralateral wrist). Three heavy manual workers were unable to return to their former occupation, while one patient developed asymptomatic radiocapitate arthritis.

For patients of this category, who frequently present cartilage defects at the head of the capitate and who are usually treated with proximal row carpectomy, the interposition of the dorsal capsule is possibly effective [41, 42].

Wrist arthrodesis is indicated in cases of generalized arthritis of the wrist, while in cases of neglected perilunate dislocations, the suggestion made by Richards and Roth [43] to perform a fusion of the distal carpal row to the radius, preceded by proximal row carpectomy, is interesting. Advantages of this method are: the simultaneous decompression of the carpal tunnel, the removal of sclerotic, and avascular bone that may delay union, the fact that arthrodesis is performed on less articular surfaces and thus reduces the risk of nonunion, that wrist malalignment (ulnar displacement and radial subluxation) is easier fixed and that the risk of ulnocarpal impaction is reduced.

For patients who appear many years after the injury (frequently for another reason) with symptoms of carpal tunnel syndrome or with flexor-tendon rupture, we usually tackle the problem alone (carpal tunnel release, tendon reconstruction), since these patients may not be candidates for surgical correction of the bony deformity [6, 9]. Although the few reports of isolated carpal bone excision agree on its lack of success, in cases where the lunate has been dislocated for years and the wrist has been adapted to its absence, excision of the lunate (because of tendon or median nerve problems) probably makes no difference (Fig. 7.1a–k).

References

1. Herzberg G (2002) Acute perilunate dislocations and fracture-dislocations. In: EFORT (ed) Surgical techniques in orthopaedics and traumatology. Elsevier, 55-370-E-10, pp 1–4
2. Garcia-Elias M (1999) Carpal instabilities and dislocations. In: Green DP, Hotchkiss RN, Pederson WC (eds) Green's operative hand surgery, vol 1. Churchill Livingstone, New York, pp 865–928
3. Garcia-Elias M, Irisarri C, Henriquez A et al (1986) Perilunar dislocation of the carpus. A diagnosis still often missed. Ann Chir Main 5:281–287
4. Herzberg G, Comtet JJ, Linscheid RL et al (1993) Perilunate dislocations and fracture dislocations: a multicenter study. J Hand Surg [Am] 18:768–779
5. Dhillon MS, Prabhakar S, Bali K et al (2011) Functional outcome of neglected perilunate dislocations treated with open reduction and internal fixation. Indian J Orthop 45(5):427–431
6. Inoue G, Shionoya K (1999) Late treatment of unreduced perilunate dislocations. J Hand Surg [Br] 24:221–225
7. Siegert JJ, Frassica FJ, Amadio PC (1988) Treatment of chronic perilunate dislocations. J Hand Surg [Am] 13:206–212

8. Bathala E, Murray P (2007) Long-term follow-up of an undiagnosed trans-scaphoid perilunate dislocation demonstrating articular remodeling and functional adaptation. J Hand Surg [Am] 32:1020–1023

9. Herzberg G, Cooney WP (1998) Perilunate fracture dislocations. In: Cooney WP, Linscheid RL, Dobyns JH (eds) The wrist: diagnosis and operative treatment, vol 1. Mosby, Mayo Clinic, pp 651–683

10. Stern PJ (1981) Multiple flexor tendon ruptures following an old anterior dislocation of the lunate: a case report. J Hand Surg [Am] 63:489–490

11. Tomaino MM (2002) Late management of perilunate fracture-dislocations. In: Trumble TE (ed) Carpal fractures-dislocations. American academy of orthopaedic surgeons, pp 67–74

12. Howard FM, Dell PC (1986) The unreduced carpal dislocation. A method of treatment. Clin Orthop 202:112–116

13. Gellman H, Schwartz SD, Botte MJ et al (1988) Late treatment of a dorsal transscaphoid, transtriquetral perilunate wrist dislocation with avascular changes of the lunate. Clin Orthop 237:196–203

14. MacAusland WR (1944) Perilunar dislocation of the carpal bones and dislocation of the lunate bone. Surg Gynecol Obstet 79:256

15. Kozin SH (2010) Perilunate dislocations. In: Cooney WP (ed) The wrist: diagnosis and operative treatment. Lippincott Williams and Wilkins, ch 23, pp 532–549

16. Massoud AHA, Naam NH (2012) Functional outcome of open reduction of chronic perilunate injuries. J Hand Surg [Am] 37:1852–1860

17. Takami H, Takahashi S, Ando M et al (1996) Open reduction of chronic lunate and perilunate dislocations. Arch Orthop Trauma Surg 115:104–107

18. Fisk GR (1984) The wrist. J Bone Joint Surg Br 66:396–407

19. Green DP, O'Brien ET (1978) Open reduction of carpal dislocations: indications and operative techniques. J Hand Surg [Am] 3:250–265

20. Mir BA, Dhar SA, Mir MR et al (2008) Open reduction and internal fixation in a case with transscaphoid perilunate dislocation 8 months after the injury: a patient with a 5-year follow-up. Strat Trauma Limb Reconstr 3:93–96

21. Campbell RD, Lance EM, Yeoh CB (1964) Lunate and perilunar dislocation. J Bone Joint Surg Br 46:55–72

22. Campbell RD, Thompson TC, Lance EM et al (1965) Indications for open reduction of lunate and perilunate dislocations of the carpal bones. J Bone Joint Surg Am 47:915–937

23. Inoue G, Miura T (1990) Proximal row carpectomy in perilunate dislocations and lunatomalacia. Acta Orthop Scand 61:449–452

24. Jebson PJL, Engber WD (1977) Chronic perilunate fracture dislocations and primary proximal row carpectomy. Iowa Orthop J 14:42–48

25. Neviaser RJ (1983) Proximal row carpectomy for posttraumatic disorders of the carpus. J Hand Surg [Am] 8:301–305

26. Neviaser RJ (1986) On resection of the proximal carpal row. Clin Orthop 202:12–15

27. Hastings DE, Silver RL (1984) Intercarpal arthrodesis in the management of chronic carpal instability after trauma. J Hand Surg [Am] 9:834–840

28. Wagner CJ (1956) Perilunar dislocations. J Bone Joint Surg Am 38(6):1198–1230

29. Russell TB (1949) Inter-carpal dislocations and fracture-dislocations: a review of fifty-nine cases. J Bone Joint Surg Br 31:524–531

30. Yao J, Jagadish A (2010) Carpus: perilunate and greater arc injuries. In: Slutsky DJ (ed) Principles and practice of wrist surgery. Saunders, ch 44, pp 473–486

31. Jones D, Kakar S (2012) Perilunate dislocations and fracture dislocations. J Hand Surg [Am] 37:2168–2174

32. Weir IG (1992) The late reduction of carpal dislocations. J Hand Surg [Br] 17:137–139

33. Fernandez DL (1993) Technique and results of external fixation of complex carpal injuries. Hand Clin 9:625–637

34. Garcia-Elias M (2004) Perilunar injuries including fracture dislocations. In: Berger R, Weiss AP (eds) Hand surgery, vol 1. Lippincott Williams & Wilkins, pp 511–524

35. Mizuseki T, Tsuge K, Kajitani N et al (1999) Open reduction of chronic perilunate dislocation with the aid of external fixator. J Jpn Soc Surg Hand 16(1):113–115

36. Sousa HP, Fernandes H, Botelheiro JC (1995) Pre-operative progressive distraction in old transcapho-peri-lunate dislocations. J Hand Surg [Br] 20:603–605

37. Vegter J (1987) Late reduction of the dislocated lunate. J Bone Joint Surg Br 69:734–736

38. Vo DP, Mohler LR, Trumble TE (2002) Lunate and perilunate dislocations. In: Trumble TE (ed) Carpal fracture-dislocations. American Academy of Orthopaedic Surgeons, ch 4, pp 27–35

39. Kailu L, Zhou X, Fuguo H (2010) Chronic perilunate dislocations treated with open reduction and internal fixation: results of medium-term follow-up. Int Orthop 34(8):1315–1320

40. Rettig ME, Raskin KB (1999) Long-term assessment of proximal row carpectomy for chronic perilunate dislocation. J Hand Surg [Am] 24:1231–1236

41. Eaton RG (1997) Proximal row carpectomy and soft tissue interposition arthroplasty. Techn Hand Upper Extrem Surg 1:248–254

42. Tomaino MM, Delsignore J, Burton RI (1994) Long-term results following proximal row carpectomy. J Hand Surg [Am] 19:694–703

43. Richards RS, Roth JH (1994) Simultaneous proximal row carpectomy and radius to distal carpal row arthrodesis. J Hand Surg [Am] 19:728–732

44. Apergis E (2004) καταγματα-εξαρθρήματα του καρπου. Konstantaras Medical Books, Athens

Radiocarpal Dislocations or Fracture-Dislocations

8

Emmanuel Apergis and Anna Palamidi

8.1 Introduction

Until the description of the fractures of the distal radius by Claude Pouteau in 1783, the radiocarpal (RC) dislocations were the only known carpal injuries. Dupuytren was the first, who in 1834 recognized their rarity. The RC dislocation injury was first recognized and described by Malle in 1838, when he identified a volar RC fracture-dislocation. Shortly thereafter, Marjolin and Voillemier identified and reported dorsal RC fracture-dislocations. All these observations were made from examination of postmortem specimens [1, 2]. Destot [3] reported the first radiographically documented case of a RC fracture-dislocation in 1926.

RC fracture-dislocations are relatively rare injuries, whose exact frequency is unknown. Gui [4] reported that these dislocations represent 0.2 % of all dislocations (quoted by Rosado [5]), while Dunn [6], from 112 fracture-dislocations of the wrist, reported 6 RC dislocations, i.e., a percentage of 5.3 (quoted by Bilos et al. [7]). However, it was later disputed, whether three of those cases actually belonged to the category of RC dislocations [8]. Moneim et al. [9] reported that within a 13-year period, he treated 7 cases of RC dislocations and that this number represented 20 % of all carpal

dislocations, encountered during that period. Between these two extremes (0.2–20 %), Ilyas' et al. [10] estimation of 2.7 % (12 out of 438 patients with distal radius fracture or wrist dislocation) and 0.46 % with pure ligamentous dislocations, seems to be more realistic. We will probably never find out the true incidence of these injuries, since there is no consensus as to which injuries should be named RC fracture-dislocations.

Due to the rarity of the injury of most references, describe a relatively small number [7, 9, 11–15] or isolated cases [16–34]. At present only a few reports involve more than 10 patients: the report by Nyquist and Stern [35] with 10 cases, by Mudgal et al. [36] with 12 cases, by Girard et al. [37] with 12 cases, and by Dumontier et al. [38] with 27 cases throughout a 23-year period.

The literature reveals that pure RC dislocations are rare injuries, while the RC fracture-dislocations involving radial styloid fractures are the most frequent. In addition, the dorsal RC fracture-dislocations are much more common than their palmar counterpart [36, 38, 39], although it seems the opposite is true for pure RC dislocations. By reviewing the literature, Table 8.1 shows the number of cases of pure dislocations (dorsal, volar, and multidirectional) that have been reported so far and the subtype of volar dislocations associated with the ulnovolar fragment of the distal radius.

As for more violent traumas, these injuries have been reported mainly in males and usually of young age. In our series of 26 patients, the average age was 33.7 (range, 19–60) and only

E. Apergis (✉) · A. Palamidi
Red Cross Hospital, Evagelistrias 13, 15342,
Athens, Greece
e-mail: apergis@gmail.com

E. Apergis, *Fracture-Dislocations of the Wrist*,
DOI: 10.1007/978-88-470-5328-1_8, © Springer-Verlag Italia 2013

Table 8.1 Pure dorsal, pure volar, pure volar with associated ulnovolar fragment and multidirectional RC dislocations, as reported in the literature

	Author	Years	Cases
Pure dorsal RC dislocations	Hardy [54]	1999	1
	Varodompun [119]	1985	1
	Dumontier [32]	2001	1
	Berschback [14]	2012	1
	Bohler [16]	1930	2
	Rosado [101]	1966	1
	Dunn [33]	1972	2
	Fehring [34]	1984	1
Pure volar RC dislocations	Moneim [83]	1985	1
	Moore [84]	1988	1
	Howard [59]	1997	1
	Naranja [91]	1998	1
	Mudgal [87]	1999	1
	Dumontier [32]	2001	1
	Mourikis [86]	2008	2
	Bellinghausen[9]	1983	2
	Penny [96]	1988	1
	Thomsen [118]	1989	1
Volar RC dislocations + Ulnovolar fragment	Apergis [6]	1996	1
	Dumontier [32]	2001	1
	Takase [114]	2004	1
	Freeland [40]	2006	1
	Hofmeister [58]	2008	1
	Obafemi [93]	2012	1
Multidirectional pure ligamentous RC dislocations	Fennel [35]	1992	1
	Our series	2012	2

one was a woman, while in Dumontier's [38] series the percentage male/female was 4/1.

8.2 Restraints of the Radiocarpal Joint

We know that wrist motion along the transverse plane (pronation-supination) is only possible if the wrist is not loaded. The range of passive rotational motion between radius and carpus varies from 40° to 45° [40–43] and extrinsic tendon loading affects significantly the rotational stability of the wrist: the passive pronosupination laxity of the RC and midcarpal joint decreases from 45° to 10° by clenching the fist [40].

Many daily manual tasks are performed by rotation of the forearm. To perform these rotational tasks adequately, the relative motion between the radius and the carpus must be constrained within a limited amount of laxity. These constraints to rotation (which at the same time provide stability to the RC joint) consist of *the concavity of the radial fossas,the dorsal and palmar capsuloligamentous structures* that link the forearm to the carpus, and *the extrinsic tendons* that cross the RC joint.

8.2.1 Ligamentous Structures

Ligamentous structures provide constraints in both rotational (pronosupination between radius and carpus) and translational (dorsopalmar and ulnar) displacement of the wrist.

8.2.1.1 Rotational Constraints

Ritt et al. [41] stated that ligamentous structures, having a proximal-radial to distal-ulnar course on the dorsal side (DRC ligament) and a proximal-ulnar to distal-radial course on the palmar side (UL, UT ligaments), provide resistance to passive supination of the radiocarpal joint. On the contrary, ligamentous structures having a proximal-radial to distal-ulnar course on the volar side (RSC, LRL, and SRL ligaments) provide resistance to passive pronation of the RC joint with the RSC ligament being the primary pronation constraint. The author supported that ulnarly located structures changed their major constraint contribution with forearm orientation, whereas those with a radial origin had a constant contribution independent of forearm rotation.

Rotational motion between radius and carpus is obviously not restricted to the RC joint alone. The midcarpal joint contributes as well. Gupta and Moosawi [44] stated that active RC pronosupination occurs predominantly at the midcarpal joint with the RC joint contributing only

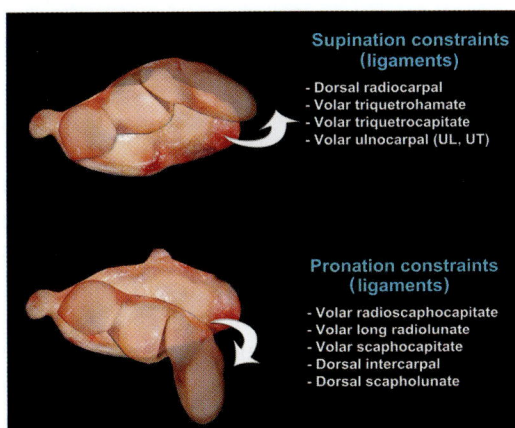

Supination constraints (ligaments)
- Dorsal radiocarpal
- Volar triquetrohamate
- Volar triquetrocapitate
- Volar ulnocarpal (UL, UT)

Pronation constraints (ligaments)
- Volar radioscaphocapitate
- Volar long radiolunate
- Volar scaphocapitate
- Dorsal intercarpal
- Dorsal scapholunate

Fig. 8.1 Supination and pronation constraining ligaments

18 % to supination and 31 % to pronation. In that case, the stabilizing ligaments of the midcarpal joint (SC, TH, TC ligaments) must also contribute significantly to the rotational motion between radius and carpus. Hence, the concept of anti-pronation and anti-supination slings [45] running in opposite directions, could be the main restraining ligamentous construction stabilizing the RC unit during rotational motion (Fig. 8.1).

8.2.1.2 Dorsopalmar Translation Constraints

The integrity of the palmar RC capsuloligamentous structures seems crucial to RC stability. Katz et al. [46] using fresh-frozen cadaver specimens, found that palmar structures (RSC, LRL, and SRL ligaments) provided greater restraint (61 %) to dorsal translation of the carpus than did dorsal structures (DRC ligament) (2 %). The palmar structures also provided a greater restraint (48 %) to palmar translation of the carpus than did the dorsal structures (6 %). In particular, the SRL ligament is considered by some [11, 47] as the primary soft-tissue restraint against volar translation of the carpus.

Interestingly, the remaining structures (radial and dorsal capsule and UC ligaments) provided 37 % restraint to dorsal translation and 46 % restraint to palmar translation.

8.2.1.3 Ulnar Translation Constraints

The RC ligaments, both volar (RSC, LRL, SRL ligaments) and dorsal (DRC), having an oblique direction (lateral to medial), constrain the natural tendency of the carpus to slide down the ulnopalmarly inclined distal articular surface of the radius [46, 48, 49]. The extent of ligament injury necessary for an ulnar translation to occur, although not exactly known, is quite substantial [50, 51] and certainly greater than previously reported [52]. In partial injuries, the carpus may translate palmarly rather than ulnarly [50]. Viegas et al. [50] found experimentally that, while the RSC ligament alone was not adequate to stabilize the wrist against ulnar translation, the UC ligaments alone, were. Ilyas and Mudgal [2] stated that ulnar translation in conjunction with loss of the ulnolunate ligaments led to progression of the injury from ulnar translocation to multidirectional instability of the wrist.

The importance of the volar ulnocarpal ligaments (UL, LT, UC) on ulnocarpal stability, has been emphasized in the literature. Munk et al. [53] noted that the rupture of these ligaments produced significant instability not only in deviation but also in rotation of the wrist, while Wiesner et al. [54] stated that sectioning of these ligaments increased significantly the displacement of the carpus in the palmar direction. It has also been reported that the ulnocarpal ligaments can prevent abnormal radioulnar translation of the carpus [55, 56]. Moritomo et al. [57] found that ulnocarpal ligaments are at risk with the wrist in radial extension or hyperextension when associated with axial loading or forearm rotation (or both), a mechanism which has been implicated in RC dislocations.

8.2.2 Extensor Compartments

Extensor compartments contribute markedly to resisting both pronation and supination at the RC joint [41]. Iwamoto et al. [58] investigated the mechanical strength of each septal attachment on the radius and each of the 6 compartments of the extensor retinaculum. He found that septa 1/ 2 and 2/3 had the highest stiffness and failure forces, while compartment 3 had the highest stiffness and compartment 2 had the highest failure force. He concluded that large bony attachment sites and a wide breadth of retinaculum fibers may attest to the high stiffness and failure loads of the first 3 compartments.

8.2.3   Extrinsic Tendons

Capsuloligamentous structures are considered as passive, while extrinsic tendons as dynamic constraints of joints. The interaction between passive and dynamic constraints is now well documented in recent publications that have identified the presence of mechanoreceptors in the joint capsule and carpal ligaments [59]. The neurophysiological mechanisms triggering contraction of certain muscles in order to protect the joint against external forces, have also been defined [60–62]. When a ligament is about to fail, a neuromuscular reflex is triggered that hampers further injury, either by direct contraction of some muscles or by inhibition of some other.

Salva-Coll et al. [63] categorized muscles into two groups: the muscles that pronate the midcarpal joint, (mainly the ECU and in a lesser extent the FCR) and those that supinate the midcarpal joint (the FCU, the ECRL and APL).

8.3   Correlation Between Articular Fracture Fragments and Ligamentous Attachments

Only few reports are dealing with the association between articular fracture fragments and the attachments of the RC ligaments to the radius [64–66]. Siegel and Gelberman [65] studied the damage that can be caused to the palmar RC ligaments during radial styloidectomy, but they described the regions of ligament origin in absolute dimensions, without taking into account

that the areas of origin of the RC ligaments vary in their width when comparing wrists of different sizes. They performed three types of styloidectomies: the short oblique (equated to a fracture of the tip of the radial styloid) corresponds to the interruption of the radial collateral ligament; the vertical oblique (compared to a fracture through the middle of the scaphoid fossa) corresponds to disruption of the RSC ligament origin; and the horizontal styloidectomy (representing a fracture line exiting at the interfacet prominence, proximal to the SL joint) corresponds in addition, to interruption of a major portion (av. 46 %) of the long radiolunate ligament. Hence, in RC dislocations associated with a fracture of only the tip of the radial styloid, the reconstruction of the palmar RC ligaments is mandatory [38]; in RC fracture-dislocations with a fracture of the radial styloid exiting at the level of the SL joint, fixation of the fragment, which contains a major part of the palmar RC ligaments, could probably restore the stability of the wrist.

Berger and Amadio [64] attempted to correlate the size and location of the intraarticular fracture fragments of the distal radius with the palmar RC ligament injuries, while Mandziak et al. [66] by reviewing CT scans of intraarticular distal radius fractures, analyzed the relationship of fracture line locations to known ligament attachments. They found that fracture lines were significantly more likely to occur at the intervals between the ligament attachments than at the ligament attachments themselves and concluded that the ligaments can contribute to the fracture pattern in at least 2 ways: either the intact ligaments avulse the bone fragments or ligaments are shielding the underlying bone. They also noted that the mode of failure depends on patient age. As age increases, so does the modulus of elasticity, stiffness, ultimate tensile strength, and ultimate load, making avulsion-type injuries potentially more common in younger groups and mid-substance tears more likely in older groups.

8.4   Association Between the Location of an Intraarticular Fracture Fragment and the Stability of the Radiocarpal Joint

The intraarticular fractures of the distal radius, do not equally destabilize the RC joint. Giunta et al. [67] analyzed the subchondral mineralization of the RC joint, by using CT-osteo-absorptiometry. In most cases, two density maxima were found on the articular radial surface, one corresponding to the scaphoid and one to the lunate. These matched the positions of pressure peaks described in reports of research on mechanical models. The density maximum on the articular surface of the radius opposing the scaphoid is, however, rather more dorsally placed, whereas that opposing the lunate lies palmar to the radioulnar midline. This practically means that the volar half of the lunate fossa receives a considerable amount of loads applied to the RC joint and its absence (e.g., after a fracture) would greatly destabilize the RC joint. It is also possible that different anatomical elements contribute to the stability of the RC articulation, in each quarter of the distal articular surface of the radius. At the volar half of the lunate fossa and the dorsal half of the scaphoid fossa, stability is mainly of bone origin, while in the dorsal half of the lunate fossa and the volar half of the scaphoid fossa stability is mainly ligamentous (Fig. 8.2).

It is known that the short radiolunate ligament inserts at the palmar rim of the radius correspondingly to the lunate fossa. The exact

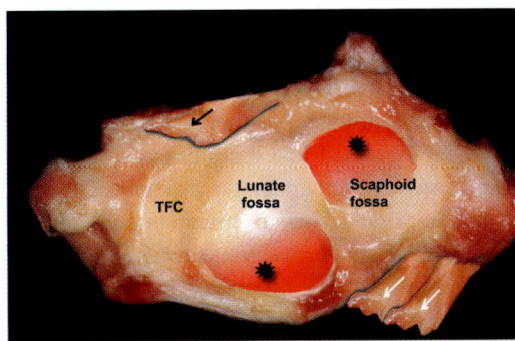

Fig. 8.2 (Electronically processed image) The stability of the RC joint at the volar half of the lunate fossa and the dorsal half of the scaphoid fossa is mainly of bone origin (*asterisks*), while in the dorsal half of the lunate fossa and the volar half of the scaphoid fossa the stability is mainly ligamentous (*arrows*). With permission from [127]

functional significance of this ligament is not well known, although it is believed to contribute to the stability of the radiolunate joint [47]. Indirectly, however, its importance is highlighted in fractures of the ulnovolar radial rim where this ligament inserts and which, if not treated, results progressively in volar wrist subluxation (Fig. 8.3a–b).

8.5   Mechanism of Injury

RC dislocations are high-energy injuries (fall from a height, traffic or industrial accidents) and therefore the patients rarely remember the exact mechanism of injury.

This injury is a product of several factors: the anatomy of the articulating units, the strength and elasticity of the RC ligaments, the strength of the

Fig. 8.3 Fractures of the ulnovolar radial rim destabize the RC joint in volar direction (**a**, **b**)

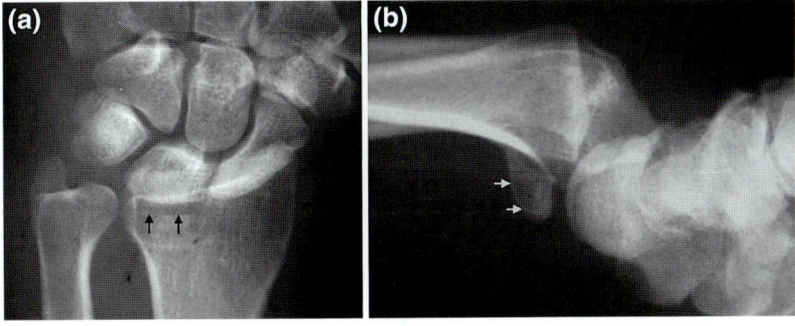

bony structures, the magnitude, rate of loading, and position of the RC joint at impact [68, 69].

Bohler [70] in 1930, who originally postulated the mechanism of injury for dorsal RC fracture-dislocations, stated that a compressive and rotational force occurs against a hyperextended and pronated wrist. This mechanism was subsequently confirmed by Weiss et al. [71] in a cadaveric study. They found that a torsional element is essential, since an axial load alone causes fractures of the scaphoid with or without midcarpal dislocations or fractures of the distal radius.

Freeland et al. [23] supported that shear forces at the palmar or dorsal edges of the RC joint, often accompanied by excessive reciprocal rotation force combined between the wrist and forearm, have been implicated as the principal mechanisms causing RC dislocation and instability. The ulnar head appears to act as a fulcrum for the rotational forces. The wrist is typically hyperextended on impact, although hyperflexion [19, 25] or distraction [26] has been cited.

Dorsal dislocation of the RC joint occurs when a torsional force is applied to a hyperextended and ulnarly deviated wrist, while the forearm is fixed in hyperpronation [1, 71, 72].

Dumontier et al. [8] supported that the high frequency of an associated fracture of the ulnar styloid, may indicate that these injuries start to develop from the ulnar side of the wrist, but most authors believe that failure begins on the radial side and progresses to the ulnar side of the wrist [28, 73].

Possibly the magnitude and direction of the rotational force and the axial compression will determine the variable amount of bony and soft-tissue injuries encountered in different forms of dislocations or fracture-dislocations. The compressive and torsional component appears in many cases, where the proximal chondral surfaces of the proximal carpal row bones were stripped-off of the cartilage and the osteochondral fragments were found in various positions intra- or extraarticularly (Figs. 8.4a–c, 8.5a–c).

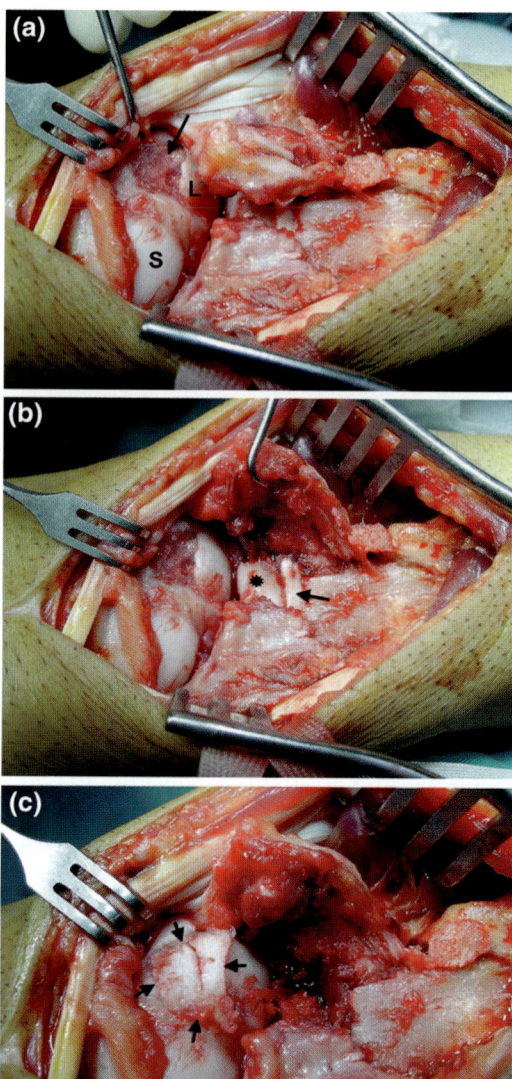

Fig. 8.4 The compressive and torsional component needed to produce a RC fracture-dislocation is evident in this dorsal RC fracture-dislocation, where the *arrow* indicates an osteochondral defect from the dorsal surface of the lunate (**a**); by elevating the fractured dorsal radius fragment, an impacted articular fragment of the distal radius is seen (*asterisk*), while the *arrow* indicates the missing osteochondral fragment originating from the dorsal lunate (**b**); the osteochondral fragment is relocated to its original position (**c**). With permission from [127]

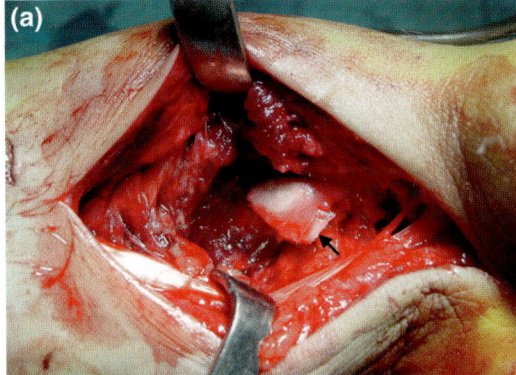

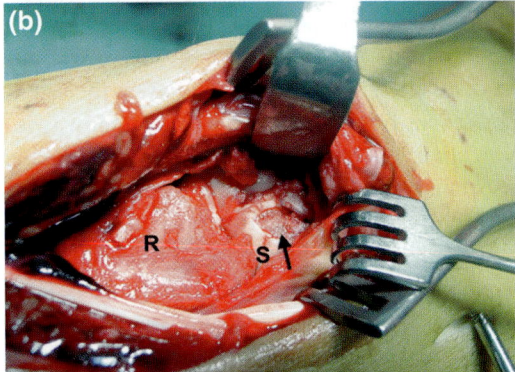

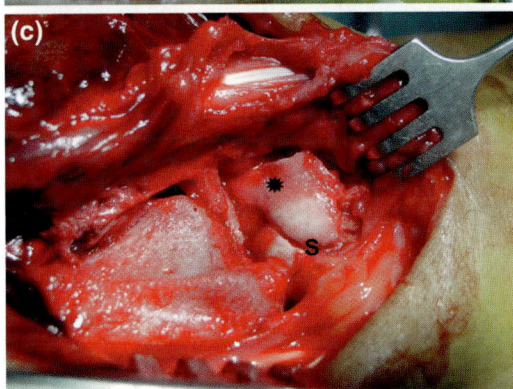

Fig. 8.5 During palmar approach for open reduction of a dorsoulnar RC dislocation, an osteochondral fragment was found (*arrow*) (**a**); the dorsal approach revealed an osteochondral defect mainly of the dorsal scaphoid, comprising also the dorsal SL ligament and a small chondral piece of the dorsal lunate (**b**); relocation of the osteochondral fragment (**c**) (*asterisk* dorsal SL ligament, *S* scaphoid, *R* radius) (The case is continued in Figs. 8.11, 8.33). With permission from [127]

It is very possible, that independently of their direction, the pivotal separation of the wrist-forearm toward opposite directions is responsible. Specifically, when at the time of injury the forearm is fixed in pronation and the wrist is violently supinated, a dorsal RC dislocation may develop. Conversely, with the hand being fixed in pronation and the forearm violently supinated, a palmar RC dislocation may develop.

Apart from the rotation and the axial compression which are major components of the mechanism of injury, dorsiflexion and ulnar deviation [29, 31, 68], dorsiflexion and radial deviation [38, 74], or volarflexion and radial deviation [25] of the wrist, have all been implicated in the formation of injury. However, in many cases the mechanism of injury is extremely complex and hard to explain.

Anatomical characters of the wrist joint, such as the negative ulnar variance [52], the degree of inclination of the distal articular surface of the radius [55] or DISI deformity [34], could play an important role in the development of RC instability.

8.6   Terminology

RC fracture-dislocations are the most debatable of carpal dislocations. The term RC fracture-dislocation has been incorrectly used in a considerable number of cases previously reported [75]. Thus, many questions arise concerning their incidence, terminology, and classification. In a strict manner of speaking, dislocations of the RC joint should be either pure ligamentous injuries or dislocations associated with bony avulsions of ligamentous attachments.

There is agreement on terminology, only for pure ligamentous RC dislocations. Confusion exists concerning the various types of fractures of the distal radius associated with dislocation of the RC joint. Thomsen and Falstie-Jensen [33] critically reviewed past reports of 35 cases with RC dislocations or fracture-dislocations and gave credit to only 13 cases. Similarly, Watanabe and Nishikimi [75] considered reliable only 45 of 124 cases that had been reported in the literature.

Dumontier et al. [38] stated that most of the seventy cases reported in the nineteenth century, were not RC dislocations but intracarpal dislocations, epiphyseal injuries or very displaced wrist fractures.

Various authors adopted different criteria to include injuries to the RC fracture-dislocation group: Dumontier et al. [38] considered as RC fracture-dislocations, patients whose entire carpus had been dislocated volarly or dorsally to the radius, with fractures of the radial styloid more than one-third of the width of the scaphoid fossa, provided that the ulnar half of the distal part of the radius was intact; carpal translations associated with a fracture of the volar or dorsal margin of the radius were excluded. On the contrary, others [2, 9, 68, 73, 75, 76], under the term RC fracture-dislocations comprised injuries characterized by dislocation of the RC joint in either dorsal or volar direction, which can be associated with radial and ulnar styloid as well as marginal rim fractures of the distal radius.

The main injury, from which RC fracture-dislocation must be differentiated, is the shearing marginal articular fractures of the distal radius (Type B according to AO classification or type II according to Fernandez classification) (Table 8.2). This type of injuries includes: volar Barton's fracture (Fig. 8.6a) [77], Schauffeur's fracture (Fig. 8.6b) [78], and the sizable ulnopalmar (Fig. 8.3a, b) or radiopalmar (Fig. 8.6c, d) fracture fragments of the distal radius, when accompanied by carpal translation [16, 79, 80]. These injuries should not be confused with true RC fracture-dislocations, since, the fractured fragment containing significant ligamentous attachments, remains in contact with the proximal carpal row and its fixation restores the stability of the RC joint. However, most importantly they constitute one-sided injuries by definition, since the opposite cortex and the extrinsic RC ligaments must be intact [69, 81–83]. Thus, the distinction should not be based on the size of the osseous fragment alone, which either way is a subjective criterion, but whether there is an associated injury opposite the osseous fragment side. On the contrary, fractures of the dorsal radial rim associated with dorsal RC subluxation (frequently referred to as dorsal Barton) merit particular attention, as they are more related to RC fracture-dislocations. Lozano-Calderon et al. [84] examined 20 such patients and found that 18 of them also had a wide spectrum of opposite volar injuries.

The term "transstyloid radiocarpal dislocation" which has been used by some authors [75, 85] is just an indication of the coexistence of a fractured radial styloid with dislocation of the RC joint.

RC fracture-dislocations must also be differentiated from patterns of perilunate ligamentous injuries that have a radial styloid component

Table 8.2 Differences between RC fracture-dislocations and shearing fractures with wrist subluxation

	RC fracture-dislocation	Shearing fractures + wrist subluxation
Mechanism	Mainly rotational injury	Mainly compressive or axial load injury
Pathoanatomy	Injury at both sides of the RC joint (ligamentous or osseoligamentous)	One side injury (osseous)
Relation of osseous fragments with PCR	Fragments with no or only partial contact with PCR	Fragment in contact with PCR contains stabilizing ligaments
Reduction	Ease of reduction insecure maintenance	Reduction and fixation of the sizable osseous fragment ensure joint stability

PCR proximal carpal row

Fig. 8.6 A RC fracture dislocation must be differentiated from shearing type of fractures, the reduction and fixation of which suffice to restore the RC joint stability: volar Barton's (**a**); Schauffeur's (**b**); shearing fracture of the palmar part of the scaphoid fossa (**c, d**). With permission from [127]

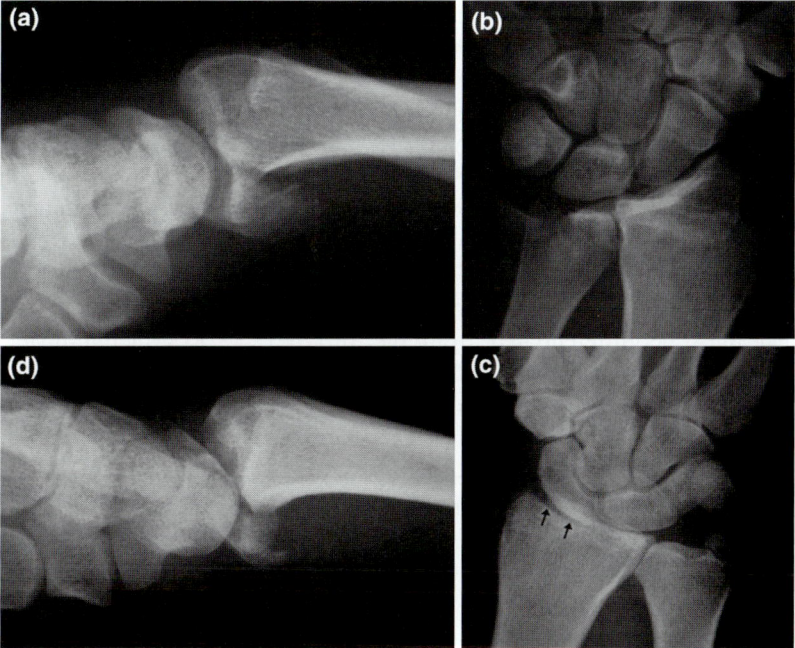

[68], since they have a different mechanism of injury, pathoanatomy, treatment, and prognosis.

Therefore, we believe that the prerequisite to consider these injuries as *radiocarpal dislocations* is the dislocation of the entire carpus volar or dorsal to the distal radius without fracture or with avulsion fractures at the insertion site of the ligaments (e.g., tip of the radial styloid, small ulnovolar fragment). Under the term *radiocarpal fracture-dislocations* we should include patients: (a) with dislocation of the RC joint associated with fractures which involve: the marginal cortical radial rims (volar and/or dorsal), the radial styloid or both, while there must be injuries (osseous and/or ligamentous) to both sides of the RC joint (dorsal and volar), (b) whose radius metaphysis and the main portion of articular surface of the distal radius are intact, and (c) with no associated intercarpal dislocations (the head of the capitate retains normal alignment with the distal lunate).

Idler [86] defined RC dislocation "as loss of articular contact between the proximal carpal row and distal radius not in association with a biomechanically significant fracture of the distal radius". Although the expression "biomechanically significant" raises much debate, we believe that the definition would be more accurate if the phrase: "and which also requires injury of at least both sides of the RC joint" is also added at the end.

However, there will always be cases in the gray area or questionable cases as to where they belong. These are the cases presented by Capo et al. [87], where the whole proximal carpal row dislocated volarly and disengaged from both the radius and distal carpal row or the case presented by Klein et al. [88], where the dorsally dislocated carpus was associated with a dorsal perilunar dislocation.

Pure RC dislocations are classified as nondissociative instabilities (CIND) that involve rupture of the extrinsic RC ligaments. In two cases of RC dislocations, the instability is described as complex (Carpal Instability Complex-CIC): in type II RC dislocations according to Moneim et al. [9] and in type II ulnar translocation of the wrist according to Taleisnik [39], where in addition, rupture of the interosseous ligaments of the proximal carpal row is involved. In these cases, the instability is considered as a combination of dissociative (CID) and non-dissociative type (CIND).

In the AO classification, the only type close to RC fracture-dislocations is the B2.3 subtype, which however, involves only the dorsal RC dislocations while dislocations of other directions (palmar, ulnar, radial) are not represented in any subgroup. In the classification by Fernandez et al. [68], based on the mechanism of injury, RC dislocations belong to the IV type and must be differentiated from the II type, which involves the shearing fractures that are associated with carpal subluxation.

8.7 Pathologic Anatomy of the Injury

Understanding the pathologic anatomy of RC dislocations or fracture-dislocations is dependent on findings at surgical exposure. Since, only few cases have been treated operatively with detailed description of their osseoligamentous injuries, the magnitude and spectrum of injuries are not exactly known. As a result, the extent of tissue compromise is often underestimated, leading to undertreatment and inferior results.

Many authors based on clinical observations [11, 52, 75, 86] or cadaveric studies [50, 89] supported that, dislocation of the proximal row of the carpus from the distal radius and ulna requires complete disruption of the volar RC ligaments in addition to capsuloperiosteal avulsion of the dorsal RC ligaments.

Arthroscopic evaluation, despite the limitations, has been attempted in few cases allowing a precise intraarticular observation [25, 90].

Dumontier et al. [38] presumed that in pure RC dislocations or those accompanied by fracture of the tip of the radial styloid, all volar RC ligaments were torn or presented avulsion fractures at the insertion site of the ligaments. Dorsally, the ligamentous injury presented most often as a capsuloperiosteal avulsion rather than as a rupture of the dorsal RC ligaments. In RC fracture-dislocations, the volar RC ligaments are probably intact and remain attached to the fractured radial fragment, which is probably secondary to impaction of the carpus into the radius. This fracture usually includes all of the scaphoid fossa and may continue on the dorsal margin.

Freeland et al. [23] supported that the specificity, sequence, and extent of extrinsic RC and ulnocarpal traumatic ligament disruptions are not fully understood, vary with injury severity and may differ in cases of dorsal as opposed to palmar subluxation or dislocation.

RC fracture-dislocations are frequently associated with ulnar-sided injuries and only a few cases have been reported in the literature, where this injury was associated with dislocation of the distal radioulnar joint [7, 22, 38, 71, 85]. Fourteen of 27 patients reported by Dumontier et al. [38] presented with an injury of the ipsilateral distal radioulnar joint and one of them had an irreducible dislocation due to the interposition of the flexor digitorum profundus of the small finger. Extensor carpi ulnaris [85], the dorsal part of the sigmoid notch where the dorsal radioulnar ligament is attached [71], or the flexor profundus tendons and the ulnar nerve and artery [22], have all been implicated as possible causes obstructing the reduction. Graham [73] supported that the association of RC dislocation with ulnar-sided injuries, indicates even more severe tissue trauma and that the path of injury propagates from the radial to ulnar side with the forces not fully dissipated to the RC joint, ongoing ulnarly and producing the ulnar-sided injuries. He also stated that ulnar-sided injuries were more common in the small fragment variant compared to the large fragment fractures, in almost a 2:1 ratio. Since, the ulnocarpal ligaments do not have proximal osseous insertion but take origin from the volar radioulnar ligament, they either rupture in their mid-substance or avulse with or without osseous fragments from their insertion at triquetrum or lunate bones.

It is generally accepted that there are four distinct fracture types of the ulnar styloid process (tip, midportion, base horizontal, and base oblique) and the level of the styloid fracture is relevant to the risk of instability development of the DRUJ [91]. Nakamura et al. [92] assessed the relevance of each of the four levels of ulnar styloid fracture

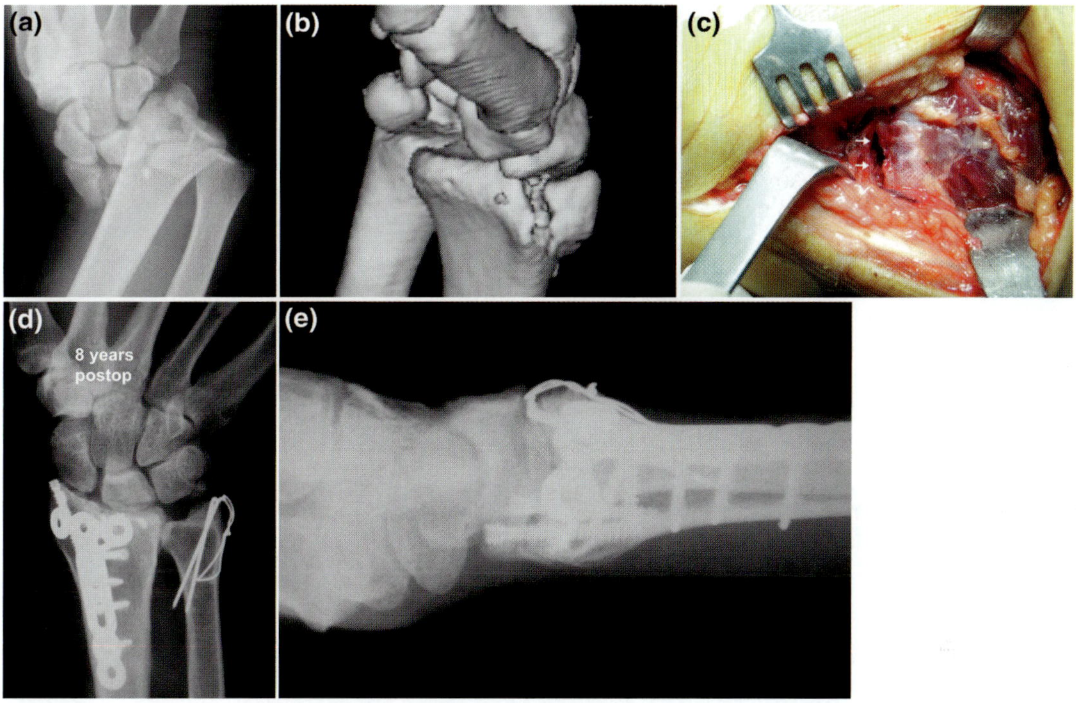

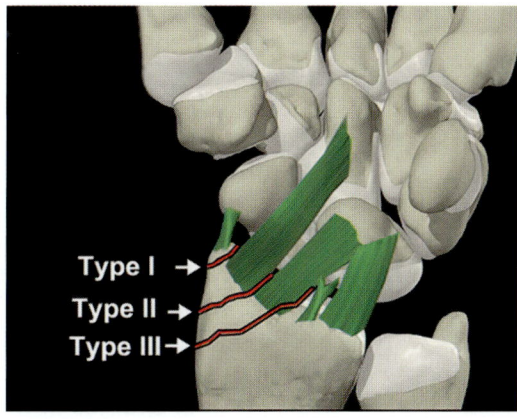

Fig. 8.7 A seemingly entire radial styloid fracture in a dorsal RC fracture dislocation (**a**) concerned only the dorsal part (**b**), while volarly the RC ligaments deracinated from the volar radial rim (*arrows*) (**c**); 8 years after open reduction and internal fixation with combine approach, stenosis of the radiolunate joint was noticed (**d, e**)

Fig. 8.8 Correlation between the 3 types of radial styloid fractures with the ligamentous attachments of the volar RC ligaments. With permission from [127]

on DRUJ stability in cadaveric wrists and found no instability in the styloid tip or midportion fractures, up to a 20 % loss of stability in basal horizontal fractures, while basal oblique fractures produced up to 70 % loss of stability, as it is more likely to disturb the foveal attachment of the radioulnar ligaments. Wide displacement of any type of ulnar styloid fracture was also recognized as a significant risk for development of DRUJ instability [91, 93]. However, it is believed that the presence of an ulnar styloid fracture is no longer considered an absolute indicator of DRUJ instability regardless of the fragment size and displacement [94, 95], but only as a risk factor [96]. Atzei and Luchetti [97] classified the peripheral tears of the TFCC (of the deep and the superficial limbs of both dorsal and palmar radioulnar ligaments) and their relation to the fractures of the ulnar styloid. A small number of cases has been reported in the literature where RC dislocation was associated with dislocation of the distal radioulnar joint [7, 18, 22, 71, 85].

By excluding patients treated with methods that preclude the ability to describe the pathoanatomy of the injury, i.e., conservative treatment

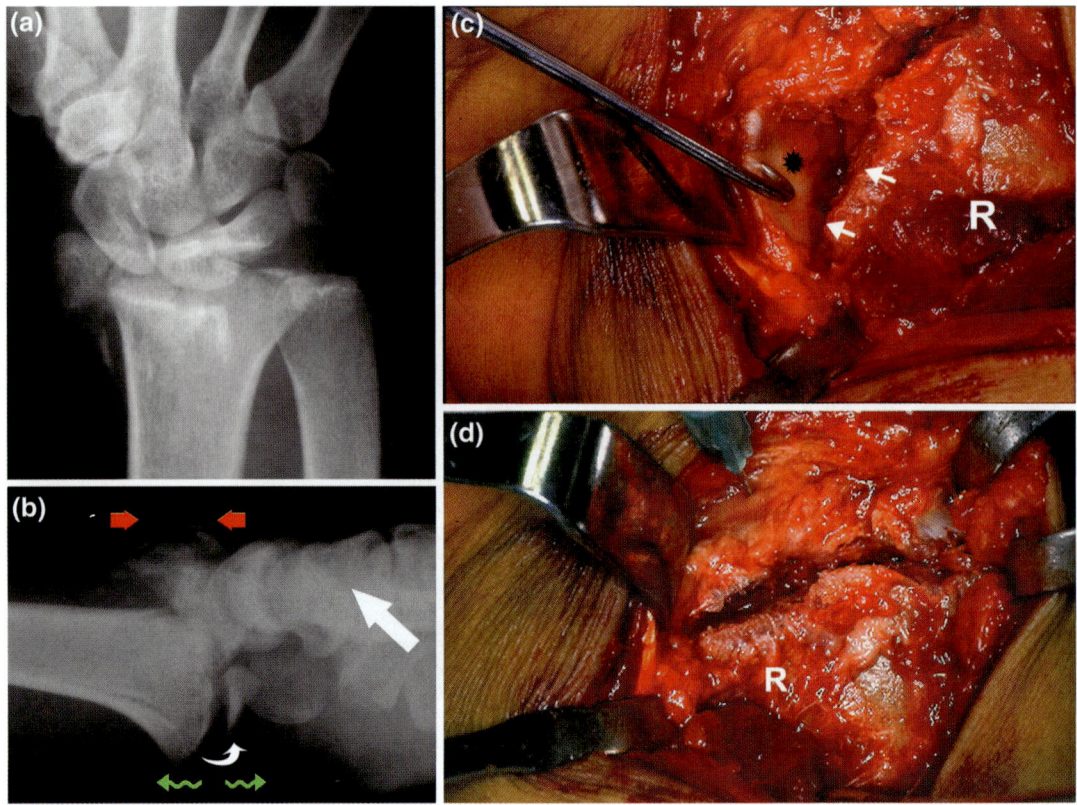

Fig. 8.9 A dorsally directed RC fracture-dislocation produced compression to the dorsal radial rim, while the distracted volar radial rim was rotated by 180° (*curved arrow*) (**a**, **b**), so that the articular cartilage was facing the fractured surface of the distal radius (*asterisk*) (**c**); derotation of the fragment (**d**); postoperative radiographic appearance indicated the wire-loop fixation, used for the stabilization of the rotated ulnovolar fragment (**e**, **f**); final x-rays 9 years postoperatively (**g**, **h**). With permission from [127]

(5 patients) or closed reduction, percutaneous wires and/or external fixation (4 patients), twenty six patients were treated operatively, mostly with combined approach and their surgical findings were recorded. A single approach (1 volar and 1 dorsal) was used in 2 patients, a double approach (dorsal and volar) in 18, and a triple approach (dorsal, volar, ulnar) in 6 patients.

Four patients presented RC dislocations and 22 patients were of RC fracture-dislocation type. According to the direction of the dislocation, there were 19 dorsal (12 pure dorsal, 4 dorsoradial, 3 dorsoulnar), 5 volar, and 2 multidirectional dislocations. All were closed injuries.

8.7.1 Surgical Findings

1. In all cases, the ligamentous or osseo-ligamentous injuries involved both the dorsal and volar sides of the RC joint.
2. Of 22 patients with RC fracture-dislocations, 19 had fractures of the radial styloid, two patients had an osseous avulsion of the dorsoulnar corner of the distal radius and one patient had a combination of the above injuries.
3. Of 20 patients with fractures of the radial styloid, no one had fractured the entire radial styloid in dorsovolar dimension,

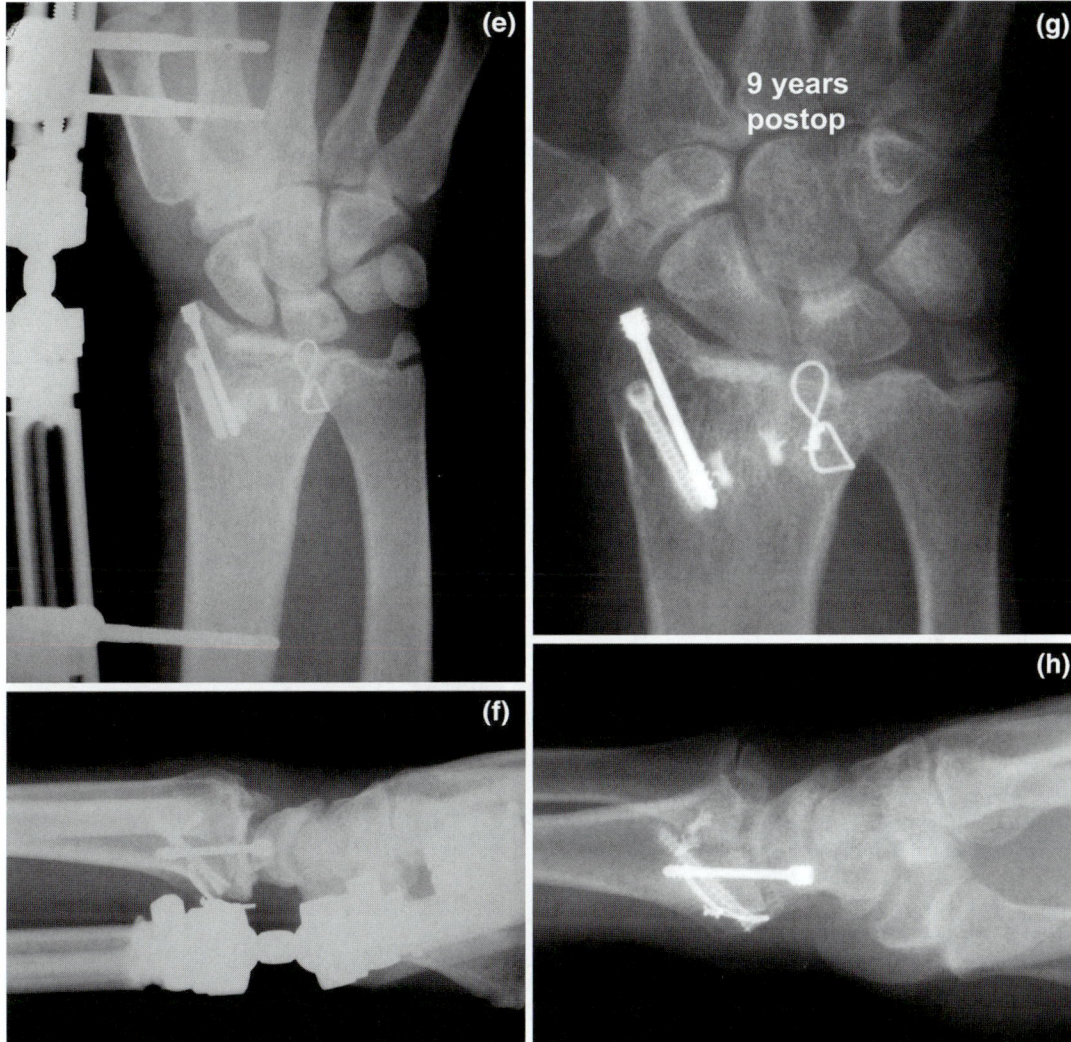

Fig. 8.9 (continued)

independently of its width. The dorsal styloid segment was involved in 6 patients, the
volar styloid segment in 3 patients, and a
combination of both segments was found in
11 patients (Fig. 8.7a–e). It was difficult to
detect radiographically the combined segments of the fractured radial styloid; it was
feasible only operatively. Concerning the
size of the radial styloid fragment we considered as: Type I the fracture of the tip of
radial styloid, type II the fracture through
the scaphoid fossa, and type III the fracture
exiting at the level of the scapholunate

interval. Postreduction X-rays (PA view)
revealed that in the dorsal styloid segment
fracture type there were 5 type III and 1 type
II fractures, in the volar styloid segment
fracture type all three fractures were of type
II and in the combined segments group there
were 4 type II and 7 type III fractures
(Fig. 8.8).

4. Fractures of radial rims were either of
compression or avulsion type depending on
the direction of the dislocation. The direction of the dislocation coincided with the
compression side of the radial rim, while the

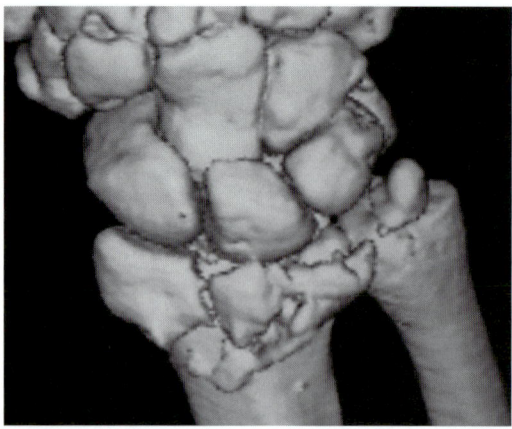

Fig. 8.10 In dorsal RC fracture dislocations, the osseous injury is frequently comprised of a larger fragment, which corresponds to the dorsal part of the radial styloid and a smaller, simple, or comminuted fragment concerning the dorsoulnar radial rim. With permission from [127]

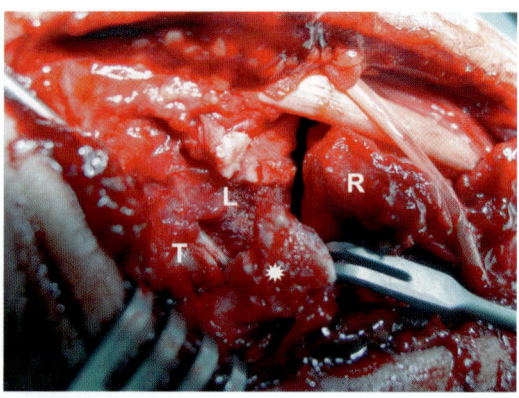

Fig. 8.12 Male, 28 years old. In a volar RC fracture dislocation the dorsal approach disclosed an osteochondral fragment from the dorsal surface of the LT complex, comprising the dorsal LT ligament (*asterisk*) (*T* triquetrum, *L* lunate, *R* radius) (The case is also illustrated in Fig. 8.25)

Fig. 8.11 Male, 27 years old, polytrauma patient with a dorsoulnar RC dislocation. White arrows indicate an avulsed osseous fragment from the dorsal rim of the sigmoid notch, while *black arrows* indicate an osteochondral fragment originating from the dorsal surface of the SL complex (see Fig. 8.5) (**a**, **b**); the dorsal approach revealed the avulsed fragment from the dorsal sigmoid notch (*asterisk*), while the black arrow indicates the ulnar head (**c**); postop x-ray (**d**). With permission from [127]

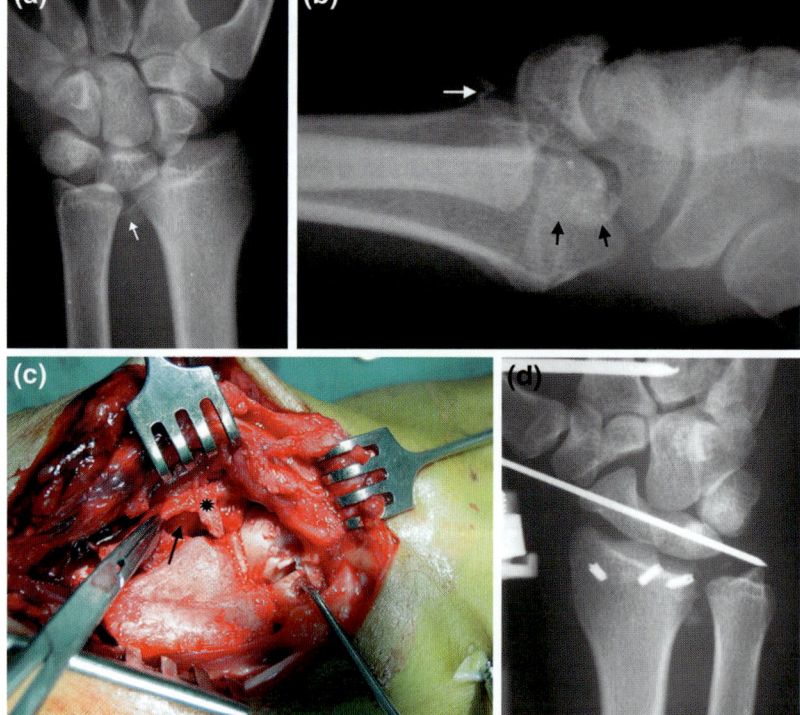

opposite radial rim had an avulsion type of fracture (Fig. 8.9a–h). Usually the osseous injury of the dorsal radial rim was double: there was a larger sized fragment from the dorsal half of the radial styloid and a smaller sized simple or comminuted fracture of the radial rim, ulnar to the Lister's tubercle which involves the attachment of the DRC ligament (Fig. 8.10). In 3 of our cases, the wrist was displaced in dorsal and ulnar direction and in all 3 cases, apart from other injuries, an avulsed osseous fragment was noticed, originating from the dorsal rim of the sigmoid notch, causing serious derangement of the DRUJ (Fig. 8.11a–d). The osseous fragments from the volar radial rim were sometimes rotated by 90°–180°, since the volar are shorter than the dorsal RC ligaments (see Fig. 8.9b). There were 10 dorsal rim fractures, 4 volar and 4 combined dorsal and volar rim fractures.

5. A wide range of injuries of the proximal carpal row was noticed in 11 patients (42 %), all of which were discovered intra-operatively: (a) Osteochondral defects of adjacent bones of the proximal carpal row comprising the interosseous ligaments (3 patients; two at scapholunate junction and one at lunotriquetral junction) (Figs. 8.12, 8.5c), (b) isolated rupture of the interosseous ligaments (4 patients; two of scapholunate and two of lunotriquetral ligament) (Fig. 8.13a–c), (c) chondral defects of isolated bones (2 patients; at proximal scaphoid and at proximal lunate respectively) (Figs. 8.13a–c, 8.4a), (d) fractured bones (2 patients; lunate and triquetrum respectively) (Fig. 8.14a–k).

6. In six patients, free osteochondral fragments were found intra- or extraarticularly, originating either from carpal bones or from the distal radius. In 2 cases of dorsal RC fracture-dislocations, during radiological examination, two sizable fragments were detected at the volar surface of the joint. Indeed, the palmar approach revealed the existence of osteochondral fragments at the level of the RC joint; however, detection of their source was difficult. The dorsal approach in both cases revealed that these osteochondral fragments originated in one case from the dorsoulnar rim of the distal radius (Fig. 8.15a–g), while in the other case from the dorsal surface of the scapholunate complex (see Figs. 8.5, 8.11). The fact that dorsal anatomical structures were found palmarly (also the opposite possibly applies), is on one hand of surgical interest, but on the other hand, it is indicative of the amplitude of the applied forces and of the complexity of the mechanism of injury.

7. The RC ligaments were usually avulsed from the volar or dorsal radial rims, but in 7 patients they were avulsed from carpal bones with or without small osseous fragments. Specifically, the short radiolunate ligament was avulsed from the lunate (5 patients) and the dorsal RC ligament was avulsed from the triquetrum (2 patients) (Fig. 8.16a–g).

8. In 3 patients (2 with volar and 1 with multidirectional dislocation) there was an extensive rupture of the floor of the dorsal retinaculum (Fig. 8.17a–f), while in the patient with the multidirectional dislocation, the extensor and abductor pollicis longus were ripped-off from their musculotendinous junction (Fig. 8.18a–h), a finding indicative of the rotational component of the mechanism of injury.

9. Seventeen patients (65.3 %) had associated injury of DRU joint (fracture through the base of the ulnar styloid in 14 patients, an osseous avulsion from the dorsal sigmoid notch of the dorsal radioulnar ligament in 3 patients, and a Type IV rupture of the TFC in 1 patient).

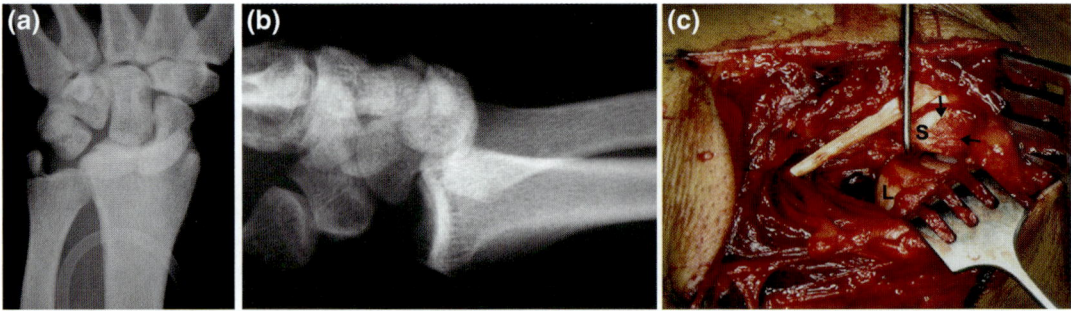

Fig. 8.13 Male, 24 years old with a dorsal RC dislocation (**a**, **b**); the dorsal approach revealed a ruptured SL
ligament and a chondral defect from the dorsal scaphoid
(*arrows*) (*S* scaphoid, *L* lunate) (**c**). With permission from
[127]

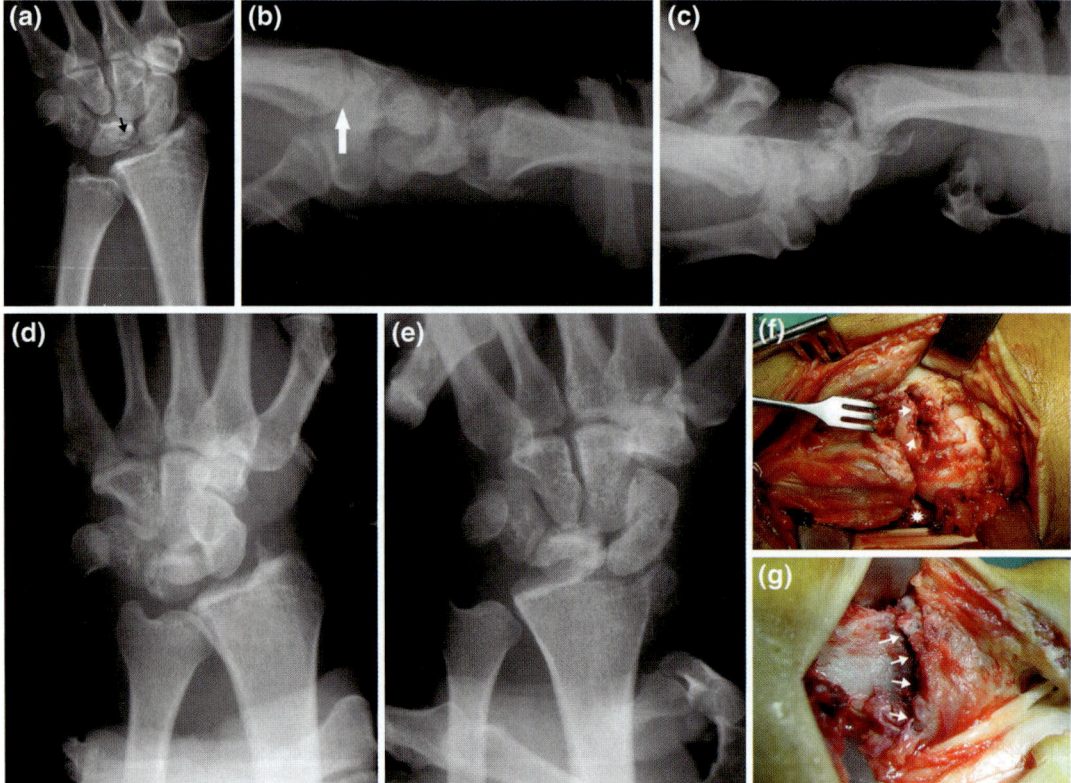

Fig. 8.14 Male, 21 years old, polytrauma patient. PA
view of a reduced volar RC fracture dislocation. The
arrow indicates a dubious fracture of the lunate(**a**);
different stress views revealed that the RC joint was
stable only in dorsal direction (**b**), while in volar (**c**),
ulnar (**d**), and radial direction (**e**) the instability of the
joint was apparent; during dorsal approach, a
comminuted fracture of the lunate was found (*arrows*)
in association with a fracture of the radial styloid
(*asterisk*) (**f**); the palmar approach revealed a comminuted fracture of the volar radial rim (*arrows*) (**g**);
postoperative radiographic views (**h**, **i**); the final x-ray
views 4 years later (**j**, **k**)

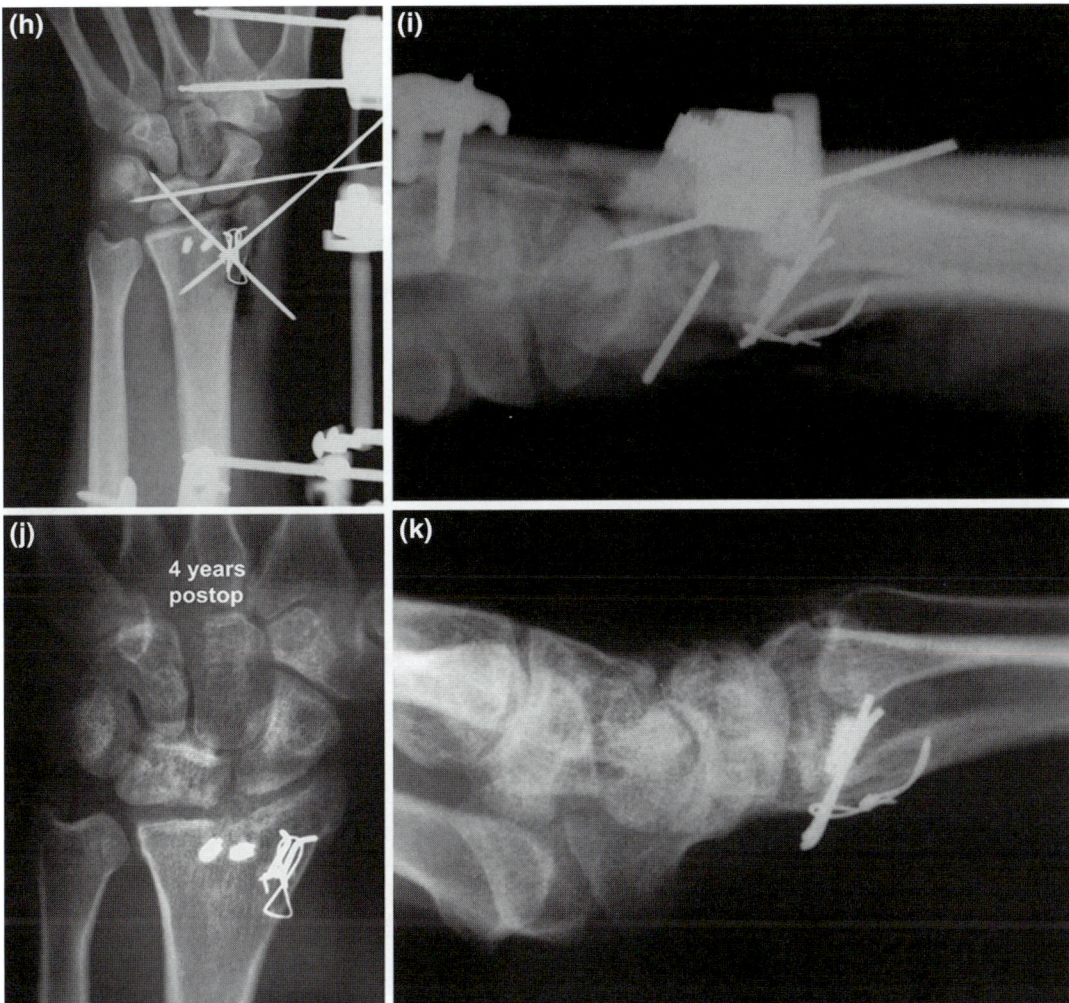

Fig. 8.14 (continued)

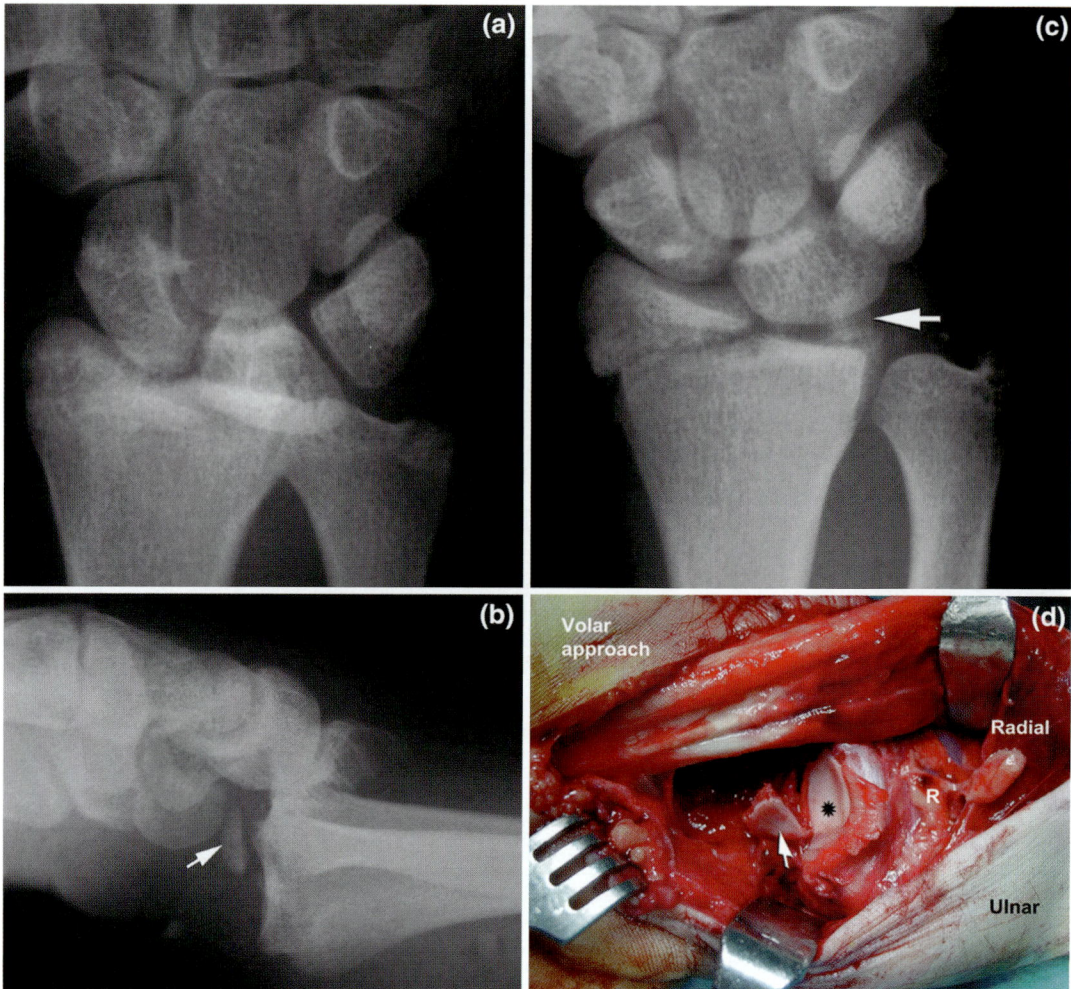

Fig. 8.15 Male, 23 years old, with a dorsal RC fracture dislocation. An osseous fragment of unknown origin (*arrow*) and a fracture of the radial styloid were apparent in the initial (**a**, **b**) and reduced (**c**) x-ray views; the volar approach with the joint dislocated showed the osteochondral fragment (*arrow*) located distal to the lunate fossa (*asterisk*) (**d**); dorsally, a large fractured fragment of the radial styloid and two smaller osseous fragments of the dorsoulnar radial rim were apparent. The *arrow* indicates the fragment that was found volarly after its relocation (**e**); postoperative x-rays (**f**, **g**). With permission from [127]

10. The two multidirectional and one volar dislocation had in addition a complete rupture of the volar ulnocarpal ligaments (Fig. 8.19).

Based on our surgical findings, we could define the pattern of osseo-ligamentous disruption as follows (Fig. 8.20):

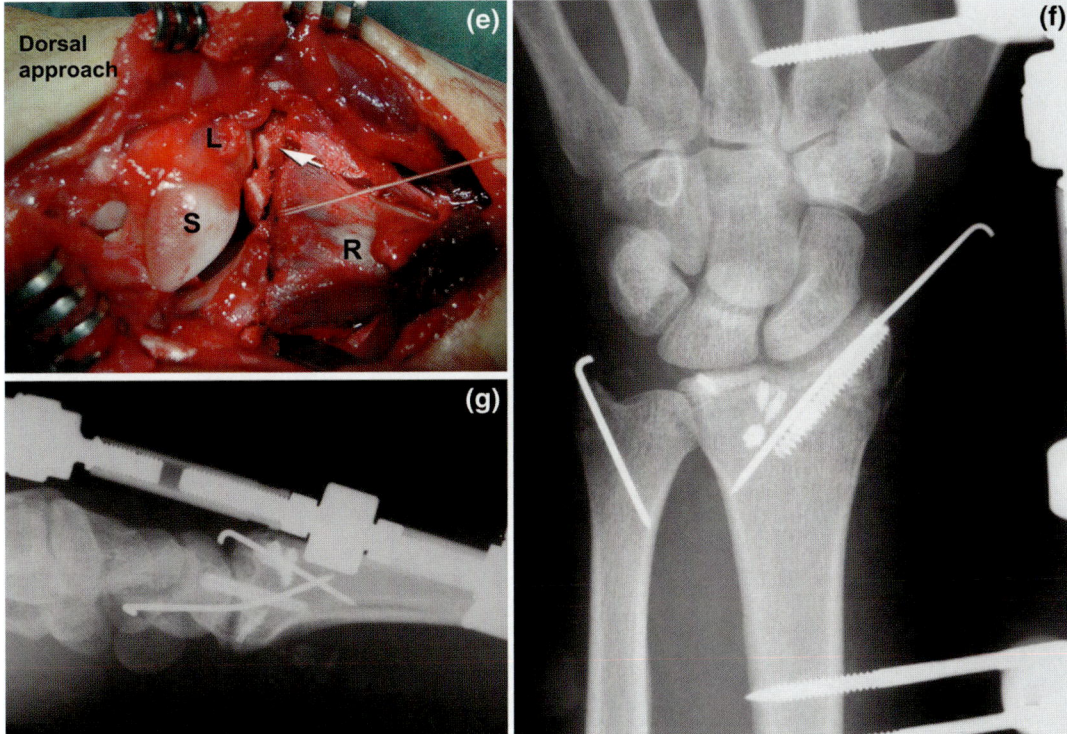

Fig. 8.15 (continued)

In **dorsal dislocations**, there were roughly 4 types of injuries:

Type I
(4 cases)
Dorsally, a double osseous injury (separate fragments, radially and ulnarly to Lister's tubercle) and volarly a purely ligamentous injury

Type II
(7 cases)
Dorsally a double osseous injury and volarly a double osseoligamentous injury. Usually the RC ligaments were detached from the ulnar side of the volar radial rim, while the radial side showed an avulsion fracture fragment. Less often, the reverse was true

Type III
(3 cases)
Double osseous or comminution on both dorsal and volar sides

Type IV
(5 cases)

Dorsal and volar, mainly ligamentous injuries, which were sometimes associated with small osseous fragments of avulsion type, originating from the radial styloid (either side) or from the dorsoulnar side of the radius

In **volar dislocations** we found 2 types of injuries:

Type I
(4 cases)
Dorsally, purely ligamentous and volarly a double or comminuted osseous injury

Type II
(1 case)
Purely ligamentous injuries on both sides

In the 2 cases with **multidirectional dislocations**, we found a purely ligamentous injury on both sides with rupture of the ulnocarpal

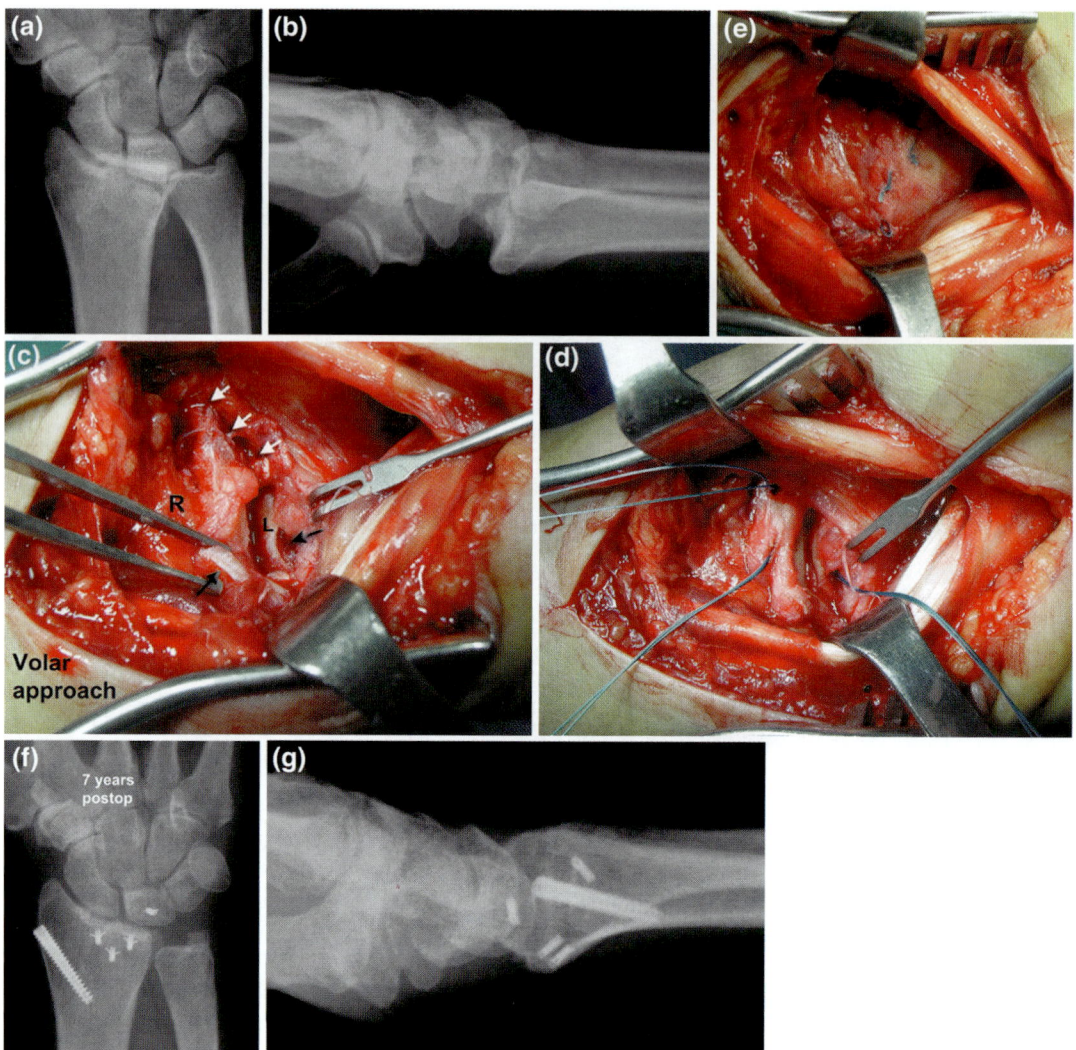

Fig. 8.16 Male, 56 years old, with a dorsal RC fracture dislocation (**a**, **b**); volarly the radiocarpal ligaments were deracinated from their attachments to the distal radius (*white arrows*), while the short RL ligament was avulsed with an osseous fragment from the lunate (*black arrows*) (**c**) (*R* radius, *L* lunate); bone anchors were used for reconstruction (**d**, **e**); radiographic appearance after 7 years (**f**, **g**). With permission from [127]

ligaments. One of those cases exhibited fracture of the tip of the radial styloid.

8.8 Classification

Two classification schemes have been discussed extensively in the literature: Dumontier et al. [38] classified RC dislocations into two types: type 1 included pure dislocations with or without fracture of only the tip of the radial styloid, a fracture involving less than one-third of the width of the scaphoid fossa, postulating that the RC ligaments were torn off the radius; type 2 included dislocations with associated fracture of the radial styloid involving more than one-third of the scaphoid fossa, postulating that most of the RC ligaments were still intact and attached to the radial styloid fragment.

Moneim et al. [9] classified these injuries into type 1 and type 2 according to the integrity of the intracarpal ligaments. In type I dislocation, the

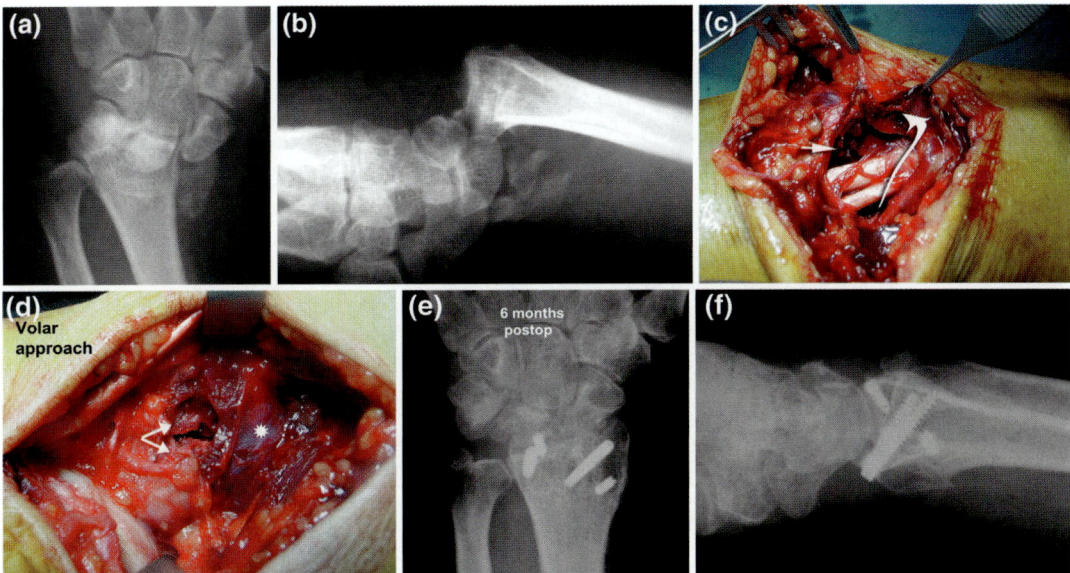

Fig. 8.17 Female, 60 years old, polytrauma patient. In a volar RC fracture dislocation (**a**, **b**); the dorsal approach revealed an osteoperiosteal avulsion from the 1st extensor compartment (*curved arrow*) that resulted in exposition of the corresponding tendons, while the DRC ligament was avulsed from the dorsal radial rim (*small arrow*) (**c**); the volar radial rim was comminuted (*arrows*) (*asterisk* pronator quadrates) (**d**); radiographic appearance 6 months later (**e**, **f**). With permission from [127]

carpus moves as one unit on the distal radius whereas in type II, an associated intercarpal dislocation is also present. He presented 7 cases and 3 of them were characterized as type II dislocations. According to the author, type II dislocations represent a more complex pattern, with a graver prognosis. It should however, be noted, that all 3 cases characterized as type II RC dislocations were in fact trans-styloid perilunate injuries with volar dislocation of the lunate, from which RC fracture dislocations must be differentiated.

The frequent occurrence of intracarpal injuries along with a RC dislocation is undeniable, but they are just associated injuries and do not deserve to constitute a particular type of injury. Besides, all these injuries from our series were discovered intraoperatively and none was recognizable by the preoperative x-rays.

Since both the aforementioned classifications are based on radiographic findings and do not take into account the pattern of osseoligamentous injuries, the direction of the dislocation or the ulnar-sided pathology, it is obvious that both must be modified.

A third classification was that of Graham [73] who considered RC dislocations as "inferior arc" injuries, in addition to the existing injury patterns: the "greater" and "lesser arc" injuries. He stated that RC dislocations could be classified as: (a) purely ligamentous disruptions, (b) dislocations with a "large fragment" styloid fracture, starting in the area of the previous physeal scar and entering the joint near the crista separating the scaphoid and lunate fossae, and (c) dislocations with a "small fragment" fracture, which represents avulsion or impaction injuries of the volar or dorsal margins of the distal radius.

Bilos et al. [7] classified these injuries into four general types: dorsal, volar, radial, and ulnar, depending on the direction in which the carpus is displaced.

Bozentka and Beredjiklian [98] commented on the need to include in the classification schemes other important factors, such as the direction, the presence of associated neurovascular injury, and the presence of associated intercarpal ligamentous injuries.

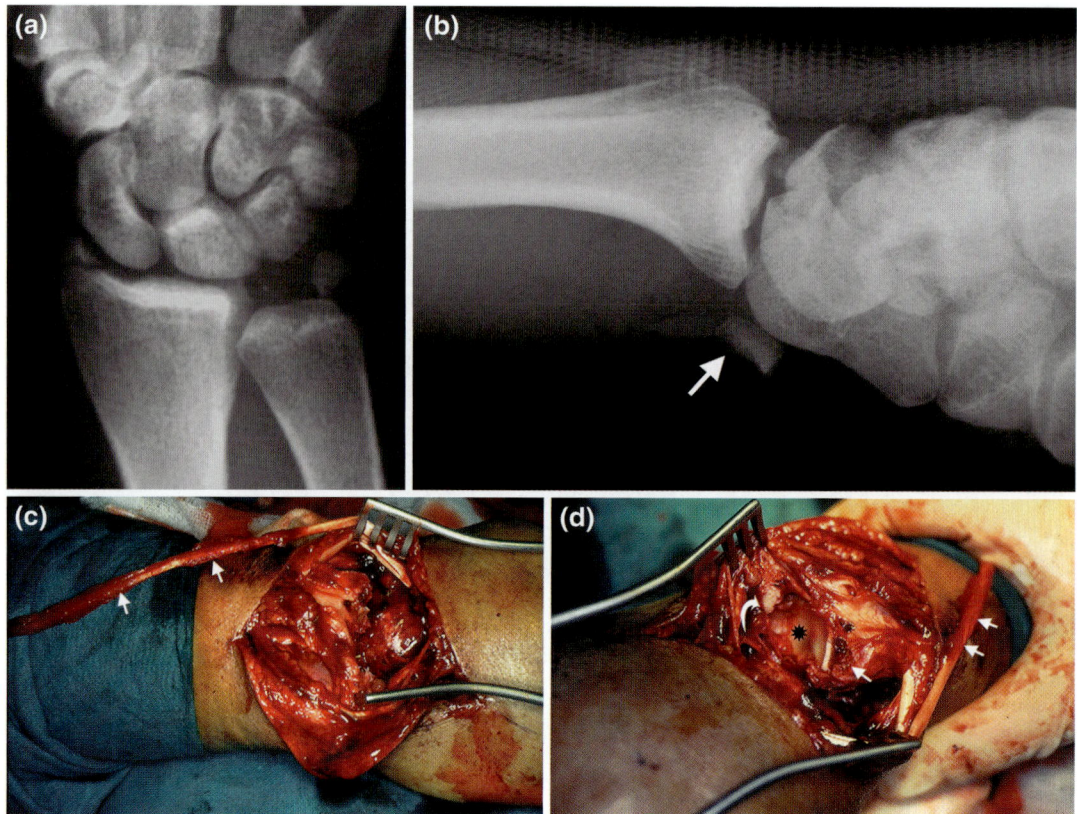

Fig. 8.18 Male, 57 years old. Multidirectional closed RC dislocation, produced in an effort to release the hand that was trapped in an agricultural machine. The PA view showed avulsion fractures of both radial and ulnar styloids and overlapping of the LT joint (**a**); the L view demonstrated that the wrist was displaced volarly and a sizeable osseous fragment that was proven to have come from the dorsal surface of the triquetrum (**b**); the dorsal approach revealed that the EPL and APL extensor tendons were ripped-off their musculotendinous junction (*arrows*) (**c**); the RC joint was unstable in all directions; the osseous fragment from the dorsal side of the triquetrum (*curved arrow*), the fracture of the radial styloid (*small arrow*), the ripped-off tendon (*double arrows*), and the articular surface of the distal radius (*asterisk*), were demonstrated through the dorsal approach (**d**); postoperative x-rays (**e**, **f**); the final radiographic appearance 13 years later (**g**, **h**). With permission from [127]

Mainly relying on surgical findings we propose a new classification based on five parameters (chronicity, pathoanatomy, direction, associated wrist injuries, and complexity). Using this classification, a RC dislocation or fracture-dislocation should be presented with information on all five parameters (Table 8.3).

Chronicity: RC dislocations or fracture-dislocations are differentiated into acute and gradually developed. The latter group includes ulnar translation as sequelae of an already treated RC dislocation or a remote consequence after a subtle RC ligament rupture. Special mention deserve those cases presented in the literature, where the RC subluxation or dislocation was associated with a small fragment from the ulnovolar articular surface of the distal radius [11, 16, 23, 30, 33, 99, 100]. Since all these cases were closely reduced and after a period of time the subluxation recurred, they could belong to the gradually developed group (Fig. 8.21a–l).

Pathoanatomy. RC dislocations are differentiated into purely ligamentous or equivalent, which include, the tip of the radial styloid or a small ulnovolar fragment. RC fracture-dislocations are differentiated according with the

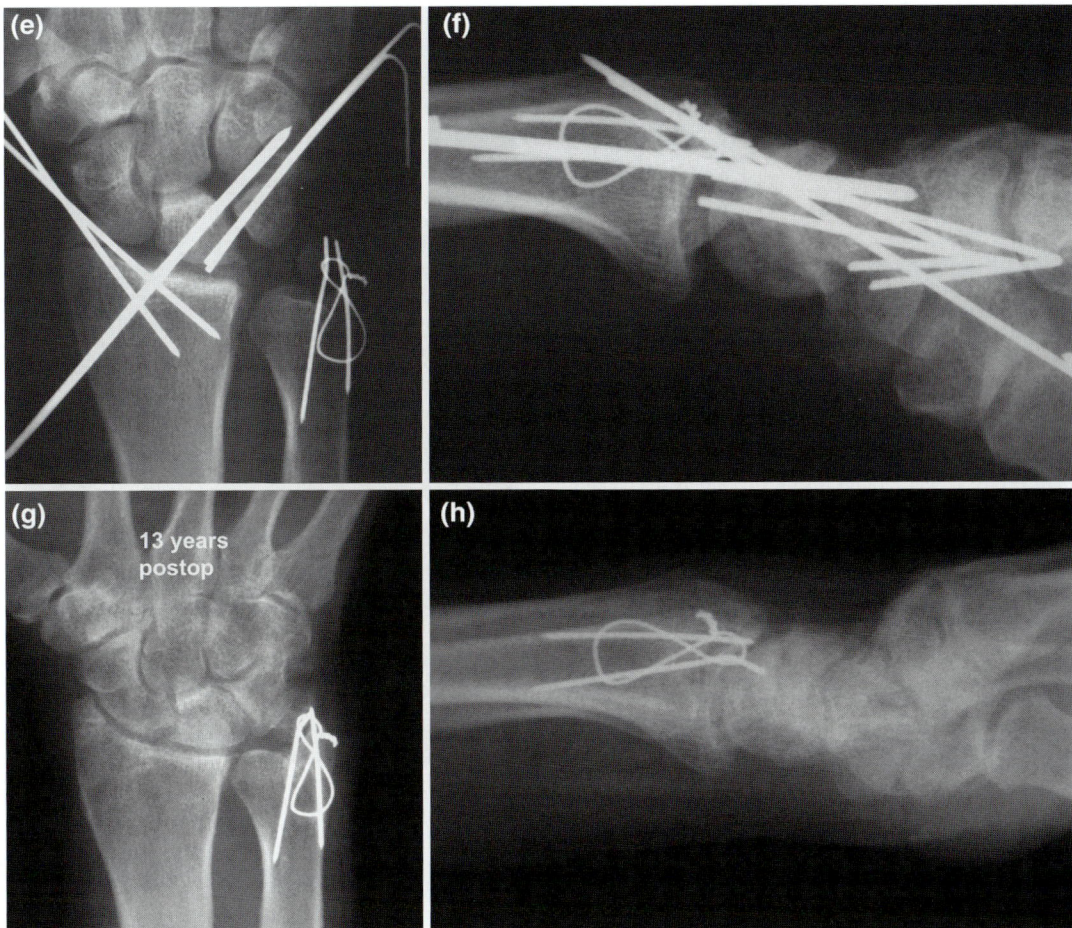

Fig. 8.18 (continued)

location of the fracture into: radial styloid (dorsal or volar part or combinations), radial rim (dorsal or volar or combined rims), and dorsoulnar fragment.

Direction. The direction of the dislocation allows us to assume in a great extent the underlying lesions. Thus, these injuries are divided into dorsal, volar, ulnar, combinations (dorsoradial, dorsoulnar, radiovolar, or ulnovolar), and multidirectional.

Associated injuries. These are related to concomitant injuries located in the vicinity of the dislocated wrist. They may concern: DRUJ, ulnocarpal or interosseous ligaments, osteochondral fragments, fractured carpal bones, ruptured tendons or muscles, neurovascular injuries, and the status of the dorsal retinaculum.

Complexity. This parameter clarifies if the dislocation is reducible or not and if the dislocation is open or closed.

8.9   Diagnosis

As for most violent traumas, these injuries have been reported mainly in males and usually of young age.

The patient with RC dislocation typically presents with a painful, swollen, and deformed wrist. The unreduced RC dislocation results in a significant deformity, with the wrist and hand being displaced dorsally or volarly in relation to the forearm axis (Fig. 8.22). Most commonly these injuries are the result of high-energy

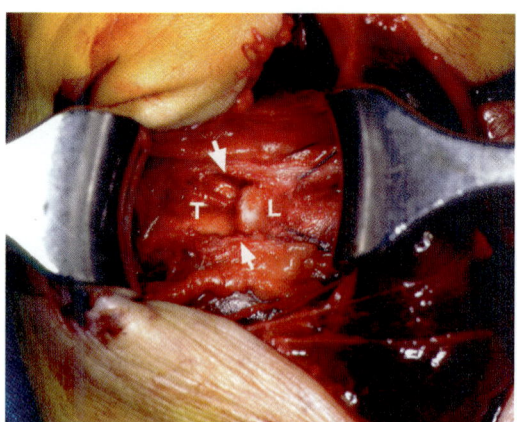

Fig. 8.19 The rupture of the ulnocarpal ligaments (*arrows*) that was found in 3 of our cases (mainly multidirectional dislocations) (*T* triquetrum, *L* lunate). With permission from [127]

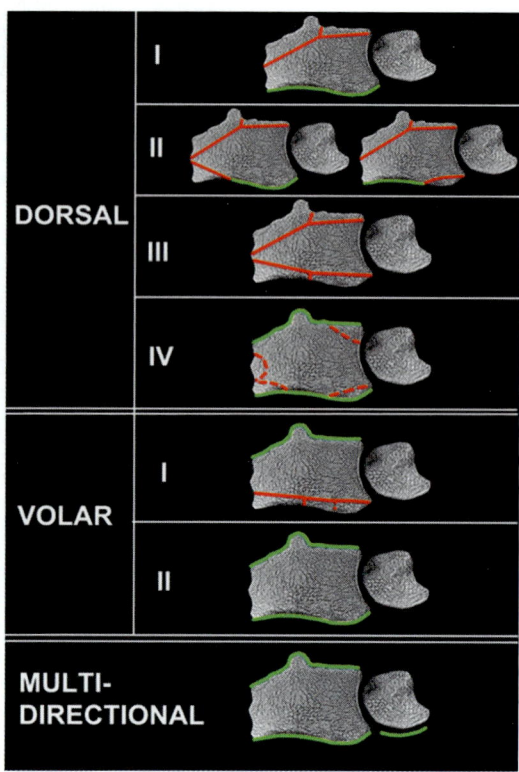

Fig. 8.20 The pattern of osseous (*red lines*) and ligamentous (*green lines*) disruption that was found in different types of dorsal, volar, and multidirectional dislocations (see text for details)

injuries (fall from height, traffic accidents, industrial injuries).

Graham [73] highlighted three basic physical findings in a reduced RC dislocation: the amount of swelling, pain on both the radial and ulnar sides of the wrist, and a semi-supinated posture of the wrist-hand unit at rest.

For radiological diagnosis the P-A and the L neutral rotation views seem to be sufficient. The characteristic findings in the P-A projection are the carpus overlapping the distal radius and the frequent occurrence of fractures of the radial and/or ulnar styloids (see Fig. 8.18a). The L view demonstrates the direction of the RC dislocation while marginal rim fractures are best evaluated on the L view.

Although the dislocated wrist reveals the magnitude of the injury and is treated with the utmost significance, particular attention must be drawn to those cases that were spontaneously reduced and are in danger to be treated superficially with the application of a simple splint. In such cases the injury must be suspected based on the history and clinical findings, while the presence of palmar carpal subluxation and/or ulnar translation are an indication of the magnitude of such an injury. On the P-A view, alignment of the wrist is evaluated by examining the position of the lunate relative to the radius, with a minimum of two thirds of the lunate

articulating with the distal radius [2]. Any disruption of the three Gilula's arcs [101] must be recorded and properly evaluated.

Periarticular rim fractures of the distal radius and/or radial and ulnar styloid avulsion fractures may also be present [73], as well as residual subluxation of the wrist. Distraction films under local or general anaesthesia will better reveal the magnitude of the injury (Fig. 8.23).

Although not mandatory, a CT scan can assist in the evaluation of cortical rim fractures, fracture depression of the articular surface, and the configuration of the DRUJ.

8.10   Associated Injuries

Since these injuries are usually the result of high-energy injuries, open wounds [3, 7, 15, 22,

Table 8.3 Classification of RC dislocations or fracture-dislocations

Chronicity	Pathoanatomy		Direction	Associated injuries	Complexity
a. Acute	*RC dislocations*		a. Dorsal	a. DRUJ	a. Reducibility
b. Gradually developed	a. Pure ligamentous		b. Volar	b. UC ligaments	b. Open or closed
	b. Equivalent:	Tip of radial styloid	c. Ulnar	c. Interosseous ligaments of PCR	
		Ulnovolar fragment	d. Combinations	d. Osteochondral fragment	
	RC fracture-dislocations		e. Multidirectional	e. Carpal bone fractures	
	a. Radial styloid:	Dorsal part		f. Tendons–muscles	
		Volar part		g. Neural or vascular	
		Combination		h. Retinaculum	
	b. Radial rim:	Dorsal rim			
		Volar rim			
		Both rims			
	c. Dorsoulnar fragment				

DRUJ distal radioulnar joint, *PCR* proximal carpal row, *UC* ulnocarpal ligaments

34–36], and associated injuries (often life-threatening) to other organ systems are common. The percentage of such injuries in the literature ranges between 41.6 and 80 % [9, 35, 36, 38]. Associated injuries within the same limb are not uncommon [7, 19, 74]. In our series 38.4 % (10 of 26) of the patients had associated injuries from other organs and 11.5 % (3 of 26) had associated injuries of the same limb.

Usually the median and less common the ulnar nerve may be involved [7, 9, 12, 15, 18, 22, 28, 31, 34, 35, 68, 71], but following reduction, they are usually fully restored [7, 9]. Even acute hand ischemia [7, 12, 15, 28, 35] and compartment syndromes of the hand and forearm [102] have also been reported.

The magnitude of rotational force required for RC dislocations may be of such amount, that it may result in tendon rupturing or detachments. Le Nen et al. [12] reported ruptures of the extensor carpi ulnaris and of the corresponding extensor of the little finger. Others [22, 35] presented a case of flexor tendon rupture or even a case with detachment of the pronator quadratus

[15]. In one of our cases, the extensor and abductor pollicis longus were deracinated from their musculotendinous junction (see Fig. 8.18c).

8.11 Management

There have been reports of successful treatment with: closed reduction and casting [11, 20, 29, 38, 103], closed or open reduction and percutaneous pinning [5, 9, 15, 21, 31, 38], open reduction and casting [34, 104], open reduction and internal fixation with ligamentous repair [7, 9, 12, 16, 38, 52, 71, 75, 102]. Due to the rarity of these injuries, there is no unanimously accepted method for their management.

The majority of these dislocations are relatively easy to reduce, there are therefore cases that, being spontaneously reduced, escape diagnosis. The reported cases of a non-reducible dislocation are rare. In one case there was tendon interference [22], whereas in two other cases there was bone fragment interference [32, 71].

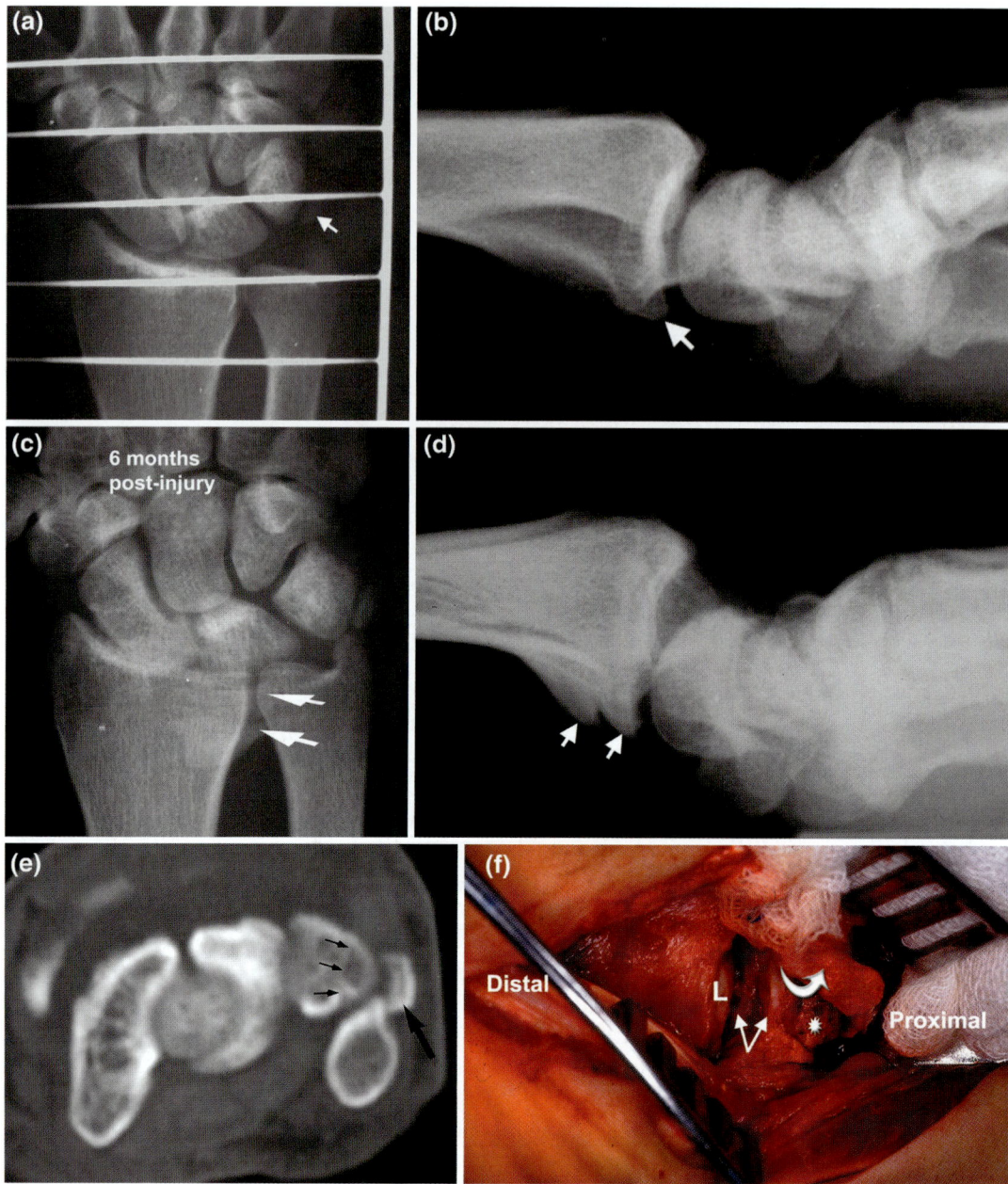

Fig. 8.21 Male, 32 years old, motorcycle injury. A case of a gradually developed RC subluxation after fracture of the ulnovolar radial rim. The PA view demonstrated an avulsed fragment from the triquetrum (**a**); L view showed an undisplaced fracture of the volar radial rim (**b**); he was treated initially with a splint for 3 weeks. The symptoms persisted after splint removal and physiotherapy was recommended. Six months post-injury, the PA view showed radiocarpal joint overlapping, volar RC subluxation, and new bone formation in association with the displaced ulnovolar fragment was detected (*double arrows*) (**c**, **d**); a CT-scan showed the displaced fragment from the triquetrum (**e**); the volar approach revealed the articular step-off (*double arrows*), the new bone formation (*asterisk*), and the raised capsuloligamentous flap (*curved arrow*) (**f**); with intraarticular osteotomy the ulnovolar fragment was raised (*curved arrow*) (**g**); it was reduced and fixated using 2 K-wires (**h**); the RC joint was reduced and stabilized with a transfixing pin and the wrist joint immobilized with an external fixator; postoperative x-rays (**i**, **j**); final radiographic appearance 18 months later (**k**, **l**). With permission from [127]

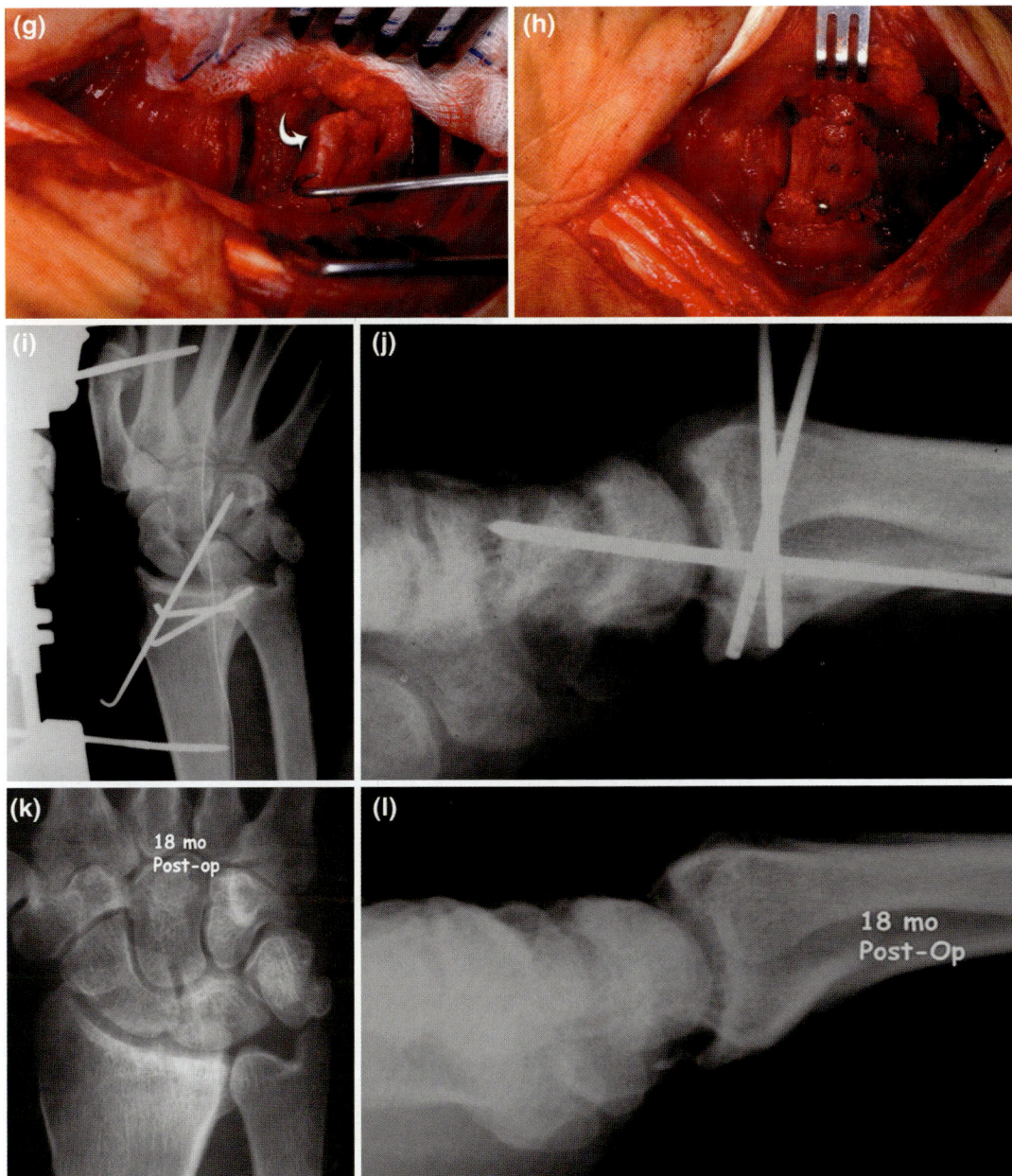

Fig. 8.21 (continued)

Inability to perform closed reduction in 4 out of 6 cases, due to interference of ligamentous or bone origin has also been reported [15].

In several literature reports, mostly of isolated cases, closed reduction, and cast immobilization are advised [9, 11, 20, 29, 33], in dorsiflexion for the dorsal and in palmarflexion for the palmar dislocations [33, 39]. However, RC dislocations treated nonsurgically have been reported to develop palmar subluxation, ulnar translation DISI or VISI instabilities [11, 14, 17, 20, 21, 26, 29, 30, 75]. Certainly everyone

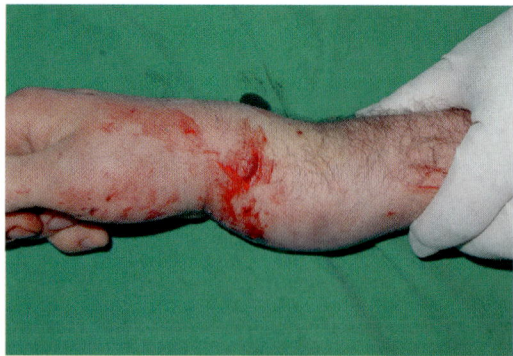

Fig. 8.22 The dislocated RC joint showed considerable deformation. With permission from [127]

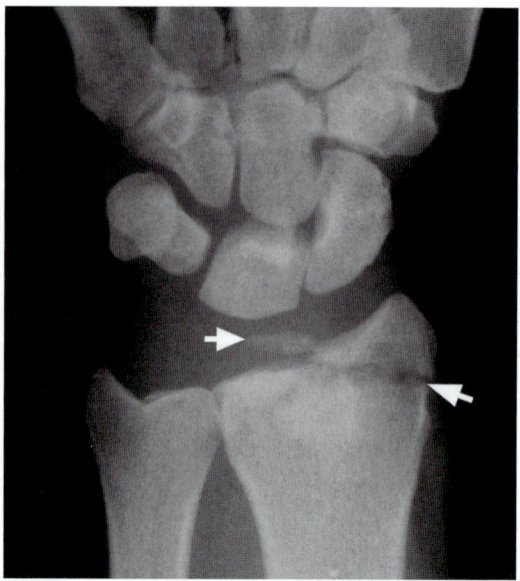

agrees that open, non-reducible dislocations and those accompanied by neurovascular injury must be managed with open reduction [1, 15]. Moneim et al. [9] suggests the attempt of closed reduction and casting for type I injuries and open reduction, internal fixation, and ligamentous repair for type II injuries. However, many reports [35, 36, 38, 68, 105–107], plead for open

Fig. 8.23 The distraction view provides useful information for the injury. Excessive widening of the RC joint indicates the magnitude of the RC ligaments' injury, while arrows indicate the fracture of the radial styloid and an osseous fragment from the volar radial rim

Fig. 8.24 A dorsal RC fracture-dislocation which was treated with closed reduction and cast application (**a**, **b**), resulted in VISI malalignment (**c**, **d**)

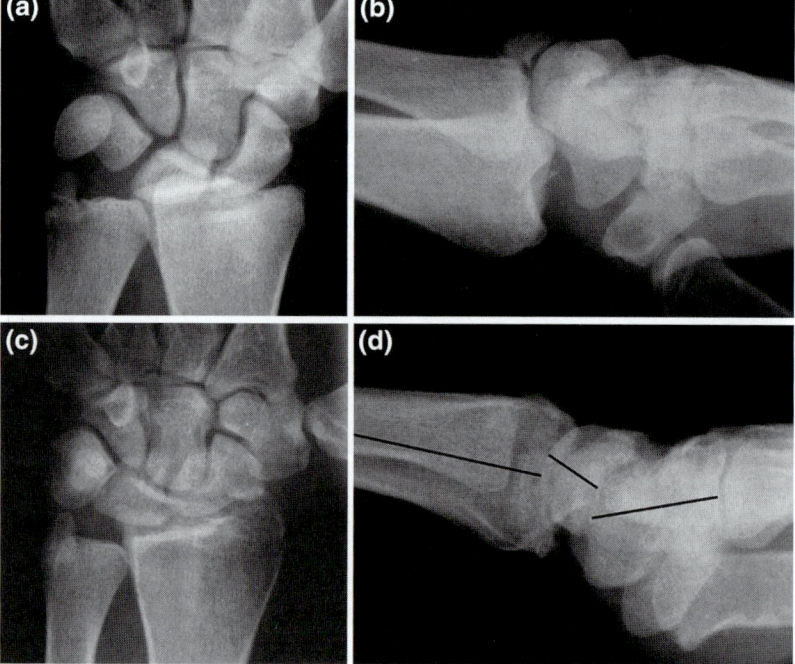

reduction since, if the RC ligamentous mechanism is not repaired, wrist function will be severely compromised with instability and/or subluxation later [102].

The concern whether these injuries should be managed conservatively or surgically, is directly related to the unstable nature of these injuries (Fig. 8.24a–d). There are many cases in the literature that were initially managed with closed reduction and casting, but the wrist was subluxated early or late [9, 15, 21, 38]. In our series 7 out of 26 patients lost their reduction and were treated operatively with a delay of 4–20 days. Schoenecker et al. [15], supports that even with open reduction, maintaining the anatomical reduction is difficult, especially when a compressive fracture of the dorsal radial rim coexists. Conversely, Fernandez et al. [68] rationale was based on the fact that rupture of the palmar RC ligaments predisposes the wrist to ulnar translocation, which will be observed if there is no ligamentous repair. In addition, one more reason supporting surgical management is for the removal of small cartilaginous and osteochondral fragments, which frequently interfere in the joint and obstruct its reduction.

If for any reason closed reduction is chosen, a basic requirement is to ensure that during the healing period, the anatomical alignment of the bones and joints will be preserved, in order for intraarticular fractures to be united without articular incongruity and most importantly, the RC joint to be axially aligned so that the ruptured ligaments can heal with proper tensioning. Prerequisites for the above are: frequent radiological control, good application of the cast, prompt identification of wrist displacement (palmar, ulnar or dorsal), detection of possible injuries of the interosseous ligaments, and sufficient time for immobilization (6–8 weeks). Alternatively, following closed reduction and once we have ensured that the RC joint has been anatomically reduced, we can immobilize the joint using K-wire or external fixation.

There is no consensus as to which is the most appropriate approach for open reduction. The approach should be dictated by the direction of the dislocation, the fracture pattern, the

associated carpal bone injuries, the presence of neurovascular injury and if we are dealing with an open or closed injury. Moneim et al. [9] for cases necessitating open reduction proposed combined approaches. Mudgal et al. [36] advised the use of palmar approach in the presence of a neurological defect, dorsal approach if the dorsal radial rim is involved and ulnar approach when the ulnar styloid requires fixation. Dumontier et al. [38] believed that group 1 patients should be treated with reattachment of the ligaments through a volar approach. In group 2 patients, the ligaments are still attached to the radial fragment and in this group of patients, exact articular reduction should be performed through a dorsal approach. Lipton and Jupiter [102] supported an extended palmar approach in cases of dorsal RC dislocation with neurovascular compromise, in order to repair in addition the volar ligaments, whereas if there are dorsal avulsion fractures or if the dislocation is volarward, then the surgical approach is through an extensive dorsal approach. The Mayo clinic group, as quoted by Idler [86], has recommended palmar and dorsal approaches for ligament repair of the radiocapitate, long radiolunate, ulnocarpal, and dorsal radiotriquetral ligaments.

Considering that by definition, RC dislocations or fracture-dislocations constitute doublesided injuries and that structures important for wrist stability are located both dorsally and volarly, we regard the combined approach as the most appropriate. In any case of an acute dislocation or fracture dislocation, regardless of its direction, we consider the palmar approach most important in order to repair the volar RC and ulnocarpal ligaments as well as any fractures of the volar radial rim, since these structures are crucial for wrist stability. In the majority of cases dorsal approach is also required, especially in cases of compressive fractures of the dorsal radial rim, for the fixation of a potential dorsal part of a fracture of the radial styloid or to evaluate the integrity of proximal carpal row bones. Sometimes, when dorsally the injuries are purely ligamentous or are associated with small avulsed fragments or with subperiosteal

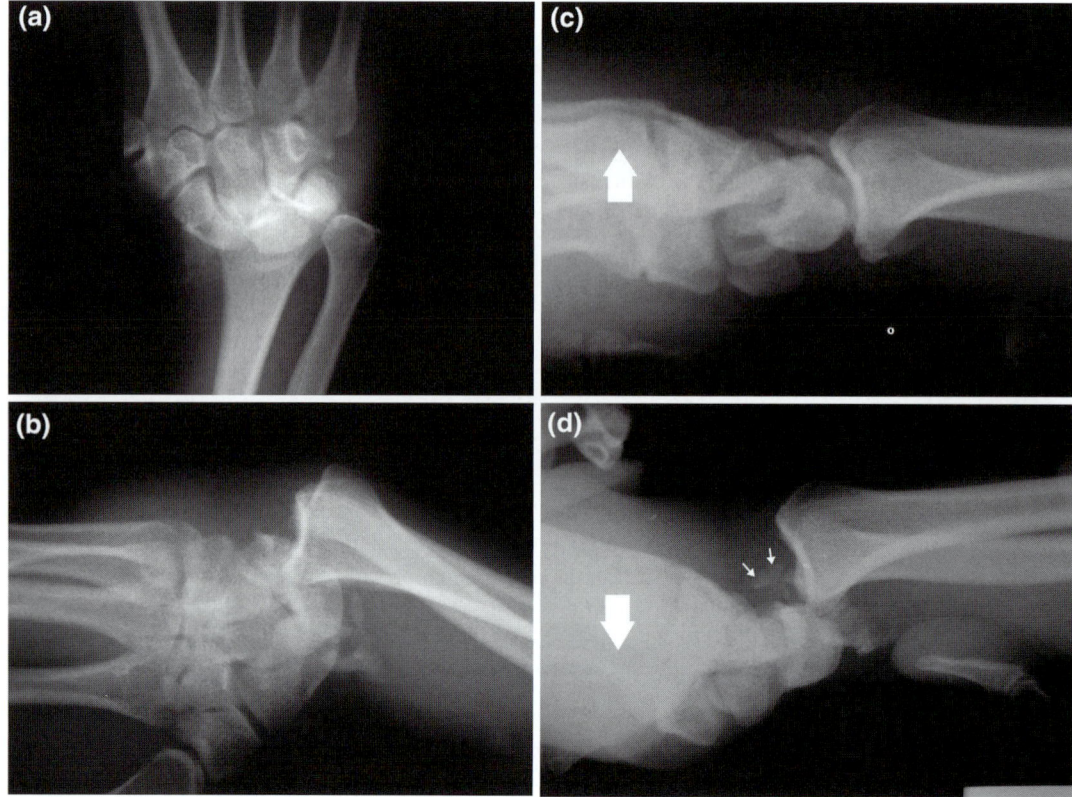

Fig. 8.25 Male, 28 years old. Volar RC fracture-dislocation (**a**, **b**); stress views in different directions showed that the RC joint was stable only in dorsal direction (**c–f**); in volar displacement view, the osseous fragment indicated with *arrows*, was shown to have originated from the dorsal LT complex (see Fig. 8.12); postoperative X-rays (**g**, **h**)

detachment of the dorsal extensor compartments, then dorsal approach may be avoided, on the premise that the volar structures have been restored and the RC joint is maintained reduced and properly aligned for 6–8 weeks.

In cases of DRUJ instability or of a displaced fracture at the base of the ulnar styloid, a separate ulnar approach is frequently necessary.

Based on the literature and on personal experience, we consider the following steps as necessary for open reduction:

- The patient is positioned supine on the operating table. An arm table is positioned beneath the affected extremity and the procedure is performed under tourniquet control. During anesthesia, useful information concerning the magnitude and direction of dislocation can be acquired under image intensifier, through manipulation of the wrist (longitudinal traction and dorsal, volar, radial, and ulnar displacement) with the forearm stabilized (Fig. 8.25a–h). In addition, PA and L radiographs with the RC fracture dislocation reduced are recommended.

- Depending on the nature and the time elapsed from injury, an external fixator may be applied from the initial stages of operation, so that the wrist is kept in gross alignment and mild distraction, as it facilitates the exposure of the capsuloligamentous structures. The more delayed the injury's treatment is, the greater the need for the application of the external fixator at the initial stages of the operation. Its placement on the radial side of the wrist does not obstruct the impending approach.

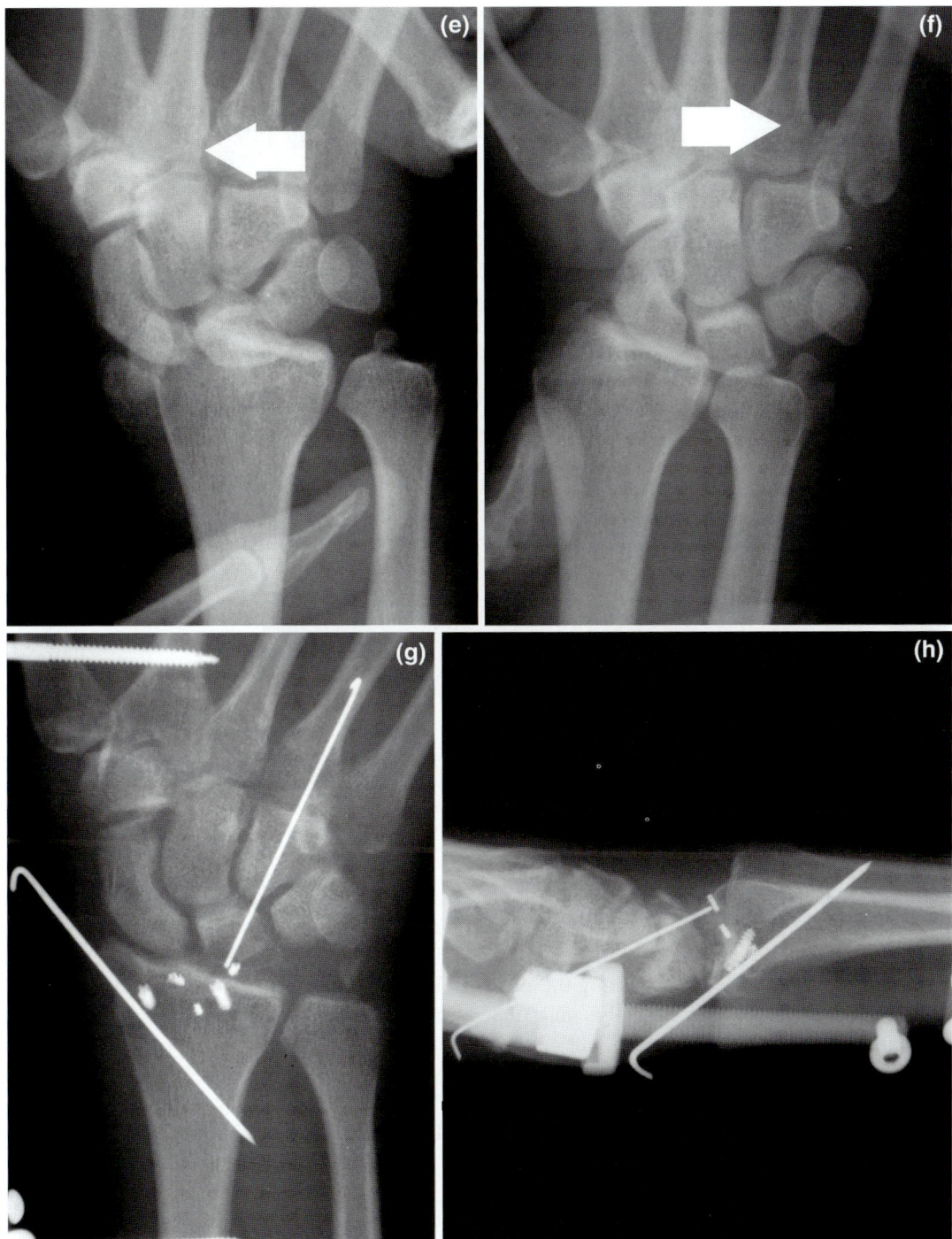

Fig. 8.25 (continued)

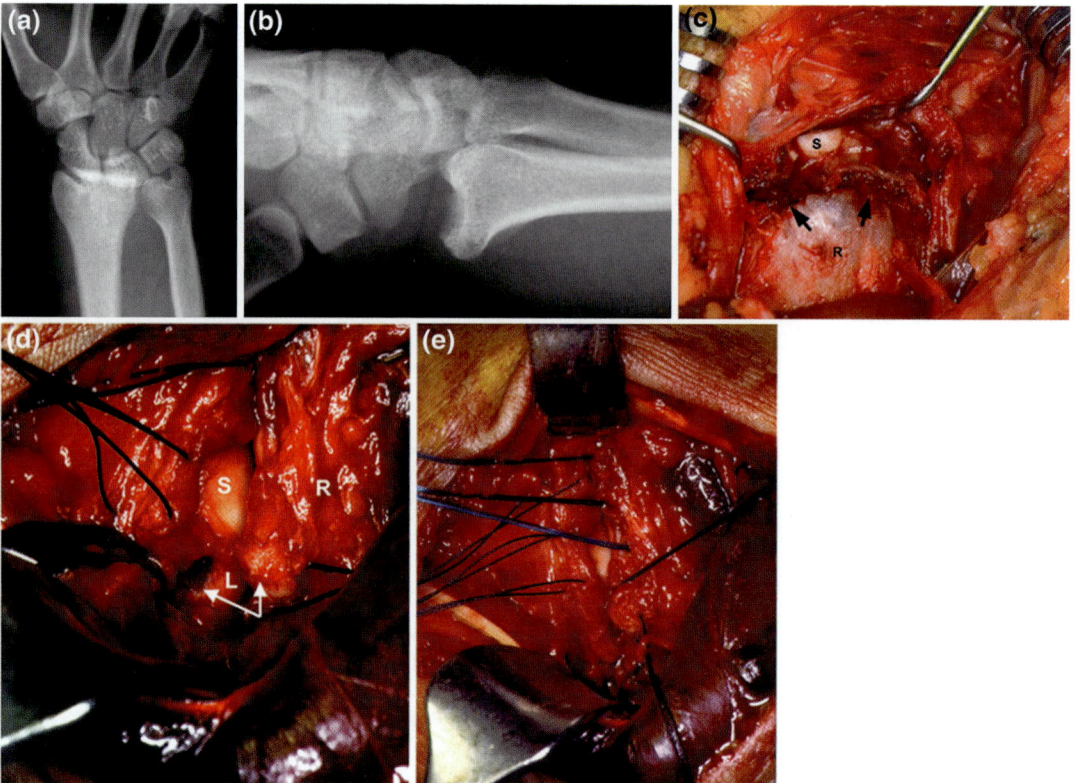

Fig. 8.26 Male, 31 years old. Dorsal RC fracture-dislocation (**a**, **b**); with the dorsal approach, a double osseous injury of the dorsal radial rim (*arrows*) was evident after raising the dorsal capsuloligamentous flap (**c**); volarly, the RC ligaments were deracinated from the volar radial rim, except for the short RL ligament that was detached with an osseous fragment from the lunate (*arrows*) (**d**); reconstruction was accomplished using bone anchors (**e**, **f**); final x-rays 1 year later (**g**, **h**). With permission from [127]

- The extended carpal tunnel approach is used to decompress both the carpal tunnel and Guyon canal if needed and to fully evaluate the radio-volar injuries by displacing the FPL and the median nerve radially and the remaining flexor tendons ulnarly. The ulnovolar injuries are assessed by displacing the flexor tendons radially. Less often and depending on the extent of injuries, Henry's approach is sufficed. The joint is irrigated and the osseoligamentous lesions are recorded in detail. The palmar RC ligaments are either detached from their insertions to the volar radial rim or from carpal bones (usually the lunate) or avulsed with a small osseous fragment from their insertions. The reattachment of ligaments is achieved using nonabsorbable sutures through transosseous holes or bone anchors that are inserted at the sites where the ligaments were detached (Fig. 8.26a–h). Depending on the size of the fractured fragments of the volar rim, their fixation is achieved using K-wires, small plates, or a wire-loop [108] (Figs. 8.27a, b and 8.9g–h). The possibility of fragmentation of the bone fragments must always be kept in mind, both during manipulation and stabilization.

In cases where the healing capacity of the volar RC ligaments is questionable, especially in delayed cases, augmentation using tendon grafts is an option. Originally Rayhack et al. [52] and more recently Maschke et al. [89] described a cadaveric model for reconstructing the radioscaphocapitate using the brachioradialis tendon,

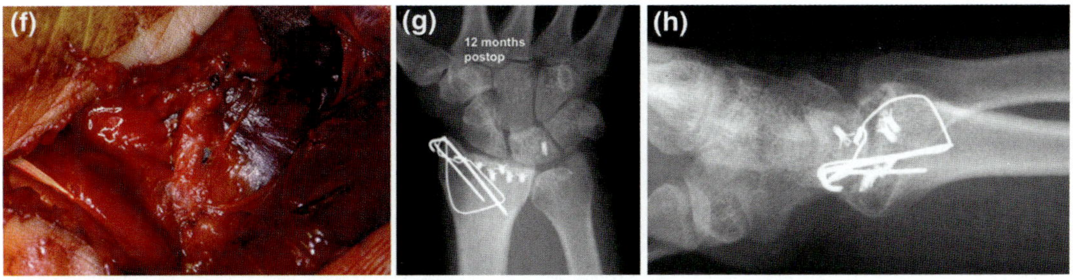

Fig. 8.26 (continued)

Fig. 8.27 The wire-loop technique which was used for the fixation of an avulsed small ulnovolar fragment (*arrow*)

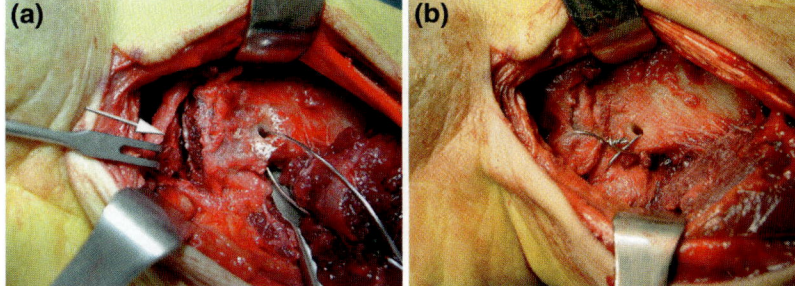

while Obafemi and Pensy [109] applied the same technique in a patient with palmar RC dislocation, in order to reconstruct the radioscaphocapitate ligament and to reinforce the dorsal capsular repair.

- The dorsal approach is longitudinal over Lister's tubercle, the third compartment is exposed if intact and the EPL tendon is displaced radially. The integrity of the dorsal retinaculum is recorded; if it is intact, subperiosteal elevation of the second and fourth compartments allow for a full evaluation of the dorsal injuries, since the dorsal capsule is already ruptured. At this stage and after joint irrigation, the injuries of the dorsal surface of the radius (from radial to ulnar) and the integrity of the chondral surfaces and the interosseous ligaments of the proximal carpal row bones are evaluated. Any entrapped chondral or osteochondral fragments are debrided or preserved for later transfixation. The integrity of the dorsal RC ligament must be checked throughout its course. In cases of compressive fractures of the dorsal radial rim, the insertion of cancellous bone grafting is

necessary to support the articular surface, using small buttress plates for fixation [36, 102, 110] (Fig. 8.28a–d). In cases with purely ligamentous injuries, small osseous fragments or subperiosteal detachment of the dorsal cortex, there are many alternative stabilizing methods including K-wires, bone anchors, screws or tension band wiring (Fig. 8.29a–d). Any injury of the proximal carpal row bones is treated accordingly and stabilized with K-wires.

- As we previously noted, the fracture at the base of the ulnar styloid may indicate a destabilization of the DRUJ. This however is not absolute, as it is not certain that the fracture of the tip of the radial styloid has no effect on joint stability. Consequently, at the end of a stable reconstruction of the RC joint, the stability of the DRUJ is assessed. This information will be provided with passive anteroposterior glide of the distal ulna relative to the distal radius in positions of neutral rotation, full pronation and full supination, and whether the ballottement test demonstrates or not a hard end point. Thus, in cases

Fig. 8.28 A dorsal RC fracture dislocation (**a, b**); the sizable dorsal osseous fragments were reduced and fixated using 2 small buttress plates (**c, d**). With permission from [127]

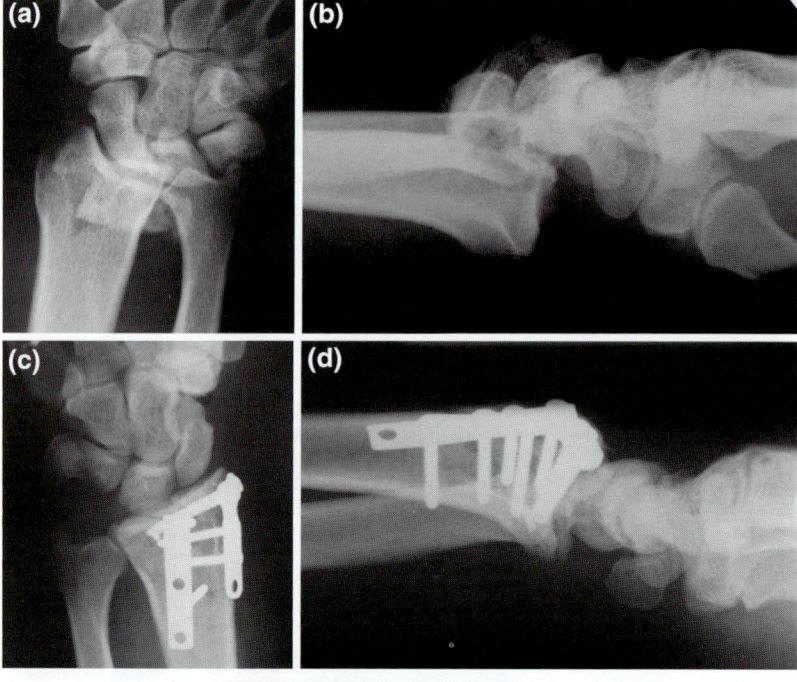

Fig. 8.29 Male, 23 years old. Motorcycle injury. A dorsal RC fracture-dislocation (**a, b**); a cannulated screw; and bone anchors were used for stabilization after combined approach (**c, d**)

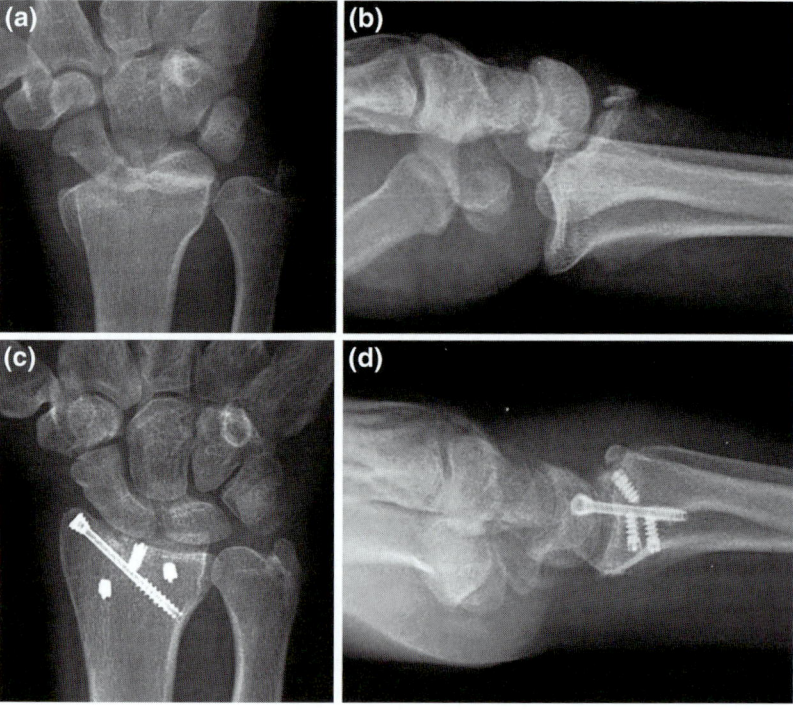

of DRUJ instability or displaced fracture of the base of the ulnar styloid, tension band wiring, or TFCC suturing are recommended [36, 102]. An additional type of fracture which is always associated with instability of the DRUJ and need to be fixated, is an avulsion fracture of the dorsal sigmoid notch, which pertains the TFCC (usually accompanies the dorsoulnar RC dislocations). In such cases a radioulnar transfixing pin is required.

- It is necessary, using the external fixator, to maintain the RC joint in a reduced position throughout the healing process for 6–8 weeks and to protect the reconstructed RC ligaments from slackening. In highly unstable injuries or when the reconstruction is suboptimal, an additional RC pinning is essential and is usually inserted percutaneously or through a small incision (protecting the sensory branches of the radial nerve), from the radial aspect of the radius and through the lunate towards the wrist (Fig. 8.30a–i).
- The immobilization of the RC joint is maintained for 6–8 weeks and physiotherapy consisting of active and passive wrist mobilization, must be initiated.

8.12 Outcome

The conclusions concerning the outcome of these injuries present three drawbacks: First, there are no large series with patients with RC dislocations; second, the existing studies are dealing with mixed type of injuries, which are treated with various methods; and third, there are no long-term follow-up reports on the outcome.

Despite being complex injuries, favorable clinical results have been reported with both methods, closed or open. However, there is discrepancy between clinical and radiological results, with the latter being clearly worse, something which renders unknown the long-term consequences. The anatomical reduction and maintenance of the proper alignment of the RC joint throughout the healing process, are the factors that will ensure a good functional result, regardless of the method chosen.

Factors predictive of an inferior clinical and/or radiological outcome include: open injuries, associated severe nerve injuries, purely ligamentous dislocations, intercarpal ligamentous injuries that are initially missed and remain untreated and associated DRUJ injuries. The compressive type of fractures of the radial rims have worse prognosis than avulsion fractures, since the former, could be associated with articular cartilage injury or collapsing due to comminution or osteonecrosis, because of devascularization of small fragments (Fig. 8.31a–k). In addition, fracture fragments associated with unfavorable results if ignored or inadequately treated, are the ulnovolar (Fig. 8.32a–k) and the dorsoulnar fragments of the distal radius. Both are implicated in ulnar translocation and the latter in DRUJ subluxation.

Large series in the literature indicate that an overall 30–40 % decrease in total arc of wrist flexion–extension and 20–30 % of grip strength, can be expected following open treatment [2, 35, 38]. Howard et al. [26] highlighted the possibility of weakness development in pronation and supination, which may be the result of residual global laxity of the extrinsic wrist ligaments.

Dumontier et al. [38] concluded that patients with pure RC dislocations (group I) present with good mid-term results, but long-term results are doubtful, since the majority of these patients presented with varying severity of ulnar translocation of the wrist, regardless of the method applied for their management. Conversely, in patients with RC fracture-dislocations (group II), ulnar or palmar displacement of the wrist does not seem to constitute a problem, while long-term results depend upon the quality of fracture reduction.

Schoenecker et al. [15] reported 4 patients out of 6 with arthrosis at 3-year follow-up. The results of Le Nen's et al. [12] patients showed that 5 out of 6 patients had some narrowing of the RC interval with a follow-up ranging from 3 months to 11 years. Fernandez et al. [68] reported a series of 12 patients treated operatively and after a follow-up of 36 months, 3 of them had radiographic evidence of grade I arthritic changes. Mudgal et al. [36] reporting on a series of 12 patients and after a mean follow-up

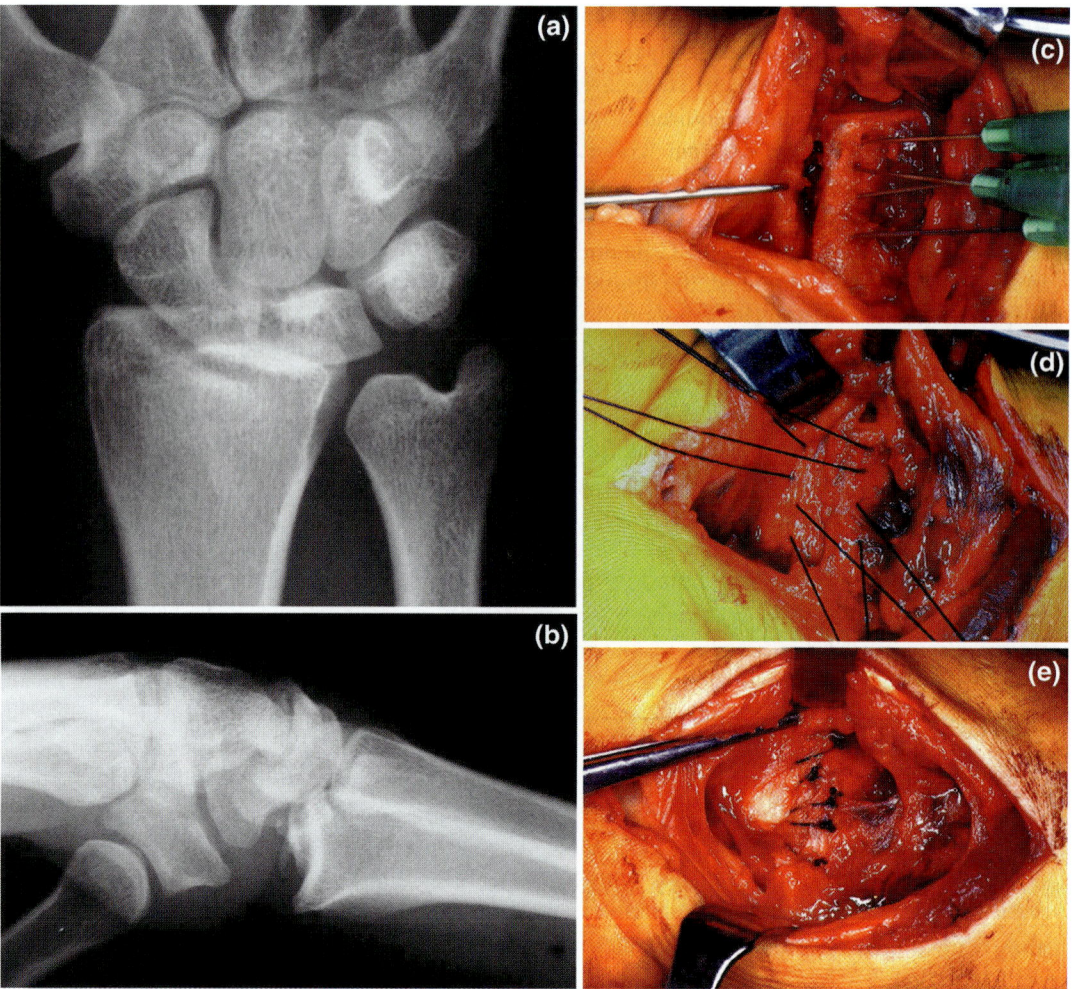

Fig. 8.30 Male, 32 years old, with a dorsal RC fracture-dislocation (**a**, **b**); the uprooted volar RC ligaments were reattached with transosseous sutures (**c**, **d**, **e**); the RC joint was stabilized using RC pinning (**f**, **g**); final x-rays after 2 years (**h**, **i**). With permission from [127]

of 36 months, identified 3 patients as presenting evidence of RC arthritis. Dumontier et al. [38] reported that 6 out of 18 patients that were followed-up for 44 months average, developed RC arthritis (1 out of 5 patients belonging to group I and 5 of 13 patients belonging to group II). Patee and Thomson [111] after a follow-up of 3.2 years reported that 13 of 20 patients (65 %), who were treated with a variety of methods, presented with roentgenographic evidence of posttraumatic arthritis.

Oberladstatter et al. [76] examined 8 patients (9 cases) with Moneim I RC fracture dislocations, who were treated operatively. After an average follow-up of 4.1 years and using the classification system described by Knirk and Jupiter [112], 5 patients (56 %) had stage 1 arthritic changes, three (33 %) had stage 2 arthritis, and 1 patient (11 %) had stage 3 arthritis with total loss of the RC joint space.

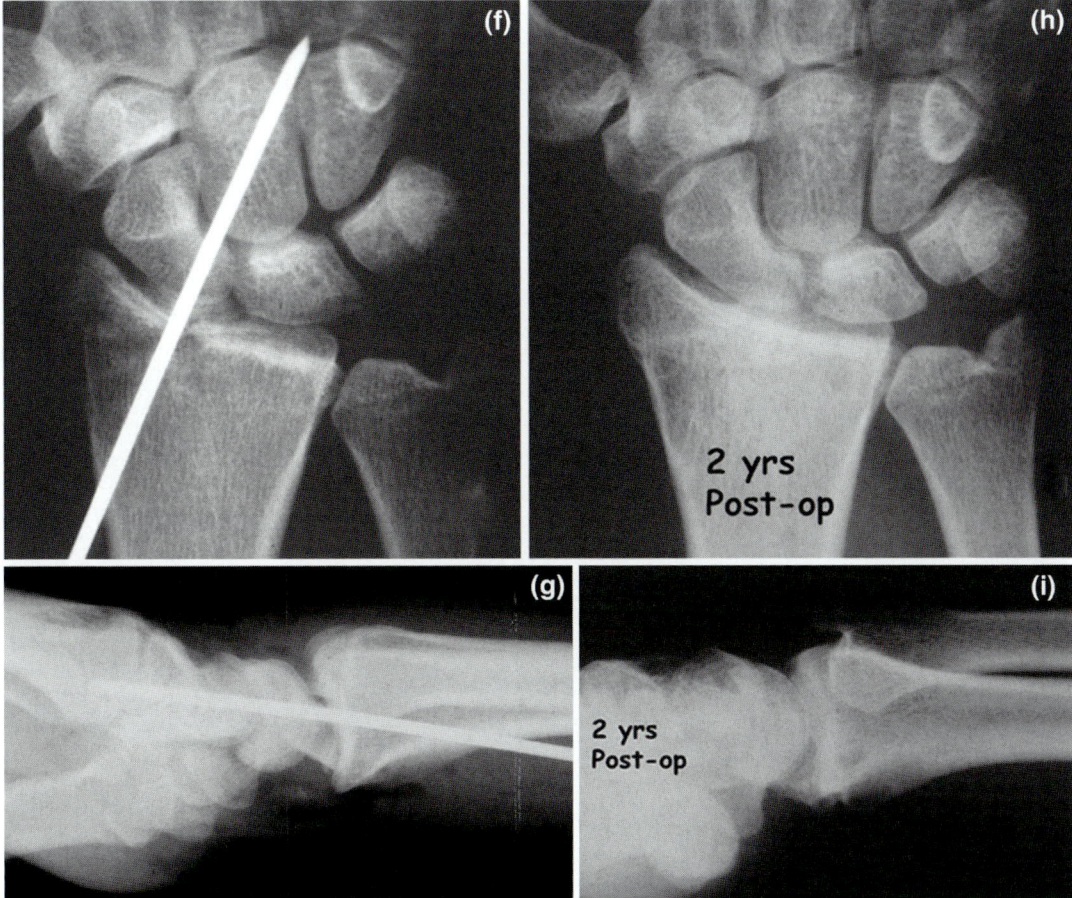

Fig. 8.30 (continued)

Twenty of 26 patients in our series returned for evaluation at a mean of 57.6 months (range, 12–158.8 months). All of them had returned to their original jobs. Eight patients were free of pain, 7 had cold weather symptoms, and 5 patients noted mild pain only with heavy labor. The mean grip strength was 82.7 %, and the flexion–extension arc was 80 % of the contralateral healthy wrist. Four patients had grade 1 arthritic changes (3 with dorsal and 1 with volar RC fracture-dislocations) (Fig. 8.33a, b), 3 patients developed mild ulnar translation (1 with multidirectional dislocation and 2 with dorsal RC fracture-dislocations) (Fig. 8.34a, b), 1 patient developed mild radial translation due to malalignment of the radial styloid, and 1 patient developed VISI malalignment due to disruption of the LT joint.

8.13 Complications

Limitations in the range of motion and reduction in grip strength are common occurrences regardless of the treatment method applied for these injuries. In addition, posttraumatic arthritis, instability findings and residual volar, dorsal, or ulnar subluxation of the wrist, have been reported as possible complications after the management of these injuries [2, 15, 38, 86].

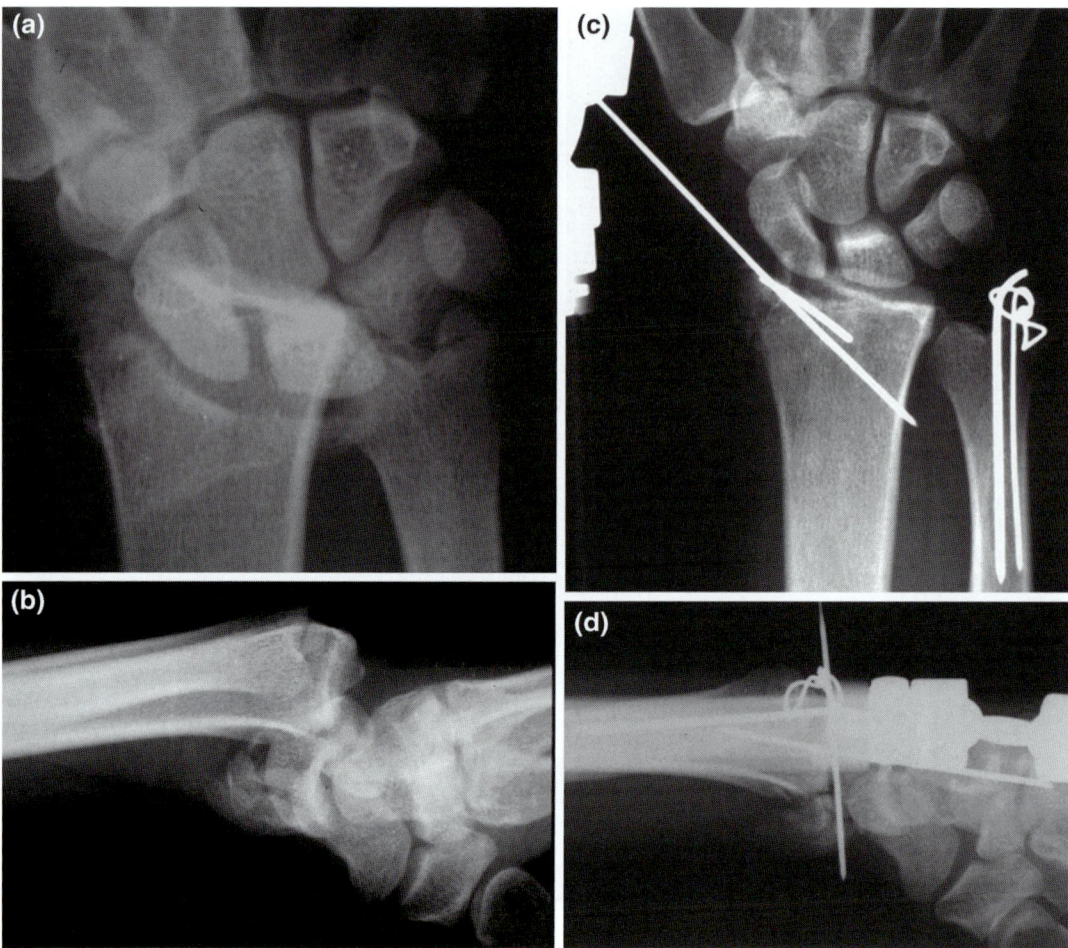

Fig. 8.31 Male, 26 years old, after a motorcycle injury with a volar RC fracture-dislocation (**a, b**). He was treated elsewhere with a dorsal approach, while K-wires were used in an effort to fixate the fractured fragments. In addition a tension band wire was used for the minimally displaced ulnar styloid fracture. On the 3rd postop day and despite the external fixation, the RC joint displayed volar subluxation and the patient was sent for further treatment (**c, d**); with palmar approach the fractured fragments were reduced and fixated using K-wires. An additional K-wire was used percutaneously for a suspected SL ligament injury (**e, f**). 12 years later the x-rays showed fragmentation and osteonecrosis of the radial styloid (**g, h**), while the patient had a satisfactory ROM with only cold weather symptoms (**i–k**). With permission from [127]

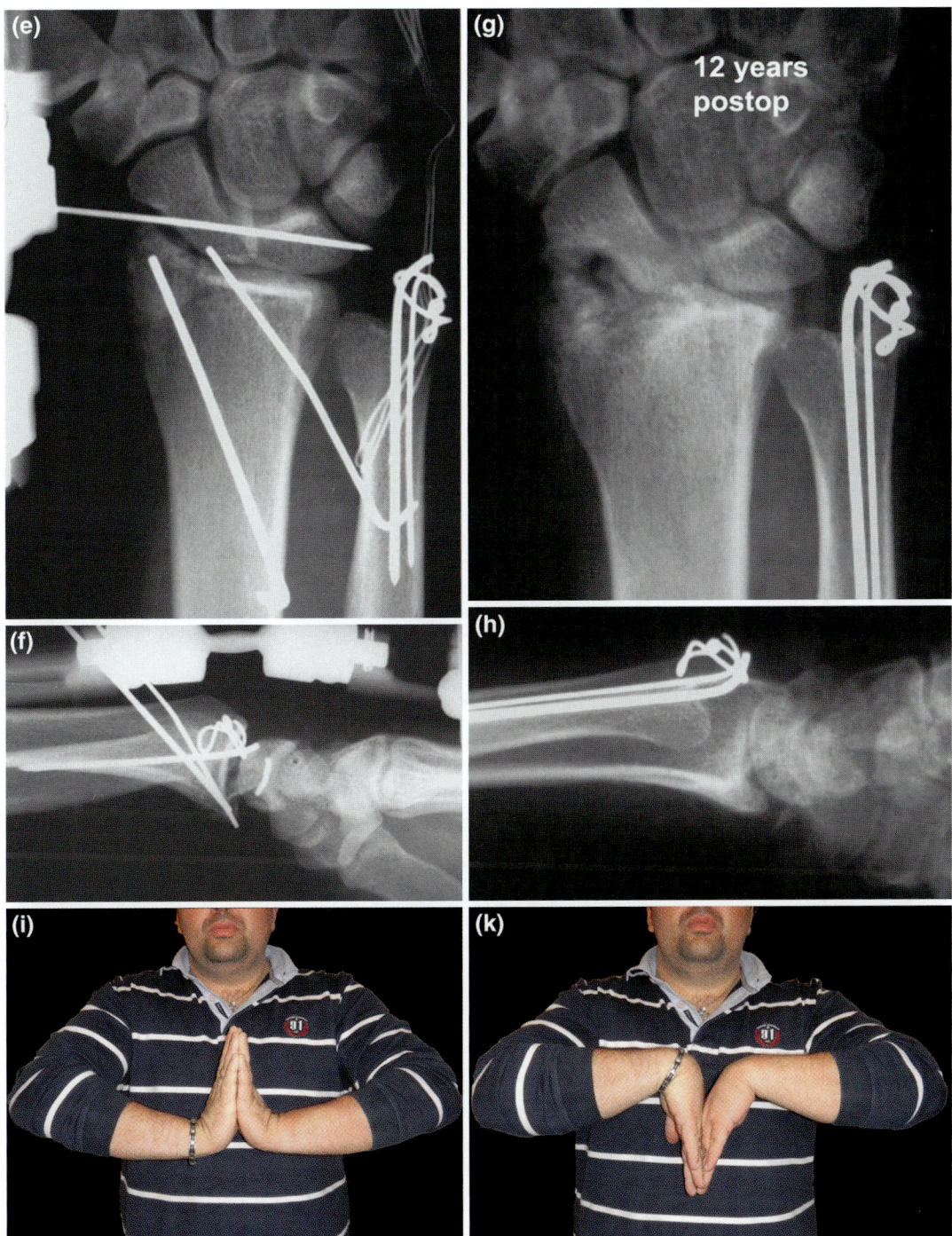

Fig. 8.31 (continued)

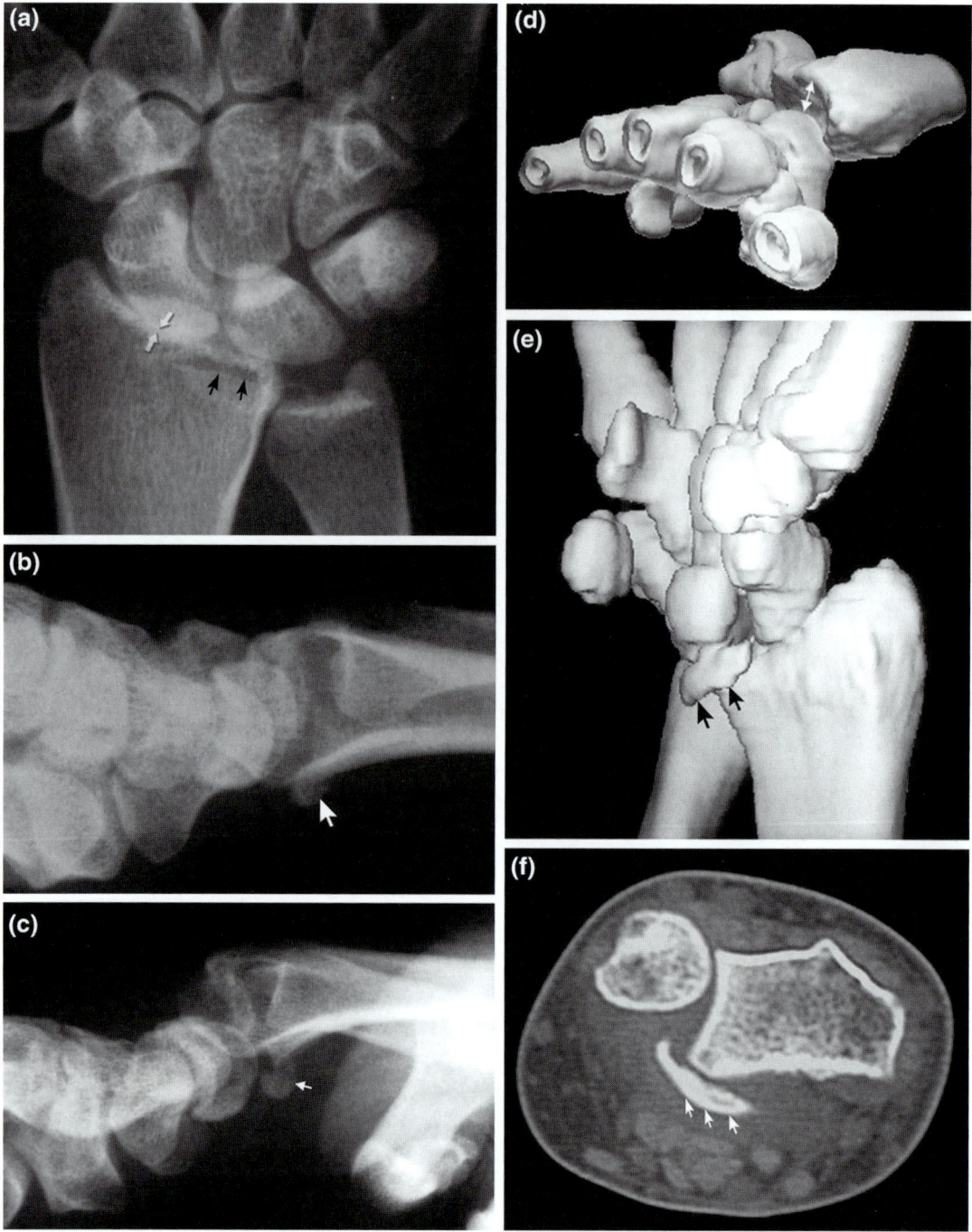

Fig. 8.32 Female, 27 years old. Car accident. Despite the initial radiographs which were indicative of RC joint instability (overlapping of radioscaphoid joint and fracture of the ulnovolar fragment) (*arrows*) (**a**, **b**), she was treated with a below elbow cast for 3 weeks. Three months later the volarly subluxated RC joint and the displaced ulnovolar fragment (*arrows*) were depicted in x-rays (**c**), 3D CT-scan (**d**, **e**) and CT-scan (**f**); the palmar approach revealed that the short RL ligament (*asterisk*) was attached to the ulnovolar fragment (*arrow*), which was detached (**g**) and reconstructed with 2 bone anchors (**h**); an external fixator was used for stabilization of the RC joint for 6 weeks (**i**); final x-rays 2 years postoperatively (**j**, **k**). With permission from [127]

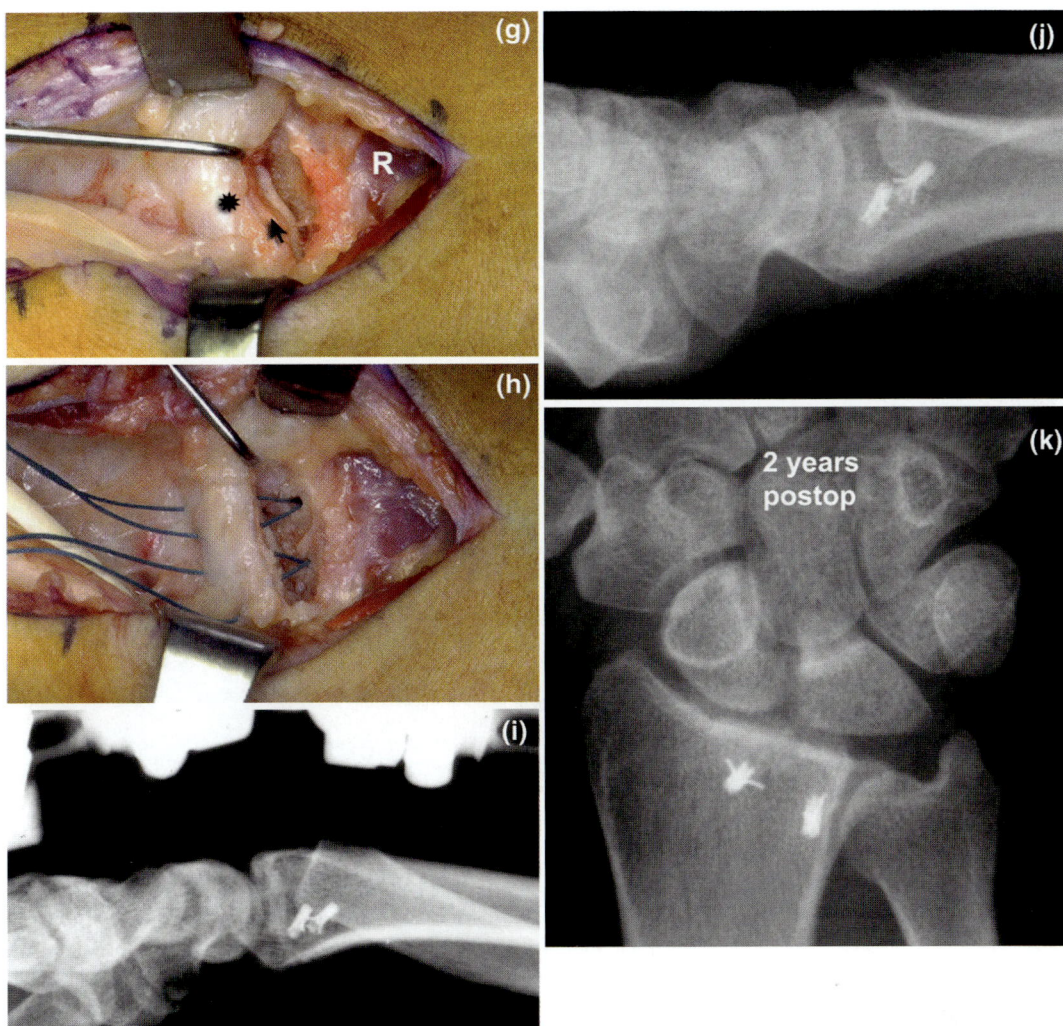

Fig. 8.32 (continued)

Fig. 8.33 **a,**
b Radiocarpal irregularities
and signs of arthritis
3 years postoperatively of
the case illustrated in
Fig. 8.25. With permission
from [127]

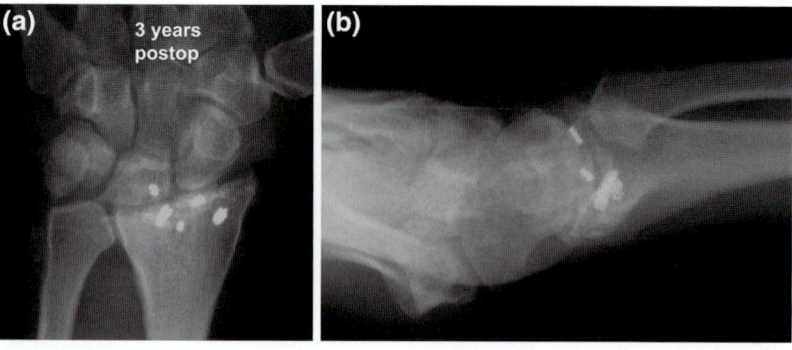

Fig. 8.34 **a, b** The final
radiographic appearance
6 years postoperatively of
the case illustrated in
Fig. 8.11, showed ulnar
translocation of the RC
joint. With permission
from [127]

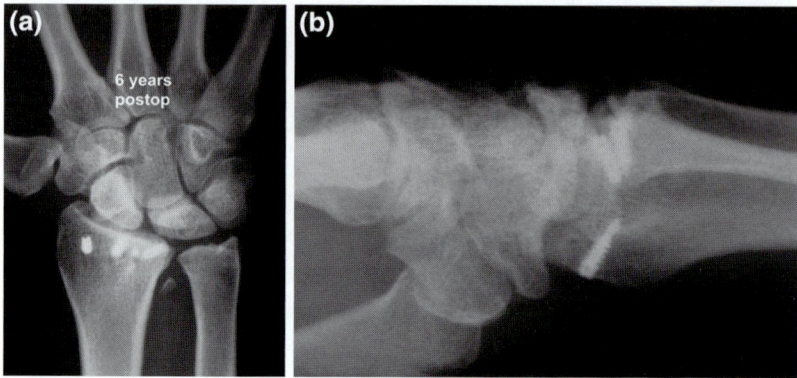

8.13.1 Ulnar Translation or Ulnar Translocation

Ulnar Translation [113] or Ulnar Translocation [39] is observed in cases of serious and generalized ligamentous injuries of both the palmar and dorsal sides of the wrist. It could be manifested as either pure ulnar translocation [17, 52, 90, 114, 115] or as sequelae of reduced palmar [23, 26, 30] or dorsal [27] RC dislocations, which were treated with closed or open reduction and inadequate reconstruction of the volar RC and ulnocarpal ligaments (Fig. 8.35a–k). Ulnar translocation of the wrist is more common with purely ligamentous injury patterns [21, 26, 30, 33, 38], while excessive minus variance of the ulna with deficient ulnar buttressing by the TFCC, may be a predisposing factor [52, 116].

Taleisnik [39] distinguished 2 types of ulnar translocation: In type I, the entire carpus, including the scaphoid, is displaced and the distance between the radial styloid and the scaphoid is widened. In type II, the relationship between the distal row, the scaphoid, and the radius remains normal; the scapholunate space is widened and the lunate-triquetrum complex is ulnarly translocated. The distinction between the two types is essential since type I ulnar translocation constitutes a CIND type of instability, while type II is a combination of CIND and CID (SL dissociation) type of instabilities, hence a complex (CIC) type of instability. In type I injuries the failure concerns all RC ligaments, while in type II translocation the radioscaphocapitate ligament is intact but there is complete disruption of the scapholunate and radiolunate ligaments [117].

Fig. 8.35 Male, 22 years old. Motorcycle accident that resulted in hip dislocation and a wrist injury with an initially normal PA view (**a**); during examination the wrist was found unstable in multiple directions (**b, c, d**); the volar RC ligaments (**e**) and the dorsal capsule including the DRC ligament (**f**) were deracinated from the radial rims, while the ulnocarpal ligaments were also ruptured (*arrows*) (**g**); three absorbable bone anchors were placed volarly and one metallic bone anchor was introduced dorsally, while a small external fixator was used to stabilize the RC joint leaving the midcarpal joint unobstructed for early initiation of dart-throw motion (**h, i**); 5 years later, the patient although symptoms-free, displayed radiographically ulnar translation (**j, k**)

Schernberg [116] identified four grades of ligamentous lesions leading to complete ulnar translocation. In grade I injury there is only partial disruption of the involved ligament and the joint remains stable under dynamic radiographic examination. A grade II injury corresponds to complete disruption of the involved ligament but does not cause any displacement of the wrist and standard radiographs remain normal. Only passive stress views must be used to reveal this abnormality. Grade III lesions consist of complete disruption of the relevant ligament(s) and permanent displacement of the wrist, which is obvious in the standard radiographs. As there is some contact between the remaining articular surfaces, this condition is also called subluxation. Finally, Grade IV injuries present with dislocation, i.e., complete loss of joint contact between the involved carpal elements. Grade II injuries represent a dynamic pattern of ulnar translocation, while grades III and IV represent static patterns of the instability. Such dynamic patterns of ulnar translocation have been reported [118–120]. A seemingly minor dynamic ulnar translation pattern may progress with time to a major static displacement, as it was clearly demonstrated in at least 3 out of 8 cases presented by Rayhack et al. [52].

Palmar translation of the wrist was found with less ligament disruption than that required for ulnar translation, whereas in all cases of ulnar translation, there was a component of palmar wrist displacement [50, 117].

Different methods of assessing ulnar translation have been reported. The methods using the center of the capitate head [121–123] as a carpal reference should not be used in type II injuries, because only the lunate-triquetrum complex is significantly displaced in these cases. In contrast, when using the lunate as a reference [124–126], if the wrist is slightly radially or ulnarly deviated, the measurements may be unreliable [117].

The diagnosis of ulnar translation is usually delayed and this renders a difficult problem to be effectively treated [52]. In acute injuries and using a combined approach, the RC ligaments (both palmar and DRC) are repaired or reattached to the distal radius or to the carpal bones using bone tunnels or suture anchors. The palmar ulnocarpal ligaments must also be repaired and during the healing process, i.e., 6–8 weeks, the alignment of the RC joint is maintained by pinning of the radioscaphoid and radiolunate articulation. An additional external fixator may be necessary.

Delayed ligament repairs usually have disappointing results. In such cases ligament repair alone is insufficient to prevent recurrent ulnar translation, while radiolunate fusion after reduction of the carpus, has been described as the most effective form of treatment [39, 52, 68, 116] (Fig. 8.36a–f). However, in patients whose deformity can be passively corrected and without arthritic changes, ligaments augmentation with a tendon strip can be carried out [115]. Maschke et al. [89] using a brachioradialis tendon tried to recreate the stabilizing effect of the RSC ligament in cadavers while Obafemi and Pensy [109] applied the same technique in a patient with a palmar, 2 weeks old RC dislocation, in order to augment the reconstructed palmar and dorsal RC ligaments. Both authors used the same technique (with minor modifications) in which the brachioradialis tendon was stripped proximally of its muscle, leaving the distal insertion at the radial styloid intact. Then a 3.5 mm drill hole was created in the center of the capitate, with passage of the tendon graft through this drill hole from palmar to dorsal and

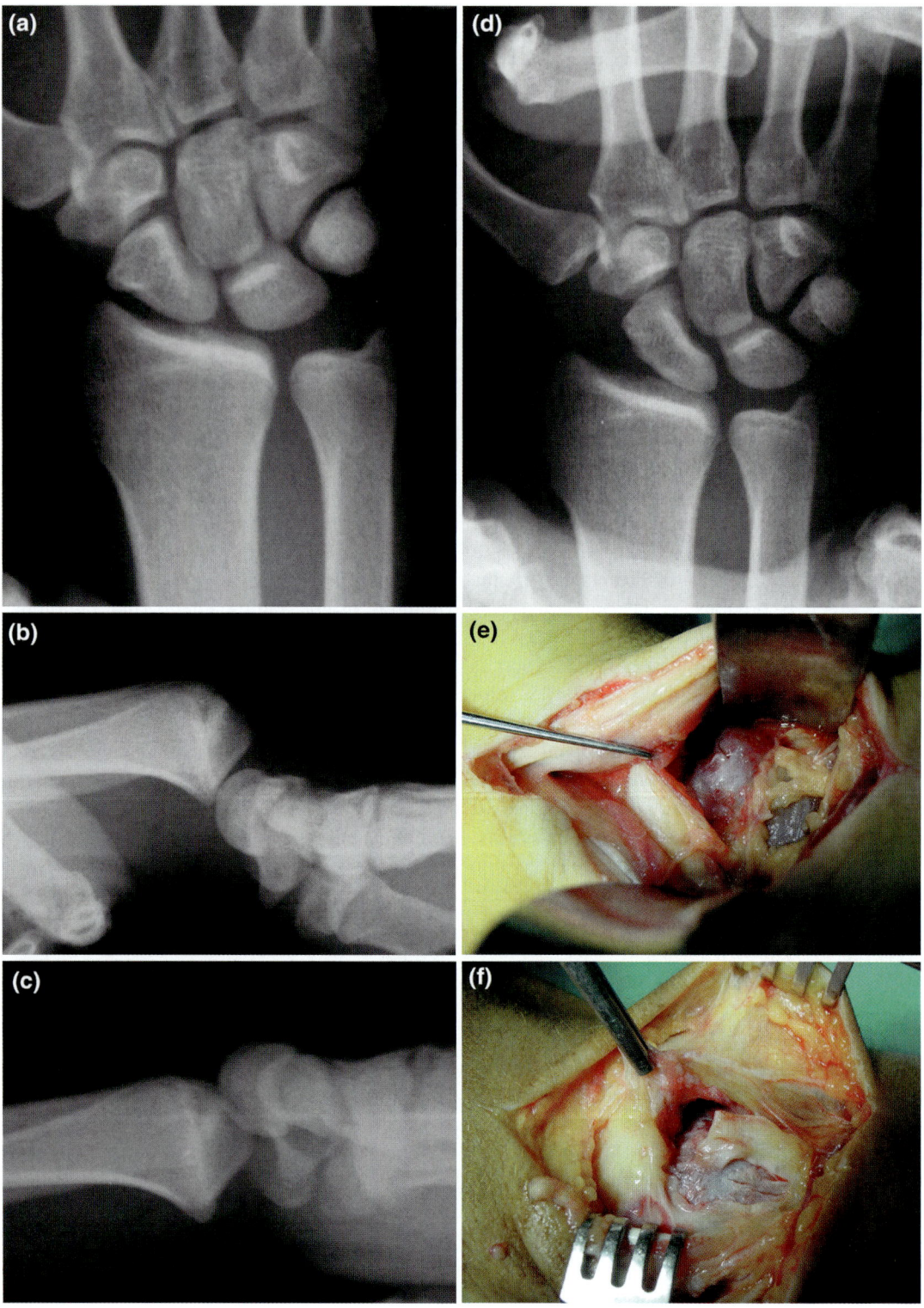

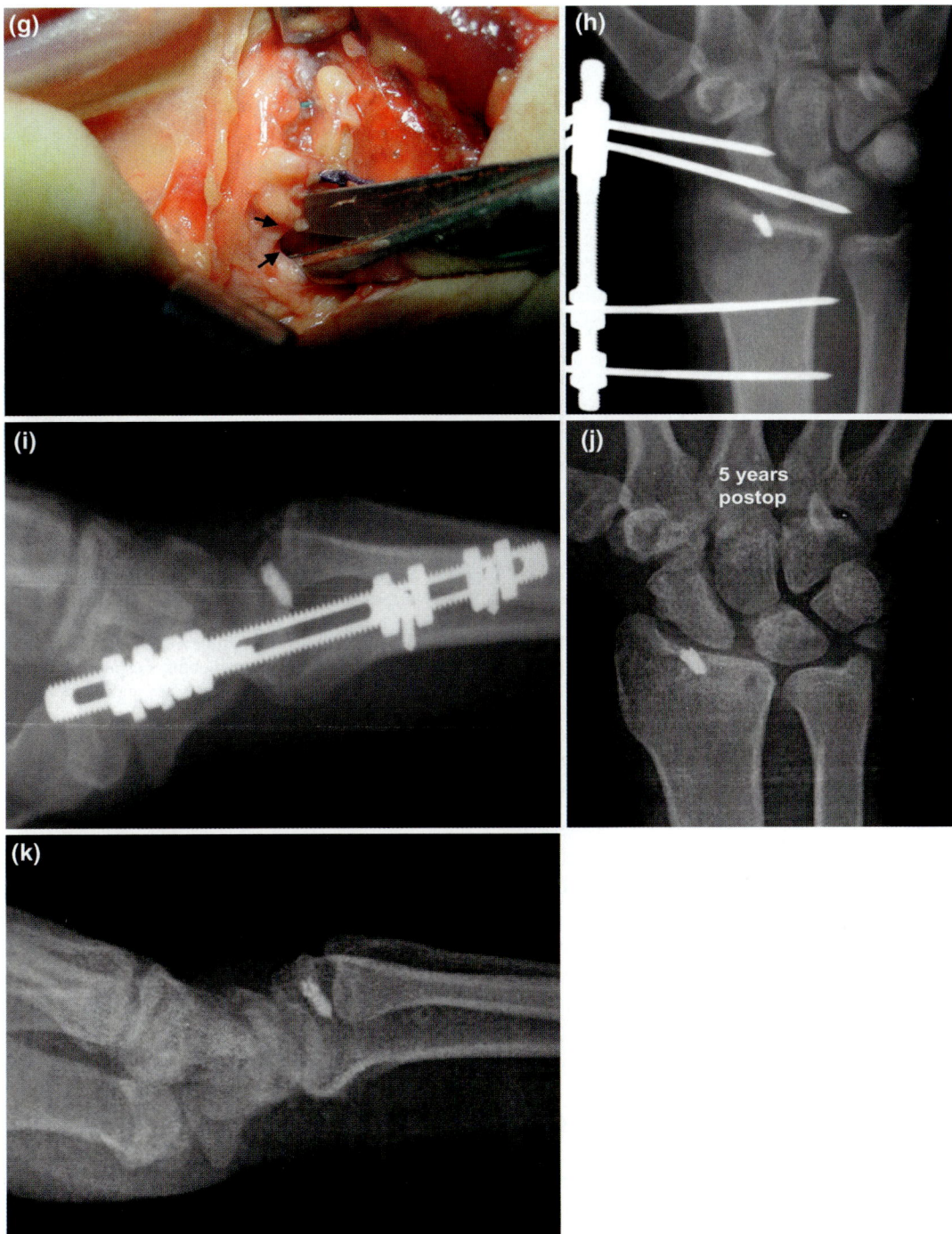

Fig. 8.35 (continued)

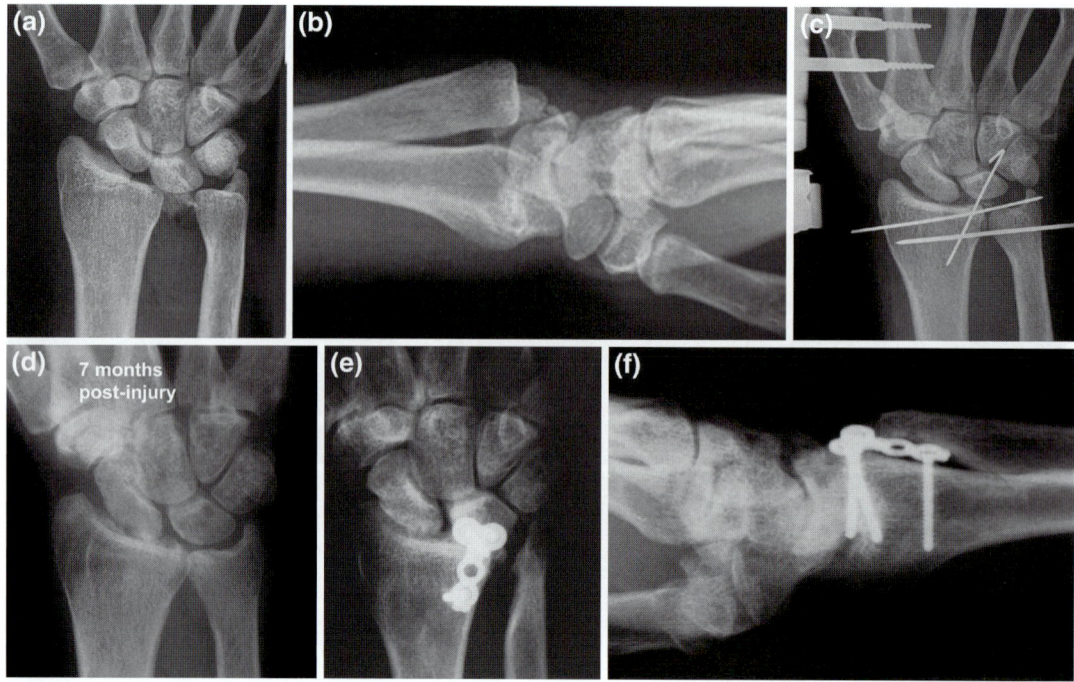

Fig. 8.36 Male, 31 years old, with injury by a press machine. A dorsoulnar RC fracture dislocation with a sizeable fragment comprising the dorsal part of the lunate fossa and the dorsal sigmoid notch, while the DRUJ was subluxated (**a**, **b**); he was treated elsewhere with closed reduction, percutaneously inserted K-wires under image intensifier to stabilize the fractured fragment and an external fixator (**c**); seven months postinjury he was referred to us for pain, wrist stiffness and restriction of forearm supination (**d**); the patient was treated with radiolunate fusion, associated with matched distal-ulnar resection

secured to the dorsum of the distal radius with a 4.5 mm suture anchor just distal to Lister's tubercle.

We used a modification of this technique in cadavers using the brachioradialis tendon to recreate the stabilizing effect of the DRC, palmar LRL, and the palmar ulnocarpal ligaments, using the triquetrum instead of capitate as the anchored bone for the tendon graft (Fig. 8.37a–f). In the first version the tendon graft exiting from the volar triquetrum was inserted into a bony tunnel created at the radiovolar surface of the distal radius. In the second version and given that the proximal stump of the brachioradialis tendon

graft is wide enough, we splitted the exited graft from the volar triquetrum in one radial and one ulnar component. The radial part, substituting the LRL ligament, was inserted into the above mentioned bony tunnel of the distal radius, while the ulnar part, substituting the volar UC ligaments, was inserted into a bony tunnel created at the ulnar fovea, where the UC ligaments are mainly attached.

By manually testing the stability of the RC joint, particularly the second version of the above-mentioned tenodesis proved to be effective, but further studies are needed (Fig. 8.38a, b).

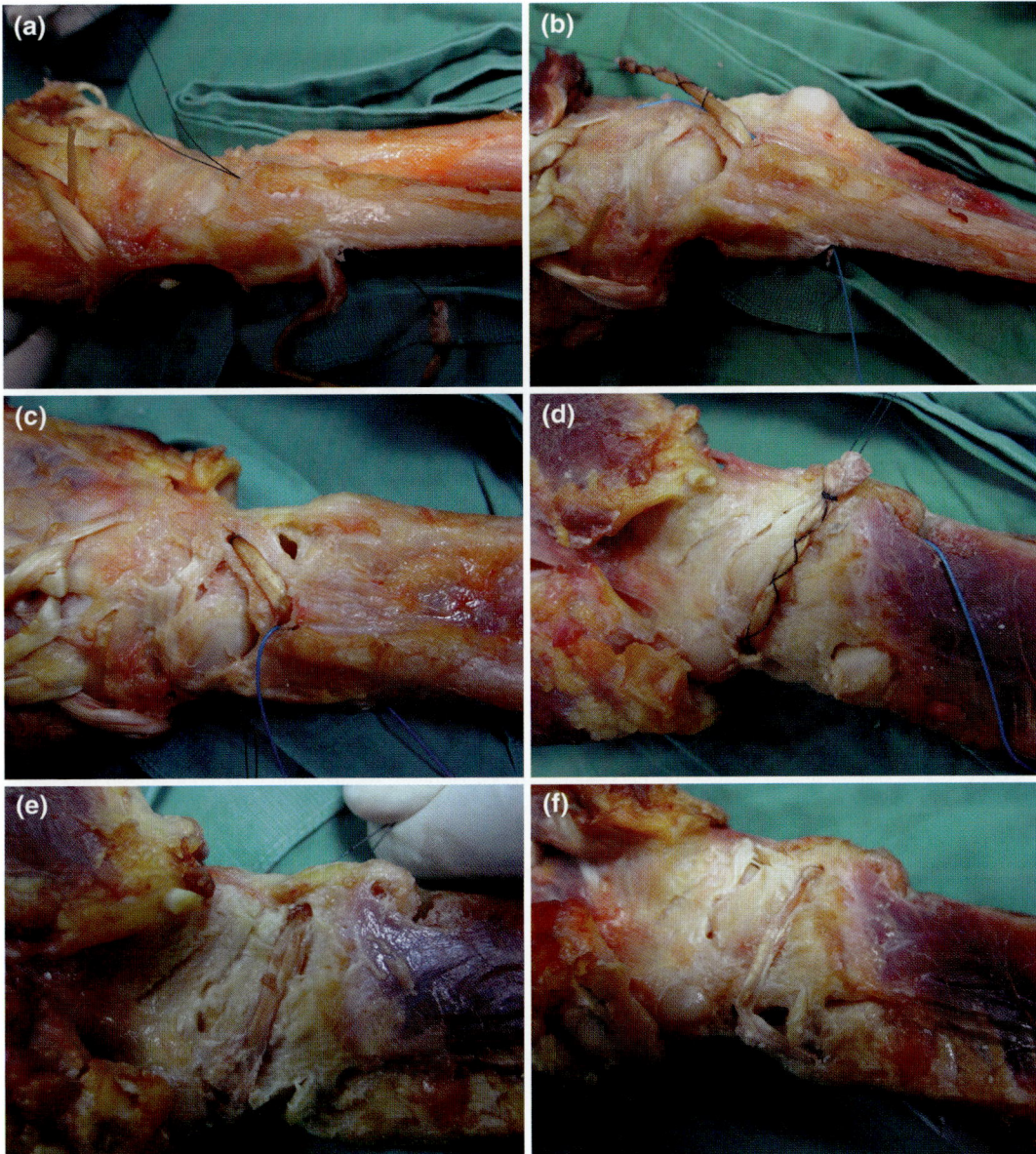

Fig. 8.37 A bony tunnel was created just proximal to the brachioradialis insertion exiting dorsally, where the DRC ligament is attached to the radius (**a**); the tendon graft was passed through the tunnel exiting ulnar to Lister's tubercle (**b**); the tendon graft was inserted into a bone tunnel created at the triquetrum dorsally to volarly (**c**); the graft exiting from the volar surface of the triquetrum (**d**); in the first version, the tendon graft was inserted into a bony tunnel created where the LRL ligament attaches to the radius (**e**); in the second version the graft was splitted and its radial part was inserted as previously mentioned, while its ulnar part was inserted and fixed into a bone tunnel at the ulnar fovea (**f**)

Fig. 8.38 The wrist was manually translated in ulnar direction after sectioning of the DRC, volar RC, and volar UC ligaments (**a**); the wrist stability seemed to be restored after rerouting the brachioradialis tendon (second version) (**b**)

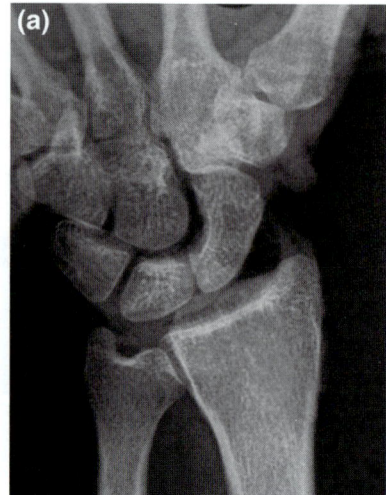 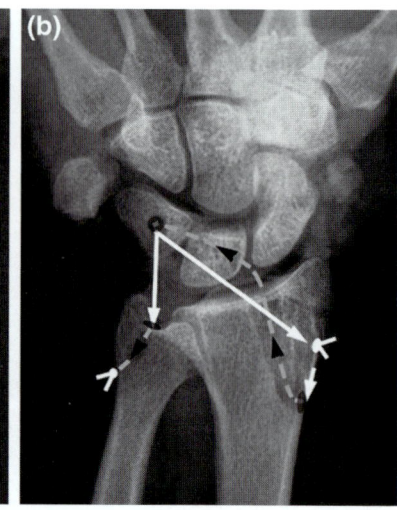

References

1. Fernandez DL, Jupiter JB (2002) Fracture of the distal end of the radius: a historical perspective. In: Fernandez DL, Jupiter JB (eds) Fractures of the distal radius. A practical approach to management, Chap 1, 2nd edn. Springer, New York, pp 1–22
2. Ilyas A, Mudgal C (2008) Radiocarpal Fracture-dislocations. J Am Acad Orthop Surg 16:647–655
3. Destot E (1926) Injuries of the wrist: a radiological study. Hoeber, New York
4. Gui L (1957) Fratture e lussazioni. Edizioni scientifiche Instituto Ortopedico toscano, Firenze, p 510
5. Rosado AP (1966) A possible relationship of radiocarpal dislocation and dislocation of the lunate bone. J Bone Joint Surg Am 48:504–506
6. Dunn AW (1972) Fractures and dislocations of the carpus. Surg Clin North Am 52:1513–1518
7. Bilos ZJ, Pankovich AM, Yelda S (1977) Fracture-dislocation of the radiocarpal joint. J Bone Joint Surg Am 59:198–203
8. Dumontier C, Lenoble E, Saffar P (1995) Radiocarpal dislocations and fractures-dislocations. In: Saffar P, Cooney WP (eds) Fractures of the distal radius. Martin Dunitz, London, pp 267–278
9. Moneim MS, Bolger JT, Omer GE (1985) Radiocarpal dislocation–classification and rationale for management. Clin Orthop 192:199–209
10. Ilyas AM, Williamson C, Mudgal CS (2011) Radiocarpal dislocation: is it a rare injury? J Hand Surg [Eur] 36(2):164
11. Bellinghausen HW, Gilula LA, Young LV et al (1983) Post-traumatic palmar carpal subluxation. Report of two cases. J Bone Joint Surg Am 65:998–1006
12. Le Nen D, Riot O, Caro P et al (1991) Luxation-fractures of the radiocarpal joint. Clinical study of 6 cases and general review. Ann Chir Main Memb Super 10:5–12
13. Mourikis A, Rebello G, Villafuente J et al (2008) Radiocarpal dislocations: review of the literature with case presentations and a proposed treatment algorithm. Orthopedics 31:386
14. Naranja RJ, Bozentka DJ, Partington MT et al (1998) Radiocarpal dislocation: a report of two cases and a review of the literature. Am J Orthop 27(2):141–144
15. Schoenecker PL, Gilula LA, Shively RA et al (1985) Radiocarpal fracture-dislocation. Clin Orthop 197:237–244
16. Apergis E, Dimitrakopoulos K, Chorianopoulos K (1996) Late management of post-traumatic palmar carpal subluxation: A case report. J Bone Joint Surg Br 78:419–421
17. Arslan H, Tokmak M (2002) Isolated ulnar radiocarpal dislocation. Arch Orthop Trauma Surg 122:179–181
18. Ayekoloye CI, Shah N, Kumar A et al (2002) Irreducible dorsal radiocarpal fracture dislocation with dissociation of the distal radioulnar joint: a case report. Acta Orthop Belg 68(2):171–174
19. Dodd CA (1987) Triple dislocation in the upper limb. J Trauma 27:1307
20. Fehring TK, Milek MA (1984) Isolated volar dislocation of the radiocarpal joint. A case report. J Bone Joint Surg Am 66:464–466
21. Fennell CW, McMurtry RY, Fairbanks CJ (1992) Multidirectional radiocarpal dislocation without fracture: a case report. J Hand Surg [Am] 17:756–761
22. Fernandez DL (1981) Irreducible radiocarpal fracture-dislocation and radioulnar dissociation with entrapment of the ulnar nerve, artery and

flexor profundus II-V-case report. J Hand Surg
[Am] 6:456–461
23. Freeland A, Ferguson CA, McCraney WO (2006)
Palmar radiocarpal dislocation resulting in ulnar
radiocarpal translocation and multidirectional
instability. Orthopedics 29(7):604–608
24. Freund LG, Ovesen J (1977) Isolated dorsal
dislocation of the radiocarpal joint. J Bone Joint
Surg Am 59:277
25. Hardy P, Welby F, Stromboni M et al (1999) Wrist
arthroscopy and dislocation of the radiocarpal joint
without fracture. Arthroscopy 15(7):779–783
26. Howard RF, Slawski DP, Gilula LA (1997) Isolated
palmar radiocarpal dislocation and ulnar
translocation: a case report and review of the
literature. J Hand Surg [Am] 22(1):78–82
27. Jebson PJL, Adams BD, Meletiou SD (2000) Ulnar
translocation instability of the carpus after a dorsal
radiocarpal dislocation; a case report. Am J Orthop
29(6):462–464
28. Matthews MG (1987) Radiocarpal dislocation with
associated avulsion of the radial styloid and fracture
of the shaft of the ulna. Injury 18:70–71
29. Moore DP, McMahon BA (1988) Anterior radiocarpal dislocation: an isolated injury. J Hand Surg
[Br] 13:215–217
30. Penny WH III, Green TL (1988) Volar radiocarpal
dislocation with ulnar translocation. J Orthop
Trauma 2:322–326
31. Reynolds ISR (1980) Dorsal carpal dislocation.
Injury 12:48–49
32. Tanzer TL, Horne JG (1980) Dorsal radiocarpal
fracture dislocation. J Trauma 20:999–1000
33. Thomsen S, Falstie-Jensen S (1989) Palmar
dislocation of the radiocarpal joint. J Hand Surg
[Am] 14:627–630
34. Varodompun N, Limpivest P, Prinyaroj P (1985)
Isolated dorsal radiocarpal dislocation: case report
and literature review. J Hand Surg [Am]
10:708–710
35. Nyquist SR, Stern PJ (1984) Open radiocarpal
fracture-dislocations. J Hand Surg [Am] 9:707–710
36. Mudgal CS, Psenica J, Jupiter JB (1999)
Radiocarpal fracture-dislocation. J Hand Surg [Br]
24:92–98
37. Girard J, Cassagnaud X, Maynou C et al (2004)
Radiocarpal dislocation: Twelve cases and a review
of the literature. Rev Chir Orthop 90:426–433
38. Dumontier C, Zu Reckendorf GM, Sautet A et al
(2001) Radiocarpal dislocations: classification and
proposal for treatment (a review of twenty-seven
cases). J Bone Joint Surg Am 83:212–218
39. Taleisnik J (1985) The wrist. Churchill Livingstone,
New York
40. Kapandji IA (1991) Etude du carpe au scanner a
trois dimensions sous contraintes de
pronosupination. Ann Chir Main 10:36–47
41. Ritt MJPF, Stuart PR, Berglund LJ et al (1995)
Rotational stability of the carpus relative to the
forearm. J Hand Surg [Am] 20(2):305–311
42. Roux JL (1992) La rotation longitudinale radio-
metacarpienne. Thesis. Montpellier, France
43. Taleisnik J (1978) Wrist: anatomy, function, and
injury. AAOS Instr Course Lect 27:61–68
44. Gupta A, Moosawi NA (2005) How much can
carpus rotate axially? An in vivo study. Clin
Biomech 20(2):172–176
45. Heras-Palou C (2009) Midcarpal instability. In:
Slutsky DJ, Osterman AL (eds) Fractures and
injuries of the distal radius and carpus. The
Cutting edge. Saunders, Philadelphia, pp 417–423
46. Katz DA, Green JK, Werner FW et al (2003)
Capsuloligamentous restraints to dorsal and palmar
carpal translation. J Hand Surg [Am] 28(4):610–613
47. Berger RA, Landsmeer JM (1990) The palmar
radiocarpal ligaments: a study of adult and fetal
human wrist joints. J Hand Surg [Am] 15:847–854
48. Berger RA (1997) The ligaments of the wrist. Hand
Clin 13(1):63–82
49. Garcia-Elias M (1997) Kinetic analysis of carpal
stability during grip. Hand Clin 13:151–158
50. Viegas SF, Patterson RM, Ward K (1995) Extrinsic
wrist ligaments in the pathomechanics of ulnar
translation instability. J Hand Surg [Am] 20:312–318
51. Werner FW, Sutton LG, Allison MA et al (2010)
Scaphoid and lunate translation in the intact wrist
and following ligament resection: a cadaver study.
J Hand Surg [Am] 36(2):291–298
52. Rayhack JM, Linscheid RL, Dobyns JH et al (1987)
Posttraumatic ulnar translation of the carpus.
J Hand Surg [Am] 12:180–189
53. Munk B, Jensen SL, Olsen BS et al (2005) Wrist
stability after experimental traumatic triangular
fibrocartilage complex lesions. J Hand Surg [Am]
30(1):43–49
54. Wiesner L, Rumelhart C, Pham E et al (1996)
Experimentally induced ulno-carpal instability. A
study on 13 cadaver wrists. J Hand Surg [Br]
21(1):24–29
55. Allieu Y, Garcia-Elias M (2000) Dynamic radial
translation instability of the carpus. J Hand Surg
[Br] 25(1):33–37
56. Yin Y, Mann FA, Hodge JC et al (1996)
Roentgenographic interpretation of ligamentous
instabilities of the wrist. In: Gilula LA, Yin Y
(eds) Imaging of the wrist and hand. WB Saunders,
Philadelphia, pp 203–224
57. Moritomo H, Murase T, Arimitsu S et al (2008)
Change in the length of the ulnocarpal ligaments
during radiocarpal motion: possible impact on
triangular fibrocartilage complex foveal tears.
J Hand Surg [Am] 33(8):1278–1286
58. Iwamoto A, Morris RP, Andersen C et al (2006) An
anatomic and biomechanic study of the wrist
extensor retinaculum septa and tendon
compartments. J Hand Surg [Am] 31(6):896–903
59. Hagert E, Persson JKE, Werner M et al (2009)
Evidence of wrist proprioceptive reflexes elicited
after stimulation of the scapholunate interosseous
ligament. J Hand Surg [Am] 34:642–651

60. An KN, Horii E, Ryu J (1991) Muscle function. In: An KN, Berger EJ, Cooney WP (eds) Biomechanics of the wrist joint. Springer, New York, pp 157–169

61. Brand PW (1981) Relative tension and potential excursion of muscles in forearm and hand. J Hand Surg [Am] 6:209–219

62. Hagert E, Forsgren S, Ljung BO (2005) Differences in the presence of mechanoreceptors and nerve structures between wrist ligaments may imply differential roles in wrist stabilization. J Orthop Res 23:757–763

63. Salva-Coll G, Garcia-Elias M, Leon-Lopez MT (2011) Effects of forearm muscles on carpal stability. J Hand Surg [Eur] 36(7):553–559

64. Berger RA, Amadio PC (1994) Predicting palmar radio-carpal ligament disruption in fractures of the distal articular surface of the radius involving the palmar cortex. J Hand Surg [Br] 19:108–113

65. Siegel DB, Gelberman RH (1991) Radial styloidectomy: an anatomical study with special reference to radiocarpal intracapsular ligamentous morphology. J Hand Surg [Am] 16:40–44

66. Mandziak DG, Watts AC, Bain GI (2011) Ligament contribution to patterns of articular fractures of the distal radius. J Hand Surg [Am] 36(10):1621–1625

67. Giunta R, Lower N, Kierse R et al (1997) Stress on the radiocarpal joint. CT studies of subchondral bone density in vivo. Handchir Mikrochir Plast Chir 29:32–37

68. Fernandez DL, Jupiter JB, Ghillani R (2002) Radiocarpal fracture-dislocation. In: Fernandez DL, Jupiter JB (eds) Fractures of the distal radius. A practical approach to management, Chap 8, 2nd edn. Springer, New York, pp 253–264

69. Ilyas A, Mudgal C, Jupiter J (2009) Volar rim and Barton's fracture. In: Slutsky DJ, Osterman AL (eds) Fractures and injuries to the distal radius and carpus, Chap 14. Saunders Elsevier, pp 157–163

70. Bohler L (1930) Verrenkungen der Handgelenke. Acta Chir Scand 67:154–177

71. Weiss C, Laskin RS, Spinner M (1970) Irreducible radiocarpal dislocation. J Bone Joint Surg Am 52:562–564

72. Bohler L (1956) The treatment of fractures. Grune & Stratton, New York, pp 826–854

73. Graham TJ (2003) The inferior arc injury: an addition to the family of complex carpal fracture-dislocation patterns. Am J Orthop 32(9):10–19

74. Sivan M, Davies N, Archibald C et al (2005) An unusual combination of radiocarpal fracture dislocation, scaphoid fracture and posteromedial elbow dislocation. Injury Extra 36:312–315

75. Watanabe K, Nishikimi J (2001) Transstyloid radiocarpal dislocation. Hand Surg 6(1):113–120

76. Oberladstätter J, Arora R, Dallapozza C et al (2010) Radiological radio-carpal and mid-carpal motion after operative treatment of dorsal radio-carpal fracture dislocations. Arch Orthop Trauma Surg 130:77–81

77. Jupiter JB, Fernandez DL, Toh CL et al (1996) Operative treatment of volar intra-articular fractures of the distal end of the radius. J Bone Joint Surg Am 78(12):1817–1828

78. Helm RH, Tonkin MA (1992) The chauffeur's fracture. Simple or complex? J Hand Surg [Br] 17(2):156–159

79. Apergis E, Darmanis S, Theodoratos G et al (2002) Beware of the ulno-palmar distal radial fragment. J Hand Surg [Br] 27:139–145

80. Harness NG, Jupiter JB, Orbay JL et al (2004) Loss of fixation of the volar lunate facet fragment in fractures of the distal part of the radius. J Bone Joint Surg Am 86(9):1900–1908

81. Cohen MS, McMurtry RY, Jupiter JB (1998) Fractures of the distal radius. In: Browner BD, Jupiter JB, Levine AM, Trafton PG (eds) Skeletal Trauma, 2nd edn. WB Saunders, Philadelphia, p 1385

82. Fernandez DL, Jupiter JB (2002) Articular marginal shearing fractures. In: Fernandez DL, Jupiter JB (eds) Fractures of the distal radius. A practical approach to management, Chap 6, 2nd edn. Springer, New York, pp 188–212

83. King RE (1959) Barton's enigma. J Bone Joint Surg Am 41:753–769

84. Lozano-Calderón SA, Doornberg J, Ring D (2006) Fractures of the dorsal articular margin of the distal part of the radius with dorsal radiocarpal subluxation. J Bone Joint Surg Am 88(7):1486–1493

85. Stoffelen D, Fortems Y, De Smet L et al (1996) Dislocation of the distal radioulnar joint associated with a transstyloid radiocarpal fracture dislocation a case report and review of the literature. Acta Orthop Belg 62(2):52–55

86. Idler RS (2001) Carpal dislocations and instability. In: Watson HK, Weinzweig J (eds) The Wrist, vol 1. Lippincott Williams & Wilkins, pp 203–229

87. Capo JT, Armbruster ED, Hashem J (2010) Proximal carpal row dislocation: a case report. Hand 5:444–448

88. Klein A, Bohrer SP, Martin W III (1986) Dorsal dislocation of the radiocarpal joint with associated dorsal perilunar dislocation. Can Assoc Radiol J 37(3):201–202

89. Maschke S, Means KR, Parks BG et al (2010) A radiocarpal ligament reconstruction using brachioradialis for secondary ulnar translation of the carpus following radiocarpal dislocation: a cadaver study. J Hand Surg [Am] 35(2):256–261

90. Kamal RN, Bariteau JT, Beutel BG et al (2011) Arthroscopic reduction and percutaneous pinning of a radiocarpal dislocation. A case report. J Bone Joint Surg [Am] 93(15):1–5

91. Campbell DA (2009) Ulnar head and styloid fractures. In: Slutsky DJ, Osterman AL (eds) Fractures and injuries to the distal radius and carpus. The cutting edge, Chap 28. Saunders, Philadeiphia, pp 297–308

92. Nakamura T, Moy OJ, Peimer CA (2003) Relationship between the ulnar styloid fracture and DRUJ instability. J Hand Surg [Br] 28(1):48

93. Gabl M, Lener M, Pechlaner S (1993) Destabilization of the discus articularis with rupture of the ulnar styloid apex in distal radius fracture. Diagnosis with dynamic MR. Unfallchirurgie 19:108

94. Lindau T, Adlercreutz C, Aspenberg P (2000) Peripheral tears of the triangular fibrocartilage complex cause distal radioulnar joint instability after distal radial fractures. J Hand Surg [Am] 25(3):464–468

95. Souer JS, Ring D, Matschke S et al (2009) Effect of an unrepaired fracture of the ulnar styloid base on outcome after plate-and-screw fixation of a distal radial fracture. J Bone Joint Surg Am 91(4):830–838

96. May MM, Lawton JN, Blazar PE (2002) Ulnar styloid fractures associated with distal radius fractures: incidence and implications for distal radioulnar joint instability. J Hand Surg [Am] 27(6):965–971

97. Atzei A, Luchetti R (2011) Foveal TFCC tear classification and treatment. Hand Clin 27(3):263–272

98. Bozentka DJ, Beredjiklian PK (2001) Classification of radiocarpal dislocations and appropriate treatment. J Bone Joint Surg Am 83(10):1587–1588

99. Hofmeister EP, Fitzgerald BT, Thomson MA et al (2008) Surgical reconstruction of a late-presenting volar radiocarpal dislocation: a case report. Am J Orthop 37(2):96–99

100. Takase K, Yamamoto K, Yoshino S et al (2004) Palmar dislocation of the radio-carpal joint: a case report. J Orthop Surg 12(2):258–262

101. Gilula LA (1979) Carpal injuries: analytic approach and case exercises. Am J Roentgenol 133:503–517

102. Lipton HA, Jupiter J (2001) Open reduction and internal fixation of distal radius fractures. In: Watson HK, Weinzweig J (eds) The wrist. Lippincott Williams & Wilkins, pp 333–335

103. Antuna SA, Mendez JG, Paz Jimenez J (1994) Displaced radiocarpal dislocation with multiple associated fractures. Acta Orthop Belg 60:430–431

104. Lourie JA (1982) An unusual dislocation of the lunate and the wrist. J Trauma 22:966–967

105. Berger RA, Weiss AP (2004) Hand Surgery. Lippincott Williams & Wilkins

106. Cooney WP, Linscheid RL, Dobyns JH (1998) The Wrist. Diagnosis and operative treatment. Mosby, St. Louis

107. Watson HK, Weinzeig J (2001) The Wrist. Lippincott Williams & Wilkins

108. Chin KR, Jupiter JB (1999) Wire-loop fixation of volar displaced osteochondral fractures of the distal radius. J Hand Surg [Am] 24:525–533

109. Obafemi A, Pensy R (2012) Palmar radiocarpal dislocation: a case report and novel treatment method. Hand 7:114–118

110. Schweitzer G (1987) Radiocarpal fracture-dislocation [letter]. Clin Orthop 216:298–299

111. Patee G, Thomson G (1988) Anterior and posterior marginal fracture-dislocations of the distal radius.

An analysis of the results of treatment. Clin Orthop 231:183–195

112. Knirk JL, Jupiter JB (1986) Intra-articular fractures of the distal end of the radius in young adults. J Bone Joint Surg Am 68(5):647–659

113. Dobyns JH, Linscheid RL, Chao EYS et al (1975) Traumatic instability of the wrist. In: AAOS instructional course lectures, vol 24. CV Mosby, St Louis, pp 182–199

114. Berschback JC, Kalainov DM, Husain SN et al (2012) Traumatic ulnar translocation of the carpus: early recognition and treatment. J Hand Surg [Eur] 37(8):755–764

115. Mulier T, Reynders P, Broos P et al (1992) Posttraumatic ulnar translation of the carpus. Acta Orthop Scand 63(1):102–103

116. Schernberg F (1996) Ulnar translation of the carpus: a rare type of wrist instability. In: Buchler U (ed) Wrist instability, Chap 23. Martin Dunitz, Philadelphia, pp 175–179

117. Garcia-Elias M (1999) Carpal instabilities and dislocations. In: Green DP, Hotchkiss RN, Pederson WC (eds) Green's operative hand surgery,Chap 28, vol 1. Churchill Livingstone, New York, pp 865–928

118. Rettig AC, Rettig LA, Jelinek JA (2010) Ulnar translocation of the wrist in a professional quarterback: a case report. Am J Sports Med 38(3):608–612

119. Rutgers M, Jupiter J, Ring D (2009) Isolated posttraumatic ulnar translocation of the radiocarpal joint. J Hand Microsurg 1(2):108–112

120. Stabler A, Baumeister RGH, Szeimies U et al (1994) Rotatory palmar subluxation of the lunate in post-traumatic ulnar carpal translocation. Skeletal Radiol 23:103–106

121. Chamay A, Della Santa D, Vilaseca A (1983) Radiolunate arthrodesis. Factor of stability for the rheumatoid wrist. Ann Chir Main 2:5–17

122. DiBenedetto MR, Lubbers LM, Coleman CR (1990) A standardized measurement of ulnar carpal translocation. J Hand Surg [Am] 15:1009–1010

123. McMurtry RY, Youm Y, Flatt AE et al (1978) Kinematics of the wrist. II. Clinical applications. J Bone Joint Surg Am 60:955–961

124. Bouman HW, Messer E, Sennwald G (1994) Measurement of ulnar translation and carpal height. J Hand Surg [Br] 19:325–329

125. Gilula LA, Weeks PM (1978) Post-traumatic ligamentous instabilities of the wrist. Radiology 129:641–651

126. Schuind FA, Linscheid RL, An KN et al (1992) A normal data base of posteroanterior roentgenographic measurements of the wrist. J Bone Joint Surg Am 74:1418–1429

127. Apergis E (2004) καταγματα-εξαρθρήματα του καρπου. Konstantaras Medical Books, Athens

Carpometacarpal (CMC) Dislocations or Fractures-Dislocations Excluding the Thumb

9

9.1   Introduction

Malgaigne in 1855 stated that up to that time only three cases of dislocation of Carpometacarpal (CMC) joints had been reported. The first of these cases was an isolated dislocation of the base of the third MC, reported by Blandin in 1844. The second case, also an isolated dislocation of the base of the third MC, was reported by Roux in 1848; and the third case was an isolated dislocation of the base of the second MC reported by Bourguet in 1853. Vigouroux, in 1856, was the first to report a multiple CMC dislocation, involving the bases of the second, third, fourth and fifth MC; Rivington, in 1873, was the first to report a case of multiple dislocations of the bases of all five metacarpals (cited by Waugh and Yancey [1]).

In contradistinction to the thumb CMC joint, injuries of the four ulnar CMC joints are referred to as "finger carpometacarpal" [2] or as "medial four CMC" [3] injuries.

Although CMC injuries of the thumb are not uncommon, those of the base of one or more of the four medial metacarpals are rather rare. The clinical problems arising from injury of the 2nd to 5th CMC joints differ sufficiently from those of the thumb, to warrant separate consideration [4].

Dislocations of the CMC joints disrupt the normal transverse and longitudinal arches of the palm, impair grip strength, and can also affect the balance between intrinsic and extrinsic muscles when there is proximal displacement of the metacarpal. This displacement causes laxity of the extrinsic muscle tendons. Sterling Bunnell in 1944 [5] was the first to emphasize the importance of early anatomical reduction of all CMC dislocations, when he supported that "reduction is necessary to restore muscular balance and proper mechanics of the hand".

Injuries of the CMC joints are rare and represent less than 1 % of all wrist and hand injuries [6, 7]. Dobyns et al. [8] reported only 3 such injuries in a series of 1,621 fractures and dislocations of the hand and wrist over 3 years at a military hospital (0.18 %).

In cases of CMC joint injuries, the coexistence of a distal carpal row fracture is quite frequent. Garcia-Elias [9] reported that out of 50 patients with traumatic fracture-dislocation of the CMC joints, 13 (26 %) also presented major fracture of the capitate, hamate or trapezoid, which resulted in subluxation or dislocation of the respective metacarpal base.

9.2   Anatomy

The CMC joints are anatomically stable and their stability is the result of: interlocking saddle joints, complex ligamentous support and dynamic protection by the long flexor and extensor tendons and intrinsic muscles [10].

The distal row of carpal bones forms a fixed transverse arch, while the ring and little fingers on the ulnar side of this arch and the thumb on the radial side, form two mobile longitudinal arches. Both longitudinal arches provide

E. Apergis, *Fracture-Dislocations of the Wrist*,
DOI: 10.1007/978-88-470-5328-1_9, © Springer-Verlag Italia 2013

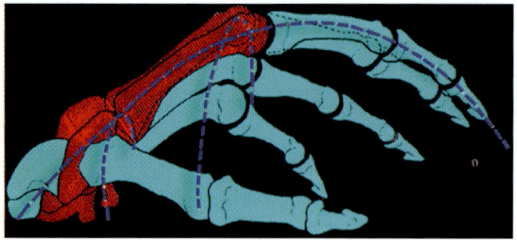

Fig. 9.1 The distal carpal row with the longitudinal arches of the index and middle fingers constitute the stable central unit of the hand. With permission from [132]

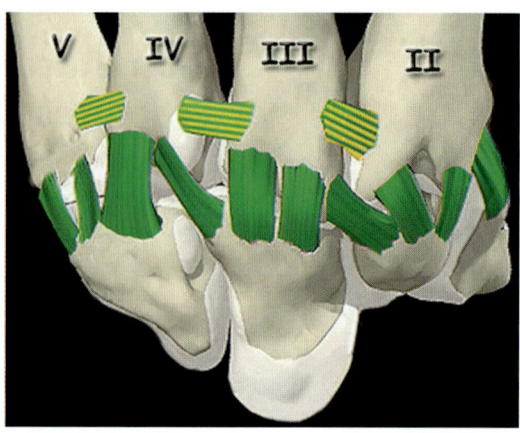

Fig. 9.2 The dorsal CMC and the three inter-metacarpal ligaments. With permission from [132]

mobility about a fixed central unit comprising the index and middle fingers, whose metacarpals are firmly fixed to the distal carpal row [6] (Fig. 9.1). These bones establish the functional transverse and longitudinal arches of the hand.

Experimental studies have indicated less than 1° of motion in the flexion–extension plane at the second ray and 3° at the third ray. Conversely, the flexion–extension motion for the 4th ray is approximately 10°–15° and 15°–30° for the 5th ray [6, 11, 12].

A kinematic analysis of the 2nd through 5th CMC joints using three-dimesional computerized imaging, revealed that the overall flexion–extension motions of the 2nd, 3rd, 4th, and 5th CMC joints, were found to be 11°, 7°, 20° and 27°, respectively; in radial-ulnar deviation 2°, 4°, 7°, and 13°, respectively and in pronation-supination motion 5°, 5°, 27°, and 22°, respectively [13]. This study moreover revealed that the range of motion of the 5th CMC joint reduces by 40 % when the 4th CMC joint is immobilized.

The anatomy of the ligaments and the formation of the articular surfaces of the CMC joints have not been sufficiently described, not only because literature reports are few, but also because there is a considerable number of anatomic varieties [6, 12, 14, 15]. Harwin et al. [12] reported seven dorsal CMC ligaments and eight palmar CMC ligaments of the 2nd through 5th CMC joint. Gurland [6] reported six dorsal CMC ligaments and six palmar CMC ligaments. Nakamura et al. [15] described nine dorsal CMC ligaments and seven palmar CMC ligaments and specifically: dorsally he reported two for the 5th, two for the 4th, three for the 3rd, and two for the

2nd CMC joint (Fig. 9.2) and volarly: one for the 5th, one for the 4th, four for the 3rd, and one for the 2nd CMC joint. Nanno et al. [16] in a three-dimensional analysis of the ligamentous attachments of the 2nd through 5th CMC joints, identified 9 dorsal and 11 palmar CMC ligaments.

Additional ligamentous restraint is provided by 3 dorsal and 3 palmar intermetacarpal ligaments that connect the bases of the metacarpals [15], while Nanno et al. [16] identified 4 dorsal and 4 palmar intermetacarpal ligaments of the 2nd through 5th CMC joints. In addition, one intraarticular ligament extending between the 3rd and 4th MC and capitate—hamate was also identified [15, 16], which secures stability even upon rupture of the dorsal and palmar ligaments. However, the role that these ligaments might play in the pathomechanics of axial disruptions and/or CMC dislocations and fracture-dislocations of the carpus has not been well described.

Of particular, importance is the pisometacarpal ligament extending between the pisiform and the ulnovolar base of the 5th metacarpal, through which the flexor carpi ulnaris exerts its effect (Fig. 9.3).

The strong periarticular ligamentous supports of the CMC joints render the anyway rare CMC fracture-dislocations, more frequent than pure dislocations. Although the dorsal ligaments are described as stronger and more distinct than their volar counterparts, dorsal dislocations are more frequent.

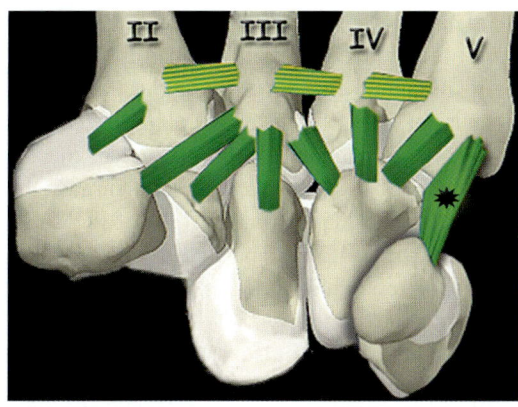

Fig. 9.3 The volar CMC and the three volar inter-metacarpal ligaments. The pisometacarpal ligament is indicated with the *asterisk*. With permission from [132]

The extensor and flexor tendons of the wrist ensure dynamic stabilization by adhering to the base of the 2nd MC (flexor carpi radialis and extensor carpi radialis longus), the base of the 3rd MC (extensor carpi radialis brevis), and the base of the 5th MC (extensor carpi ulnaris and flexor carpi ulnaris via the pisometacarpal ligament) [6, 17] (Fig. 9.4a, b).

There is more variability and often multiple distinct joint surfaces forming the articulations between adjacent metacarpals and/or adjacent distal carpal bones. Nakamura et al. [15] recognized two types of articulation between the 2nd and 3rd MC, five types of articulation between the 3rd and 4th MCs, while the articulations between the 4th and 5th MCs, between the 2nd MC and the trapezium, and between the trapezoid and the trapezium were all single articulations. The authors also noticed that the area of the 2nd and 3rd CMC joints was found to have the highest incidence (18 %) of carpal coalition. Viegas et al. [18] reported that the joint surfaces between the 4th MC and the capitate and/or the hamate were variable and recognized 5 different types of articulation: A type I, with a single dorsal projection radially, a type II with a double projection radially, a type III with a narrow radioulnar dimension without any projection, a type IV with a narrow radio-ulnar dimension of the base and a separate small articular surface dorsoradially, and finally, a type V with a broad radioulnar dimension of the articular base of the 4th metacarpal.

The base of the 2nd MC has a cuneiform configuration and articulates with the corresponding surfaces of the trapezium-trapezoid. The 3rd metacarpal base has a dorsoradial styloid process that articulates with the base of

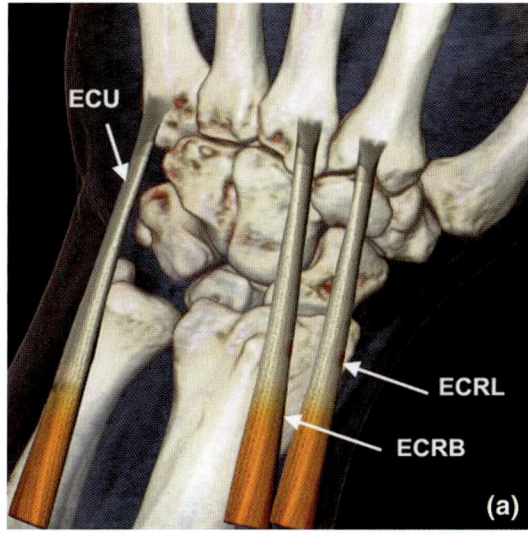
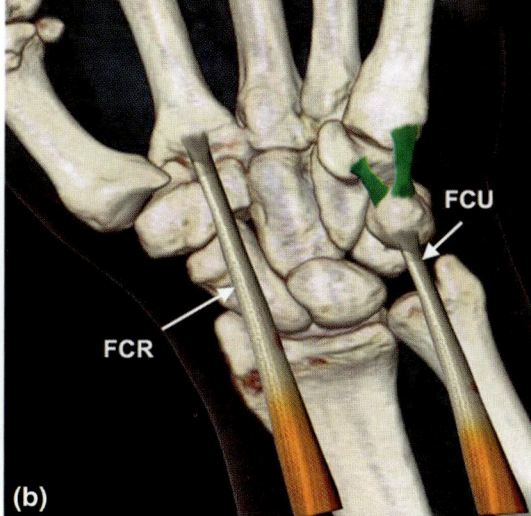

Fig. 9.4 The relation of the extensors (**a**) and flexor (**b**) tendons with the CMC joints. (*ECU* Extensor carpi ulnaris, *ECRB* Extensor carpi radialis brevis, *ECRL* Extensor carpi radialis longus, *FCR* Flexor carpi radialis, *FCU* Flexor carpi ulnaris)

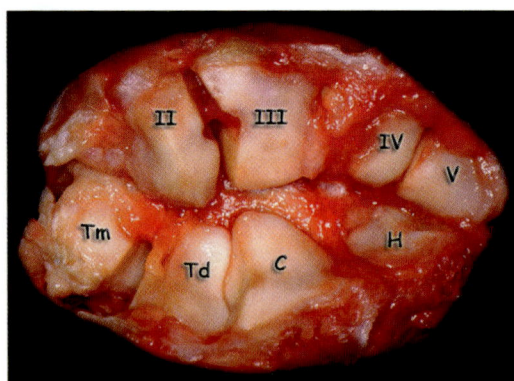

Fig. 9.5 The CMC joints opened dorsally and hinged volarly. The anatomic configuration is described in the text (*Tm* Trapezium, *Td* Trapezoid, *C* Capitate, *H* Hamate). With permission from [132]

the 2nd metacarpal, while ulnarly it has a double articular surface that articulates with the 4th MC and proximally with the capitate. The 4th and 5th metacarpals articulate with the saddle-shaped distal articular surface of the hamate. In general, CMC joints are saddle joints, where the metacarpal base is convex and the distal surface of the carpals is concave (Fig. 9.5). This relationship becomes less pronounced when progressing toward the ulnar column and is a major contributor to the decreased stability that the 4th and 5th metacarpals exhibit. This becomes a major factor in the relative frequency of CMC fracture-dislocations, with the 4th and 5th metacarpals being far more commonly involved [19].

9.3   Mechanism of Injury

Great and sudden force is required to disrupt the strong periarticular ligamentous supports of the CMC joints. The general consensus in the literature is that the dislocation of the CMC joints can occur either by a direct force on the bases of the metacarpals or by an indirect force transmitted via the metacarpal shafts [20].

These injuries are the result of traffic accidents, falls from heights or striking a hard object with a closed fist. However, a low-energy trauma has also been implicated [10, 21, 22].

In many cases, the axial force is transmitted along the metacarpal shaft, distally to proximally inducing a dislocation at the base of the metacarpal [9, 10, 17, 23–35]. This is the most likely of the mechanisms implicated in the dislocation of the 4th and/or 5th metacarpals, but also of the 2nd metacarpal [36], or of the 2nd to 4th metacarpals [37]. The actions of the ECU and the hypothenar muscles contribute to the deformity of this injury [38].

These injuries are also caused following the application of a force on the palmar surface of the wrist, while the wrist is dorsiflexed (dorsal dislocations), or the application of a force on the dorsal surface of the wrist, while the wrist is palmarflexed (palmar dislocations) [1, 2, 9, 12, 35, 39, 40].

Frequently, CMC injuries are produced after high-energy injuries (e.g., motorcycle accidents) in which, while gripping the handlebars at the time of collision, a significant amount of force is transmitted to the volar aspect of the metacarpal bases producing dorsal dislocations of the medial four CMC joints [2, 3, 20, 41]; in rare cases the handlebars act as a fulcrum causing the metacarpal base to dislocate volarly [42]. Kumar and Malhotra [43] described the need to apply a torsional force in a high-energy incident, to achieve a divergent variant of multiple CMC dislocations.

A rare type of injury, in which a palmarly dislocated 5th metacarpal is associated with a fracture of the hook of the hamate, has been described [44–48]. In this type of injury, a violent contraction of the FCU against a fixed wrist in dorsiflexion [45] or a direct mechanism of production [44, 46–48] has been implicated.

9.4   Clinical Evaluation

Clinical evaluation reveals either a blatant appearance with excessive swelling, pain, limited range of motion and signs of neurovascular dysfunction or in less severe injuries, mild swelling, and localized sensitivity above the affected joints. Sometimes splaying of the fingers is noted [49]. Waugh and Yansey [1] described the deformity of the more frequent

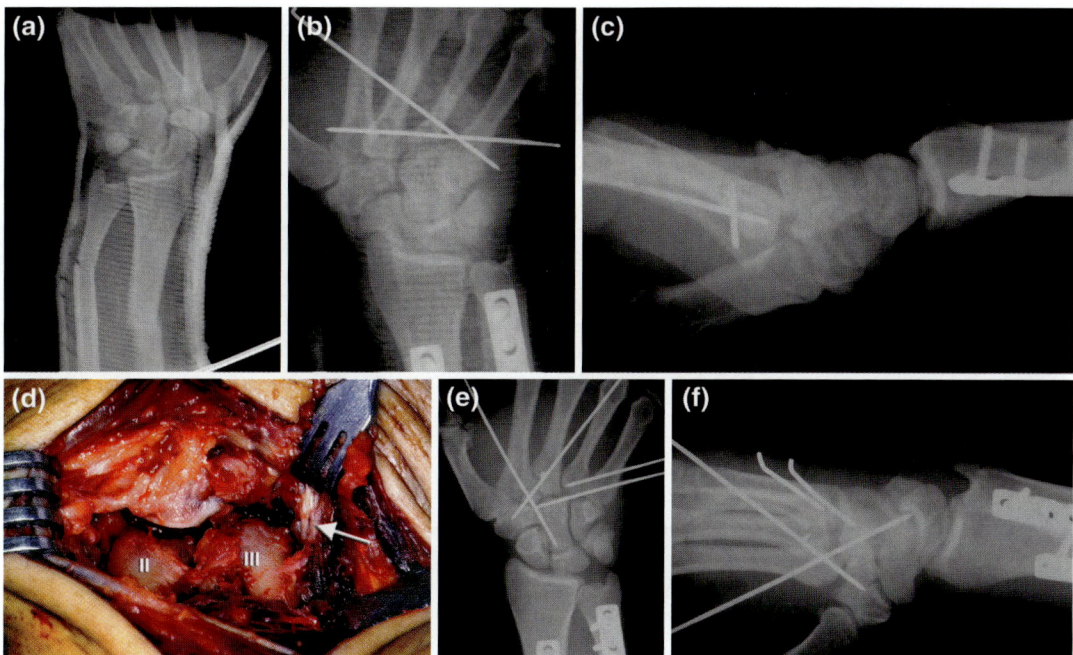

Fig. 9.6 Male, 18 years old, motorcycle accident. A forearm fracture was associated with volar dislocations of the 2nd to 5th metacarpals (**a**); after forearm reduction, the attempt for closed reduction and pinning of the CMC joints was unsuccessful (**b**, **c**); exploration through a dorsal approach revealed the avulsion of the ECRB from the base of the 3rd metacarpal (*arrow*) (**d**); a bone anchor was used for tendon reattachment and K-wires were inserted to stabilize the CMC joints (**e**, **f**). With permission from [132]

dorsal dislocations as "dinner- fork", while that of the volar dislocations as a "spade" type of deformity. Massive dorsal edema may obscure the characteristic clinical deformity and this, in combination with insufficient radiological control, are responsible for the high frequency of missed diagnosis [2, 6, 50–53]. Henderson and Arafa [27] reported that in 15 out of 21 cases with dorsal dislocations of the CMC joints, the diagnosis was missed at the emergency department, due to the swelling and use of routine radiographs. Garcia-Elias et al. [9] reported that 6 of their 13 patients had delayed or incorrect diagnosis. Shortening of the fingers, compared to the patient's healthy hand, will arise suspicion for injury of the CMC joints, once simple radiological examination rules out injury of the fingers or metacarpals (Indian salutation test [54]). With injuries to the 4th or 5th CMC joint, function of the motor division of the ulnar nerve may be affected because of that nerve's close proximity to the joint [6, 17, 52, 55–57]. This leads to weakness of the interossei and adductor pollicis, which manifests clinically as separation of the long and ring fingers when making a fist [10, 55]. Median nerve function may also be influenced in cases of palmar dislocations of the 2nd and 3rd CMC joints [9, 58], or of delayed reduction of central CMC joint dislocations or due to extensive swelling of the soft tissue. The close proximity of the deep palmar arterial arc with the palmar surface of the 3rd CMC joint must also be considered [17]. Another probable injury is the detachment of the flexor or extensor tendons of the wrist, which insert at the base of the affected metacarpal (Fig. 9.6a–f).

9.5 Radiological Evaluation

Diagnosis of CMC joint injuries is usually delayed due to insufficient initial radiological control. Gunther [3] stated that subtle findings in the overlapping articular surfaces and minor loss

Fig. 9.7 **a1–f2** Six X-ray projections fully demonstrating the CMC joints. See text for description. With permission from [132]

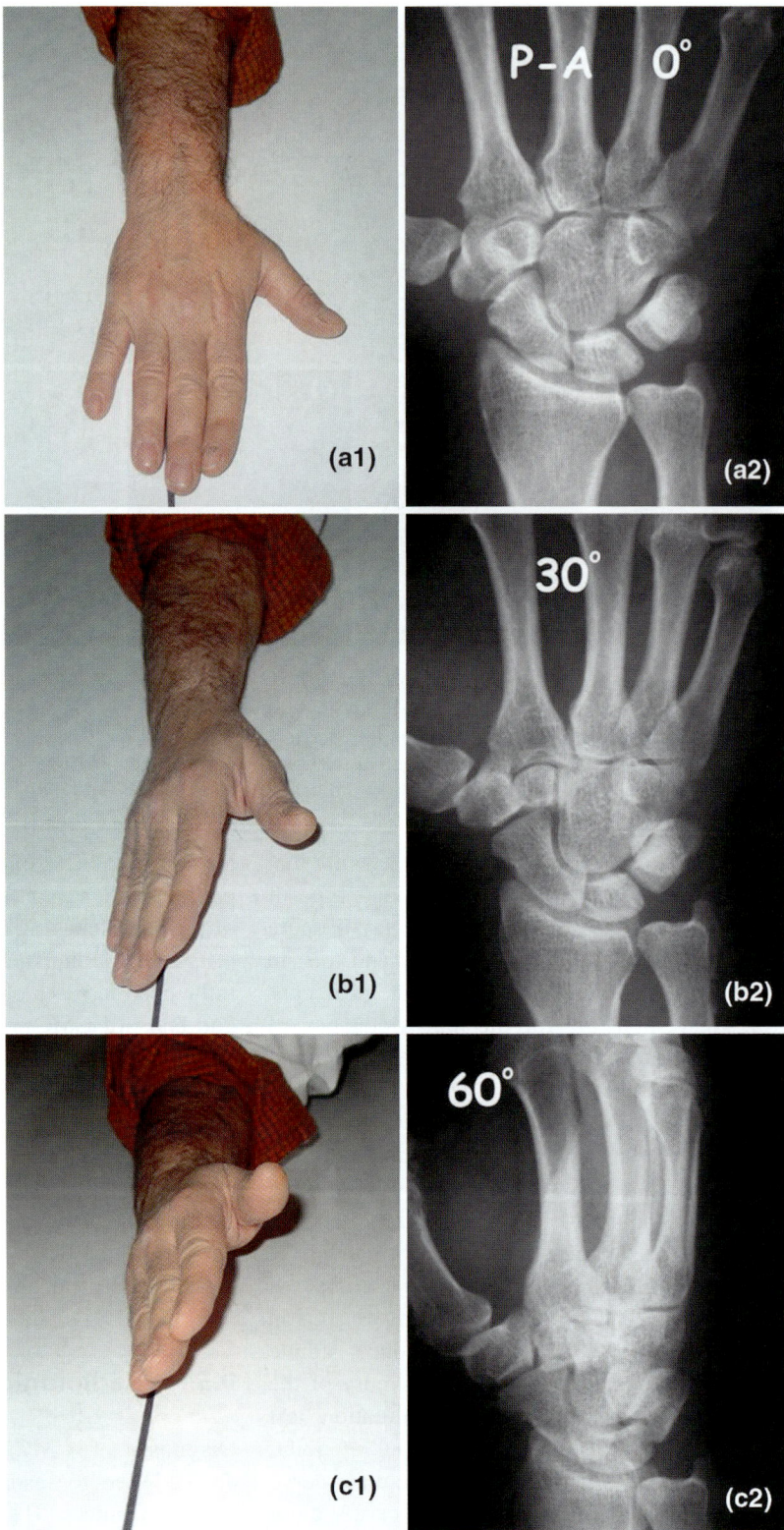

Fig. 9.7 (continued)

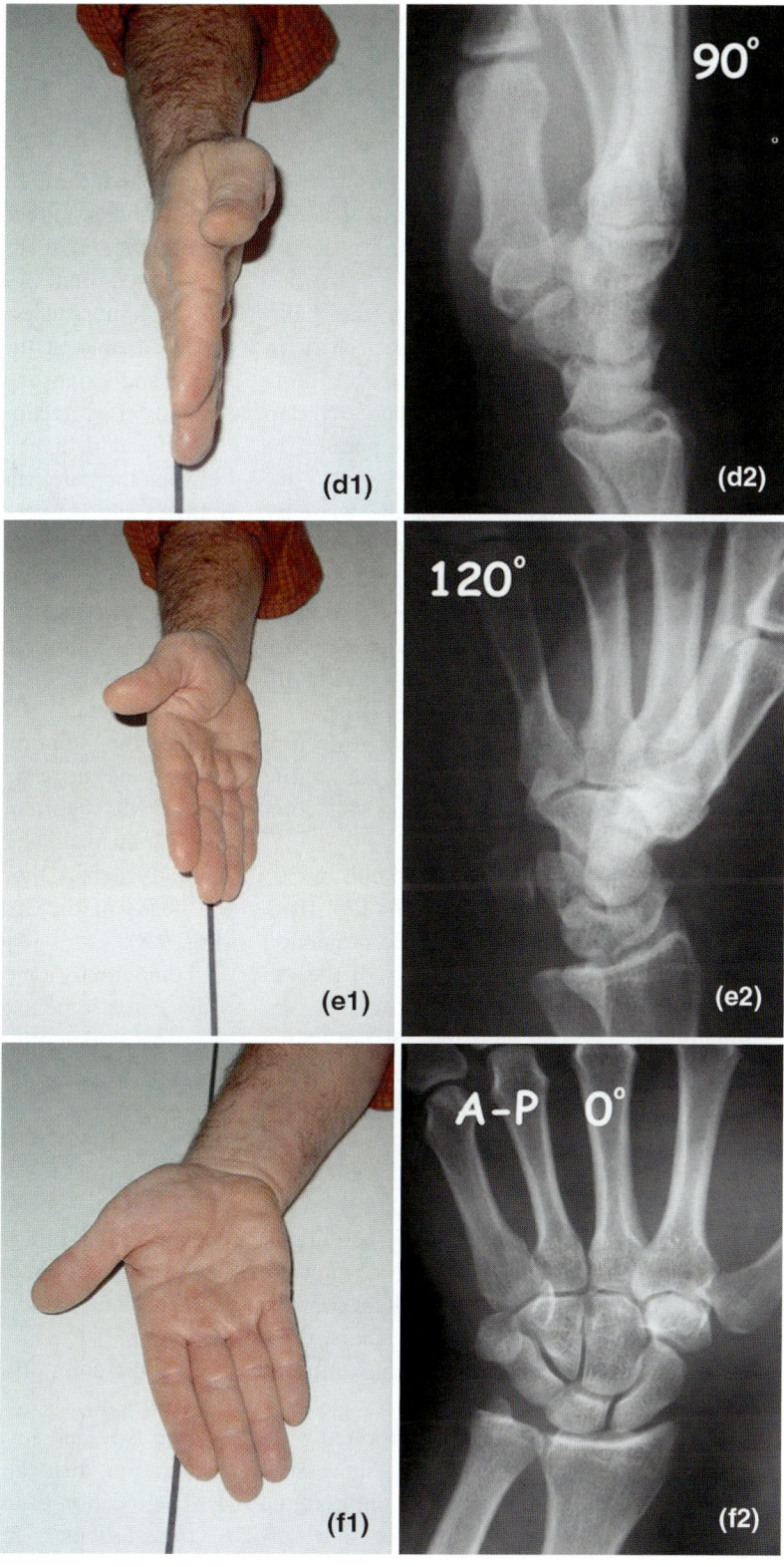

of symmetry may escape the average orthopedic surgeon. He suggested four x-ray projections as being necessary for diagnosing injuries of the CMC joints, which are performed by gradual supination of the hand and wrist, starting with the hand flat and the wrist in neutral position. To the projections mentioned above we have added two more projections to fully demonstrate the CMC joints:

1. Posteroanterior (PA) view with the palm attached to the cassette and the wrist in neutral position. The 3 medial CMC joints should be demonstrated without bony overlap and with their articular surfaces parallel to each other (Fig 9.7 a1–a2).
2. Elevation of the radial side of the wrist by 30°. This position shows the 2nd, as well as the 1st CMC joints adequately (Fig. 9.7b1–b2).
3. Elevation of the radial side of the wrist by 60° clearly shows the lateral view of the 4th and 5th CMC joints (Fig. 9.7c1–c2).
4. Further rotation to a true lateral projection and with the wrist in neutral, is in fact, a true lateral view of only the 3rd CMC joint (Fig. 9.7d1–d2).
5. Further rotation of the wrist-hand unit by 30° beyond the lateral neutral position (120° from the starting position), is a suitable projection for the anteroposterior (AP) view of the 4th and 5th CMC joints (Fig. 9.7e1–e2).
6. Finally, an AP view with the dorsum of the wrist attached to the cassette, clearly demonstrates the 2nd to 4th CMC joints in AP direction (Fig. 9.7f1–f2).

Parkinson and Paton [59] identified an increase in the angle formed by the long axis of the 2nd and 5th MC on a true lateral radiograph. In cases of dislocation of the 5th CMC joint the CMC angle is increased compared to controls (38.5° compared to 9.8°). A lesser increase in the CMC angle is suggestive of subluxation of this joint.

The PA projection must be performed with the palm attached to the cassette, since substandard positioning results in overlapping of the articular surfaces. Normally, the articular surfaces of any joint must be parallel to each other and the width of the 2nd through 5th joint spaces is uniform measuring 1–2 mm. It's been supported that on the PA radiograph two parallel lines approximating the letter M (parallel M lines) can be consistently drawn to define the normal 2nd through 5th CMC bone relationships. A break in the parallel M lines suggests an abnormality at that site [60–62]. Fisher et al. [61] stated that in simultaneous 4th and 5th CMC joint dislocations, an overlap was observed only at the 5th CMC joint since the flexor and extensor carpi ulnaris draw the dislocated 5th metacarpal proximally.

McDonald et al. [63] calculated the angles between the index and small metacarpal shaft (I-S IMA) and between the long and small metacarpal shaft (L-S IMA) in a lateral radiograph, in patients with ulnar-sided CMC fracture-dislocations. They concluded that both angles are useful screening measurements if they are greater than 10°.

Chmell et al. [64] in the PA view demonstrated the importance of the oblique line through the metacarpal heads for the evaluation of the MC shortening, which accompanies a CMC joint dislocation. This line is drawn tangentially across the distal articular surfaces of the heads of the 3rd, 4th, and 5th metacarpals (Fig. 9.8).

Tomography or computed tomography (CT) scans can also be useful, particularly when there are concomitant injuries to the carpal bones [65].

9.6   Classification

Although a generally accepted classification does not exist, injuries of the CMC joints can be classified based on different parameters, such as:

1. The number of affected rays (isolated or multiple).
2. The direction of injury (dorsal, palmar, ulnar, divergent).
3. The type and severity of injury (sprain, subluxation, dislocation, fracture-dislocation).
4. The location of the injury (MC base fracture, trans-articular, fracture of the distal carpal row or combinations).

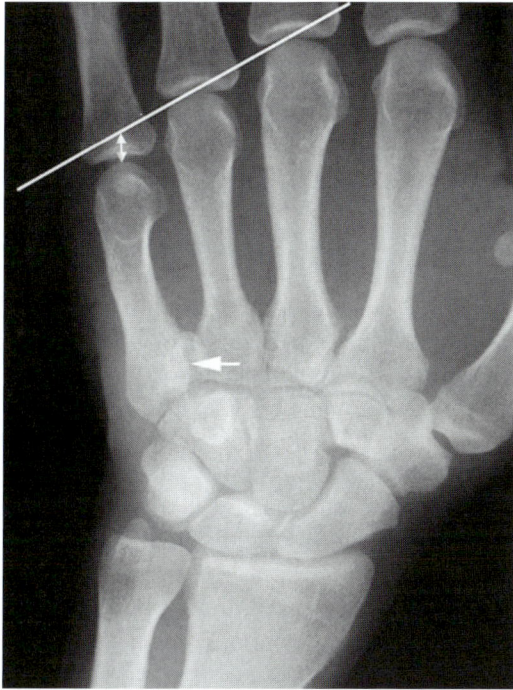

Fig. 9.8 The *oblique line* through the metacarpal heads (3rd to 5th), as described by Chmell et al. [64], for the evaluation of metacarpal shortening due to the 5th CMC joint fracture-dislocation (*arrow*). With permission from [132]

Cain et al. [23] classified injuries of the ulnar CMC joints into 4 types based on the 5th CMC joint. This classification works on the basis that the primary injury is a fracture of the 4th metacarpal and the resulting shortening leads to the hamatometacarpal dislocation. In Type IA, subluxation or dislocation of the 5th MC is accompanied by dorsal CMC ligament disruption; in Type IB the dorsal dislocation of the 5th metacarpal is associated with an avulsion fracture of the dorsal rim of the hamate; in Type II a dorsal hamate comminution is present; and in Type III a coronal splitting of the hamate is present (Figs. 9.9a–d and 9.10a–d). The authors considered Type IB as the most frequent and correlated the type of injury to the stability. They regarded that Type II and III injuries, as grossly unstable requiring open reduction, while type I injuries were reduced, tested for stability and the treatment was adjusted accordingly. The

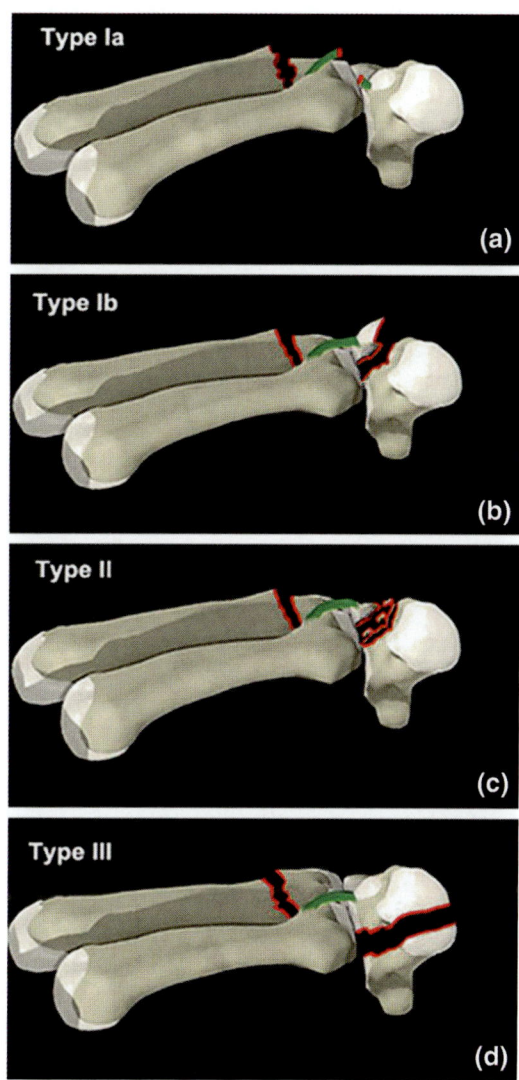

Fig. 9.9 Schematic depiction of Cain's et al. [23] classification, for injuries of the ulnar CMC joints (see text for details). With permission from [132]

main drawback of this classification is that it does not take into account the isolated dislocations of the 5th CMC joint without fracture of the 4th metacarpal.

However, since 4th and/or 5th metacarpal base intraarticular fractures are common findings that profoundly influence the treatment outcome, Lee et al. [30] recently suggested a new classification for the injuries of the ulnar CMC joints. This classification was based on the fractures of

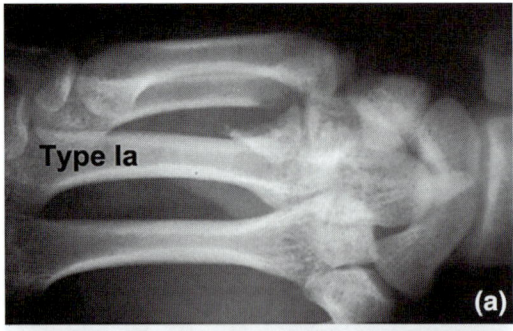

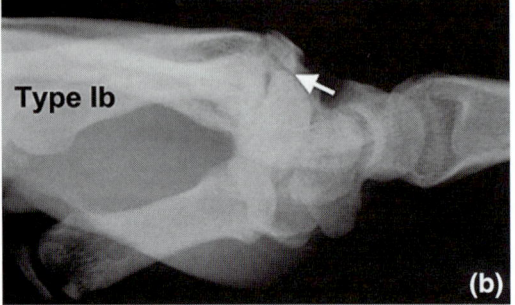

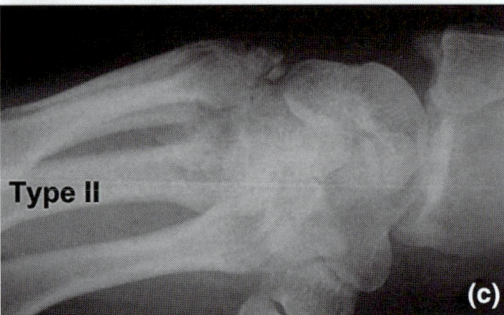

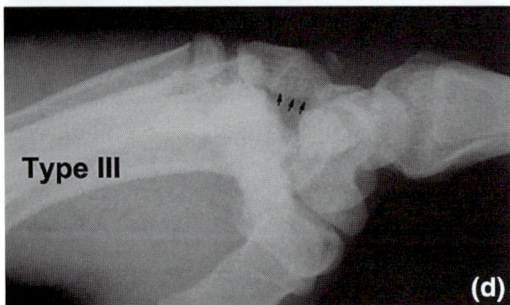

Fig. 9.10 Examples of ulnar CMC joint injuries according to the Cain et al. [23] classification. With permission from [132]

the bases of the 4th and/or 5th metacarpals and on the amount of articular surface of hamate fracture which was assumed as a fact. Three types of injuries were recognized: Type I was defined as less than one-third hamate articular surface involvement; Type II, more than one-third, and Type III, coronal splitting. Each type was divided into four subtypes: (1) absence of intraarticular MC base fracture; (2) fourth MC base fracture; (3) fifth MC base fracture; and (4) both fourth and fifth MC base fractures.

Garcia-Elias et al. [9] modified Cain's original classification system to include the radial two CMC joints and they moreover considered the stability of the injury following closed reduction as an important factor for classification. It is a common sense that prognosis of stable post-reduction injuries is much better than that of unstable injuries.

According to this classification there are three types of instabilities (Fig. 9.11a–h):

Type I (Transmetacarpal instability). Caused by fracture at the base of the metacarpal, which may be extrarticular (Ia) or intraarticular (Ib).

Type II (Carpometacarpal instability). Results after pure dislocation of the CMC joint (IIa) or a dislocation accompanied by a small chip avulsion fracture of the dorsal rim of the distal row carpal bones (IIb).

Type III (Transcarpal instability). This injury may involve only the dorsal and distal corner of the bone (IIIa) or it may be a fracture at the frontal plane of the bone affecting both the proximal and distal articulations (IIIb). Less frequently, the metacarpal along with the distal carpal row bone is dorsally subluxated with (IIIc) or without (IIId) fracture of the palmar surface of the bone. A case which could be classified as type IIId injury is illustrated in Fig. 9.12a–h.

This classification, has in addition a therapeutical importance, since type I (Ia and Ib) has been considered as a stable type and may be treated with longitudinal traction and cast support or percutaneous K-wires, while types II and III are inherently unstable and must be treated with open anatomical reduction.

It must be noted that delineation of these injuries using simple X-rays alone, is quite difficult. Tomography or CT scans at the sagittal plane are required.

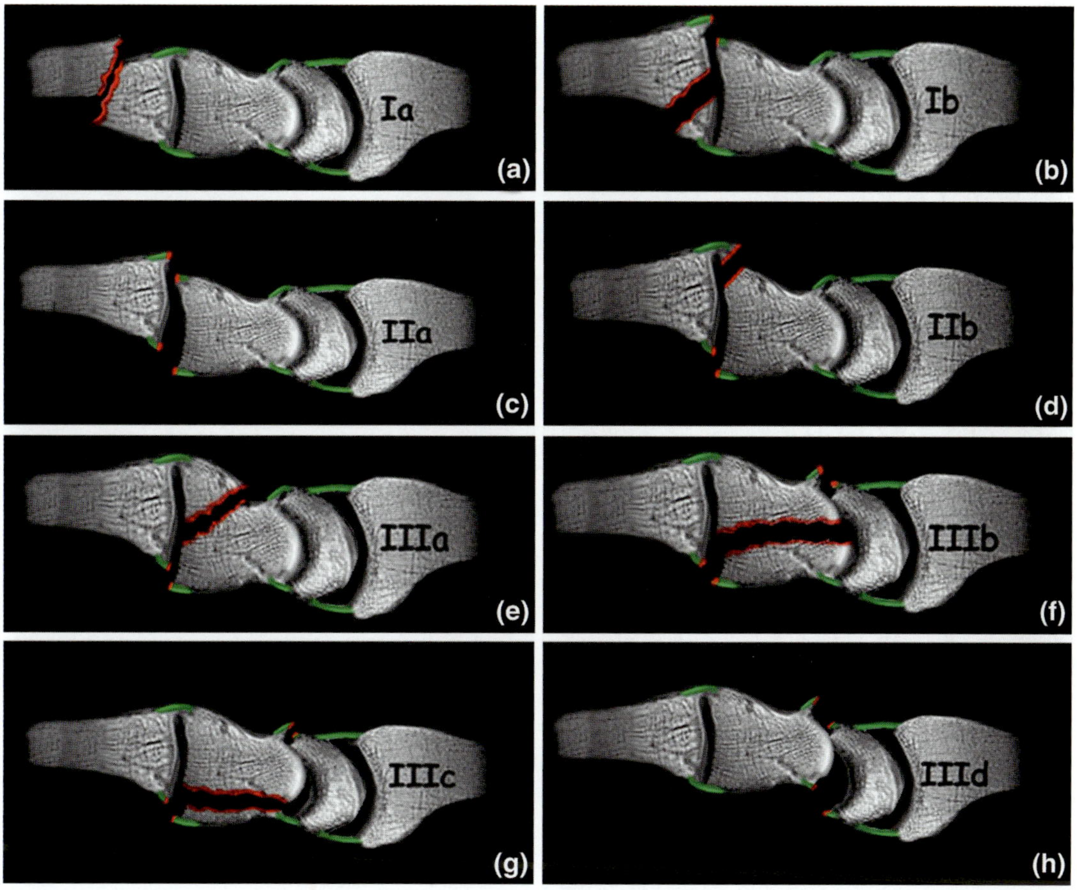

Fig. 9.11 Mayo Clinic's classification of CMC joint injuries, presented by Garcia-Elias et al. [9]. Although only the central column is depicted, it can be applied to all the affected rays. Type I injuries are considered as transmetacarpal, type II injuries as carpometacarpal, and type III injuries as transcarpal instability. With permission from [132]

9.7 Acute Injuries of the CMC Joints

Since acute injuries of the CMC joints are frequently the result of high-energy trauma, injuries to other parts of the body or even life-threatening injuries could probably coexist. In addition, complex injuries located at different levels of the same wrist (CMC, intercarpal, radiocarpal) have also been described [66, 67].

Almost every possible combination of injuries has been reported, including the divergent dislocation with some metacarpal bases being dorsally, while others being palmarly dislocated [19, 43, 68–71] (Fig. 9.13a–g). The divergence may have a different location in each case. In some cases, the divergence is localized and involves only two metacarpal bases, e.g., between 4th and 5th CMC joints [46, 72–74], while occasionally all the metacarpal bases are affected and the divergence could be located between the 2nd and 3rd [19, 43] or between the 3rd and 4th [68, 69] metacarpal bases.

Frick et al. [75] in a retrospective study of 100 CMC dislocations found that in half the cases, lesions were located only within the 5th ray, while carpal or metacarpal fractures were associated with the majority of cases (88 %).

The most common of all CMC joint injuries is considered to be the isolated injury of the 5th CMC joint, which is followed by the

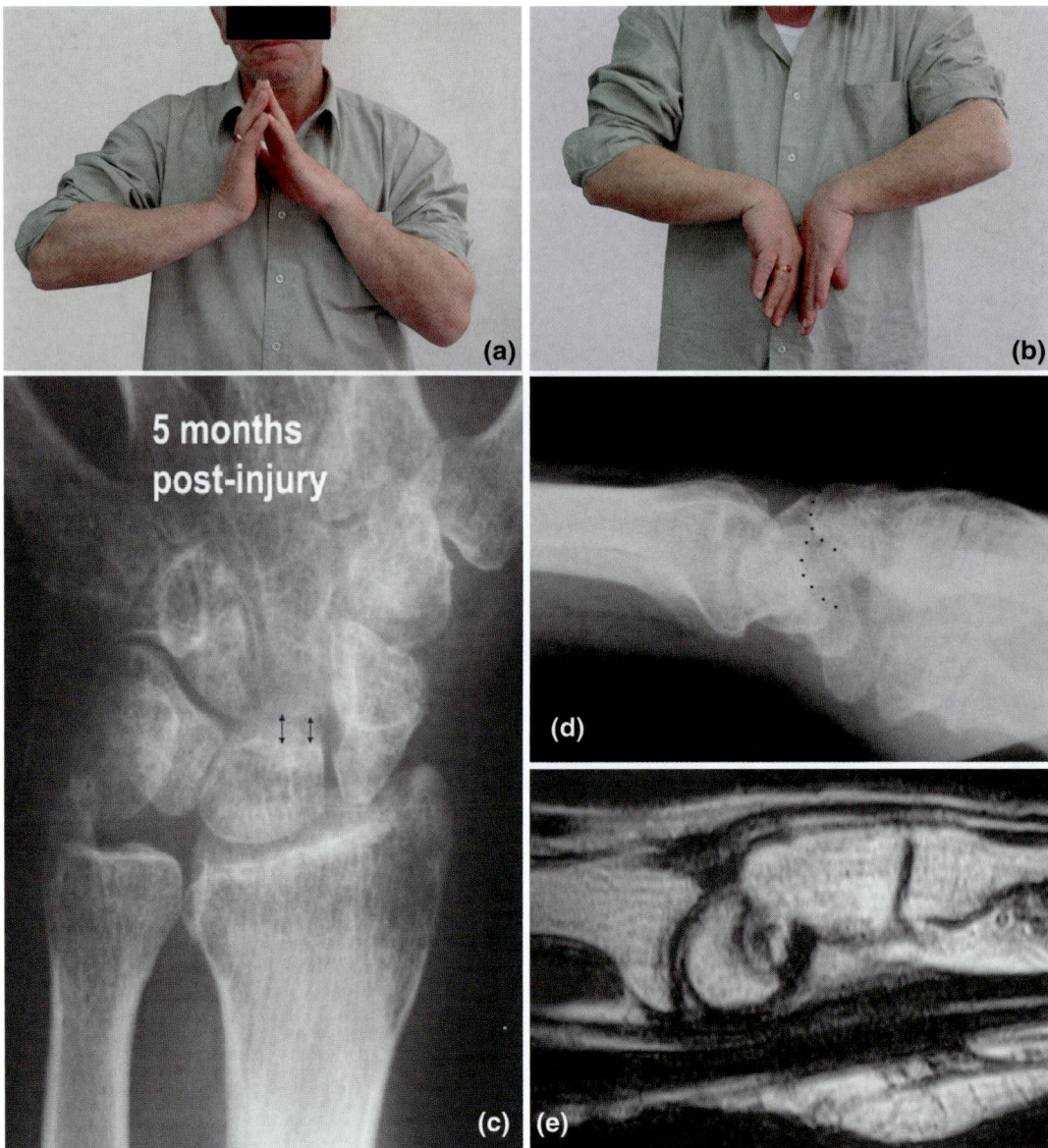

Fig. 9.12 Male, 46 years old. Five months prior to his examination he reported a left wrist injury, due to its entrapment in a garbage bin in hyperpronation position. He remained undiagnosed. Restriction of dorsal wrist extension, as well as painful osseous swelling at the dorsal side of the wrist, were noted during examination (**a**, **b**); radiological control revealed a widening of the lunocapitate joint in the P-A view (*arrows*) (**c**) and a dorsal midcarpal subluxation in the L view (**d**); MRI did not indicate further damage (**e**); dorsal approach revealed a fixed dorsal subluxation of the distal carpal row (**f**) (*C* Capitate, *L* Lunate, *S* Scaphoid); due to the difficulties of reduction and despite the good condition of the capitate head's cartilage, the patient was subjected to a scapholunocapitate fusion; the postoperative X-rays (**g**, **h**); the radiological result 1 year later (**i**, **j**). This case was considered as type IIId injury according to Mayo Clinic classification [9]

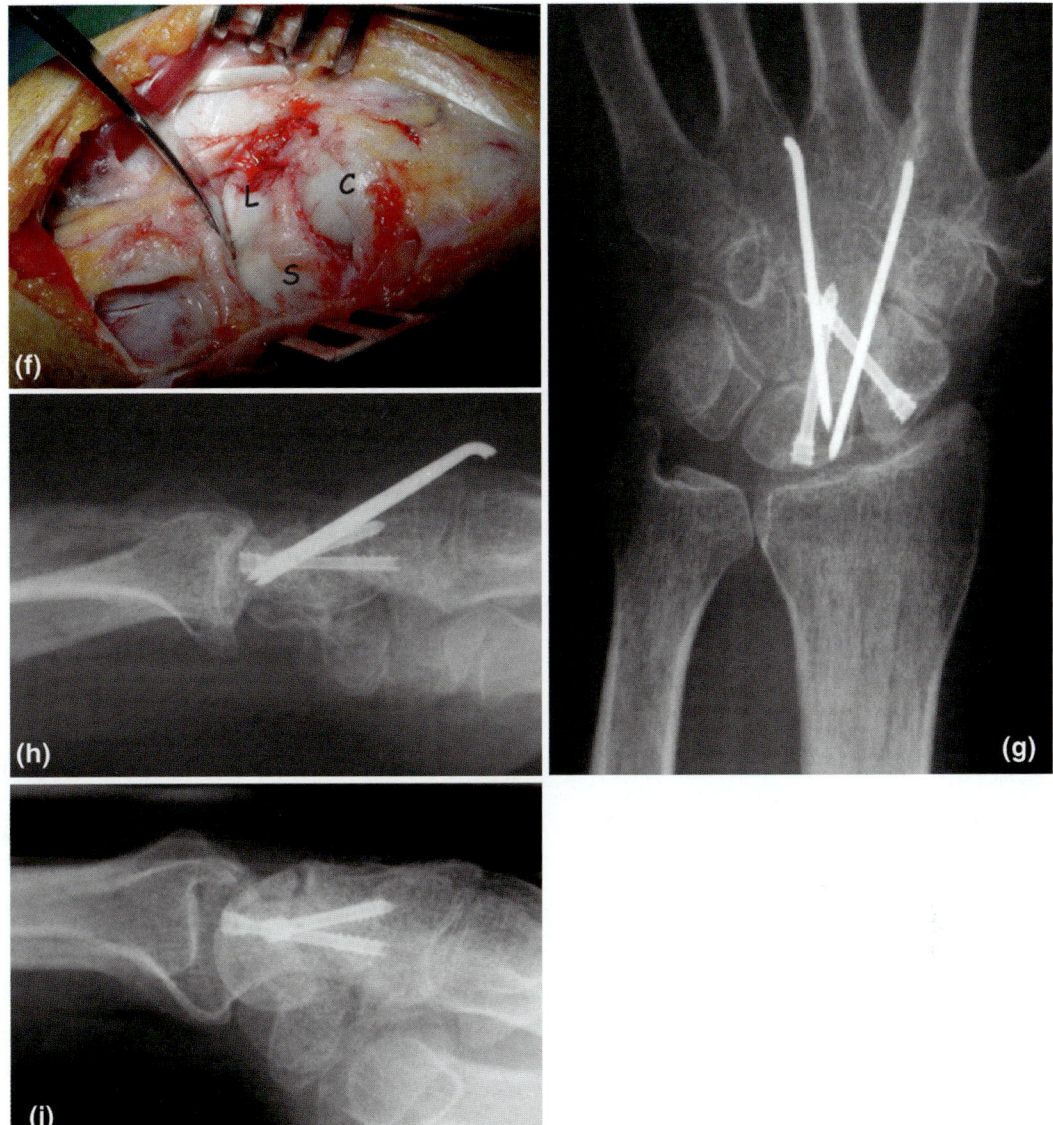

Fig. 9.12 (continued)

simultaneous injury of the 4th and 5th CMC joints (Fig. 9.14a–d).

The early recognition of these injuries is essential for satisfactory outcomes. The disability of the hand is severe in untreated cases or in those where treatment is delayed.

Management options include closed reduction and cast immobilization, closed reduction and K-wire fixation, or open reduction and internal fixation. The choice of treatment depends on the severity and stability of the CMC joints and the expertise of the attending physician [10].

9.7.1 Localized Injuries

Excluding the thumb, the most frequently injured CMC joints are the bases of the ring and small fingers, frequently described as hamato-metacarpal fracture-dislocations [9, 23, 35, 76].

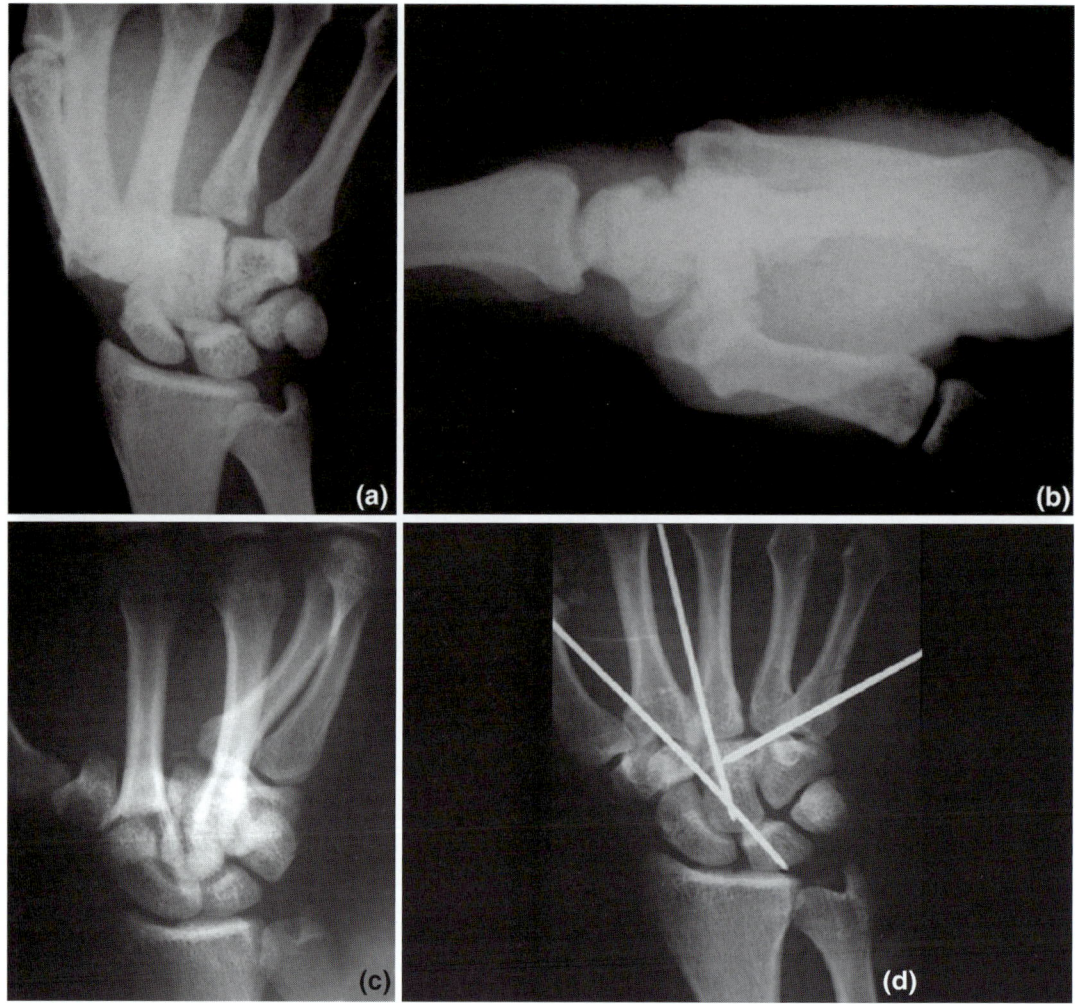

Fig. 9.13 Male, 28 years old, car accident. Divergent dislocations with the 2nd and 3rd metacarpals being dorsally dislocated, while the ulnar metacarpals were volarly displaced (**a, b, c**). With two longitudinal skin incisions dorsally, the dislocations were reduced and stabilized with K-wires (**d, e**); final radiographic appearance 6 months later (**f, g**). With permission from [132]

A limited number of pure dislocations of the 4th to 5th MC in dorsal [26, 61, 77, 78] (Fig. 9.15a, b) or in volar direction [49] or of a divergent type in different directions [46, 72–74] have been reported. Another rare combination of injuries is the coronal fractures of the body [29] or the dorsal pole of the hamate [25, 31, 76, 79–83] associated with injuries of the bases of the 4th and/or the 5th CMC joints (Fig. 9.16a–g).

The most frequently affected isolated CMC joint is the 5th, which is mainly characterized as a dorsal fracture-dislocation. The displacement is analogous to a Bennett's fracture of the thumb. Despite the fact that 4 types of intraarticular fractures at the base of the 5th MC have been described [33], the most common type involves a radiovolar bone fragment of different size, which remains attached with the 4th metacarpal through the intermetacarpal and palmar CMC ligaments, while the remainder of the 5th metacarpal is displaced ulnarly and dorsally to a varying degree, due to the action of extensor carpi ulnaris and the opponent digiti minimi muscle (Fig. 9.17a, b).

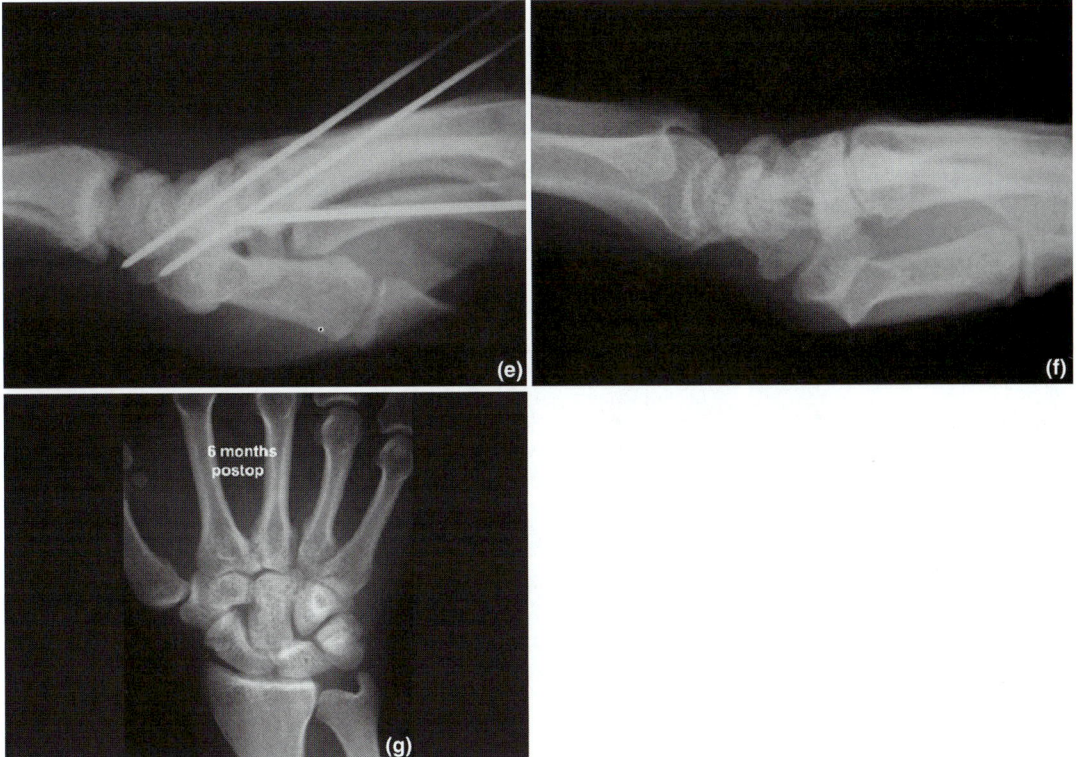

Fig. 9.13 (continued)

In addition, there are reported cases of iso-lated dislocations of the 5th CMC in dorsal [28, 84–88], or more rarely, in volar direction [45, 48, 60, 89] (Fig. 9.18a, b). There are two types of volar dislocations: radial and ulnar. In the radial type, which is the most common, all of the ligamentous and tendinous attachments are torn and usually open reduction is required using a volar-ulnar surgical approach. In the ulnar type, the pisometacarpal ligament remains intact pre-venting excessive displacement of the fifth metacarpal, which however overlaps the hamate and shortens the digit, due to the action of the flexor and extensor carpi ulnaris and the hypo-thenar muscles. Sometimes, the intact piso-metacarpal ligament prevents excessive displacement, thus rendering stress radiographs necessary for correct diagnosis [89]. In this type of injury, the problem is usually not the reduc-tion itself, but rather maintaining the reduction [6], thus percutaneous K-wire fixation of the joint is necessary.

Closed reduction is accomplished with local or general anesthesia, longitudinal traction of the finger(s), direct pressure at the bases of the affected metacarpals and dorsal extension of the head of the MC, if the most common dorsal dislocations of the CMC joints are considered. Although successful stabilization of the wrist after the reduction has been suggested only with plaster [7, 90, 91], most authors advocate using percutaneous K-wires fixation. K-wires are per-cutaneously inserted from the base of the metacarpal to the hamate or the adjacent 4th metacarpal, from the dorsal and ulnar surface of the wrist, while taking care not to disrupt the function of the extension mechanism. Recently, Mozaffarian et al. [92] described a safe corridor for pinning of the 5th CMC joint to prevent iatrogenic injury to the ulnar nerve and tendons;

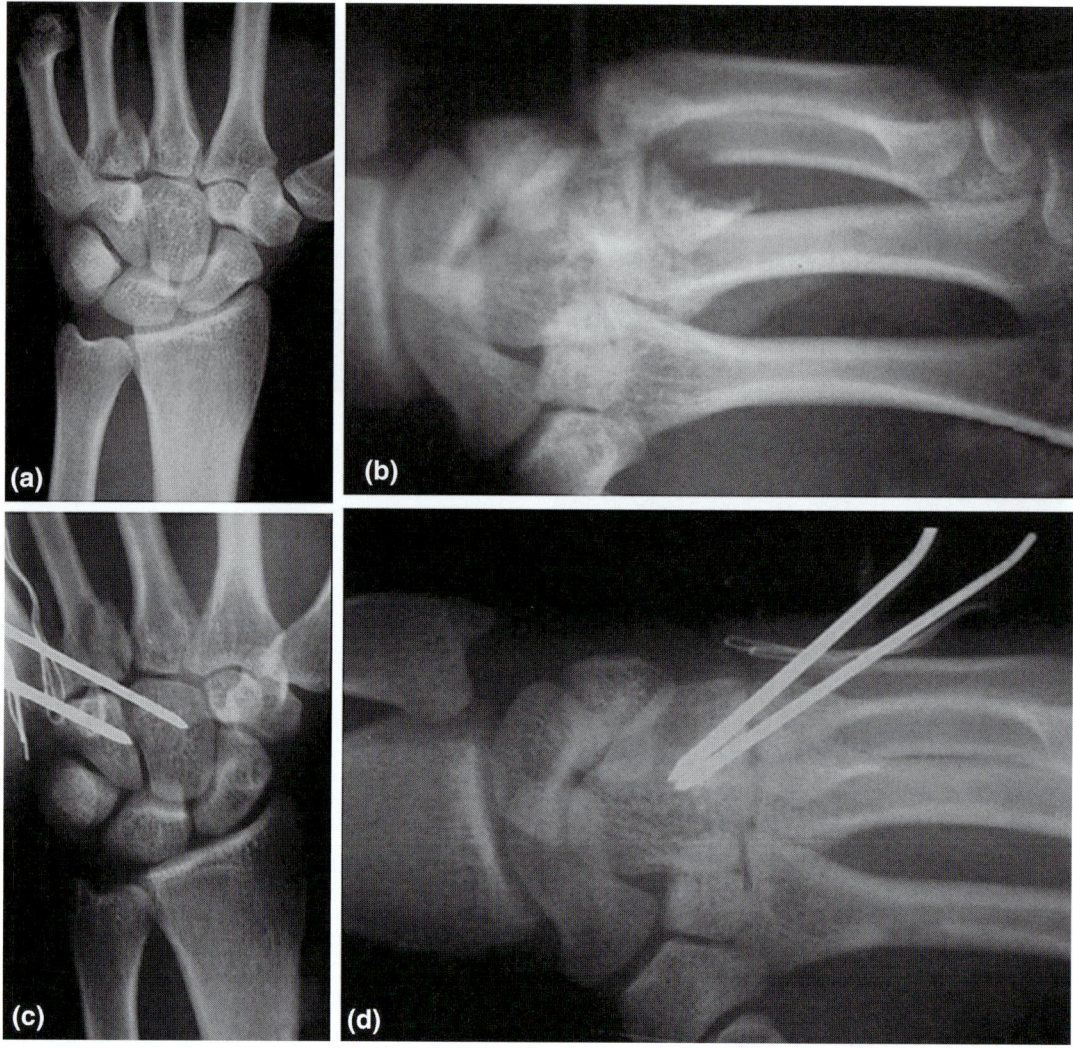

Fig. 9.14 Case with fracture of the base of the 4th metacarpal and dislocation of the 5th CMC joint (**a**, **b**); closed reduction and percutaneous fixation with K-wires (**c**, **d**). With permission from [132]

it is located 2 cm distal to the joint at an angle of 20°–30° to the coronal plane, from 10° volar to dorsal to 20° dorsal to volar direction in the saggital plane. Once stable reduction has been achieved, a direct, active, and passive mobilization of the fingers and wrist must commence within 1–2 weeks. The K-wires will be maintained for at least 6 weeks, although keeping them for up to 12 weeks has also been suggested [11]. After the K-wires are removed, the patient starts grip strengthening exercises. The importance of early controlled mobilization has been

emphasized [93] for reducing postinjury complications (stiffness of hand joints, tendon adhesions, and intrinsic muscle weakness).

Slutsky [94] described an arthroscopic technique for reduction and percutaneous fixation of 5th CMC fracture-dislocations. The technique is considered useful especially in cases where the articular fracture fragment is volar and difficult to visualize and reduced using a dorsal approach.

Rarer are the isolated injuries of the 2nd and/ or 3rd CMC joint. In literature there are reported cases of dorsal [36, 95–97] or palmar dislocation

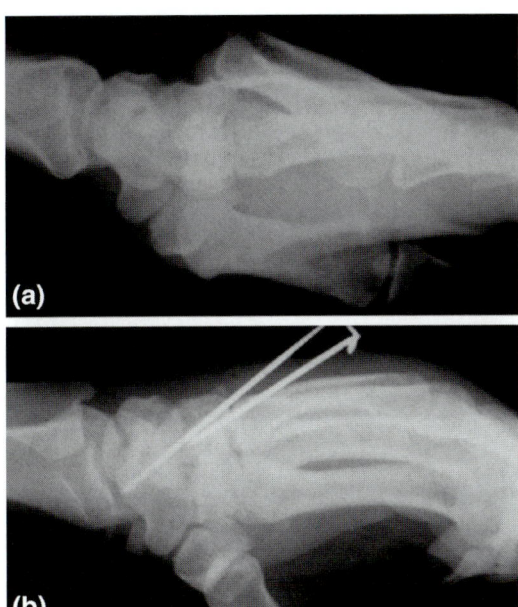

Fig. 9.15 Pure dorsal dislocations of the ulnar CMC joints (**a**), treated with closed reduction and stabilization with two K-wires (**b**). With permission from [132]

[98, 99] of the 2nd CMC joint, dorsal non-reducible dislocation of the 2nd CMC joint due to interference of the extensor carpi radialis brevis [100, 101] and finally, palmar dislocations of the 2nd to 3rd CMC joint [12, 42, 58]. Although K-wire fixation is recommended to prevent recurrent dislocation, it has been suggested that it is not always necessary because of the intrinsic stability of the joint [101].

Open reduction and internal fixation, are clearly indicated in the following cases:

1. Unsuccessful closed reduction.
2. Irreducible dislocations due to interposed soft tissue or fracture fragments.
3. In cases of delayed diagnosis, where the contraction of soft tissues hinders closed reduction.
4. Complex fracture-dislocations.

Incision of the skin for the isolated injury of a CMC joint is usually dorsal curvilinear or of S type, with the transverse part of the incision located above the joint.

9.7.2 Multiple Injuries

In general, multiple injuries of the CMC joints cause significant swelling of soft tissue that obstructs closed reduction, which even if achieved, is difficult to maintain. The inability to achieve closed reduction is sometimes due to interposed joint capsule in the CMC joints [102]. There have been reported cases of dislocations or fracture-dislocations of all five CMC joints [103–112], dorsal dislocations of the 2nd to 5th CMC joint [22, 54, 67, 102, 113–118] (Figs. 9.19a–d and 9.20a–d), palmar dislocations of the 2nd to 5th CMC joint [90, 119–121], palmar dislocations of the 2nd to 4th CMC joint [122], or fracture of the base of the 3rd and dorsal dislocations of the 4th and 5th CMC joints [51].

Garcia-Elias [2] stated that the treatment of choice for the relatively stable type II injuries (according to his classification) is early closed reduction, distal-to-proximal pin fixation, and specific cast support. Types I and III, by contrast, because of the presence of a displaced intraarticular fracture, are inherently unstable, thus open treatment, which allows identification and treatment of small osteochondral fractures, debridement of debris in the joints, accurate reduction and proper stabilization, is the method of choice. Rare cases have been reported with coronal fractures through the capitate and hamate [123] or through the capitate, hamate, and trapezoid [124], both of which necessitated a CT-scan for diagnosis. Both these cases probably constitute a type IIIb injury (according to Garcia-Elias classification) and were treated with open reduction and internal fixation.

A major distal carpal row bone fracture is frequently associated with CMC dislocations [9, 125] and in such cases open reduction and fixation of the fractured bone with K-wire(s) or with a compression screw is considered the treatment of choice (Fig. 9.21a–f).

The dislocated joints are usually approached from the dorsal side and the skin incision may be longitudinal [17, 126] or transverse [46, 50, 69,

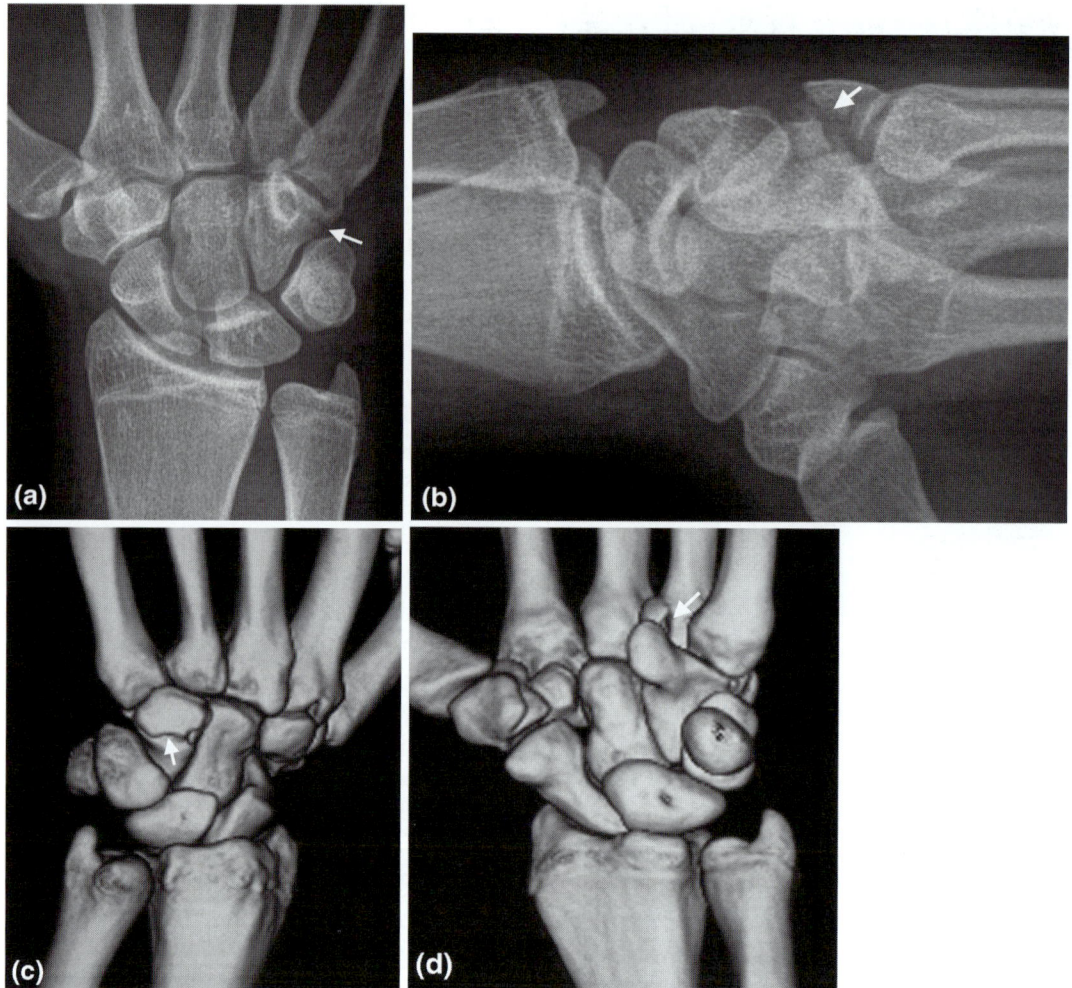

Fig. 9.16 Male, 15 years old. Subluxation of the 5th CMC joint with a coronal fracture of the dorsal pole of the hamate (**a, b**); 3D CT-scan reconstruction images disclosed the extent of the injury (*arrows*) (**c–d**), while CT images disclosed the fracture of the hamate (*arrows*) (**e–f**) and in addition a fracture of the volar base of the 4th metacarpal (*arrow*) (**g**). The patient refused any further treatment

70, 115]. Alternatively, we may approach all 4 bases of the metacarpals, using two longitudinal skin incisions (between 2nd to 3rd and 4th and 5th CMC joint). Cutaneous nerves are protected and the extensor tendons are retracted to gain access to the dislocated joints. Reconstruction of the transverse carpal row starts with the reduction and stabilization of the base of the 3rd [6, 10, 39, 43, 121] or of the 2nd [67] metacarpal. When all 4 metacarpals are dislocated,

stabilization of each joint separately is not necessary, as some of the interosseous ligaments usually remain intact, which helps to stabilize the adjacent metacarpal [3, 6, 68]. The wires must be placed so as to avoid the extensor tendons, since early mobilization is desirable.

The pins are removed at 4–6 weeks postoperatively. An alternative method to stabilize the dislocated joints with K-wires, avoiding the risk of damaging tendons and nerves, is the

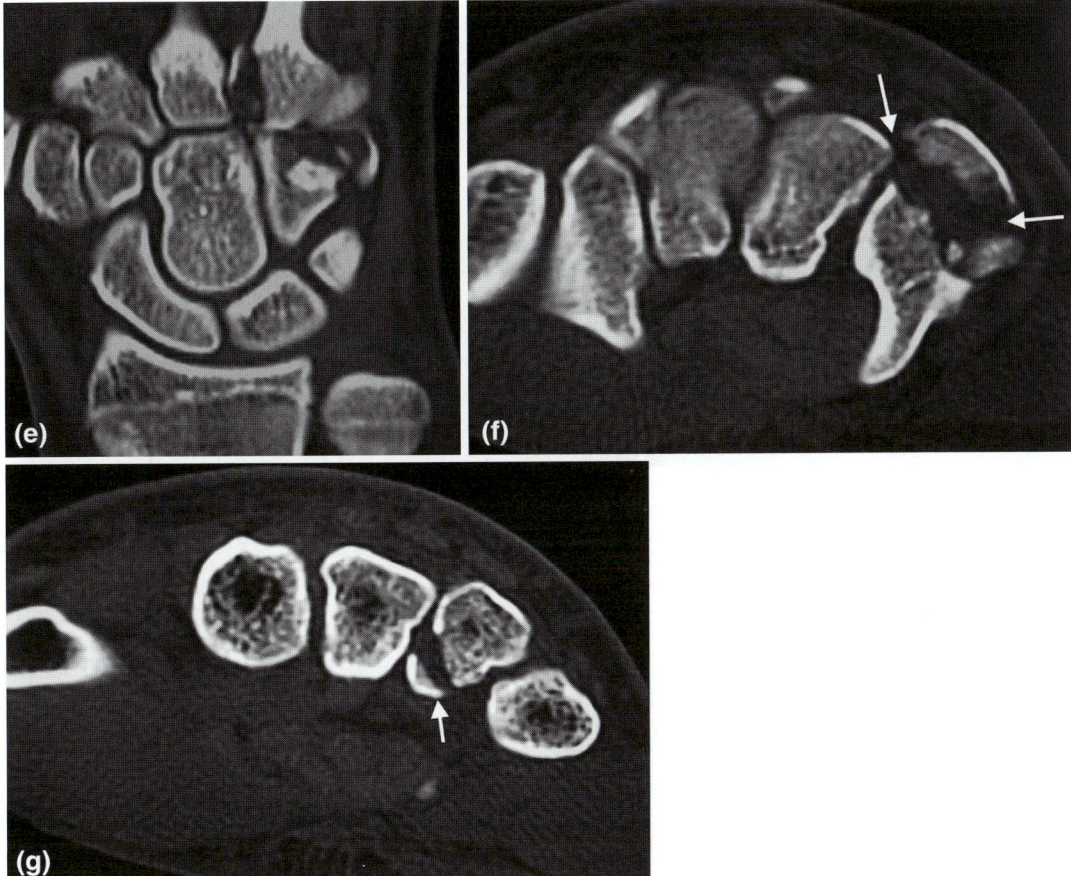

Fig. 9.16 (continued)

technique proposed by Foster [26], called "intramedullary stress sharing fixation" (originally described for ulnar CMC joints' dislocations) (Fig. 9.22a–d).

9.8 Chronic Injuries of the Carpometacarpal Joints

There is no consensus for the definition of a chronic CMC dislocation. Most authors believe that an injury dated more than 3 to 6 months is defined as chronic [17, 127], while Ahmad and Plancher [128] defined CMC dislocations as chronic when there is a delay in diagnosis and treatment of at least 6-12 weeks. Usually, chronic cases are expressed with deformity,

localized sensitivity, reduced muscle strength and in the long term, symptoms of arthritic changes (Figs. 9.23a, b and 9.24a–g).

Although there had been early reports that chronic dislocations or subluxations of the CMC joints do not result in any disability [1, 68], this view today has no advocates. Green [129] supported that injuries more than 3 weeks old do not require any treatment.

In cases with mild symptoms such as slight residual subluxation, conservative treatment is probably best [17], while in cases with marked deformity an attempt for delayed open reduction could be successful as late as 3–6 months postinjury [38]. Imbriglia [127] reported successful open reduction of the 2nd to 5th CMC joints 3 months post injury without the need for arthrodesis, due to

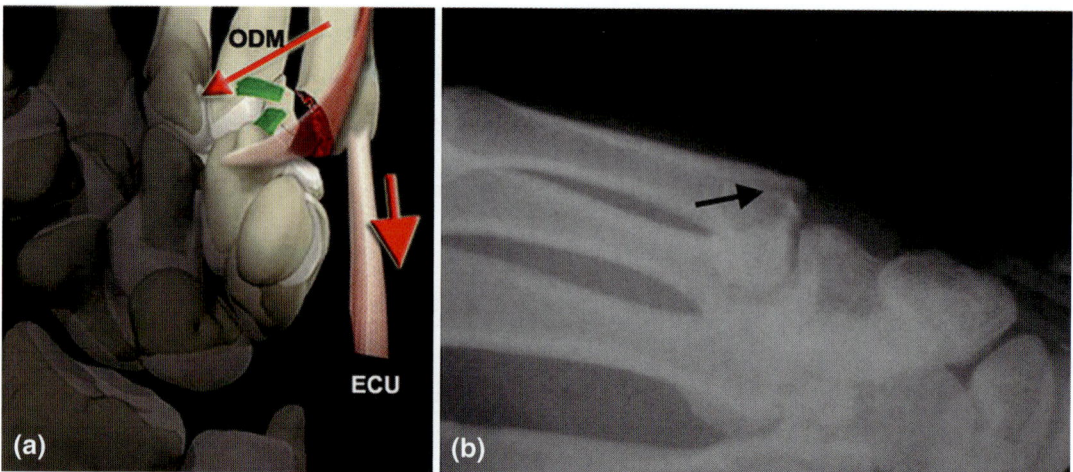

Fig. 9.17 The most common type of fracture-dislocation of the 5th CMC joint. A small ulnovolar bone fragment remains attached to the 4th metacarpal through the ligaments, while the 5th metacarpal is ulnarly and dorsally displaced due to the action of ECU tendon and the direction of pull by the hypothenar muscles (*ODM* Opponent digiti minimi) (**a**); a clinical analogue of the injury (**b**). With permission from [132]

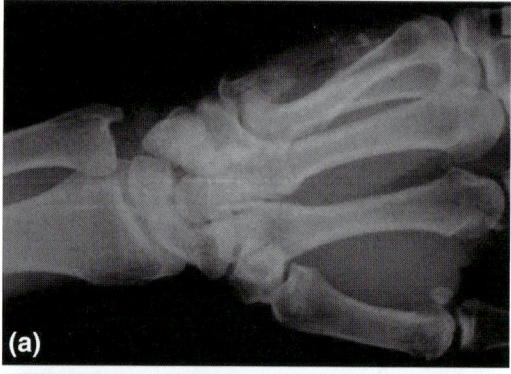

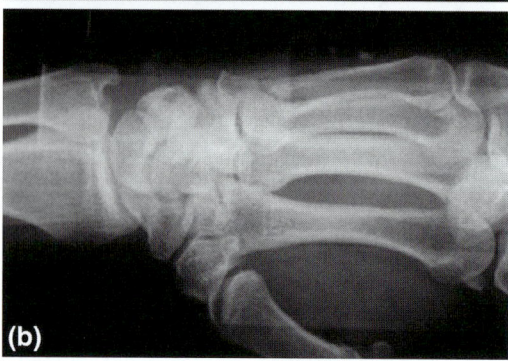

Fig. 9.18 Rare volar fracture-dislocation of the 5th CMC joint (**a**), which was treated with closed reduction (**b**). With permission from [132]

the integrity of the articular cartilage. Prokuski and Eglseder [67] stated that delay of up to 4 weeks did not adversely affect results.

In any case, regardless of the time elapsed, the management will depend on the complaints, while if operative treatment is needed, the appropriate method will depend on the reducibility of the CMC joints, and the condition of articular cartilage.

9.9   Long-Term Results

Few reports document long-term follow-up in cases of multiple carpometacarpal dislocations. However, it is uniformly accepted that with early diagnosis and prompt treatment with restoration of normal anatomical reduction, excellent results may be expected [9, 10, 35, 41]. In addition, the outcome has generally been favorable as long as the reduction is maintained.

It has been suggested [10, 121] that delayed diagnosis and treatment will usually result in an undesirable outcome of pain, reduced grip strength and degenerative arthritis and that up to

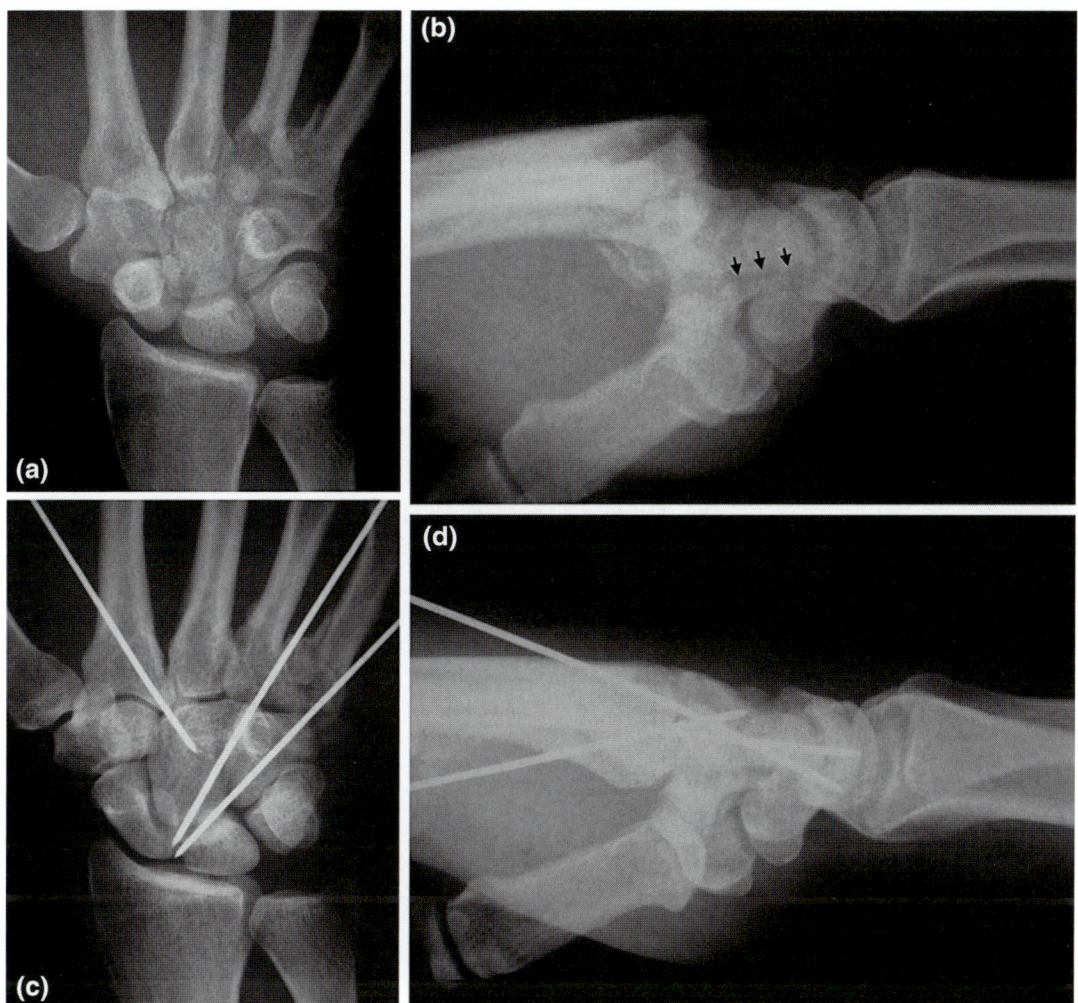

Fig. 9.19 A case of dorsal dislocations of the 2nd to 5th CMC joints associated with a fracture of the volar part of the capitate (*arrows*) (**a**, **b**); it was treated with open reduction and fixation with K-wires (**c**, **d**). With permission from [132]

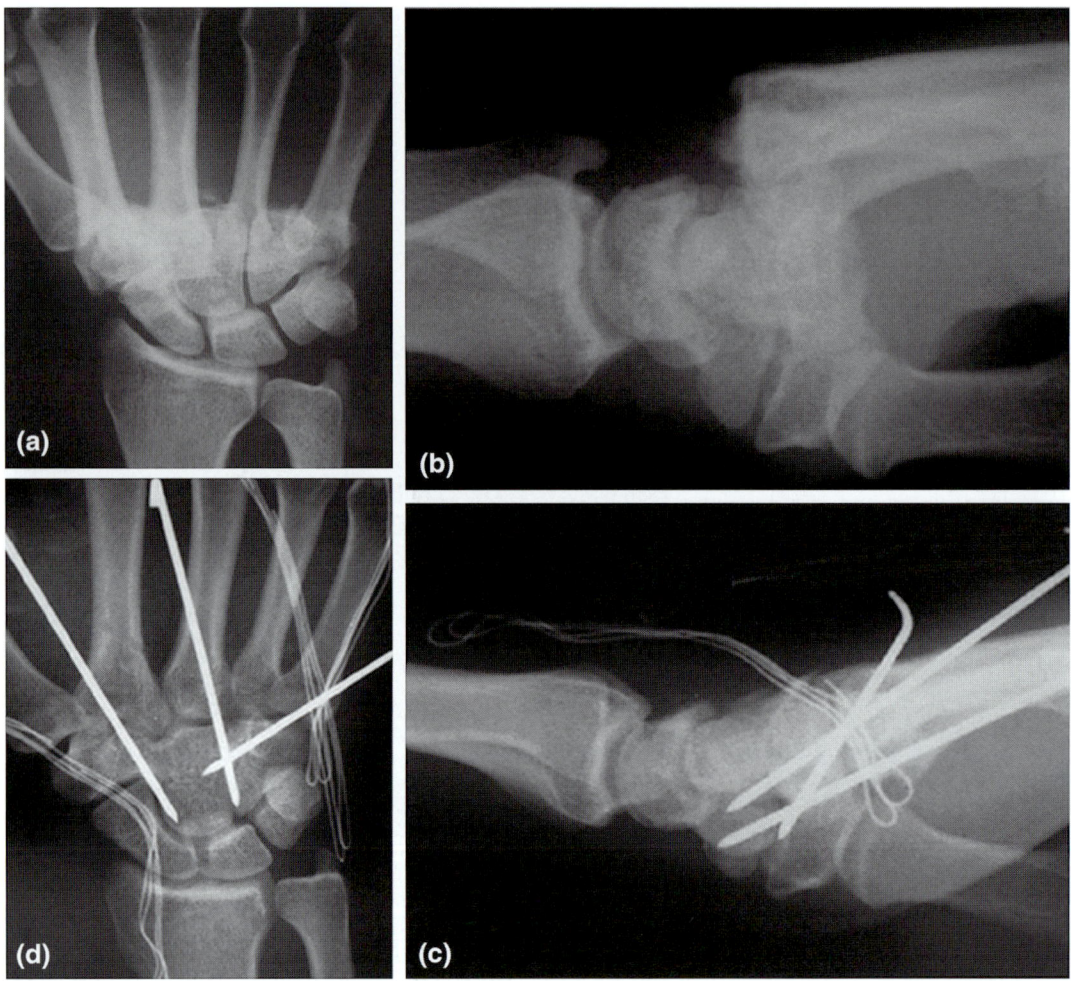

Fig. 9.20 Male, 40 years old, motorcycle accident. Dorsal dislocations of the 2nd to 5th CMC joints (**a, b**); he was treated with closed reduction and K-wires insertion, while the 4th CMC joint was reduced coincidently with the 3rd CMC joint (**c, d**). With permission from [132]

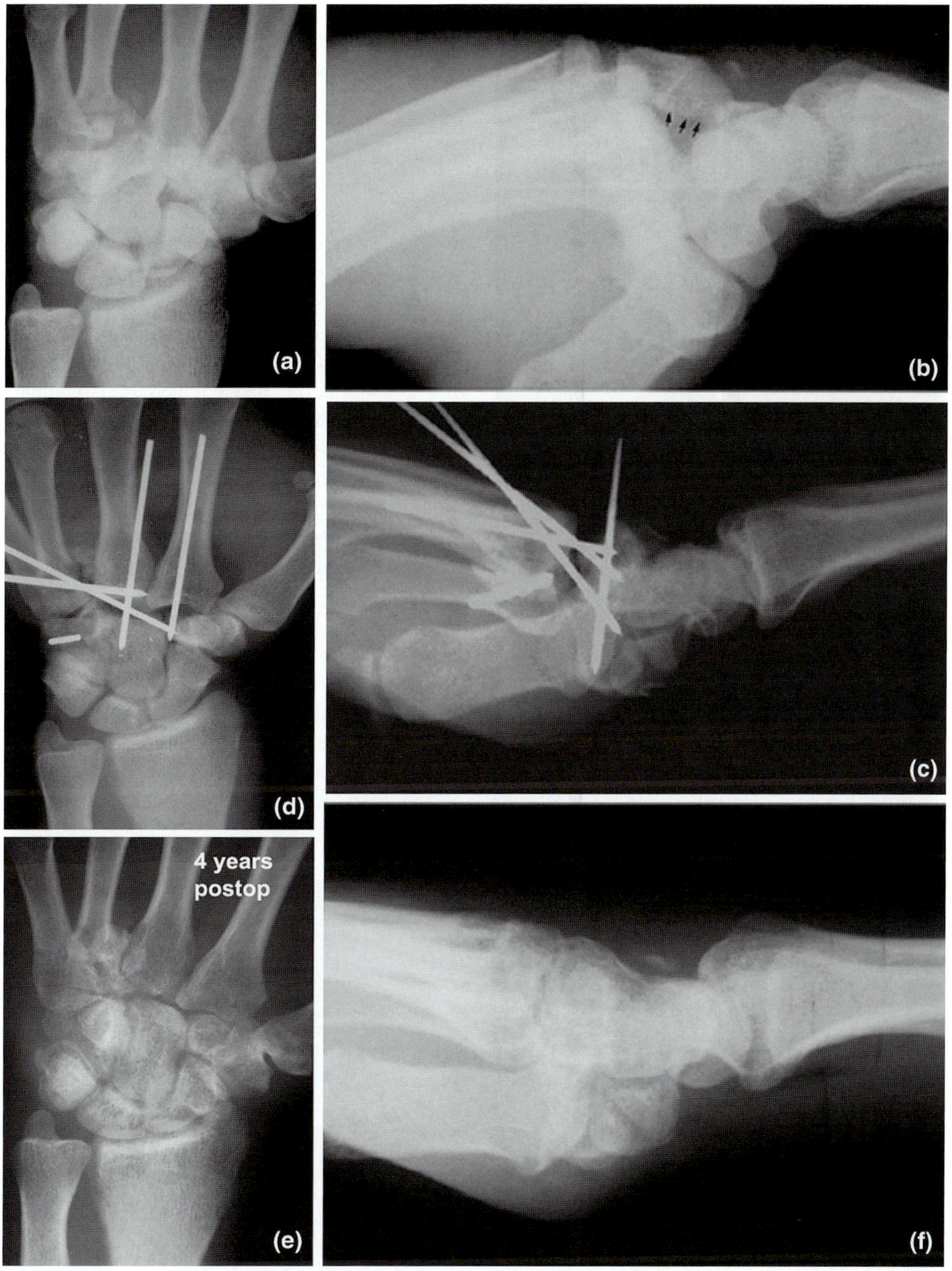

Fig. 9.21 Male, 30 years old, motorcycle accident. Dorsal dislocations of the 2nd to 5th CMC joints. The injuries of the 2nd and 3rd CMC joints were of IIa type, that of the 4th CMC joint was of Ia type and that of the 5th CMC joint was of IIIb type (associated with a fracture of the body of the hamate in the coronal plane) (*arrows*), according to the Mayo classification (**a, b**); he was treated with open reduction and K-wires stabilization including the hamate fracture (**c, d**); final radiographic appearance 4 years later (**e, f**). With permission from [132]

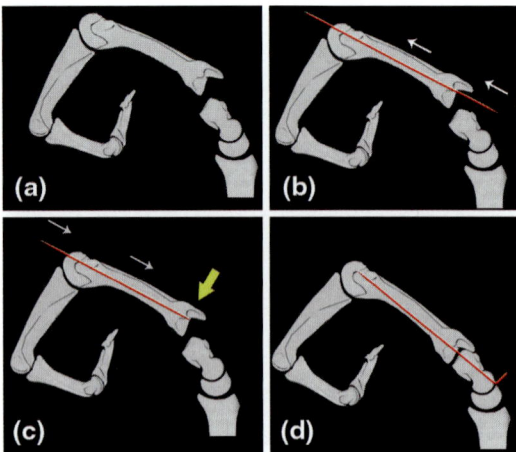

Fig. 9.22 Fosters' [26] stabilizing method of a dislocated CMC joint using intramedullary K-wire: the dislocated joint (**a**); insertion of the K-wire from the proximal to the distal side into the intramedullary canal, exiting dorsally at the flexed MP joint and through the central portion of the extensor tendon (**b**); reduction of the dislocation and proximally advancing of the K-wire into the corresponding bone of the distal carpal row after excessive wrist palmarflexion (**c**); the pin is withdrawn proximally to disengage the head of the metacarpal; its proximal portion is curved and cut below the skin level (**d**)

43 % of patients with neglected single CMC joint injuries will experience residual pain and impaired function. However, with appropriate management, up to 87 % of patients with CMC joint injuries will return to full work and sporting activities with negligible pain.

Gunther [3] stated that open reduction with K-wire fixation results in excellent hand function. Grip strength returns to normal and the only residual symptoms of the fracture-dislocation are usually mild aching during changes of weather or during extremely heavy work.

Garcia-Elias et al. [9] reported that patient satisfaction when treated in the acute phase is high; on the contrary, delayed treatment, even with bone grafting and stabilization until fracture consolidation, had an increased incidence of mild residual symptoms, including weakness of grasp or pinch and tenderness at the CMC area. In addition, delayed diagnosis may lead to fracture nonunion due to vascular or mechanical factors, with adverse consequences (muscular imbalance, reduced grip strength, and arthritis).

Lawlis and Gunther [70] suggested that most adverse results concern patients with 2nd and 3rd MC injuries or those having additional injury of the ulnar nerve.

Lundeen and Shin [33] reported clinical results of 22 patients with intraarticular fractures of the base of the 5th MC treated by closed

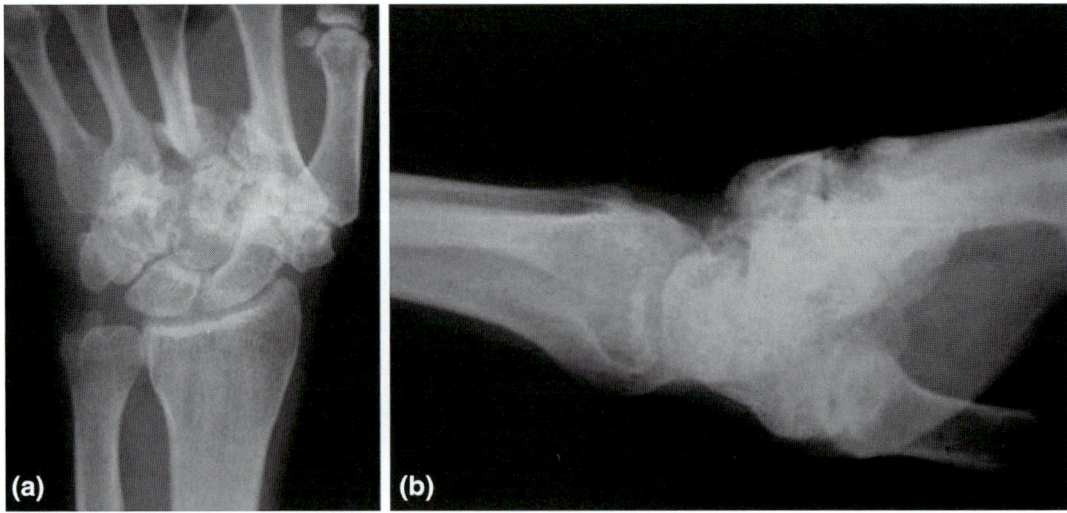

Fig. 9.23 Neglected dorsal CMC fracture-dislocations (**a**, **b**). The patient complained for dysfunction of the extensor tendons. With permission from [132]

reduction and cast immobilization. After an average follow-up of 43 months, twenty patients reported excellent or good results and two reported fair or poor results. Nine of those patients (41 %) had mild arthrosis of the CMC joint. Yildiz et al. [112] supported that mild degenerative changes in the CMC joints may be present radiographically on long-term follow-up. However, the functional results appear to be good, provided that open reduction and internal fixation of the dislocations have been achieved.

9.10 Arthrodesis of CMC Joints

In cases of chronic instability or post-traumatic arthritis of CMC joints not responding to conservative treatment, arthrodesis constitutes the operation of choice [6, 50]. Arthrodesis of the 2nd, 3rd or both CMC joints does not result in any functional deficiency, because the motion range of these joints is limited, while the method has been suggested as a primary treatment for unstable fracture-dislocations [50, 70,

126]. In addition, the need for CMC arthrodeses tends to be higher among patients with more associated injuries [67]. Even arthrodesing the mobile 4th and 5th CMC joints will not cause any problems, provided that the joints are fused in sufficient flexion to maintain the normal curvature of the distal metacarpal arch when making a fist [6]. Because mobility of the 5th CMC joint is greater than the 4th, it should be fused in greater flexion. Arthrodesis is performed with the use of a sliding inlay graft, an iliac strut graft or a corticocancellous graft from the distal radius, which is stabilized with K-wires (Fig. 9.25a–g). Fusions usually heal within 8 weeks. As an alternative to arthrodesis, resectional arthroplasty with interposition of a rolled tendon spacer has been applied [130] or if the 5th CMC joint is involved, a "stabilized arthroplasty" suggested by Dubert and Khalifa [131] can be applied. The latter technique is based on the resection of the base of the 5th metacarpal, whereas the length of the fifth digit ray is restored by fusion to the adjacent 4th metacarpal.g

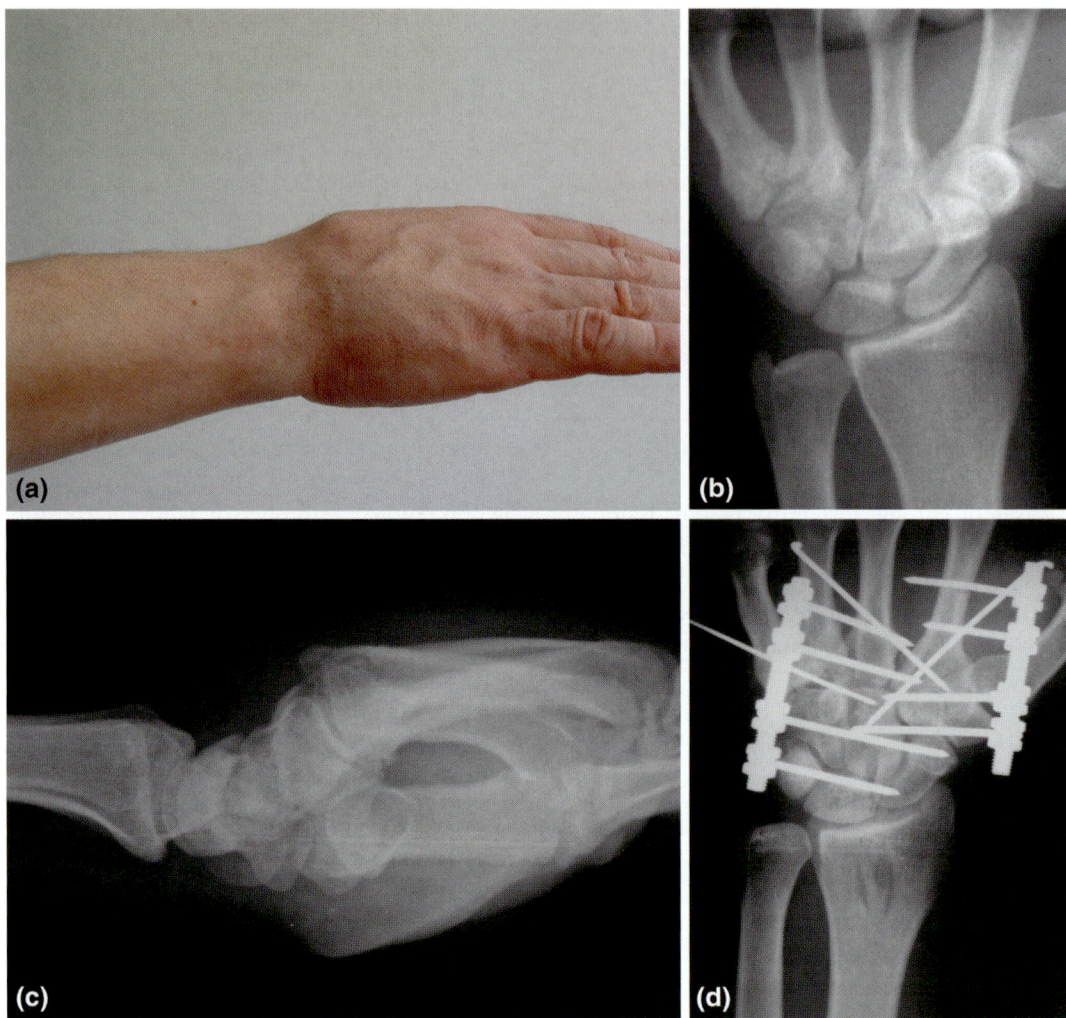

Fig. 9.24 Male, 29 years old, with a painful osseous swelling at the dorsal side of the wrist (**a**); radiographs revealed old unreduced dorsal dislocations, mainly of the 2nd to 3rd CMC joints (**b**, **c**); for the fusion of the affected joints and to regain the length of the shortened metacarpals, two small external fixators were used (**d**, **e**); radiographic appearance after the hardware removal (**f**, **g**)

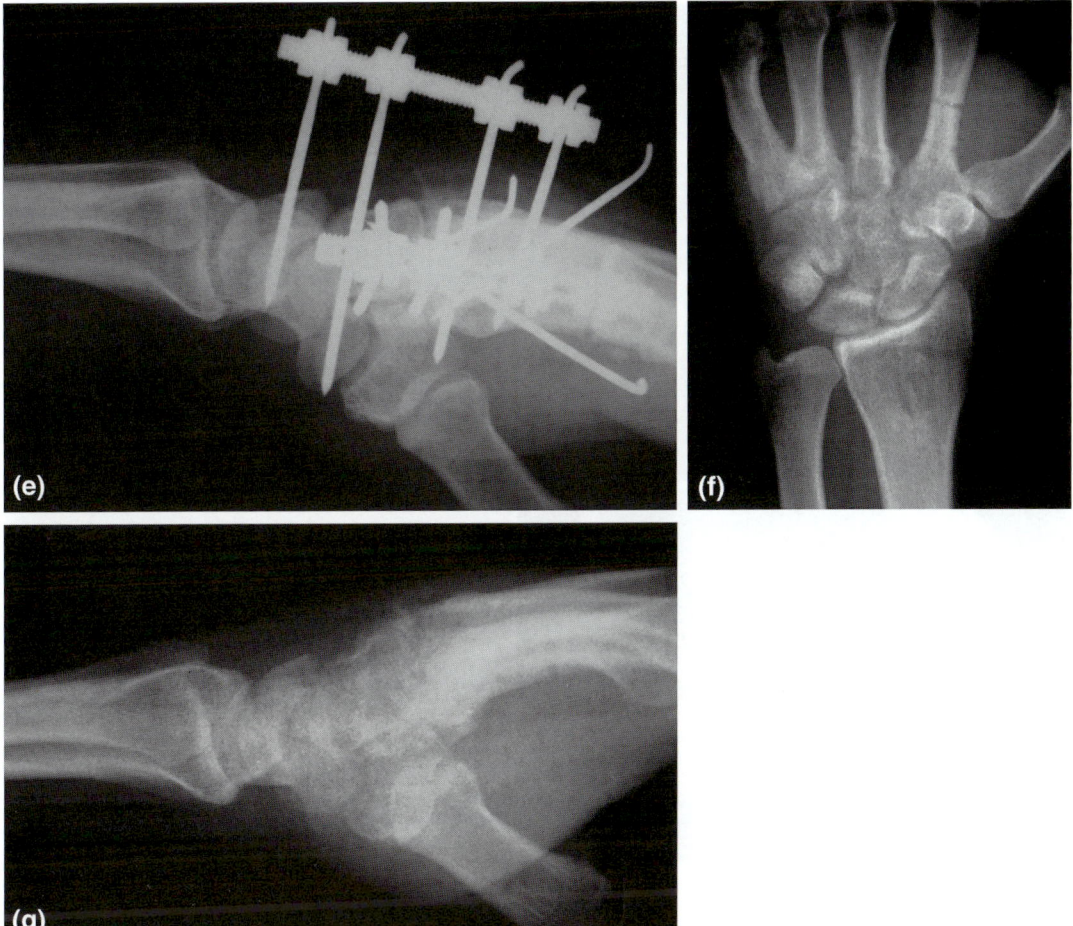

Fig. 9.24 (continued)

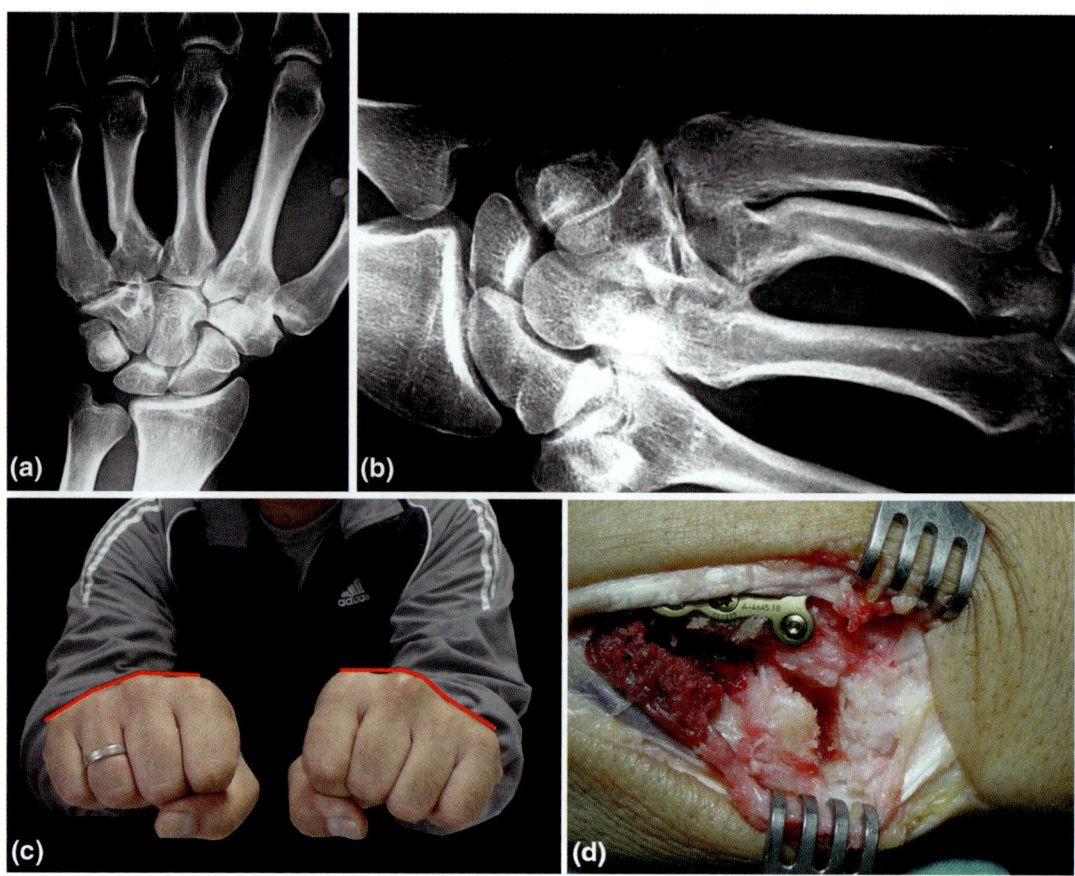

Fig. 9.25 Male, 35 years old, with a two-year-old malunion of the proximal 4th metacarpal, with arthritic changes of the dorsally subluxated 5th CMC joint (**a**, **b**); the disruption of the normal curvature of the metacarpal heads when making a fist, is showed (**c**); corrective osteotomy of the 4th metacarpal using a small plate and fusion of the 5th CMC joint (**d**, **e**); postoperative X-rays (**f**, **g**)

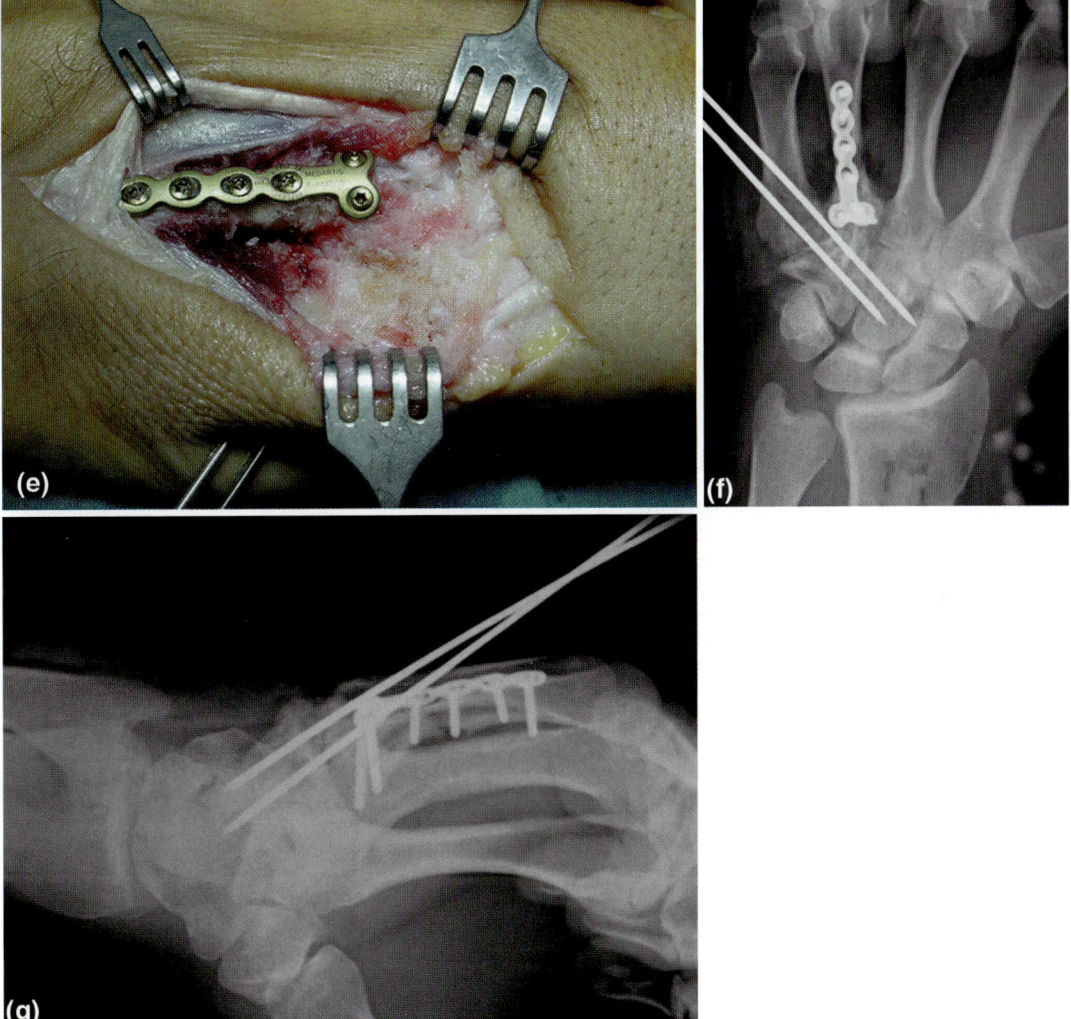

Fig. 9.25 (continued)

References

1. Waugh RL, Yancey AG (1948) Carpometacarpal dislocations. With particular reference to simultaneous dislocation of the bases of the fourth and fifth metacarpals. J Bone Joint Surg Am 30:397–404
2. Garcia-Elias M (2001) Carpometacarpal fractures and fractures dislocations. In: Watson K, Weinzweig J (eds) The wrist. Lippincott Williams & Wilkins, Philadelphia, pp 255–268
3. Gunther SF (1997) Medial four carpometacarpal joints. In: Lichtman DM, Alexander AH (eds) The wrist and its disorders, 2nd edn. WB Saunders Co, Philadelphia, pp 459–472
4. Watt N, Hooper G (1987) Dislocation of the trapezio-metacarpal joint. J Hand Surg [Br] 12(2):242–245
5. Bunnell S (1944) Fractures of metacarpals and phalanges. In: Bunnell S (ed) Surgery of the hand. JB Lippincott, Philadelphia, pp 528–531
6. Gurland M (1992) Carpometacarpal joint injuries of the fingers. Hand Clin 8:733
7. Mueller JJ (1986) Carpometacarpal dislocations: report of five cases and review of the literature. J Hand Surg [Am] 11(2):184–188
8. Dobyns JH, Linscheid RL, Cooney WP (1983) Fractures and dislocations of the wrist and hand, then and now. J Hand Surg [Am] 8:687–690
9. Garcia-Elias M, Bishop AT, Dobyns JH et al (1990) Transcarpal carpometacarpal dislocations excluding the thumb. J Hand Surg [Am] 15:531–540

10. Woon CYL, Chong KC, Low CO (2006) Carpometacarpal joint dislocations of the index to small finger: three cases and a review of the literature. Injury Extra 37:466–472
11. Gunther SF (1984) The carpometacarpal joints. Orthop Clin North Am 15:259–277
12. Harwin SF, Fox JM, Sedlin ED (1975) Volar dislocation of the bases of the second and third metacarpals. J Bone Joint Surg [Am] 57:849–851
13. El-Shennawy M, Nakamura K, Patterson RM et al (2001) Three-dimensional kinematic analysis of the second through fifth carpometacarpal joints. J Hand Surg [Am] 26:1030–1035
14. Joseph RB, Linscheid RL, Dobyns JH et al (1981) Chronic sprains of the carpometacarpal joints. J Hand Surg [Am] 6:172–180
15. Nakamura K, Patterson RM, Viegas SF (2001) The ligament and skeletal anatomy of the second through fifth carpometacarpal joints and adjacent structures. J Hand Surg [Am] 26:1016–1029
16. Nanno M, Buford WL, Patterson RM et al (2007) Three-dimensional analysis of the ligamentous attachments of the second through fifth carpometacarpal joints. Clin Anat 20:530–544
17. Rawles JG Jr (1988) Dislocations and fracture-dislocations at the carpometacarpal joints of the fingers. Hand Clin 4:103–112
18. Viegas SF, Crossley M, Marzke M et al (1991) The fourth carpometacarpal joint. J Hand Surg [Am] 16:525–532
19. Lewicky YM, Sheppard JE (2009) Closed-reduction percutaneous pinning of a complex divergent carpometacarpal fracture-dislocation involving the 4 ulnar carpometacarpal joints. Am J Orthop 38(4):191–193
20. Kirkham SG, Gray RJ (2004) Multiple carpometacarpal dislocations and an ipsilateral scapho-trapezium-trapezoid fracture-dislocation: a rare pattern of injury. J Orthop Surg 12(2):267–269
21. Griffiths MA, Moloney DM, Pickford MA (2005) Multiple carpometacarpal dislocations after a low-impact injury: a missed diagnosis. J Trauma 58(2):391–392
22. Oni O, Mackenny R (1986) Multiple dislocations of the carpometacarpal joints. J Hand Surg [Br] 11(1):47–48
23. Cain JE, Shepler TR, Wilson MR (1987) Hamatometacarpal fracture-dislocation: classification and treatment. J Hand Surg [Am] 12:762–767
24. Dunkerton M, Singer M (1985) Dislocation of the index metacarpal and trapezoid bones. J Hand Surg [Br] 10(3):377–378
25. Fakih RR, Fraser AM, Pimpalnerkar AL (1998) Hamate fracture with dislocation of the ring and little finger metacarpals. J Hand Surg [Br] 23(1):96–97
26. Foster RJ (1996) Stabilization of ulnar carpometacarpal dislocations or fracture dislocations. Clin Orthop 327:94–97
27. Henderson JJ, Arafa MA (1987) Carpometacaral dislocation: an easily missed diagnosis. J Bone Joint Surg [Br] 69:212–214
28. Laforgia R, Specchiulli F, Mariani A (1990) Dorsal dislocation of the fifth carpometacarpal joint. J Hand Surg [Am] 15:463–465
29. Langenhan R, Hohendorff B, Probst A (2011) Coronal fracture dislocation of the hamate and the base of the fourth metacarpal bone: a rare form of carpometacarpal injury. Handchir Mikrochir Plast Chir 43(3):140–146
30. Lee SU, Park IJ, Kim HM et al (2012) Fourth and fifth carpometacarpal fracture and dislocation of the hand: new classification and treatment. Eur J Orthop Surg Traumatol 22:571–578
31. Liaw Y, Kalnins G, Kirsh G et al (1995) Combined fourth and fifth metacarpal fracture and fifth carpometacarpal joint dislocation. J Hand Surg [Br] 20:249–252
32. Lilling M, Weinberg H (1979) The mechanism of dorsal fracture dislocation of the fifth carpometacarpal joint. J Hand Surg [Am] 4:340–342
33. Lundeen JM, Shin AY (2000) Clinical results of intraarticular fractures of the base of the fifth metacarpal treated by closed reduction and cast immobilization. J Hand Surg [Br] 25:258–261
34. Storm JO (1988) Traumatic dislocation of the fourth and fifth carpo-metacarpal joints: a case report. J Hand Surg [Br] 13(2):210–211
35. Topper S, Wood M (2010) Athletic injuries of the wrist. In: Cooney WP (ed) The Wrist. Diagnosis and operative treatment, 2nd edn. Wolters Kluwer/Lippincott Williams, Philadelphia, pp 1153–1186
36. Van der Lei B, Klasen HJ (1992) Dorsal carpometacarpal dislocation of the index finger: a report of three cases and a review of the English-language literature. J Trauma 32:789–793
37. Jameel J, Zahid M, Abbas M et al (2012) Volar dislocation of second, third, and fourth carpometacarpal joints: a rare and easily missed diagnosis. J Orthop Traumatol. doi: 10.1007/s10195-012-0181-3
38. Bora F, Disizian NH (1974) The treatment of injuries to the carpometacarpal joint of the little finger. J Bone Joint Surg Am 56(7):1459–1463
39. Hartwig RH, Louis DS (1979) Multiple carpometacarpal dislocations. A review of four cases. J Bone Joint Surg [Am] 61(6):906–908
40. Mullan GB, Lloyd GJ (1980) Complete carpal disruption of the hand. The Hand 12(1):39–42
41. DeBeer JV, Maloon S, Anderson P (1989) Multiple carpo-metacarpal dislocations. J Hand Surg [Br] 14:105–108
42. Kumar P (2010) Dislocation of second and third carpometacarpal joints along with fracture of first metacarpal—possible mechanisms. J Hand Microsurg 2(2):85–86

43. Kumar R, Malhotra R (2001) Divergent fracture-dislocation of the second carpometacarpal joint and three ulnar carpometacarpal joints. J Hand Surg [Am] 26:123–129

44. Chen VT (1987) Dislocation of carpometacarpal joint of the little finger. J Hand Surg [Br] 12(2):260–263

45. Garcia-Elias M, Rossignani P, Cots M (1996) Combined fracture of the hook of the hamate and palmar dislocation of the fifth carpometacarpal joint. J Hand Surg [Br] 21:446–450

46. Moriya K, Saito H, Takahashi Y et al (2011) Divergent fracture-dislocation of the hamatometacarpal joint: case report. J Hand Surg [Am] 36(1):47–51

47. North ER, Eaton RG (1980) Volar dislocation of the fifth metacarpal: report of two cases. J Bone Joint Surg Am 62:657–659

48. Tountas AA, Kwok JM (1984) Isolated volar dislocation of the fifth carpometacarpal joint. Case report. Clin Orthop 187:172–175

49. Prokopis P, Weiland A (2008) Volar dislocation of the fourth and fifth carpometacarpal joints: a case report and review of the literature. HSSJ 4:138–142

50. Carroll RE, Carlson E (1989) Diagnosis and treatment of injury to the second and third carpometacarpal joints. J Hand Surg [Am] 14:102–107

51. Gaheer RS, Ferdinand RD (2011) Fracture dislocation of carpometacarpal joints: a missed injury. Orthopedics 34(5):399

52. Guimaraes RM, Benaissa S, Moughabghab M et al (1996) Carpometacarpal dislocations of the long fingers. Apropos of 26 cases with review of 20 cases. Rev Chir Orthop Reparatrice Appar Mot 82:598–607

53. Pullen C, Richardson M, McCullough K et al (1995) Injuries to the ulnar carpometacarpal region: are they being underdiagnosed? Aust N Z J Surg 65:257–261

54. Iqbal MJ, Saleemi A (2003) Indian salutation test in acute dorsal carpometacarpal joint dislocation of the ulnar four fingers. Am J Emerg Med 21:74–76

55. Gore DR (1971) Carpometacarpal dislocation producing compression of the deep branch of the ulnar nerve. J Bone Joint Surg Am 53:1387–1390

56. Pimpalnerkar AL, Fakih R, Thomas AP (1997) Carpometacarpal dislocation producing transient motor neurapraxia of the ulnar nerve. Injury 28:397–400

57. Sreedharan S, Chew W (2008) Re: Isolated fifth carpometacarpal joint volar dislocation with ulnar neuropathy. J Hand Surg [Br] 33(2):219–220

58. Weiland AJ, Lister GD, Villareal-Rios A (1976) Volar fracture dislocations of the second and third carpometacarpal joints associated with acute carpal tunnel syndrome. J Trauma 16:672–675

59. Parkinson RW, Paton RW (1992) Carpometacarpal dislocation: an aid to diagnosis. Injury 23:187–188

60. Fischer JW, Waseem M, Gambhir A et al (2002) Ulnopalmar dislocation of the fifth carpometacarpal joint. A rare injury. Acta Orthop Belg 68:175–177

61. Fisher MR, Rogers LF, Hendrix RW (1983) Systematic approach to identifying fourth and fifth carpometacarpal joint dislocations. Am J Roentgenol 140:319–324

62. Yin Y, Mann F, Gilula LA et al (1996) Roentgenographic approach to complex bone abnormalities. In: Gilula LA, Yin Y (eds) Imaging of the wrist and hand. Saunders, Philadelphia, pp 293–318

63. McDonald LS, Shupe PG, Hammel N et al (2012) The intermetacarpal angle screening test for ulnar-sided carpometacarpal fracture-dislocations. J Hand Surg [Am] 37(9):1839–1844

64. Chmell S, Light TR, Blair SJ (1982) Fracture and fracture dislocation of ulnar carpometacarpal joint. Orthop Rev 11:73–80

65. Gehrmann SV, Grassmann JP, Schneppendahl J et al (2011) Treatment strategy for carpometacarpal fracture dislocation. Unfallchirurg 114(7):559–564

66. Nourissat G, Mudgal C, Ring D (2008) Bridge plating of the wrist for temporary stabilization of concomitant radiocarpal, intercarpal, and carpometacarpal injuries: a report of two cases. J Orthop Trauma 22:368–371

67. Prokuski L, Eglseder W (2001) Concurrent dorsal dislocations and fracture-dislocations of the index, long, ring, and small (second to fifth) carpometacarpal joints. J Orthop Trauma 15(8):549–554

68. Agarwal A, Agarwal R (2005) An unusual farm injury: carpometacarpal joint dislocations. J Hand Surg [Br] 30(6):633–634

69. Gunther SF, Bruno PD (1985) Divergent dislocation of the carpometacarpal joints: a case report. J Hand Surg [Am] 10:197–201

70. Lawlis JF III, Gunther SF (1991) Carpometacaral dislocations: long-term follow-up. J Bone Joint Surg Am 73:52–59

71. Loudyi D, Amar MF, Chbani B et al (2009) Divergent carpometacarpal joint dislocations of the ulnar four fingers (a case report). Chir Main 28(3):168–170

72. Busa R, Internullo G, Caroli A (1998) Divergent dislocation of the fourth and fifth carpometacarpal joints. J Hand Surg [Am] 23(3):529–531

73. Chalidis B, Dimitriou C (2012) Treatment of neglected divergent dislocation of hamatometacarpal complex with a circular spider plate. J Hand Surg [Eur] 37(9):897–899

74. Dillon J, Street J, Mahalingham K (2005) Divergent dislocation of the ring and little finger carpometacarpal joints–a rare injury pattern. Acta Othop Belg 71(3):353–356

75. Frick L, Mezzadri G, Yzem I et al (2011) Acute carpometacarpal joint dislocation of the long fingers: study of 100 cases. Chir Main 30(5):333–339

76. Loth TS, McMillan MD (1988) Coronal dorsal hamate fractures. J Hand Surg [Am] 13(4):616–618

77. Helal B, Kavanagh TG (1977) Unstable dorsal fracture-dislocation of the fifth carpometacarpal jont. Injury 9:138–142

78. Vandeweyer E, Botero L, Coessens BC (2002) Dorsal carpometarcarpal dislocation of ulnar fingers. A case report. Acta Chir Belg 102:279–280

79. Bonacina P, Faggioli AM, Gaetani G et al (2005) Complex fracture-dislocation of the carpometacarpal joint associated with a fracture of the hamate: a case report. J Orthop Traumatol 6(2):98–100

80. Kaneko K, Ono A, Uta S et al (2002) Hamatometacarpal fracture-dislocation: distinctive three dimensional computed tomographic appearance. Chir Main 21(1):41–45

81. Kerr HD (1992) Hamate-metacarpal fracture dislocation. J Emerg Med 10(5):565–568

82. Schrott E, Wessinghage D (1983) Course of treatment of a luxation of the 4th and 5th carpometacarpal joint with hamate involvement. Handchir Mikrochir Plast Chir 15(1):25–28

83. Syed AA, Agarwal M, Giannoudis PV et al (2002) Dorsal hamatometacarpal fracture-dislocation in a gymnast. Br J Sports Med 36(5):380–382

84. Hennig K (1986) Isolated dislocation of the 5th carpometacarpal joint. A case report. Unfallchirurg 89:574–575

85. Khodadadyan C, Hoffmann R, Moazami-Goudarzi Y et al (1995) Double dislocation of the fifth metacarpal. J Hand Surg [Br] 20:253–254

86. Tingart M, Bathis H, Bouillon B et al (2000) Dorsal carpometacarpal dislocation of the fifth finger: discussion of diagnosis and therapy on two cases. Unfallchirurg 103:76–80

87. Valente M, Saggin G, Alecci V (2009) Pure isolated dorsal dislocation of the fifth carpometacarpal joint. Chir Organi Mov 93(2):97–100

88. Vijayasekaran VS, Briggs P (2000) Isolated dorsal dislocation of the 5th carpometacarpal joint. Hand Surg 5:175–180

89. Yamakado K, Hashimoto F, Nagata S et al (2000) Isolated palmar dislocation of the fifth carpometacarpal joint diagnosed by stress X-rays. Arch Orthop Trauma Surg 120(9):529–530

90. Bajekal RA, Kotwal PP, Menon D (1992) Closed volar dislocations of the four ulnar carpometacarpal joints. Injury 23:355–356

91. Storken G, Bogie R, Jansen EJP (2011) Acute ulnar carpometacarpal dislocations. Can it be treated conservatively? A review of four cases. Hand 6(4):420–423

92. Mozaffarian K, Vosoughi AR, Hedjazi A et al (2012) The safest direction of percutaneous pinning for achieving firm fixing of the fifth carpometacarpal joint. J Orthop Sci 17(6):757–762

93. Bell T, Chinchalkar SJ, Faber K (2010) Postoperative management of carpometacarpal joint fracture dislocation of the hand: a case report. Can J Plast Surg 18(3):e37–e40

94. Slutsky DJ (2011) Arthroscopic reduction and percutaneous fixation of fifth carpometacarpal fracture dislocations. Hand Clin 27(3):361–367

95. Benoit O, Polveche G, Barbier J et al (2001) Fracture-dislocation of the second carpometacarpal joint. Case report and review of the literature. Chir Main 20(5):397–402

96. Carneiro RS, Rancatore E (2000) Dorsal dislocation of the index carpometacarpal joint. J Emerg Med 18:21–22

97. Santini AJ, Douglas DL (1998) Second carpometacarpal joint dislocation: an impossible situation? Int J Clin Pract 52:517–518

98. Schutt RC, Boswick JA, Scott FA (1981) Volar fracture-dislocation of the carpometacarpal joint of the index finger treated by delayed open reduction. J Trauma 21:986–987

99. Thomas WO, Gottliebson WM, D'Amore TF et al (1994) Isolated palmar displaced fracture of the base of the index metacarpal: a case report. J Hand Surg [Am] 19:455–456

100. Ho PK, Choban SJ, Eshman SJ et al (1987) Complex dorsal dislocation of the second carpometacarpal joint. J Hand Surg [Am] 12:1074–1076

101. Köse O, Islam C (2008) Re: irreducible dorsal dislocation of the index carpometacarpal joint. J Hand Surg [Br] 33(2):217–218

102. Peace WJ, Abrams RA (2010) Simultaneous dorsal dislocations of the carpometacarpal joints of all four fingers. Orthopedics 33(2):121–123

103. Edwards A, Pike J, Bird J (2000) Simultaneous carpometacarpal joint dislocations of the thumb and all four fingers. Injury 31:116–118

104. Fayman M, Hugo B, de Wet H (1988) Simultaneous dislocation of all five carpometacarpal joints. Plast Reconstr Surg 82:151–154

105. Hsu KY, Wu CC, Wang KC et al (1993) Simultaneous dislocation of the five carpometacarpal joints with concomitant fractures of the tuberosity of the trapezium and the hook of the hamate: case report. J Trauma 35:479–483

106. Jebson PJ, Engber WD, Lange RH (1994) Dislocation and fracture-dislocation of the carpometacarpal joints. Orthop Rev 1994:19–28

107. Kneife F (2002) Simultaneous dislocations of the five carpometacarpal joints. Injury 33:846

108. Pérez-Serna AG, Figueroa-Cal y Mayor F (2009) Multiple carpometacarpal fracture-dislocation. Acta Ortop Mex 23(3):149–152

109. Petersen MB, Nielsen PT, Nielsen LS (1992) Simultaneous occurrence of trapezium-scaphoid-trapezoid dislocation and multiple carpometacarpal

fracture dislocations. A case report. Acta Orthop Scand 63:104–105

110. Reznick SM, Greene TL, Roeser W (1985) Simultaneous dislocation of the five carpometacarpal joints. Clin Orthop 192:210–214

111. Schortinghuis J, Klasen HJ (1997) Open reduction and internal fixation of an unusual multiple carpometacarpal dislocation using one plate: a case report. Injury 28:701–703

112. Yildiz M, Baki C, Sener M (1995) Isolated dislocation of all five carpometacarpal joints. J Hand Surg [Br] 20:606–608

113. Mabee JR, Lee TJ, Halus S (1997) Dorsal dislocation of the four ulnar metacarpals. Am J Emerg Med 15:408–411

114. Mito K, Nakamura T, Sato K et al (2008) Dorsal dislocations of the second to fifth carpometacarpal joints: a case report. Hand Surg 13(2):129–132

115. Pankaj A, Malhotra R, Bhan S (2005) Isolated dislocation of the four ulnar carpometacarpal joints. Arch Orthop Trauma Surg 125:541–544

116. Pansard E, Kaba A, Peyroux LM et al (2009) Combined carpometacarpal dislocations, hand lesions and fractures of the two bones of the forearm: a report of two cases. Chir Main 28(4):250–254

117. Siddiqui YS, Zahid M, Sabir AB (2011) Multiple carpometacarpal fracture dislocation of the hand – An uncommon pattern of injury which is often missed : a case report with review of literature. JCDR 5(3):618–620

118. Smith GR, Yang SS, Weiland AJ (1996) Multiple carpometacarpal dislocations. A case report and review of treatment. Am J Orthop 25(7):502–506

119. Kleinman WB, Grantham SA (1978) Multiple volar carpometacarpal joint dislocation. Case report of traumatic volar dislocation of the medial four carpometacarpal joint in a child and review of the literature. J Hand Surg [Am] 3:377–382

120. Kumar S, Arora A, Jain AK et al (1998) Volar dislocation of multiple carpometacarpal joints: report of four cases. J Orthop Trauma 12:523–526

121. Kahlon IA, Karim A, Khan Z (2011) Multiple carpometacarpal volar dislocation. J Coll Physicians Surg Pak 21(1):49–51

122. Woo CC (1988) Traumatic volar dislocation of the second, third and fourth carpometacarpal joints: mechanism and manipulation. JMPT 11:124–129

123. Robison JE, Kaye JJ (2005) Simultaneous fractures of the capitate and hamate in the coronal plane: case report. J Hand Surg [Am] 30:1153–1155

124. Kang SY, Song KS, Lee HJ et al (2009) A case report of coronal fractures through the hamate, the capitate, and the trapezoid. Arch Orthop Trauma Surg 129:963–965

125. Hazlett JW (1968) Carpometacarpal dislocations other than the thumb: a report of 11 cases. Can J Surg 11:315–323

126. Hanel DP (1996) Primary fusion of fracture dislocations of central carpometacarpal joints. Clin Orthop 327:85–93

127. Imbriglia JE (1979) Chronic dorsal carpometacarpal dislocation of the index, middle ring and little fingers: a case report. J Hand Surg 4:343–345

128. Ahmad S, Plancher K (1996) Carpometacarpal dislocations of the fingers. Oper Techn Sports Med 4(4):257–267

129. Green DP (1990) Dislocations and ligamentous injuries of the wrist. In: Evarts CM (ed) Surgery of the musculoskeletal system, 2nd edn. Churchill Livingstone, New York, pp 449–515

130. Gainor BJ, Stark HH, Ashworth CR (1991) Tendon arthroplasty of the fifth carpometacarpal joint for treatment of post-traumatic arthritis. J Hand Surg [Am] 16:520–524

131. Dubert T, Khalifa H (2009) "Stabilized arthroplasty" for old fracture dislocations of the fifth carpometacarpal joint. Techn Hand Upper Extrem Surg 13(3):134–136

132. Apergis E (2004) καταγματα-εξαρθρήματα του καρπου. Konstantaras Medical Books, Athens

Part IV
Other Carpal Dislocations

Axial Dislocations or Fracture-Dislocations

10

10.1 Introduction

The first radiological description of a true axial dislocation of the wrist is attributed to Oberst in 1901 (cited by Shin [1]) and in the same year to Eigenbrodt [2]. The former described a case of axial-ulnar dislocation, while the latter, a case of severe crush injury to the hand that was associated with dislocation of the hamate.

The term "axial-loading dislocation" was first used by Cooney et al. [3] to emphasize that in these cases the wrist is disorganized in a direction almost parallel to the long axis of the forearm. Other terms used to describe this injury are: "carpal arch disruption" [4], "capitohamate diastasis" [5], "longitudinal disruption" [6], "crush injury of the carpus" [7], and "columnar dislocation" [8].

When the wrist is subjected to compressive high energy force in dorsopalmar direction, the resulting derangement is frequently not random, but predetermined, with the wrist being divided into two or more columns. At the same time, the metacarpals usually follow the displacement of the corresponding carpal bones causing an intermetacarpal derangement. While the transverse carpal arch widens, the transverse ligament of the wrist is either ruptured or detached from its attachments [9, 10].

Garcia-Elias et al. [8] defined axial fracture-dislocation as the longitudinal carpal and intermetacarpal derangement of the wrist, which is associated with rupture or avulsion of the flexor retinaculum. Chim et al. [11] defined axial carpal dislocation as the global disruption of the proximal (carpal) and distal (metacarpal) transverse arches of the hand with the carpus split and longitudinally displaced.

10.2 Incidence

Axial dislocations of the wrist are relatively rare injuries as, since the first radiological report in 1901 until today, approximately 72 cases have been published in the literature [12], the majority of which are case reports [11–17]. The increasing number of industrial accidents and the increased recognition of wrist injuries, will certainly result in more frequent diagnosis of such injuries.

The largest series that has been published until now, comes from Mayo Clinic with 16 cases, that is 1.4 % of all patients with fracture-dislocation of the carpus (1,140 patients) [18]. Until then, the maximum number of patients reported in a series was 4 patients [4, 6, 19]. However, in developing countries where security measures are loose and industrial accidents more frequent, this percentage increases to 2.08 % [7].

10.3 Mechanism of Injury

Most axial dislocations are industrial injuries. A crushing, explosive, or rotational mechanism usually brought upon by machinery such as a

E. Apergis, *Fracture-Dislocations of the Wrist*,
DOI: 10.1007/978-88-470-5328-1_10, © Springer-Verlag Italia 2013

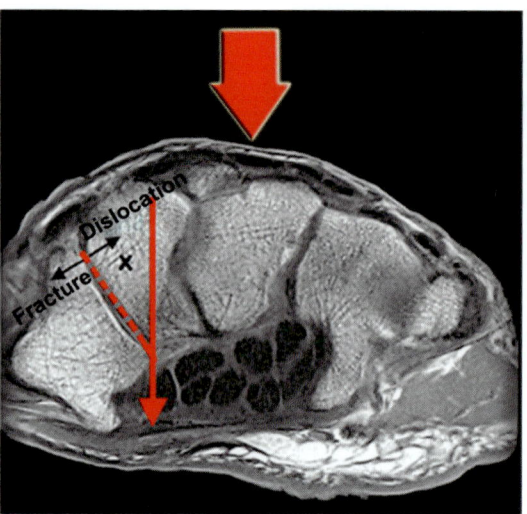

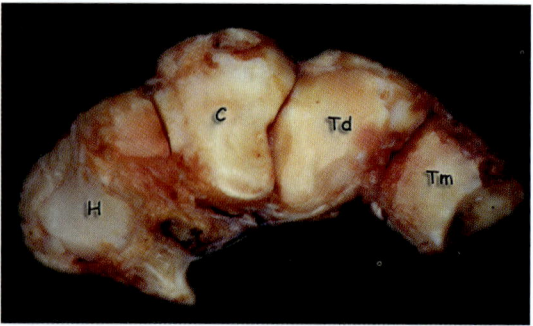

Fig. 10.2 The distal carpal row bones are positioned like stones in an arch (distal joint surfaces of the distal carpal row as seen from the side of the metacarpals). With permission from [50]

Fig. 10.1 The X angle is the angle formed between the applied force and the joint surface plane of the distal row bones. A smaller angle increases the possibility of a dislocation, while a larger angle increases the possibility of a fracture. With permission from [50]

roller or a molding press [1, 9, 20] is considered responsible for such injuries. In some cases, a direct strike by a blunt object (e.g., piston) [21] may also be implicated. The force exerted on the wrist usually has a dorsopalmar direction and the resulting injury following the application of compressive force, depends upon:

1. The angle formed by the applied force and the plane of joint surfaces of the distal carpal row. The smaller the angle, the higher the chances for a dislocation to occur, whereas the bigger the angle is, the greater becomes the possibility of a fracture at the sagittal plane [1, 10] (Fig. 10.1).
2. The magnitude, the speed, and the point of force application.
3. The relative strength of bones and ligaments.
    There are however in the literature isolated cases of combined injuries of axial disruption and perilunate wrist injuries, for which a compressive and simultaneously dorsal hyperextension mechanism is implicated [22, 23].

10.4 Biomechanics

In the transverse plane the carpal bones of the distal carpal row align in a semicircular, palmarly concave arch. The highly intrinsic stability presented by the distal carpal row is due not only to the interosseous ligaments (see Anatomy section), but also to its peculiar anatomy in which the bones fit together like stones in an arch where the capitate bone is the keystone (Fig. 10.2). Although it is subjected to a small rotational motion among the distal carpal row bones [24, 25], the distal row along with the 2nd and 3rd MC are regarded as the fixed unit of the hand.

The main stabilizing elements in the transverse coherence of the distal carpal row bones, are the interosseous ligaments and particularly the capitohamate ligament, which fails at an average of 252 N [8]. Conversely, the ultimate strength of each one of the remaining distal row interosseous ligaments ranges from 110 to 145 N. (Fig. 10.3). Since the capitohamate ligament has the highest ultimate strength, one would expect that axial disruptions would more often concern the radial side of the wrist. In the literature, however, axial disruptions of the ulnar side of the distal carpal row (between capitate-hamate) are not rare at all. On the contrary, out

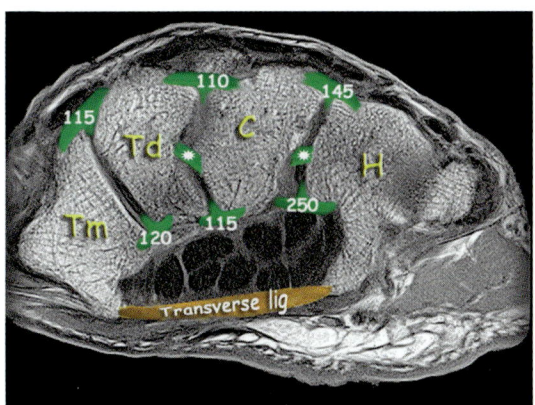

Fig. 10.3 The strength (N) of the palmar and dorsal distal carpal row ligaments (approximate values) (*Tm* Trapezium, *Td* Trapezoid, *C* Capitate, *H* Hamate). The asterisks indicate the deep part of the capitohamate and trapezoid-capitate ligaments. With permission from [50]

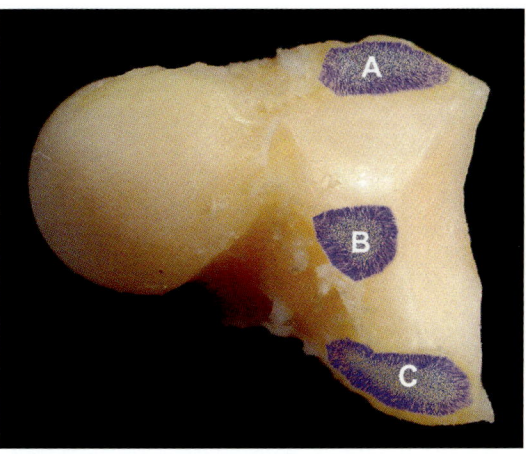

Fig. 10.4 The areas of adhesion of the capitohamate ligament at the surface of the capitate facing the hamate. **a** Dorsal part. **b** Deep part. **c** Palmar part. With permission from [50]

of the 40 cases mentioned before 1989, the 23 involved the ulnar side of the wrist [19, 26].

Ritt et al. [27] found up to 12° rotation at the capitohamate joint, which is stabilized by 3 ligaments: the dorsal, the palmar, and the deep interosseous ligaments. Failure testing showed the deep ligament was strongest at 289 N, followed by the palmar at 171 N and the dorsal at 133 N. (Fig. 10.4). The authors considered the capitohamate as the strongest joint of the wrist, supporting that it is not surprising that capitohamate dissociation was evident in only 3 out of 16 cases in the series of Garcia-Elias et al. [18].

Some authors [28, 29] have supported the crucial role of the transverse carpal ligament in the coherence of the carpal arc. Although sectioning of the transverse ligament may increase the width of the carpal tunnel (distance between the ridge of the trapezium and the hook of the hamate) up to 11 % or reduce the grip strength [30, 31], the dynamic behavior of the transverse carpal arc is not altered [30, 32]. Even though the strength of the transverse carpal ligament is greater than that of any carpal ligament (withstands 343 N), it has small axial tensile stiffness (131 N/mm) and its contribution to the

transverse coherence of the wrist does not exceed 7.5 % of the total strength [8]. Despite these, Shin [1] expressed the opinion that in cases of injury of the palmar interosseous ligaments of the distal carpal row, repairing the transverse carpal ligament can possibly restore to some extent the stability of the transverse arc.

10.5 Clinical Presentation

Patients with traumatic axial fracture-dislocations typically present severe soft tissue damage, ranging from marked swelling and tenderness, to partial or total denudation of the hand from soft tissues. Intrinsic muscles are often severely damaged; thenar muscles (more frequently) and hypothenar muscles (less commonly) are damaged at varying degrees [7]. Often extensor or flexor tendon ruptures coexist and neurovascular injuries are often present. Vascular injuries with rupture of the radial or ulnar artery or both, are not common. More frequent are nerve injuries, ranging from transient neuroapraxia to axonotmesis.

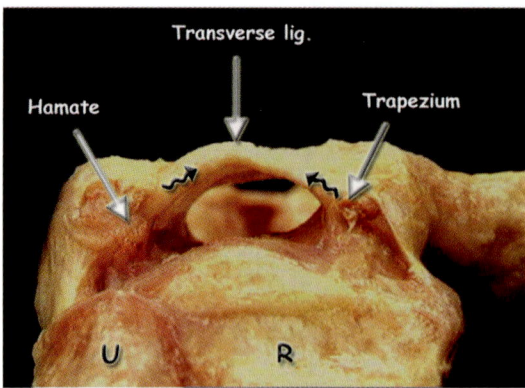

Fig. 10.5 The carpal tunnel, the transverse ligament and its attachments to the hamate and the trapezium, as seen from the proximal surface. With permission from [50]

Other frequently associated fractures are: the trapezial ridge, hook of the hamate, metacarpals, phalangeals, carpal bones or the distal radius [10, 33]. Also frequent are the dislocations of the carpometacarpal joints, while rotational deformity of the fingers is also a common clinical finding. The prevalence of acute carpal tunnel syndrome is rare, due to the traumatic decompression of the carpal tunnel that occurs with the rupture or avulsion of the transverse ligament from the hook of the hamate or the ridge of the trapezium [18] (Fig. 10.5).

Despite the rarity of reports, there certainly are cases of partial or complete rupture of distal carpal row interosseous ligaments and which manifest as chronic wrist pain due to the difficulty in diagnosing such injuries [34].

10.6 Imaging Studies

Unless there is gross disruption of the carpus, in standard radiographic views the following findings are assessed: loss of parallelism between the articular surfaces of the distal row, while diastasis or overlapping of the articular surfaces are findings suggesting subluxation or dislocation of the bones.

Breaks in Gilula's arcs are also evaluated and suggest disruption of the smooth contour of the proximal articular surfaces of the distal carpal row. It is also possible that the longitudinal axis of the affected metacarpal shafts may lack the normal parallelism to the unaffected metacarpal shafts. The lateral view reveals the direction of the dislocation and associated fractures. Traction radiographs often delineate the extent and nature of associated bony pathology [1].

Avulsion fracture of the hook of the hamate and/or the fracture of the ridge of the trapezium may be considered as indirect radiological findings indicative of the axial disruption of the wrist [33].

When in doubt, CT scans or trispiral tomography may possibly assist in the clarification of the injury.

10.7 Classification

In the classification of carpal instabilities, axial disruption of the distal carpal row belongs to the dissociative type of instabilities (CID). The spectrum of axial carpal instability ranges from acute, gross traumatic fracture dislocation with severe soft tissue trauma to chronic, dynamic instability between the axial components of the carpus [1]. In chronic cases, if the carpal derangement is evident on plane radiographs, then the case is considered as "static axial instability", while if the derangement can be diagnosed only under certain loading conditions, the term "dynamic axial instability" is used [10].

Although axial disruption of the wrist, in the majority of cases, is presented with an obvious clinical and radiological picture, in the literature at least one case of dynamic axial dissociation has been reported, due to isolated rupture of the capitohamate interosseous ligament [34]. The patient remained undiagnosed for several months complaining of ulnar wrist pain, as all examination methods were normal. The diagnosis was finally established arthroscopically (through the midcarpal ulnar portal), where a complete loss of integrity of the capitohamate interosseous ligaments was observed. The patient was treated successfully with a capitohamate fusion.

A similar case from the personal archive, involved a patient with radial wrist pain who remained undiagnosed for 6 months. It was found to be a case of dissociative instability (CID), concerning the distal carpal row and particularly the trapezium-trapezoid joint, the interosseous ligaments of which were ruptured. Clinically, a clunking associated with the appearance of a sulcus to the radial side of the wrist, during active radial deviation, was noticed (Fig. 10.6a–g).

As incomplete cases of axial dissociation of the wrist following the application of compressive forces can be considered, the avulsion of the transverse ligament from its attachments (hook of the hamate and ridge of the trapezium) as an isolated injury [35] or in combination with fracture at the body of the trapezium in the frontal plane [36] or dislocation of the hamate combined with fracture of the palmar ridge of the trapezium [37].

After reviewing the literature and adding 16 new cases, Garcia-Elias et al. [18] classified axial dissociations of the wrist into three types, according to the direction of instability:

10.7.1 Axial-Ulnar Dislocations

The carpus splits into two columns in which the radial column is stable with respect to the radius whereas the ulnar column displaces proximally and ulnarly. The fourth and fifth metacarpals are displaced along with the ulnar column. Depending on the path of injury, these injuries are adequately described by using the term "trans" to indicate fracture and the prefix "peri" to express dislocation.

The most common axial-ulnar dislocation involves the pisiform and the hamate, identified as a peri-hamate, peri-pisiform axial-ulnar dislocation [4, 16, 19, 20, 38]. Less common types of axial-ulnar dislocations that have been reported, are: the trans-hamate axial-ulnar dislocation [15], the trans-hamate peri-pisiform [16, 19], the peri-hamate dislocation with fracture of the hook of the hamate [14], the peri-

hamate, peri-pisiform, trans-triquetrum with fracture of the hook of the hamate [21], the peri-hamate trans-triquetrum fracture dislocation [13, 19, 39], and the peri-hamate, peri-triquetrum axial-ulnar dislocation [6, 10, 26]. The most common types of axial ulnar dislocation injuries and their terminology are shown in Fig. 10.7a–d.

10.7.2 Axial-Radial Dislocations

In this type the ulnar column of the wrist maintains its relation to the radius, while the radial column is displaced proximally and radially. The first or also the second metacarpal follows the displaced radial column of the wrist. The most common type of axial-radial dislocation is the peri-trapezium dislocation, followed by the peri-trapezium, peri-trapezoid, and the trans-trapezium axial dislocations (Figs. 10.8a–c, 10.9a–e). Spreading of the applied force to the proximal carpal row could injure the ligamentous support of the scaphoid, leading to a complex scaphoid dislocation [40–43].

10.7.3 Combined Axial Radial-Ulnar Dislocations

In this rare type of injuries, only the central column of the wrist maintains its relation to the radius, whereas both the radial and ulnar columns are dissociated and proximally displaced (Fig. 10.10). Only few such cases have been reported in the literature [4, 16, 18, 44–47] while the case presented by Irwin [22] was considered as a variant of the combined axial radial-ulnar disruption. In two cases from the personal records, as well as the case presented by Dobyns and Linscheid [45], the carpus separated into two columns with the central part also being dissociated (Figs. 10.11a–c, 10.12a–e). These cases possibly constitute a separate type of injuries.

Literature review by Garcia–Elias et al. [18] revealed 40 cases of axial dissociation of the wrist with adequate information about radiologic

Fig. 10.6 A 25-year old male, fell from height. He presented with radial wrist pain, which did not respond to the conservative treatment administered, while radiological imaging was negative. Six months later he was still undiagnosed with anatomic snuffbox sensitivity, while during active radial deviation he presented with sudden palmar collapse of the radial half, accompanied by a clicking sound and the appearance of a sulcus in that area. The wrist in ulnar deviation (**a**) and in radial deviation with the sulcus being evident (**b**). In comparative, under traction X-rays of the injured wrist a step between the trapezium and trapezoid was observed (**c**). With the wrist in neutral position, the subluxation of the trapezoid and rupture of the dorsal interosseous ligament were evident (**d**). With the wrist in radial deviation the subluxation was exacerbated, whereas the distal pole of the scaphoid "sunk" ulnovolarly (**e**). The patient was successfully treated with fusion of the trapezium–trapezoid bones (**f**); final radiographic appearance after 12 years (**g**). (*Tm* Trapezium, *Td* Trapezoid, *S* Scaphoid). With permission from [50]

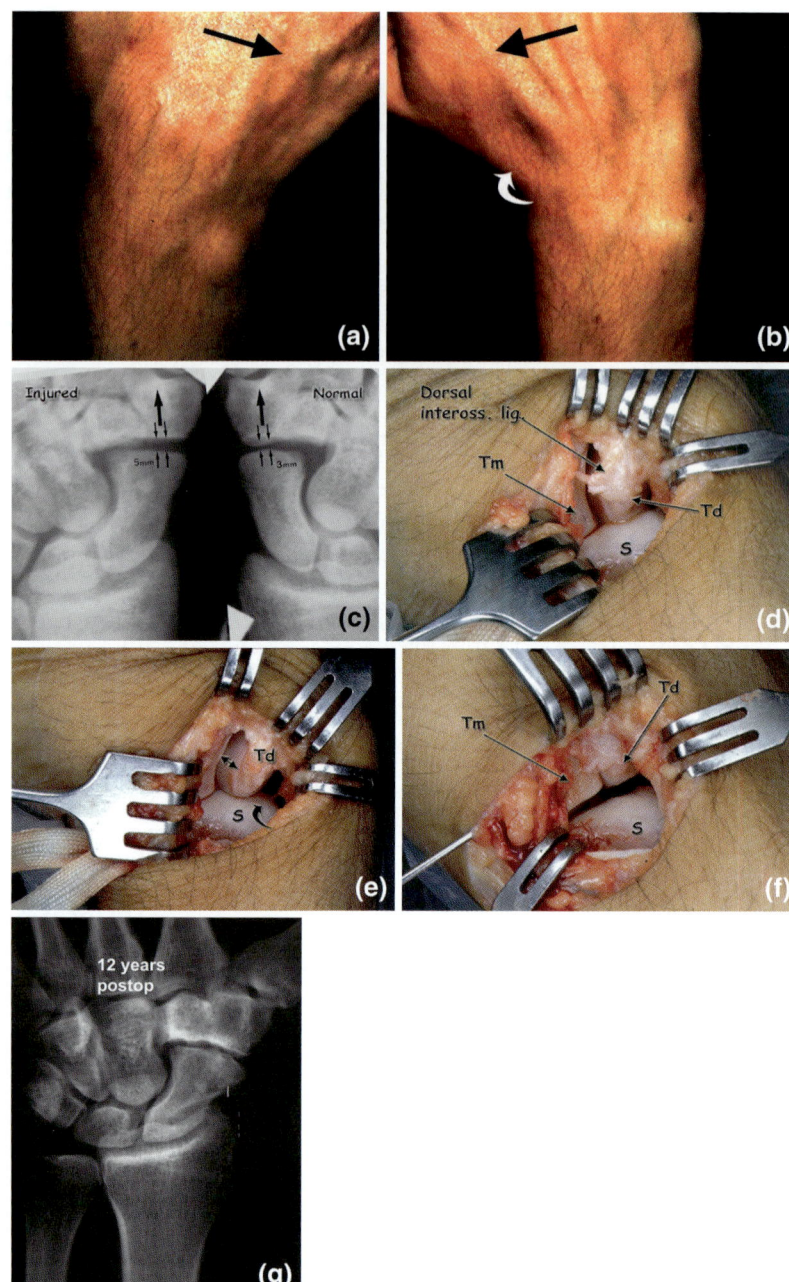

features. The same author added 16 new cases, and if we include the 13 cases presented by Pai and Wei [16], the 4 cases presented by Primiano and Reef [4] and the 2 of 3 cases presented by Norbeck et al. [6], the total of 75 cases allow us to estimate the distribution of these injuries. Thirty six of these cases were of AU type, 33 cases were of AR type and 6 cases were of combined AR-AU type. According to the above, the frequency of dissociation of the radial and ulnar columns of the wrist is approximately the same, while the combined AR-AU type is the most unusual.

Fig. 10.7 Axial-ulnar
dislocations: Peri-hamate,
Trans-triquetral (**a**); Trans-
hamate, Peri-pisiform (**b**);
Peri-hamate, Peri-pisiform
(**c**); Peri-hamate, Peri-
triquetral (**d**). With
permission from [50]

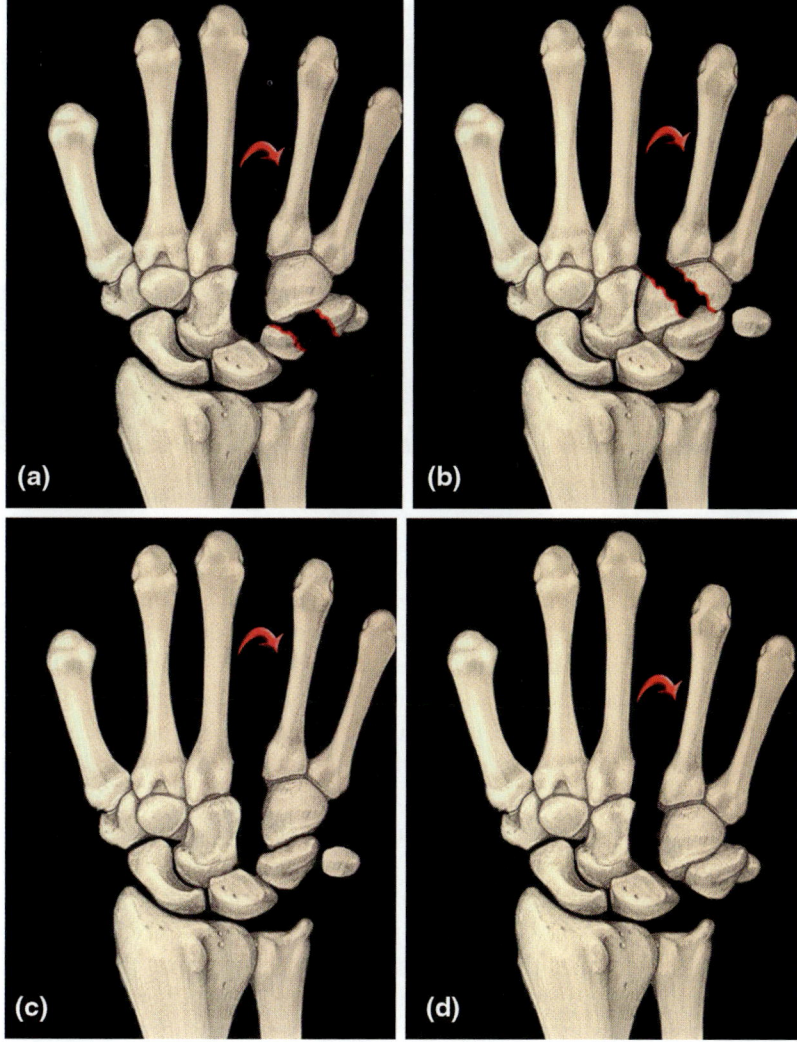

The clarification of dissociated metacarpals is necessary to be included in terminology because the path of injury, proximal to the base of the metacarpals, is not always on the same side with the metacarpals dissociation. Häcki et al. [12] reported a case with dissociation between the third and fourth metacarpals while proximally the injury progressed radially with fractures of the capitate and trapezium and dislocation of the trapezoid. A similar case was reported by Horton et al. [41] in which the dissociation between the third and fourth metacarpals was associated with disruption between capitate and hamate and proximally with scapholunate dissociation leading to a complex dislocation of the scaphoid [42]. Garcia-Elias [10] stated that this injury fulfills the criteria of an axial-radial dislocation.

A particular type of injuries are the cases reported, where the axial disruption of the wrist is associated with dislocation of the lunocapitate joint, as these cases constitute a variant between axial and perilunate dislocation [17, 23, 41, 48].

10.8 Differential Diagnosis

Differential diagnosis of axial dislocations must be made from perilunate and isolated dislocations of the carpal bones [10]. Concerning perilunate injuries the differential diagnosis is

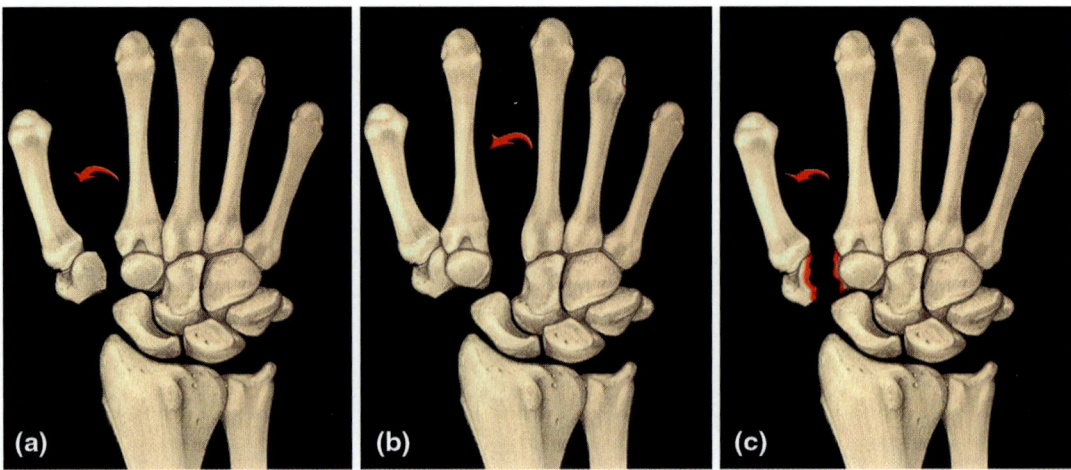

Fig. 10.8 Axial-radial dislocations: Peri-trapezium (**a**), Peri-trapezium, Peri-trapezoid (**b**), Trans-trapezium (**c**). With permission from [50]

associated with: (a) *the mechanism of injury*, where axial dislocations arise following the application of direct crushing force, while the perilunate dislocations are the result of indirect force (hyperextension, axial rotation and lateral deviation of the wrist); (b) *the path of injury*, where in axial dislocations follows a longitudinal pattern of disruption, whereas in perilunate dislocations the injury presents a progressive perilunar pattern of instability; (c) The *acute carpal tunnel syndrome* is common in perilunate injuries, while axial disruption implies a traumatic decompression that occurs with discontinuity of the flexor retinaculum. The nerve dysfunction in axial dislocations is related to the direct blow or to the associated soft-tissue swelling; and (d) *Soft tissue damage,* which is common in axial dislocations, but rare in perilunate dislocations.

Regarding isolated dislocations of carpal bones, when a localized force is concentrated over a single bone, a localized dislocation or fracture-dislocation may be caused which however is not truly an axial disruption, as there is no global carpal and metacarpal disruption and the flexor retinaculum does not appear disrupted.

10.9 Management

The majority of axial carpal dislocations are open injuries with significant associated soft tissue injuries. Treatment depends on whether the injury is open or closed and upon the extent of damage of the osseous structures and soft tissues. However, the role of nonoperative treatment in axial injuries of the carpus is limited. Careful evaluation of the condition of the neurovascular and musculotendinous units must be performed. Early and accurate diagnosis of the soft tissue and bony injuries is necessary, as delayed treatment from incorrect diagnosis is much less successful than early treatment. Injury to the soft-tissues may be severe enough to warrant fasciotomies of the volar and dorsal compartments of the forearm and hand if compartment syndrome is present or suspected throughout the perioperative period [1, 49]. We often need to put priorities in addressing these injuries. Failing to manage the osseous injuries adequately, could result in flattening of the palm, spread of the carpometacarpal arch, weakness and motion restriction [4, 45]. If soft tissue loss is significant and there is crushing, swelling,

Fig. 10.9 Male, 39 years old. Motorcycle accident. A case of peri-trapezium dislocation (**a**); the CT scan image (**b**); during exploration, the rupture of the STT ligament was apparent (*arrows*). It was reconstructed using a bone anchor inserted at the scaphoid (**c**); fixation using K-wires between trapezium-trapezoid and STT joint (**d**); final X-rays 4 months postoperatively (**e**)

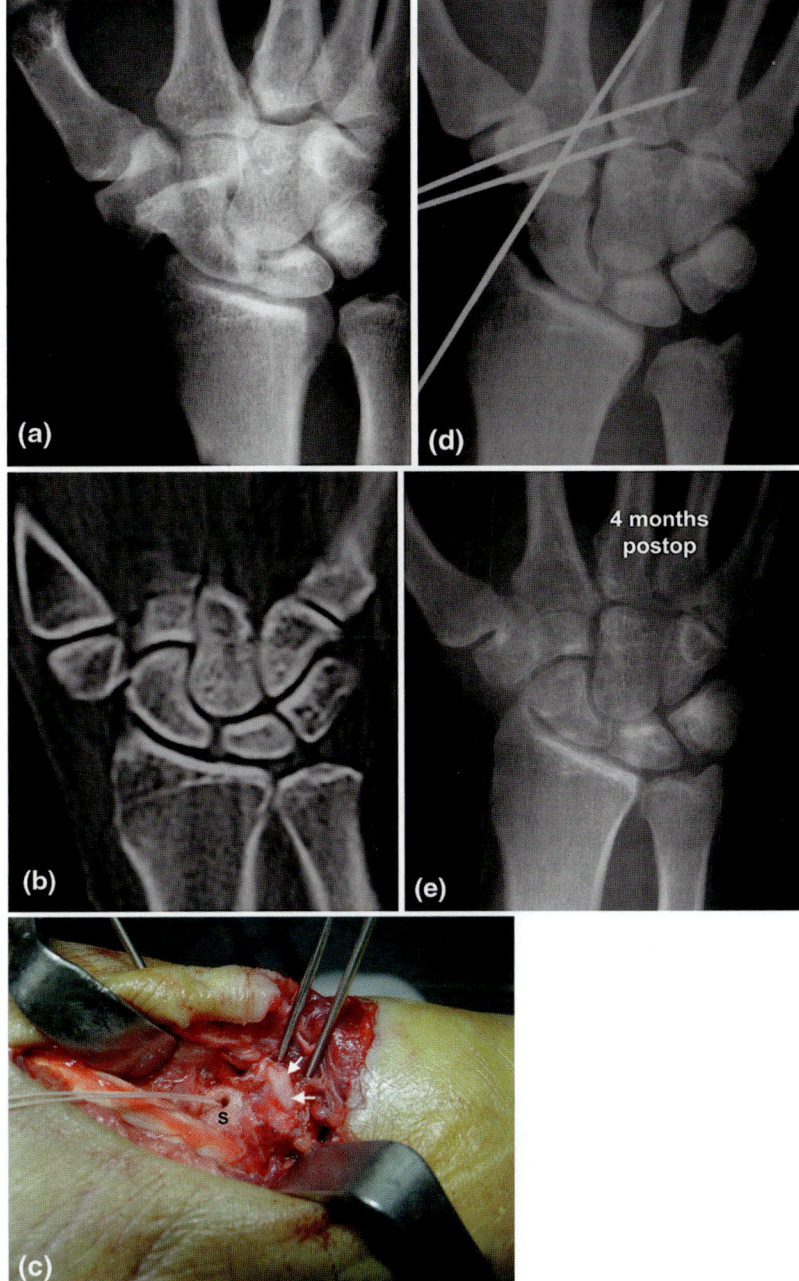

secondary contamination and infection, this may exclude the opportunity to reduce the fracture as a primary or secondary procedure [45].

Preoperatively, intravenous antibiotic and low molecular weight dextran are administered. Extensive debridement of necrotic or non-viable tissues is required, while primary suturing of the wound is rarely necessary or desirable. Surgical treatment also involves restoration of neurovascular and musculotendinous structure damage, as well as immediate skin defect coverage with local or free tissue flaps.

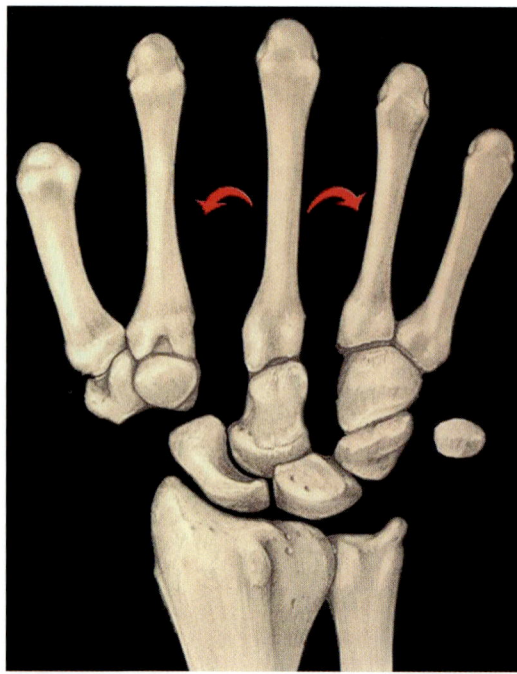

Fig. 10.10 Schematic depiction of the combined axial radial-ulnar dislocation. With permission from [50]

Closed reduction, which is usually achieved by longitudinal traction through the fingers and percutaneous fixation of the displaced bones, is an option for closed injuries and has been used for axial carpal sprains or dislocations with minimal associated injuries that are easily reduced and maintained by cast immobilization [13, 22] or

using an external fixator [26]. However, interposed soft tissue or fracture fragments may prevent anatomic reduction, necessitating open treatment [1, 49]. Only 7 out of 56 reported cases before 1989 were treated with closed reduction and cast immobilization. All of them were of the axial-ulnar dislocation type with three pure dislocations and four fracture dislocations [18].

Open reduction with combined dorsal longitudinal (for the reduction of osseous structures) and extended palmar approach through the carpal tunnel (for the evaluation and restoration of soft tissues), is more frequently used. Fixation is typically performed using K wires, while suturing the remnants of interosseous ligaments is rarely feasible. Additional fixation using screws may be considered in selected cases [12, 14]. The use of bone anchors instead of the transosseous holes is preferred, whenever possible [49]. Postoperatively, immobilization, either in a cast or with external fixation, is maintained for approximately 6 weeks depending on the extent of injuries and mobilization commences under physiotherapy supervision.

10.10 Outcome and Complications

Functional results are more dependent upon the associated injuries of soft tissues, than on the osseous injury itself [10, 18, 49].

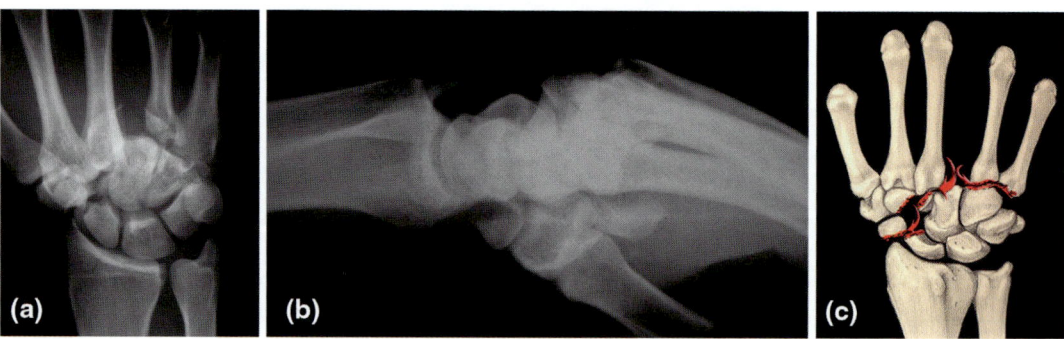

Fig. 10.11 A variant of combined axial radial-ulnar dislocation. In this case, an axial radial dislocation involving the 1st, 2nd and 3rd metacarpals, which were dislocated from the capitate in a proximal and radial direction, with fracture of the trapezoid and distal pole of the scaphoid. Concomitant injuries were the fracture-dislocations of the 4th and 5th CMC joint, where the bases of the ulnar metacarpals were ulnarly displaced (**a, b**). schematic illustration of the injury (**c**). With permission from [50]

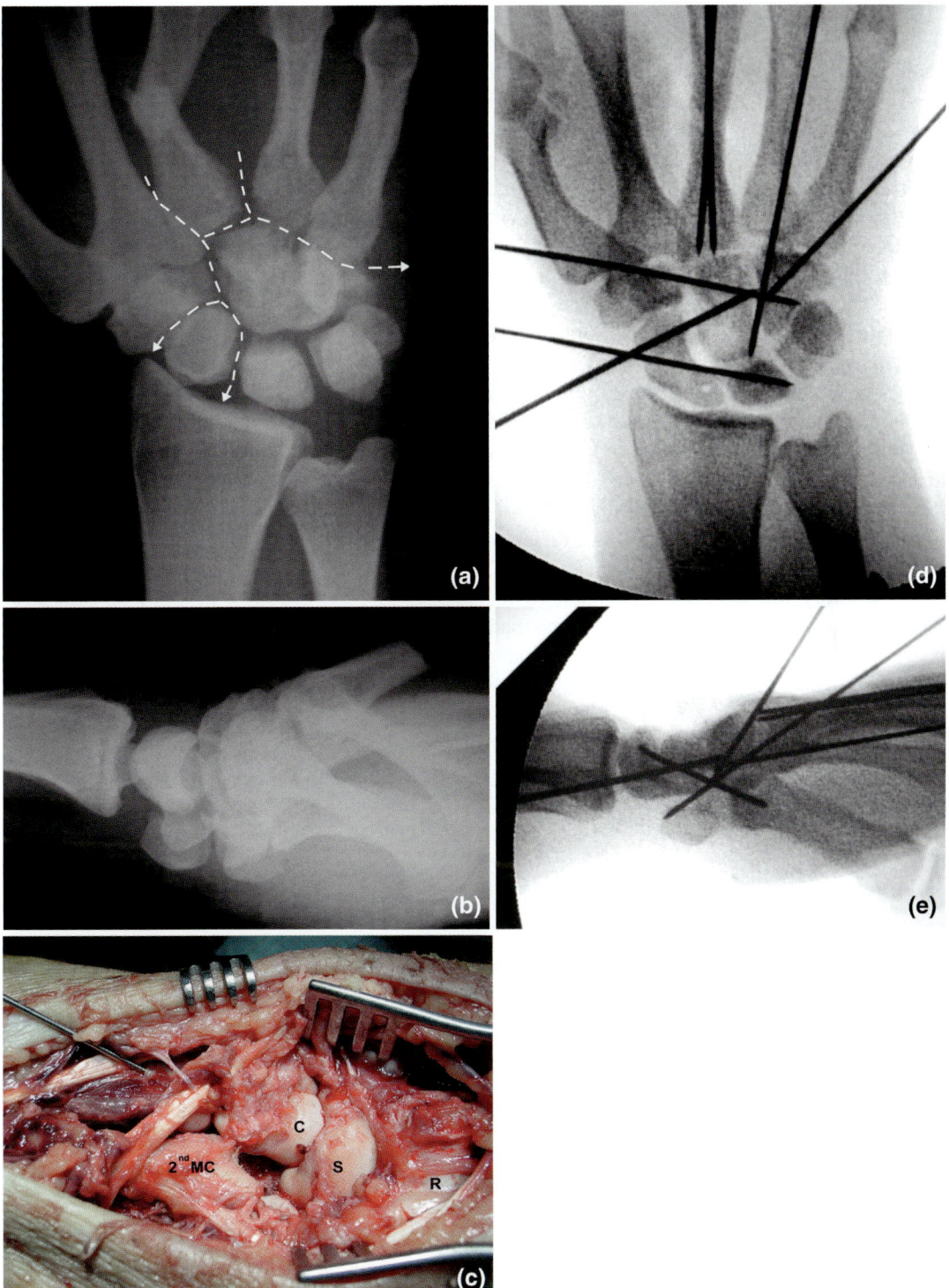

Fig. 10.12 A case of axial radial dislocation with disruption of the central column, in which the applied force is spreading to the proximal carpal row, around the scaphoid. The ulnar CMC joints are also disrupted (**a, b**), during exploration, the axial-radial injury comprising the scaphoid is apparent (*C* capitate, *S* scaphoid, *R* Radius) (**c**), internal fixation with K-wires is shown in fluoroscopy image (**d, e**)

Of the 40 cases published before 1989, 71 % of the patients presented an excellent or good result, while 29 % presented a moderate or poor result. Conversely, out of the 16 patients of the Mayo Clinic study, 73 % had a moderate or poor result and only 27 % had a good result. These adverse results were attributed to the fact that this group of patients presented more significant soft tissue injury.

Inability to reduce the transverse carpal arc will confidently lead to flattening of the palm, dissociation of the carpometacarpal joints, muscle weakness and restriction of movement [45].

The most common complications reported in the literature are: first web space contractures secondary to fibrosis of the thenar muscles, adhesion of the tendons and nerves, stiffness of the fingers, residual carpal instability, compartment syndromes and vascular insufficiency necessitating amputation of the hand [1, 18, 19].

Nerve injury was the most predictable factor in the poorer results, while patients who had axial-ulnar dislocations had a three times greater incidence of nerve injury compared with those who had axial-radial dislocations [9, 10].

References

1. Shin A (2004) Disruption of the distal carpal row: Axial carpal instability and dislocations of the carpometacarpal joint, excluding the thumb. In: Berger R, Weiss AP (ed) Hand Surgery, vol 1. Lippincott Williams & Wilkins, Philadelphia, ch 29, pp 533–547
2. Eigenbrodt (1901) Ueber isolierte luxationen der carpalknochen, spexiell des mondbeins. Beitr Klin Chir 30:805–825
3. Cooney WP, Bussey R, Dobyns JH et al (1987) Difficult wrist fractures: perilunate fracture-dislocations of the wrist. Clin Orthop 214:136–147
4. Primiano GA, Reef TC (1974) Disruption of the proximal carpal arch of the hand. J Bone Joint Surg Am 56:328–332
5. Green DP, O'Brien ET (1978) Open reduction of carpal dislocations: indications and operative techniques. J Hand Surg [Am] 3:250–265
6. Norbeck DE Jr, Larson B, Blair SJ et al (1987) Traumatic longitudinal disruption of the carpus. J Hand Surg [Am] 12(4):509–514
7. Chow SP, So YC, Pun WK et al (1988) Thenar crush injuries. J Bone Joint Surg Br 70:135–139
8. Garcia-Elias M, An KN, Cooney WP III et al (1989) Stability of the transverse carpal arch: an experimental study. J Hand Surg [Am] 14:277–282
9. Garcia-Elias M, Cooney WP (1998) Axial dislocations and fracture-dislocations. In: Cooney WP, Linscheid R, Dobyns J (ed) The wrist: diagnosis and operative treatment, vol 1. Mosby, pp 684–695
10. Garcia-Elias M (2010) Axial fracture dislocations. In: Cooney W (ed) The wrist: diagnosis and operative treatment. Wolters Kluwer/Lippincott Williams & Wilkins, ch 25, pp 579–589
11. Chim H, Yam AKT, Chin AYH (2007) Complex carpal dissociation with open, complete, and divergent trapezium, capitate, and hamate dislocation: a case report. J Hand Surg [Am] 32(9):1363–1366
12. Häcki J, Nagy L, Schweizer A (2009) Transtrapezial peritrapezoidal transcapital axial radial fracture dislocation of the carpus. Hand 4:319–322
13. Azar GA, Shaw TS, Stefanides N et al (2007) An isolated perihamate, transtriquetral fracture-dislocation: a case report. Am J Orthop 36(6):E97–E99
14. Chung US, Choi YH, Lee KH (2012) Traumatic axial-ulnar dislocation accompanied by fracture of the hook of the hamate: a case report. J Hand Surg [Eur]. doi: 10.1177/1753193412446571
15. Laing AJ, McCabe JP (2003) Axial ulnar carpometacarpal disruption. Injury 34(7):537–539
16. Pai C, Wei D (1994) Traumatic dislocations of the distal carpal row. J Hand Surg [Br] 19(5):576–583
17. Schweizer A, Kammer E (2008) Transhamate periscaphoid axial radial fracture dislocation of the carpus. J Hand Surg [Am] 33(2):210–212
18. Garcia-Elias M, Dobyns JH, Cooney WP et al (1989) Traumatic axial dislocations of the carpus. J Hand Surg [Am] 14:446–457
19. Garcia-Elias M, Abanco J, Salvador E et al (1985) Crush injury of the carpus. J Bone Joint Surg Br 67:286–289
20. Inoue G, Miura T (1991) Traumatic axial-ulnar disruption of the carpus. Orthop Rev 20(10):867–872
21. Rasmussen S (1990) Closed longitudinal splitting of the carpus. Case report. Scand J Plast Reconstr Surg Hand Surg 24:167–169
22. Irwin LR (1995) Complex carpal dislocation. J Hand Surg [Br] 20:746–749
23. Naam NH, Smith DK, Gilula LA (1992) Transtriquetral perihamate ulnar axial dislocation and palmar lunate dislocation. J Hand Surg [Am] 17:762–766
24. Berger RA, Crowninshield RD, Flatt AE (1982) The three-dimensional rotational behaviors of the carpal bones. Clin Orthop 167:303–310
25. Kobayashi M, Berger RA, Linscheid RL et al (1997) Intercarpal kinematics during wrist motion. Hand Clin 13:143–150
26. Vegter J, Bessems JH (1994) Brief reports. A new type of crush injury of the carpus. J Bone Joint Surg Br 76:330–331

27. Ritt MJPF, Berger RA, Bishop AT et al (1996) The capitohamate ligaments: a comparison of biomechanical properties. J Hand Surg [Br] 21:451–454

28. Fisk G (1984) The influence of the transverse carpal ligament (flexor retinaculum) on carpal stability. Ann Chir Main 3:297–299

29. Kaplan EB, Milford LW (1984) The retinacular system of the hand. In: Spinner M (ed) Kaplan's functional and surgical anatomy of the hand. JB Lippincott Co, ch 6:245–282

30. Gartsman GM, Kovach JC, Crouch C et al (1986) Carpal arch alteration after carpal tunnel release. J Hand Surg [Am] 11:372–374

31. Kozin SH, Pagnanelli DM (2002) Grip strength after carpal tunnel release: role of the transverse carpal ligament. Am J Orthop 31:571–574

32. Garcia-Elias M, Sanchez-Freijo JM, Salo JM et al (1992) Dynamic changes of the transverse carpal arch during flexion-extension of the wrist: effects of sectioning the transverse carpal ligament. J Hand Surg [Am] 17:1017–1019

33. Idler RS (2001) Carpal dislocations and instability. In: Watson HK, Weinzweig J (eds) The Wrist, vol 1. Lippincott Williams & Wilkins, pp 223–229

34. Shin AY, Glowacki KA, Bishop AT (1999) Dynamic axial carpal instability: a case report. J Hand Surg [Am] 24:781–785

35. Jensen BV, Christensen C (1990) An unusual combination of simultaneous fracture of the tuberosity of the trapezium and the hook of the hamate. J Hand Surg [Am] 15:285–287

36. Tracy CA (1999) Transverse carpal ligament disruption associated with simultaneous fractures of the trapezium, trapezial ridge, and hook of hamate: a case report. J Hand Surg [Am] 24:152–155

37. Ohshio I, Ogino T, Miyake A (1986) Dislocation of the hamate associated with fracture of the trapezial ridge. J Hand Surg [Am] 11:658–660

38. Matsumoto T, Tsunoda M, Yamaguchi S et al (2005) Traumatic dislocation of the hamate and pisiform: a case report and review of the literature. J Orthop Trauma 19(4):282–285

39. Wanadurongwan W, Sakkarnkosol S (1990) Triquetral fracture associated with hamate dislocation: a case report. Bull Hosp Jt Dis Orthop Inst 40:54–58

40. Connell MC, Dyson RP (1955) Dislocation of the carpal scaphoid. Report of a case. J Bone Joint Surg Br 37:252–253

41. Horton T, Shin AY, Cooney WP III (2004) Isolated scaphoid dislocation associated with axial carpal dissociation: an unusual injury report. J Hand Surg [Am] 29(6):1102–1108

42. Leung YF, Wai YL, Kam WL et al (1998) Solitary dislocation of the scaphoid. From case report to literature review. J Hand Surg [Br] 23:88–92

43. Richards RS, Bennett JD, Roth JH (1993) Scaphoid dislocation with radial-axial carpal disruption. Am J Roentgenol 160:1075–1076

44. Ali MA (1986) Fracture of the body of the Hamate bone associated with compartment syndrome and dorsal decompression of the carpal tunnel. J Hand Surg [Br] 11:207–210

45. Dobyns JH, Linscheid RL (1986) Complications of treatment of fractures and dislocations of the wrist. In: Epps CH (ed) Complications in orthopaedic surgery, vol 1. JB Lippincott Co, ch 15, pp 339–417

46. Freeland AE, Rojas SL (2001) Traumatic combined radial and ulnar axial wrist dislocation. Orthopedics 24:1161–1163

47. Tanaka Y, Ohshige T, Hanakawa S (2002) Traumatic axial dislocation of the carpus: a case report of transscaphoid pericapitate transhamate axial dislocation. J Orthop Sci 7(3):414–416

48. Chin A, Garcia-Elias M (2008) Combined reverse perilunate and axial-ulnar dislocation of the wrist: a case report. J Hand Surg [Eur] 33(5):672–676

49. Grabow R (2006) Carpal dislocations. Hand Clin 22:485–500

50. Apergis E (2004) καταγματα-εξαρθρηματα του καρπου. Konstantaras Medical Books, Athens

Isolated Dislocations of the Carpal Bones

11

Isolated carpal bone dislocations are uncommon injuries, however all the carpal bones have been reported to dislocate in an isolated fashion when a localized, direct, or indirect force is concentrated over a single bone of the wrist [1, 2]. The most common dislocation of carpal bone is that of the lunate which was examined in detail in the chapter on perilunate injuries. Less common is the dislocation of pairs of adjacent carpal bones which will be discussed in brief later on.

11.1 Scaphoid

Since the first description by Higgs in 1930 [3], only 32 [4] or 34 [5] cases of isolated scaphoid dislocation have been reported in the literature. The male to female ratio is approximately 7:1 [6, 7].

11.1.1 Evaluation

Wrist pain, swelling, and limitation of wrist motion are the usual complaints. A bony prominence is usually evident along the radial, palmar, or rarely dorsal aspect to the radius [6, 8]. Usually there are no signs of neurovascular involvement [6], but dislocations with palmar-ulnar direction could produce median nerve injury [9].

The percentage of cases with delayed diagnosis ranges between 48 and 50 % [6, 7]. Most of the delay in recognition is due to lack of awareness of this rare occurrence.

Simple radiographs are usually sufficient to make the diagnosis and are greatly facilitated by identifying the Gilula's arcs. A CT scan may be helpful when in doubt, while arthroscopy may be used as both a diagnostic and a therapeutic modality if imaging modalities are nondiagnostic [10–12].

11.1.2 Classification

Dislocation of the scaphoid bone may occur after an apparently successful reduction of a major carpal dislocation or it may occur as a primary condition [13]. Richards et al. in 1993 [14] categorized scaphoid dislocations as simple (isolated to the scaphoid) or complex (a combination of scaphoid dislocation with axial carpal dislocation). Others, characterized these injuries as Type I (isolated anterolateral dislocation of the proximal pole); and Type II (scaphoid dislocation associated with an axial derangement of the capitate-hamate joint) [1, 2, 15, 16].

Leung et al. [7] have proposed a classification scheme for isolated dislocations of the scaphoid:

1. *Primary versus secondary*: The primary type results directly from the injury. The secondary type represents a residual dislocated scaphoid after closed [5, 17] or self-reduced perilunate dislocation.
2. *Simple versus complex*: The simple type only involves the scapholunate and radioscaphoid articulation, whereas disruptions of the distal carpal row including the capitate and hamate

E. Apergis, *Fracture-Dislocations of the Wrist*,
DOI: 10.1007/978-88-470-5328-1_11, © Springer-Verlag Italia 2013

and middle/ring metacarpal articulations are classified as a complex type [11, 14, 18, 19].

3. ***Partial versus total***: Partial dislocations retain some soft tissue attachments (usually distal), while complete dislocations have lost all soft tissue attachments.

4. ***Direction of dislocation***: In partial dislocations, the proximal pole can be dislocated volarly (in ulnar, radial, or neutral direction), dorsally or purely radially.

A case of total dislocation in volar direction was reported by McNamara and Corley in 1992 [20], while one case of total dorsal dislocation of the scaphoid was reported by Amaravati et al. in 2009 [21].

Horton et al. [10] described a case of complex or type II dislocation and after reviewing the literature they found only 11 similar cases. Variants of a complex type of injury could be the combination of scaphoid dislocation with dislocation of the hamate [22] or with fracture of the hamate [23].

Lee et al. [5], after reviewing the literature, found 34 cases of isolated scaphoid dislocation. There were 26 palmar (14 in palmar-radial, 9 in neutral, 1 in proximal, and 2 in palmar-ulnar direction), 5 radial, and 3 dorsal dislocations.

Other carpal injuries that might be associated with scaphoid dislocation can be easily overlooked such as chip fractures of other carpal bones [21, 24–26].

11.1.3 Mechanism

The majority of cases result from traffic accidents especially motorcycle injuries, while the usual mechanism of injury is the application of an indirect force resulting in a dorsiflexion and ulnar deviation [8, 24, 27] or a twisting injury to the wrist [7]. Scarcer injury mechanisms reported are blast injuries [28], entrapment of the wrist [6] or following a penetrating injury with a sharp object [29]. In addition, the position of the wrist during injury, may be related to the direction of dislocation of the proximal pole of the scaphoid [7].

For type I injuries, a violent hyperpronation injury has been implicated with the wrist in dorsiflexion and ulnar deviation while grasping a fixed object, causing SL dissociation followed by the enucleation of the proximal pole of the scaphoid [1, 4, 15]. For type II injuries a high-energy axial compressive load along the 3rd and 4th metacarpals, creating enough shear stress to the capitate-hamate joint to disrupt its strong ligament attachments has been implicated [1]. Others have proposed that with hyperdorsiflexion, the proximal pole of the scaphoid slides down the volar slope of the radius and is ejected volarly. If the energy of injury is not dissipated, the capitate abuts the radial dorsal rim and the shearing force between the capitate and hamate is transmitted distally between the middle and ring metacarpals [16, 30].

Leung et al. [7] considered scaphoid dislocation as an extreme form of scapholunate dissociation representing one end of a spectrum of scapholunate injuries. Both are the result of a similar mechanism of injury and the only clinical difference between dorsal partial dislocation of the scaphoid and chronic scapholunate dissociation with DISI, is that the contact between the proximal pole of the scaphoid and the radius is lost in the former.

11.1.4 Pathoanatomy

The severity of the dislocation depends on the number of ligaments that have been disrupted. In partial palmar dislocation of the scaphoid, the SLI, RSL, and the RSC ligaments are disrupted while in total dislocation, all ligaments attached to the scaphoid are disrupted [7]. Szabo et al. [12], based on arthroscopic and surgical findings of 3 patients, postulated that the sequence of ligamentous failure in scaphoid dislocations begins in the radiopalmar aspect of the proximal pole of the scaphoid with the RSC and SLI ligaments failing first, followed by the LRL and ultimately by the ST ligament (Fig. 11.1a–n).

In complex or type II dislocations the ligamentous injuries are more extensive, including mainly the intercarpal capitohamate, the SLI, DRC, DIC, RSC, and LRL ligaments [10].

11.1.5 Treatment

Treatment ranges from closed reduction and casting, to percutaneous fixation after closed or open reduction and to open reduction and ligament reconstruction with internal fixation. Closed reduction is usually accomplished in most cases when treated acutely, by traction and direct manual pressure of the scaphoid with the wrist being ulnarly deviated. However, unsuccessful attempts for closed reduction have been reported, necessitating open reduction [4, 6, 7, 12, 26, 31]. In cases of incomplete reduction, ligamentous material (usually the SLI ligament) invaginated into the SL interval is blocking the reduction [12].

Case reports have described successful treatment with closed reduction and immobilization in a cast as definitive treatment, in cases of partial dislocation of the scaphoid detected early [18, 23, 24, 26, 27, 32, 33]. A scaphoid plaster is usually applied for 4–6 weeks. Closed reduction, percutaneous K-wires fixation, and cast application have also been reported, although these methods were not always successful [34]. However, many publications have advocated an open reduction, ligament repair, and internal fixation through a dorsal [1, 12, 26, 34–37] or volar approach [4, 6–9, 19, 20, 38]. In contrast to treatment for simple scaphoid dislocation, which is frequently treated with closed reduction, in cases with complex dislocations, reduction of the scaphoid alone is insufficient to stabilize the carpus with associated axial carpal disruption. Open reduction is necessary to fix the unstable radial half of the carpus to the stable ulnar half [11].

Most reported cases, have achieved good to excellent results [15]. The patients have returned to their prior activities with only moderate limitations, while there is a nearly universal loss of range of wrist motion [10].

The most significant risk factors in poor prognosis are delayed diagnosis and treatment, particularly if more than 2–3 weeks, although successfully treated delayed cases have recently been described [35]. Excision of scaphoid [37], proximal row carpectomy [13, 21], or partial wrist fusion [9] have been applied in cases of late diagnosis. The longer the delay, the worse the prognosis will be. Potential complications following an isolated scaphoid dislocation are residual carpal instability [19, 20, 31], stiffness and posttraumatic arthrosis.

Although transient radiological features of early avascular necrosis have occurred, in none of the cases reported has there been any evidence of permanent avascular necrosis [1, 7, 10, 24]. In partial dislocations, vascularity of the scaphoid is partly maintained by intact distal soft tissue attachments, while in cases of complete dislocation it is proposed that there are intact intraosseous channels inside the intact scaphoid bone that allow rapid revascularization from the surrounding soft tissues [7]. However, Szabo et al. [12] reported that one out of three of their patients showed avascular necrosis with fragmentation of the proximal pole of the scaphoid after 20 months follow-up.

11.2 Triquetrum

Dislocation of the triquetrum has rarely been described in the context of perilunar injuries [39, 40]. These cases probably constitute a variant of reverse perilunar instability, where the force is applied to the hypothenar area and the disruption propagates around the triquetrum disrupting the ligaments from its distal (triquetrohamate), proximal (ulnotriquetral) and radial (lunotriquetral) articulation.

Both dorsal [40–43] and volar dislocations [44, 45] of the triquetrum have been documented. With so few cases, the exact mechanism of injury remains obscure. Usually, a major fall, a motor vehicle accident, or a crush injury has been implicated. During the frequently mentioned mechanism, with a fall on the outstretched hand and the wrist in dorsiflexion and

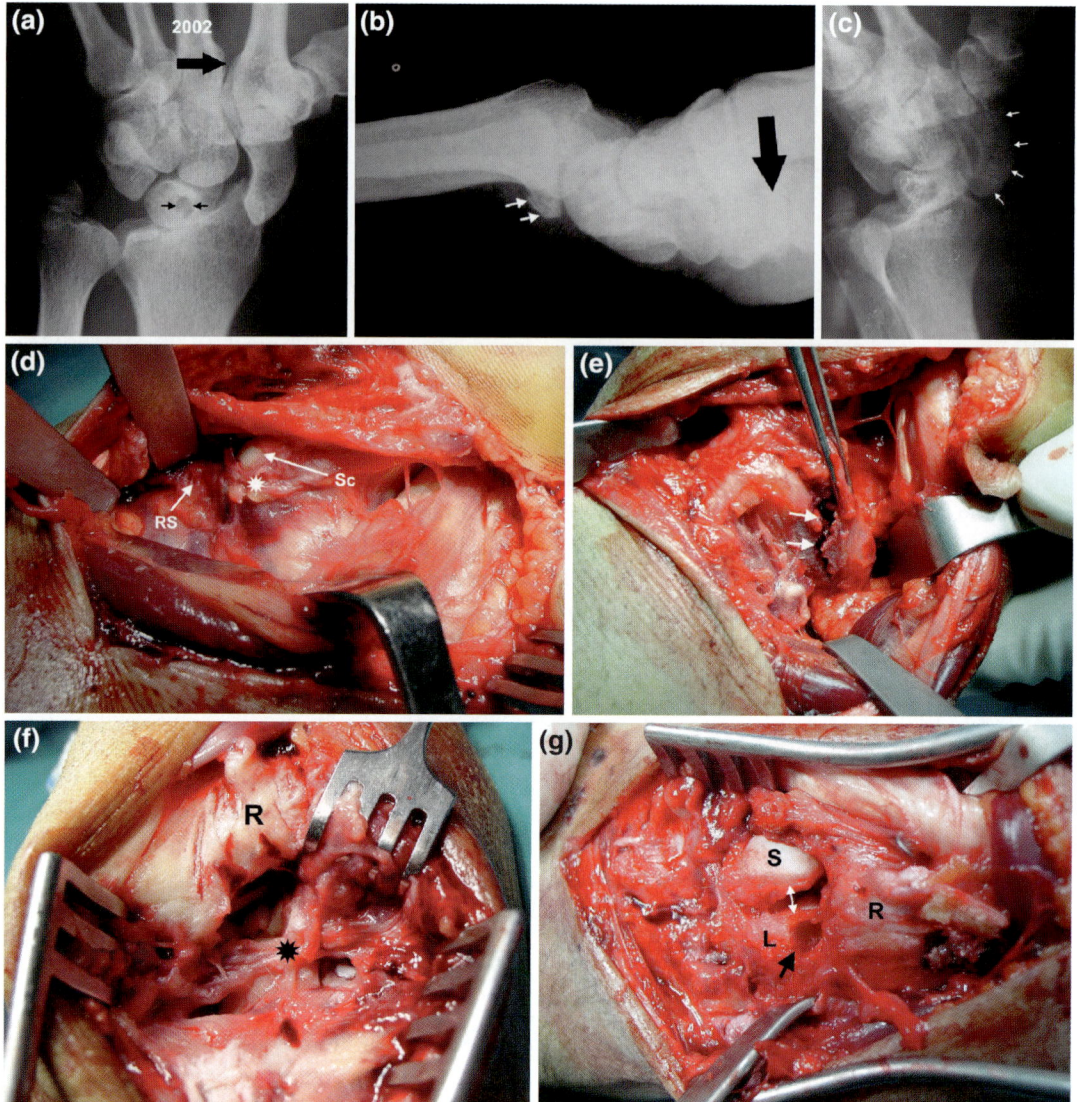

Fig. 11.1 Male, 54-years old, car accident. A case of primary, simple, partial volar-radial scaphoid dislocation was recognized (**a**, **b**, **c**). The wrist was radially and volarly displaced. An accidental, unrelated cyst in the lunate was obvious (*arrows*) (**a**); and a concomitant fracture of the ulnovolar radial rim was indicated (*arrows*) (**b**); the volar approach revealed the dislocation of the proximal pole of the scaphoid in radiovolar direction and the ruptured volar RSC and LRL ligaments (*asterisk*) (*RS* radial styloid, *Sc* scaphoid) (**d**); *arrows* indicate the fractured ulnovolar fragment (**e**); dorsal approach revealed the attenuated dorsal intercarpal ligament which was detached from the dorsal scaphoid (*asterisk*), while the wrist was volarly displaced (*R* radius) (**f**); the dorsal approach also indicated the rupture of the SL ligament (line with *arrows* on each end) and the evacuated cyst of the lunate (*arrow*) (*S* scaphoid, *L* lunate, *R* radius) (**g**); a wire-loop was used to fixate the ulnovolar fragment (**h**); bone anchors were used for the reattachment of the SL ligament and the volar RC ligaments to the radius; the scaphoid was stabilized with K-wires to the lunate and capitate; cancellous bone grafts were placed to the lunate cyst. Postoperative X-rays (**i, j**). Two years later, the patient was pain free with good ROM, while the radiologic appearance was satisfactory (**k, l**); 7 years postoperatively, stenosis of the scapho-capitate joint was obvious, while the patient was complaining for weather-change symptoms (**m, n**)

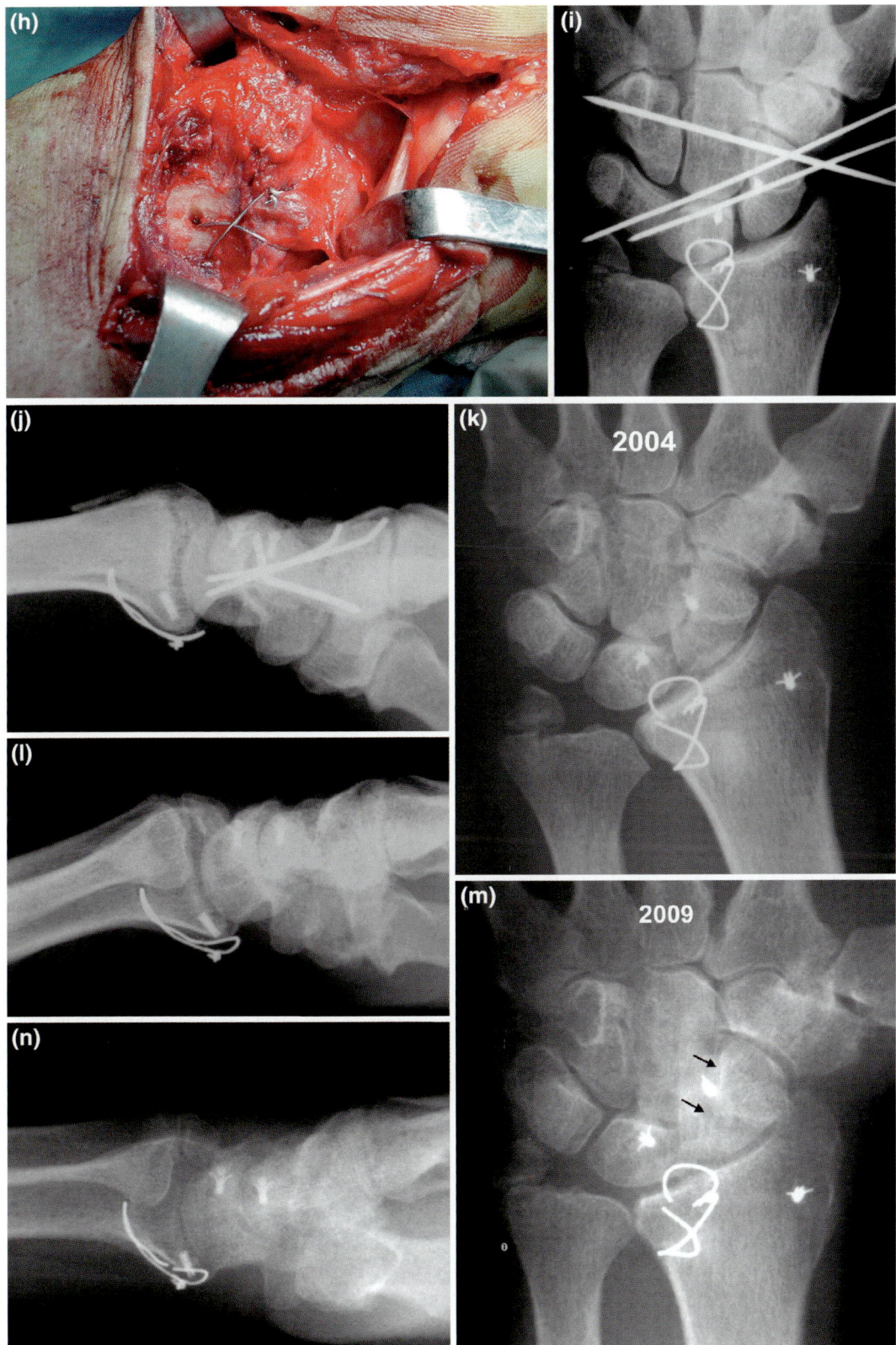

Fig. 11.1 (Continued)

ulnar deviation, the triquetrum is thought to become covered by the lower end of the ulna, avoiding dorsal displacement and favoring volar dislocation [42]. In addition, with forced wrist hyperextension, the proximal pole of the hamate rides dorsally on the triquetrum, exerting a palmar force leading to a palmar dislocation of the triquetrum [45]. However, the higher frequency of dorsal dislocations makes more likely the mechanism of injury to be the direct impact to the hypothenar area. Dorsal dislocation may also be produced by wrist hyperflexion and pronation [43], secondary to a perilunar dislocation or a variant of an ulnar axial loading injury [40].

In many of the reported cases the diagnosis was delayed [41, 44, 45]. On examination, swelling will be noted about the ulnar aspect of the wrist and if the dislocation is dorsal, it may be possible to palpate the displaced triquetrum. The volar displacement is associated with transient median nerve compression [15, 44, 45]. Usually, PA lateral and oblique views are adequate for radiographic evaluation, with the lateral view providing information on the direction of the dislocation.

Treatment has included triquetrum excision [44, 45], open reduction and internal fixation [40, 41, 43], and closed reduction without fixation [42], all with reasonably good clinical results, although in two cases signs of instability (VISI [43] and ulnar translation [45]) were found. In any case, excision of the triquetrum must be avoided, since significant stabilizing ligaments are attached to the bone, which in addition, has an important proprioceptive role. Although closed reduction and percutaneous pinning could be attempted, we believe that open reduction is required. The approach is dictated by the direction of dislocation, although combined palmar and dorsal approaches may be necessary, followed by K-wire fixation of the reduced triquetrum with ligament repair. There have been no reported cases of avascular necrosis following treatment for a triquetral dislocation [28].

11.3 Pisiform

Pisiform dislocation is an extremely rare injury and has been reported in isolation [46, 47], in combination with distal radial fractures [48, 49] or with hamate dislocation [50–52]. The possible relationship between pisiform subluxation and distal radius fractures has also been mentioned [53]. In children, two cases of pisiform dislocation associated with a distal radius fracture have been reported [48, 54]. Displacement of the pisiform has been reported distally, ulnarly, and proximally [15, 36, 55].

Since the pisiform has a flat articular surface articulating with the triquetrum, it relies mainly on its many soft tissue attachments for stability. These include: the attachment of flexor carpi ulnaris tendon, abductor digiti minimi, extensor retinaculum, transverse carpal ligament, pisometacarpal and pisohamate ligaments, and the joint capsule to the triquetrum (Fig. 11.2). Mechanical testing has showed the soft tissues around the pisotriquetral joint to be strongest proximally and distally and weakest medially [56]. The ulnar nerve and the volar branch of the ulnar artery are located in the immediate vicinity to the pisiform with the nerve being medial to the artery and closer to the pisiform.

Two possible mechanisms have been postulated [15, 28, 46, 54]. One is a direct blow to the ulnar aspect of the wrist and the other is strong eccentric contraction on the flexor carpi ulnaris with the wrist in extension. Fall from height, traffic accidents, and lifting heavy objects have been implicated. Pulling of the FCU, as well as forced wrist hyperextension can disrupt the thin capsule of the pisotriquetral joint, and the FCU tendon's distal continuation or the pisohamate and pisometacarpal ligaments. If these ligaments are damaged, the function of the FCU becomes impaired, with the pisiform retracting proximally [57].

The diagnosis should be based on the injury mechanism and the presentation of pain, swelling, and tenderness over the ulnar border of the wrist, while a painful restriction of all wrist movements is a usual finding. Frequently a characteristic depression is found at the base of the hypothenar eminence, where the pisiform bone should lie [46, 55]. Ulnar neuropathy may also be caused by pisotriquetral joint instability [55, 56].

Posteroanterior, lateral, and oblique radiographs are usually adequate for diagnosis. X-ray features of the pisotriquetral joint including parallelism, width of the joint space and symmetry have been suggested to be diagnostically relevant [53]. Oblique view is taken with the ulnar side of the wrist placed against the plate, with the forearm in about 15° of supination. Comparison films with the contralateral wrist may be needed.

Treatment includes immobilization after a closed reduction [48, 55, 58], open reduction with internal fixation, closed reduction and pinning [59], and resection of the pisiform either initially [46, 57, 60–63] or secondarily in cases of persistent pain or recurrent dislocation [47].

The manipulation for closed reduction usually requires maximum wrist flexion with direct pressure to relocate the bone [28, 58]. The reduction can be aided by placing the forearm in pronation [55]. There are some differences in opinion regarding the position of the wrist immobilization. The following variants have been proposed: a below elbow cast with the wrist in 30–40° of dorsiflexion and slight radial deviation for 3–4 weeks [58], a radially deviated short arm cast for a minimum of 3 weeks [46], a dorsal splint holding the wrist flexed and the forearm pronated for 3 weeks [55] or a long arm plaster splint in 25° of dorsiflexion for 3 weeks [59].

It has been stated [64] that excision of the pisiform decreases wrist flexion strength without functional deficit or loss of range of motion and that the soft tissue's confluence over the pisiform allows for subperiosteal pisiform excision and repair of the tissues without disturbing the FCU insertion. Excision of the pisiform is consistently the most successful treatment for pain without functional deficit [47, 65, 66].

11.4 Trapezium

The trapezium may dislocate in isolation or together with the thumb metacarpal. Incomplete dislocation, in which the trapezium remains attached to the base of the first metacarpal should be categorized as a peritrapezium axial-radial dislocation [1]. True volar isolated dislocations of the trapezium are very rare and are thought to be caused by a direct blow to the dorsolateral aspect of the wrist or as a consequence of a hyperextension-supination injury to the radial-deviated wrist [1, 15]. Dorsal radial dislocations are described as the result of hyperflexion of the first metacarpal combined with an axial compression force [67, 68]. Crush injuries and motor vehicle accidents are the most commonly reported causes of these injuries.

Palmar and dorsal radial dislocations have been described [68–71]. However, Garcia-Elias [72] after reviewing the literature, found that only six cases have been reported of true isolated dislocations with complete enucleation of the bone and were all palmarly displaced.

Clinically, depending on the mechanism an open wound may be present at the thenar area [73–75]. With isolated dislocation, a palpable mass may be present at the base of the thumb. Pain, instability, and limited range of motion of the first CMC joint may be noted [28]. Palmar dislocation of the trapezium has been associated with avulsion of the recurrent motor branch of the median nerve [75]. Diagnosis is best confirmed by radiographs, while the posteroanterior axial oblique view is used to evaluate the trapezium with the surrounding bones [76].

In acute cases, open reduction and K-wire fixation are thought to be the treatment of choice [68, 69, 74, 75, 77] and whenever possible, repair of the periarticular ligamentous structures should be accomplished [28]. Closed reduction and percutaneous pinning could also be attempted or in cases of delayed diagnosis, excision of the trapezium has been applied [70, 78].

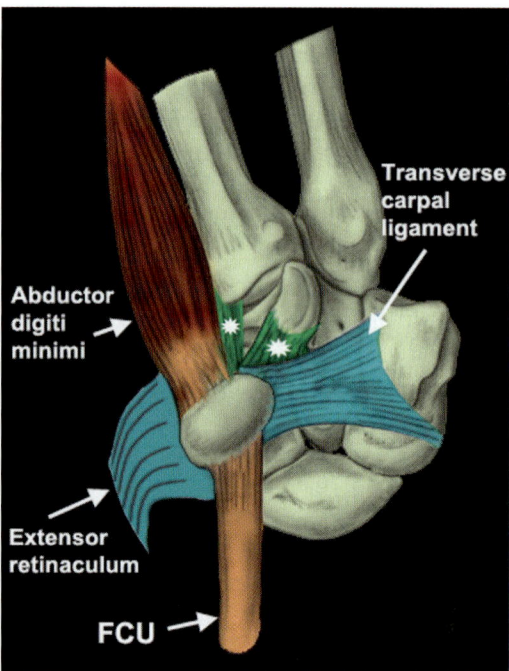

Fig. 11.2 The soft tissues stabilizing the pisiform to the flat articular surface of the triquetrum (*asterisks* pisohamate and pisometacarpal ligaments, *FCU* flexor carpi ulnaris)

Since the trapezium receives its blood supply from nutrient arteries entering the bone from three surfaces and has consistent intraosseous anastomoses, the risk of avascular necrosis is negligible.

11.5 Trapezoid

The trapezoid has been described as the keystone of the proximal carpal arch with its palmar surface narrower than the dorsal, while it is attached to the surrounding bones by strong ligaments. It has been stated [36, 79] that Gay in 1869 was the first to describe a case of trapezoid dislocation and since that time there have been 25 [79] or 26 [36] reported cases in the literature, while a literature review by De Tullio [80] revealed only 24 published cases since 1962. Frequently, the dislocation of the trapezoid is

associated with other fractures or dislocations of the hand or constitutes a part of the axial-radial dislocations of the wrist [81]. Both palmar [80, 82, 83] and dorsal [84–86] isolated dislocations of the trapezoid have been reported. Less than 10 of these dislocations were displaced volarly with one having caused an attritional rupture of flexor tendons in a case whose diagnosis was missed for 4 months [82] and another presented with acute carpal tunnel syndrome [79].

There is no clear explanation as to how a wedge-shaped bone which is wider dorsally, dislocates palmarly, but a direct blow to the dorsum of the wrist has been implicated [1]. The more common dorsal dislocations may be produced by direct trauma or indirectly from a blow to the second metacarpal with the wrist flexed [28].

In acute cases, pain, considerable swelling, and limited motion of the fingers are noticed, while vascular or neurological damage has not been reported. With dorsal dislocation an osseous prominence is palpated at the base of the index finger metacarpal, while a palmar dislocation will not have such an obvious presentation [28]. Diagnosis of trapezoid dislocation is confirmed by standard posteroanterior, lateral, and oblique radiographs looking for an empty space at the base of the second metacarpal. When necessary, tomograms or a CT scan may be necessary.

Treatment for dorsal dislocation of the trapezoid has included closed reduction [87, 88] or open reduction with a dorsal approach [84, 86] and pinning with K-wires.

Closed reduction of a palmar dislocation is ineffective because of the shape of the trapezoid [82, 83], thus open reduction is always necessary with combined [79] or with only dorsal approach [80, 83]. Few cases were treated with excision of the trapezoid [81, 82], which resulted in the proximal migration of the second MC and the development of degenerative changes to the midcarpal joint. A reasonable alternative in difficult cases is a primary limited fusion [82, 89]. The trapezoid has nutrient vessels that enter its palmar

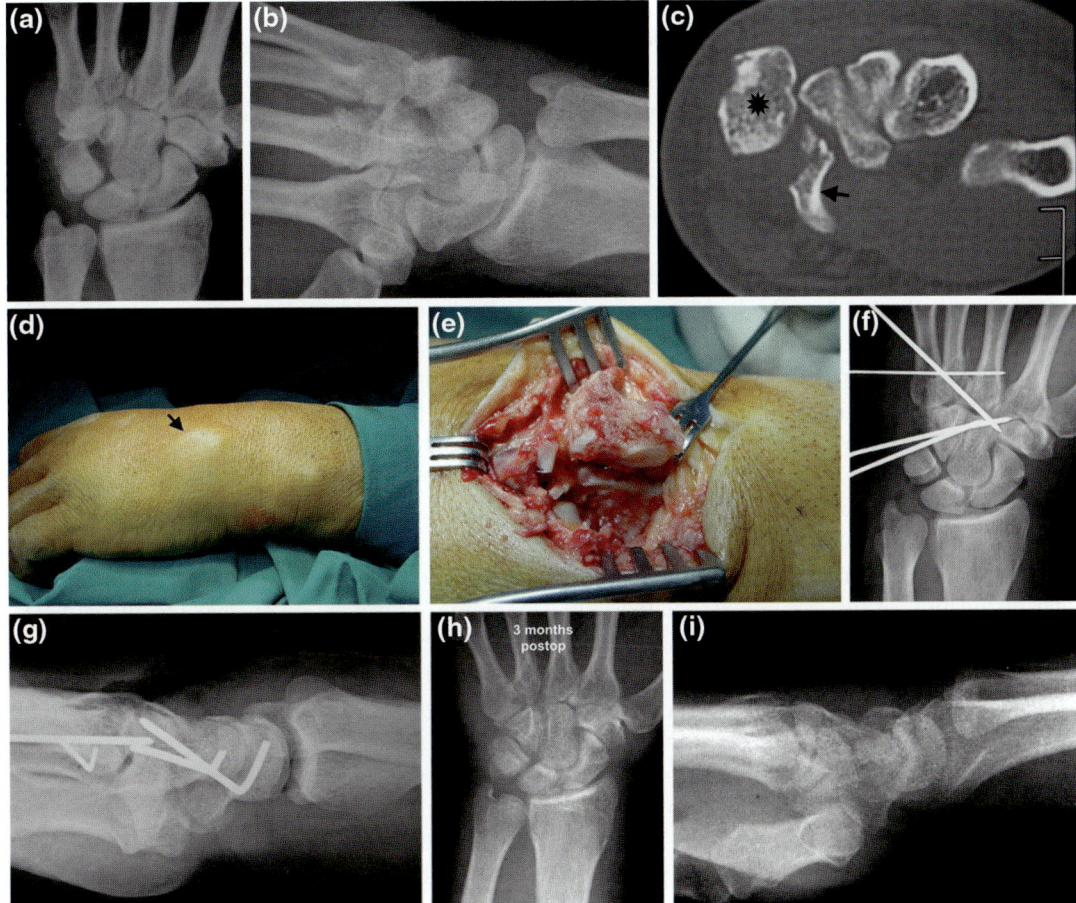

Fig. 11.3 Male, 62-years old, car accident. The wrist injury remained initially undiagnosed and was treated with a below elbow splint. Routine examination of the X-rays 10 days later revealed a dorsal dislocation of the hamate, associated with proximal migration of the 5th metacarpal (**a, b**); a CT scan indicated the dorsal dislocation of the main portion of the hamate (*asterisk*) with a fractured hamulus (*arrow*) (**c**); a painful osseous swelling of the dorsum of the wrist was apparent (*arrow*) (**d**); during exploration the main portion of the hamate was found beneath the subcutaneous tissue, devoid of any soft tissue attachments (**e**); postoperative X-rays (**f, g**); radiographic appearance 3 months later (**h, i**)

and dorsal surfaces, while there are no intraosseous anastomoses between the palmar and dorsal systems. Thus, the trapezoid is at risk in cases of dislocation and cases with findings of avascular necrosis have been reported [15, 82, 86].

11.6 Capitate

True isolated dislocation of the capitate is an extremely rare injury. It requires disruption of the interosseous ligaments to the adjacent trapezoid and hamate, disruption of the ligaments of the third CMC joint distally, and disruption of the radiocapitate and capitotriquetral ligaments proximally [28]. To our knowledge, only one such case has been reported by Cherucci et al. [90], who described a total volar dislocation of the capitate after a crush injury of the hand in a metal press. In the majority of the reported cases, the dislocated capitate is associated with other carpal injuries. Most commonly the capitate dislocates in a volar direction [90–94] and in one case only it dislocated in dorsal direction [95].

Lowrey et al. [93] reported a case of volar capitate dislocation associated with other multiple carpal injuries. Hirata et al. [91] described a case with dorsal dislocation of the third CMC joint, associated with volar rotational subluxation of the capitate from its distal (CMC), and proximal (LC) articulation. This case constitutes a combination of types IIa and IIId injuries, according to Garcia-Elias's classification for CMC injuries. Walker and Pradhan [95] described a case with dorsal dislocation of the capitate and the third metacarpal. This case could be a type IIId injury according to previous classification for CMC injuries. Ruijters and Kortmann [94] reported a volar dislocation of the capitate associated with a fracture of the lunate in the coronal plane, constituting a case of volar perilunate injury. Lee et al. [92] described a case of volar dislocation of the capitate associated with dislocation of the ulnar side of the carpometacarpal joint.

Dislocation of the capitate usually resulted after a crush injury [90, 91] or a motorcycle accident [93, 95]. Clinical findings are dependent on the mechanism of injury while the diagnosis is sometimes difficult to establish using standard radiographs. In the case presented by Checcucci et al. [20], a definitive diagnosis was obtained only after a CT scan.

The majority of cases presented in the literature were treated with open reduction and fixation with K-wires, except for the case presented by Walker and Pradhan [95], which was reduced with closed manipulation under general anesthesia and immobilization in a below elbow cast for 8 weeks. Short-term results were generally good but early development of degenerative changes [93] or instability findings [91] have been reported.

11.7 Hamate

Isolated dislocation of the hamate bone is an extremely rare injury, with only eight cases reported in the literature since the first description by Buchanan in 1882 [96]. Most cases of hamate dislocation have been described as part of more complex injuries or in association with other carpal bones' dislocation [22, 50, 97] or constituting cases of axial-ulnar derangements, with the hamate being displaced along with the 4th and 5th metacarpals [98] (Fig. 11.3a–i). Dislocation of the hamate requires disruption of the triquetrohamate ligament, pisohamate ligament, and capitohamate interosseous ligament as well as disruption of the 4th and 5th CMC joints.

Both volar [96, 99, 100] and dorsal [101, 102] dislocations of the hamate have been reported. The usual mechanism of injury is a direct impact by a sharp tool or indirect trauma by hyperextension [15, 28, 36].

On physical examination, there is painful palmar or dorsal swelling on the ulnar aspect of the wrist, with or without a palpable bony prominence. Nerve damage does not seem to be common, however, given that the ulnar neurovascular bundle is in close proximity, injury to this structure might be anticipated [28, 101].

Diagnosis is usually made by conventional X-ray examination. Posteroanterior (PA) and lateral neutral rotation views of the wrist are adequate for diagnosis. In the PA view, most noticeable is a gap distal to the triquetrum, while the lateral view reveals the direction of the dislocation. A CT scan is usually necessary to unveil the true extent of the damage e.g., fracture of the hook of the hamate [96]. Since 50 % of hamates lack an intraosseous anastomosis of its nutrient vessels, the risk of avascular necrosis is a possible complication, although it has not been reported so far.

Treatment alternatives include: closed reduction [99, 102], closed reduction and percutaneous fixation [98], open reduction with [96, 100] or without internal fixation [101] and excision [103, 104]. The small number of cases reported does not allow inferences about the best treatment. However, closed reduction (when feasible) with percutaneous pinning under image intensifier, open reduction with the approach depending on the direction of the dislocation, and pinning of the hamate to the metacarpals, the capitate and triquetrum, seem to be the indicated methods of treatment.

11.8   Pairs of Dislocated Wrist Bones

Carpal dislocation may occur in units of adjacent bones. These unusual patterns of dislocation are most likely the result of direct trauma [28]. When adjacent bones of the proximal carpal row are dislocated, they probably constitute variants of perilunate dislocations or reverse perilunate dislocations. On the contrary, when adjacent bones of the distal carpal row are dislocated, they possibly represent cases of axial dislocations. The most common pattern is combined dislocation of scaphoid and lunate. Other reported patterns of adjacent bone dislocations are: triquetrum and lunate [39], hamate and pisiform [50–52], capitate and hamate [97], trapezium and trapezoid [105], trapezoid and capitate [106]. A case of dislocation of non-adjacent carpal bones (scaphoid and hamate) has been reported by Sakada et al. [22]. Extremely rare are cases of three carpal bone dislocations, such as: trapezium, capitate and hamate [107] or lunate, triquetrum and hamate [108].

Scaphoid and lunate: Domeshek et al. [109] in a review of the literature found only 17 reported cases that involved simultaneous dislocation of the scaphoid and lunate. In 11 of these cases, the two carpal bones dislocated as a unit, while in 6 cases the dislocation was of divergent type. All reported cases had dislocated in a palmar direction, sometimes producing symptoms from the median nerve [110–112]. Most of the cases resulted from high-energy injuries (fall from height or motor vehicle accident) and the mechanism of injury is thought to be extreme dorsiflexion with ulnar deviation [109, 111, 113, 114]. A direct blow to the dorsum of the wrist has also been reported [115]. Various treatment methods have been applied: closed reduction and casting [116], closed reduction and percutaneous pinning [115], open reduction and cast immobilization, open reduction, ligamentous repair and percutaneous pinning [110, 111, 117]. Late wrist malalignment [116, 118–120] and avascular necrosis [112, 120] are the main concerns of these injuries. The recommended treatment is open reduction with combined approach, repair of the volar LT ligament and the SLI ligament (in divergent type of dislocation), and stabilization with K-wires of the scapholunate, scaphocapitate and lunotriquetral joints.

References

1. Garcia-Elias M (2011) Isolated carpal bone dislocations. In: Wolfe SW, Hotchkiss RN, Pederson WC, Kozin SH (eds) Green's operative hand surgery, chap 15, 6th edn. Elsevier Churchill Livingstone, Philadelphia, pp 519–520
2. Melsom DS, Leslie IJ (2007) Carpal dislocations. Curr Orthop 21:288–297
3. Higgs SL (1930) Two cases of dislocation of the carpal scaphoid. Proc R Soc Med 23:1337–1339
4. Kiliç M, Kalali F, Ünlü M (2012) Isolated carpal scaphoid dislocation. Acta Orthop Traumatol Turcica 46(1):68–71
5. Lee BJ, Kim SS, Lee SR et al (2010) Palmar scaphoid dislocation associated with dorsal Perilunate Dislocation: case report. J Hand Surg [Am] 35(5):726–731
6. Chloros GD, Themistocleous GS, Zagoreos NP et al (2006) Isolated dislocation of the scaphoid. Arch Orthop Trauma Surg 126:197–203
7. Leung YF, Wai YL, Kam WL et al (1998) Solitary dislocation of the scaphoid. From case report to literature review. J Hand Surg [Br] 23(1):88–92
8. Amamilo S, Uppal R, Samuel A (1985) Isolated dislocation of carpal scaphoid. J Hand Surg [Br] 10(3):385–388
9. Takami H, Takahashi S, Ando M (1992) Dislocation of the carpal scaphoid associated with median nerve compression. J Trauma 33:921–924
10. Horton T, Shin AY, Cooney WP III (2004) Isolated scaphoid dislocation associated with axial carpal dissociation: an unusual injury report. J Hand Surg [Am] 29(6):1102–1108
11. Sides D, Laorr A, Greenspan A (1995) Carpal scaphoid: radiographic pattern of dislocation. Radiology 195:215–216
12. Szabo RM, Newland CC, Johnson PG et al (1995) Spectrum of injury and treatment options for isolated dislocation of the scaphoid. A report of three cases. J Bone Joint Surg Am 77(4):608–615
13. Thompson TC, Campbell RD, Arnold WD (1964) Primary and secondary dislocation of the scaphoid bone. J Bone Joint Surg Br 46(1):73–82
14. Richards RS, Bennett JD, Roth JH (1993) Scaphoid dislocation with radial-axial carpal disruption. Am J Roentgenol 160:1075–1076

15. Grabow R (2006) Carpal Dislocations. Hand Clin 22:485–500
16. Polveche G, Cordonier D, Thery D et al (1995) A rare variety of dislocation of the carpus. External vertical dislocation: a case report and review of the literature. Ann Chir Main 14(3):159–166
17. Yamabe E, Nakamura T, Matsumura T et al (2008) Palmar dislocation of the scaphoid with dorsal perilunate dislocation. J Hand Surg [Br] 33(5):682–683
18. Buzby BF (1934) Isolated radial dislocation of carpal scaphoid. Ann Surg 100:553–555
19. Somford MP, Sturm MFAM, Vroemen JPAM (2010) Reconstruction of isolated scaphoid dislocation with carpal dissociation, associated with a carpal anomaly. Strat Trauma Limb Recon 5:105–110
20. McNamara MG, Corley FG (1992) Dislocation of the carpal scaphoid. An 8 year follow-up. J Hand Surg [Am] 17(3):496–498
21. Amaravati RS, Saji MJ, Rajagopal HP et al (2009) Neglected dorsal dislocation of the scaphoid. Indian J Orthop 43(2):213–215
22. Sakada T, Ninomiya S, Ohmori M (1998) Simultaneous dislocation of the scaphoid and hamate bone. J Hand Surg [Br] 23(1):93–95
23. Taylor A (1969) Dislocation of the scaphoid. Postgrad Med J 45:186–192
24. Connell M, Dyson R (1955) Dislocation of the carpal scaphoid. Report of a case. J Bone Joint Surg Br 37(2):252–253
25. Fishman MC, Dalinka MK, Osterman L (1985) Case report 309. Skeletal Radiol 13:245–247
26. Inoue G, Maeda N (1990) Isolated dorsal dislocation of the scaphoid. J Hand Surg [Br] 15(3):368–369
27. Kuth J (1939) Isolated dislocation of the carpal navicular. A case report. J Bone Joint Surg Am 21(2):479–483
28. Idler R (2001) Carpal dislocations and instability. In: Watson HK, Weinzweig J (eds) The Wrist. Lippincott Williams & Wilkins, London, pp 203–229
29. Antuna SA, Antuna-Zapico JM (1997) Open dislocation of the carpal scaphoid: a case report. J Hand Surg [Am] 22(1):86–88
30. Andre S, Feuilhade de Chauvin P, Candau B et al (1981) Luxation radio-dorsale du scaphoide. A propos d'un cas. [Posterior dislocation of the scaphoid: report of one case.]. Rev Chir Orthop Reparatrice Appar Mot 67(5):577–580
31. Murakami Y (1977) Dislocation of the carpal scaphoid. The Hand 9(1):79–81
32. Maki NJ, Chuinard RG, D'Ambrosia R (1982) Isolated complete radial dislocation of the scaphoid. J Bone Joint Surg Am 64:615–616
33. Milankov M, Somer T, Jovanovic A et al (1994) Isolated dislocation of the carpal scaphoid: two case reports. J Trauma 36(5):752–754
34. Kennedy JG, O'Connor P, Brunner J (2006) Isolated carpal scaphoid dislocation. Acta Orthop Belg 72(4):478–483

35. Akinci M, Yildirim AO, Kati YA (2012) Late-presenting, isolated, complete radial dislocations of the scaphoid treated with the Szabo technique. J Hand Surg [Eur] 37(9):901–903
36. Ruby L (1998) Isolated carpal dislocations. In: Cooney WP, Linscheid RL, Dobyns JH (eds) The Wrist. Diagnosis and operative treatment, vol 1. Mosby, ch 29, pp 696–708
37. Wani IH, Guptha N, Guptha R et al (2008) Isolated dislocation of carpal scaphoid: a case report. IJOS 10:1. doi:10.5580/156c
38. Engkvist O, Ekenstam F (1986) Closed dislocation of the scaphoid. A case report and review of the literature. Scand J Plast Reconstr Surg 20:239–242
39. Fowler JL (1988) Dislocation of the triquetrum and lunate: Brief report. J Bone Joint Surg Br 70(4):665
40. Ikpeme JO, Hankey S (1995) Dorsal dislocation of the triquetrum: a rare complication of perilunate dislocation. Injury 26(7):497–499
41. Bieber E, Weiland AJ (1984) Traumatic dorsal dislocation triquetrum: a case report. J Hand Surg [Am] 9(6):840–842
42. Goldberg B, Heller A (1987) Dorsal dislocation of the triquetrum with rotary subluxation of the scaphoid. J Hand Surg [Am] 12(1):119–122
43. Inoue G (1992) Dorsal dislocation of the triquetrum: a case report. Ann Chir Main Memb Super 11(3):233–236
44. Frykman E (1980) Dislocation of the triquetrum: case report. Scand J Plast Reconstr Surg 14:205
45. Soucacos PN, Hartofilakidis-Garofalidis GC (1981) Dislocation of the triangular bone. Report of a case. J Bone Joint Surg Am 63(6):1012–1014
46. Immerman WE (1948) Dislocation of the pisiform. J Bone Joint Surg Am 30:489–492
47. Minami M, Yamazaki J, Ishii S (1984) Isolated dislocation of the pisiform: a case report and review of the literature. J Hand Surg [Am] 9(1):125–127
48. Ashkan K, O'Connor D, Lambert S (1998) Dislocation of the pisiform in a 9-year-old child. J Hand Surg [Br] 23(2):269–270
49. Wagoner G (1930) Dislocation of the pisiform associated with fracture of the head of the radius and the styloid process of the ulna. J Bone Joint Surg Am 12(1):170–171
50. Gainor BJ (1985) Simultaneous dislocation of the hamate and pisiform: a case report. J Hand Surg [Am] 10:88–90
51. Pai CH, Wei DC, Hu ST (1993) Carpal bone dislocation: an analysis of twenty cases with relative emphasis on the role of crushing mechanisms. J Trauma 35:28–35
52. Matsumoto T, Tsunoda M, Yamaguchi S et al (2005) Traumatic dislocation of the hamate and pisiform: a case report and review of the literature. J Orthop Trauma 19(4):282–285
53. Vasilas A, Grieco RV, Bartone NF (1960) Roentgen aspects of injuries to the pisiform bone and pisotriquetral joint. J Bone Joint Surg Am 42:1317–1328

54. Cohen I (1922) Dislocation of the pisiform. Ann Surg 75:238–239
55. Sharara KH, Farrar M (1993) Isolated dislocation of the pisiform bone. J Hand Surg [Br] 18:195–196
56. Penvy T, Rayan GM, Egle D (1995) Ligamentous and tendinous support of the pisiform: anatomic and biomechanical study. J Hand Surg [Am] 20:299–304
57. Goriainov V, Bayne G, Warwick DJ (2010) Traumatic dislocation of the pisiform: a case report. J Orthop Surg 18(3):389–390
58. Singh A, Kumar V, Jain G et al (2010) Isolated dislocation of pisiform bone—a rare case. IJMU 5(2):65–67
59. Kwon O, Choi SP, Won HY (2007) Acute isolated pisiform dislocation. A case report. J Korean Orthop Assoc 42:688–691
60. Ishizuki M, Nakagawa T, Itooh S et al (1991) Positional dislocation of the pisiform. J Hand Surg [Am] 16(3):533–535
61. Levante S, Ebelin M (2002) Traumatic dislocation of the pisiform bone: a case report and review of the literature. Chir Main 21(4):264–268
62. McCarron RF, Coleman W (1989) Dislocation of the pisiform treated by primary resection. A case report. Clin Orthop 241:231–233
63. Muniz AE (1999) Unusual wrist pain: pisiform dislocation and fracture. Am J Emerg Med 17(1):78–79
64. Arner M, Haberg L (1984) Wrist flexion strength after excision of the pisiform bone. Scand J Plast Reconstr Surg 18:241–245
65. Carroll RE, Coyle MP (1985) Dysfunction of the pisotriquetral joint: Treatment by excision of the pisiform. J Hand Surg [Am] 10:703–707
66. Gómez CL, Renart IP, Pujals JI et al (2005) Dysfunction of the pisotriquetral joint: degenerative arthritis treated by excision of the pisiform. Orthopedics 28(4):405–408
67. Boe S (1979) Dislocation of the trapezium (multangulum majus): a case report. Acta Orthop Scand 50(1):85–86
68. Sherlock DA (1987) Traumatic dorsoradial dislocation of the trapezium. J Hand Surg [Am] 12(2):262–265
69. Brewood AF (1985) Complete dislocation of the trapezium: a case report. Injury 16(5):303–304
70. Goldberg I, Amit S, Bahar A et al (1981) Complete dislocation of the trapezium (multangulum majus). J Hand Surg [Am] 6(2):193–195
71. Ichikawa T, Inoue G (1999) Complete dislocation of the trapezium. Case report. Scand J Plast Reconstr Surg Hand Surg 33(3):335–337
72. Garcia-Elias M, Geissler WB (2005) Carpal instability. In: Wolfe SW, Hotchkiss RN, Pederson WC, Kozin SH (eds) Green's operative hand surgery, chap 14, 5th edn. Elsevier Churchill Livingstone, Philadelphia, pp 535–604
73. Mumtaz MU, Drabu NA (2009) Open complete dislocation of trapezium with a vertically split fracture: a case report. Cases Journal. doi: 10.1186/1757-1626-2-9092
74. Seimon LP (1972) Compound dislocation of the trapezium. A case report. J Bone Joint Surg Am 54(6):1297–1300
75. Siegel MW, Hertzberg H (1969) Complete dislocation of the greater multangular (trapezium). J Bone Joint Surg Am 51(4):769–772
76. Yin Y, Mann FA, Gilula LA (1996) Positions and techniques. In: Gilula LA, Yin Y (eds) Imaging of the wrist and hand, chap 5. WB Saunders, Philadelphia, pp 93–158
77. Ahmad MH, Midha VP (1991) Dislocation of the trapezium: open reduction by the dorsal approach. Injury 22(5):410–411
78. Peterson CL (1950) Dislocation of the multangulum majus or trapezium (and its treatment in two cases with extirpation). Arch Chir Neerlandicum 2:369–376
79. Larson BJ, DeLange LC (2005) Traumatic volar dislocation of the trapezoid with acute carpal tunnel syndrome. Orthopedics 28(2):165–167
80. De Tullio V, Celenza M (1992) Isolated palmar dislocation of the trapezoid. Int Orthop 16:53–54
81. Lewis HH (1962) Dislocation of the lesser multangular. Report of a case. J Bone Joint Surg Am 44(7):1412–1414
82. Inoue G, Inagaki Y (1990) Isolated palmar dislocation of the trapezoid associated with rupture of the flexor tendon. A case report. J Bone Joint Surg Am 72(3):446–448
83. Kopp JR (1985) Isolated palmar dislocation of the trapezoid. J Hand Surg [Am] 101:91–93
84. Ostrowski DM, Miller ME, Gould JS (1990) Dorsal dislocation of the trapezoid. J Hand Surg [Am] 15(6):874–878
85. Peterson TH (1940) Dislocation of the lesser multangular: report of a case. J Bone Joint Surg Am 22(1):200–202
86. Stein AH (1971) Dorsal dislocation of the lesser multangular bone. J Bone Joint Surg Am 53(2):377–379
87. Bendre DV, Baxi VK (1981) Dislocation of trapezoid. J Trauma 21:899–900
88. Meyn MA, Roth AM (1980) Isolated dislocation of the trapezoid bone. J Hand Surg [Am] 5(6):602–604
89. Goodman ML, Shankman GB (1984) Update:Palmar dislocation of the trapezoid: a case report. J Hand Surg [Am] 9:127–131
90. Checcucci G, Bigazzi P, Zucchini M et al (2011) Isolated complete volar dislocation of the capitate: a case report. Hand Surg 16(3):353–356

91. Hirata H, Sasaki H, Ogawa A et al (1997) Rotary dislocation of the capitate: a case report. J Hand Surg [Am] 22(1):89–90

92. Lee JH, Ehara S, Furumachi K (1999) Volar dislocation of the capitate. Radiat Med 17(5):363–364

93. Lowrey DG, Moss SH, Wolff TW (1984) Volar dislocation of the capitate: report of a case. J Bone Joint Surg Am 66:611–613

94. Ruijters R, Kortmann J (1988) A case of translunate luxation of the carpus. Acta Orthop Scand 59:461–463

95. Walker RW, Pradhan R (2000) Dorsal dislocation of the capitate. J Hand Surg Br 25(4):403–405

96. Simunovic F, Jurk V, Stark GB et al (2012) Volar dislocation and hook fracture of the hamate: a case report. Hand Surg 17(3):387–390

97. Rosh AJ, Schwartz DT (2012) Isolated capitate and hamate dislocation. J Emerg Med 42(6):151–152

98. Awan BA, Robertson GA (2000) Hamate bone dislocation: a case report. J KAU Med Sci 8:117–123

99. Duke R (1963) Dislocation of the hamate bone. Report of a case. J Bone Joint Surg Br 45(4):744

100. Gunn RS (1985) Dislocation of the hamate bone. J Hand Surg [Br] 10:107–108

101. Geist DC (1939) Dislocation of the hamate bone. Report of a case. J Bone Joint Surg Am 21(1):215–217

102. Zieren J, Agnes A, Müller JM (2000) Isolated dislocation of the hamate bone. Case report and review of the literature. Arch Orthop Trauma Surg 120:535–537

103. Ferraro C (1974) Su un caso di lussazione dell'uncinato. Clin Ortop 25:274–276

104. Johannsen S (1926) Ein fall von luxation des os hamatum. Acta Radiol 7:9

105. Clarke SE, Raphael JR (2010) Combined dislocation of the trapezium and the trapezoid: a case report with review of the literature. Hand 5:111–115

106. Ho RW, Chang CS, Lam F et al (1990) Palmar dislocation of the trapezoid and the capitate. A case of traumatic peritrapezoid pericapitate axial dislocation of the carpus. J Med Sci 10(6):385–390

107. Chim H, Yam AKT, Chin AYH et al (2007) Complex carpal dissociation with open, complete, and divergent trapezium, capitate, and hamate dislocation: a case report. J Hand Surg [Am] 32(9):1363–1366

108. Lundkvist L, Larsen CF, Juul SM (1991) Dislocation of the lunate, triquetral, and hamate bones. Case report. Scand J Plast Reconstr Surg Hand Surg 25(1):83–85

109. Domeshek LF, Harenberg PS, Rineer CA et al (2010) Total scapholunate dislocation with complete scaphoid extrusion: case report. J Hand Surg [Am] 35:69–71

110. Arora J (2005) Transulnar styloid palmar scapholunate dislocation with median nerve injury. Arch Orthop Trauma Surg 125:120–123

111. Chalidis B, Dimitriou C (2010) Palmar dislocation of the scapholunate bone-ligament-bone complex. J Hand Surg [Br] 35(4):322–324

112. Coll GA (1987) Palmar dislocation of the scaphoid and lunate. J Hand Surg [Am] 12:476–480

113. Brown R, Muddu B (1981) Scaphoid and lunate dislocation: a report on a case. The Hand 13(3):303–307

114. Komura S, Yokoi T, Suzuki Y (2011) Palmar-divergent dislocation of the scaphoid and the lunate. J Orthop Traumatol 12:65–68

115. Raemisch ME, Rotman MB (2004) Palmar dislocation of the scaphoid and lunate as a unit. Orthopedics 27(11):1199–1201

116. Sarrafian SK, Breihan JH (1990) Palmar dislocation of scaphoid and lunate as a unit. J Hand Surg [Am] 15(1):134–139

117. Healey DC, Giachino AA, Conway AF (2002) Periscaphoid perilunate dislocation of the wrist. J Bone Joint Surg Am 84(7):1201–1204

118. Baulot E, Perez A, Hallonet D et al (1997) Scaphoid and lunate palmar divergent dislocation. Apropos of a case. Rev Chir Orthop Reparatrice Appar Mot 83:265–269

119. Gordon SL (1972) Scaphoid and lunate dislocation: report of a case in a patient with peripheral neuropathy. J Bone Joint Surg Am 54(8):1769–1772

120. Kupfer K (1986) Palmar dislocation of scaphoid and lunate as a unit: case report with special reference to carpal instability and treatment. J Hand Surg [Am] 11:130–134

Index

E. Apergis, *Fracture-Dislocations of the Wrist*,
DOI: 10.1007/978-88-470-5328-1, © Springer-Verlag Italia 2013

Printing and Binding: Stürtz GmbH, Würzburg